F
C   d
Ports of Call
Daniel and Sally Grotta

Copyright © 1993
by Fodor's Travel Publications, Inc.

Fodor's is a registered trademark of Fodor's Travel Publications, Inc.

All rights reserved under International and Pan-American Copyright Conventions. Published in the United States by Fodor's Travel Publications, Inc., a subsidiary of Random House, Inc., New York, and simultaneously in Canada by Random House of Canada Limited, Toronto. Distributed by Random House, Inc., New York.

No maps, illustrations, or other portions of this book may be reproduced in any form without written permission from the publishers.

ISBN 0–679–02511–1

"At One with the Sea," by John Maxtone-Graham, reprinted with permission from *Travel & Leisure,* October 1987. Copyright © (1987) American Express Publishing Corporation. All rights reserved.
"How to Talk Like an Old Salt — or a Salt Substitute," by Henry Beard, reprinted with permission from *Travel & Leisure,* October 1987. Copyright © (1987) American Express Publishing Corporation. All rights reserved.
"What to Read at Sea — If Anything" from *The Treasurer's Report and Other Aspects of Community Singing,* by Robert Benchley. Copyright © 1930 by Robert Benchley. Copyright renewed 1958 by Gertrude Benchley. Reprinted by permission of Harper & Row, Publishers, Inc.

Fodor's Cruises and Ports of Call

Editor: Andrew Collins
Contributors: Nigel Fisher, Donnë Florence, Mary Anne Hemphill, Graham Hughes, Wendy Luft, Honey Naylor, Marcy Pritchard, M. T. Schwartzman, Julie Ann Sipos, Lisa Skriloff, Heidi Waldrop
Creative Director: Fabrizio La Rocca
Cartographer: David Lindroth
Technical Illustration: Christopher A. Wilson
Illustrator: Karl Tanner
Cover Photograph: Harvey Lloyd/The Stock Market
Cover Design: Tigist Getachew
Design: Vignelli Associates

Special Sales

Fodor's Travel Publications are available at special discounts for bulk purchases for sales promotions or premiums. Special editions, including personalized covers, excerpts of existing guides, and corporate imprints, can be created in large quantities for special needs. For more information, contact your local bookseller or write to Special Markets, Fodor's Travel Publications, 201 East 50th Street, New York, NY 10022; Random House of Canada, Ltd., Marketing Dept., 1265 Aerowood Drive, Mississauga, Ontario L4W 1B9; Fodor's Travel Publications, 20 Vauxhall Bridge Road, London, England SW1V 2SA.

MANUFACTURED IN THE UNITED STATES OF AMERICA
10 9 8 7 6 5 4 3 2 1

Contents

On Board *39*

2 Portraits of Cruising   *49*

3 Cruise Lines and Ships   *65*

Foreword

Somewhere out there is a cruise ship that offers exactly the services and amenities you want, goes to the ports and places you have always longed to visit, and can be booked at a price within your budget.

The purpose of this book is to help you find that particular ship, prepare for your cruise, and learn what to expect at the various destinations at which your ship calls.

Rating cruise ships is a popular practice with some cruise guides, but not a particularly useful method through which to convey the specific flavor of an individual ship. Furthermore, what one type of passenger finds excellent another might consider mediocre. So, instead of awarding numbers or stars, we prefer to describe exactly what each ship offers, state our impressions of each cruise line, and discuss what type of person might enjoy each ship and itinerary.

The multibillion-dollar cruise industry is changing so rapidly — with companies being bought and sold, ships being built and scrapped, and sailing schedules so frequently being modified — that it's virtually impossible to keep up with it all. While every reasonable attempt has been made to ensure the accuracy and timeliness of all the information in this guidebook, some of the details may not remain correct. For that reason, the publisher cannot accept responsibility for any errors that may occur. We strongly suggest that you confirm all prices, sailing schedules, and other relevant details with your travel agent or cruise line before booking your cruise.

We wish to express our gratitude to the following contributors for their assistance in the preparation of this guide: the Bermuda Department of Tourism, the Cruise Line Industry Association (CLIA), Susan Farewell, Ian Glass, Joan Iaconetti, Karl Luntta, Sue McManus, Carolyn Price, Jordan Simon, the Venezuelan Consulate General, and John Wade.

Fodor's wishes to know about your cruise ship experiences, pleasant or otherwise. If a particular ship does not meet or match the printed description, or if service is not what you expected to find, let us know and we will investigate the complaint and revise our entries where the facts warrant it.

Send your letters to the editors of Fodor's Travel Publications, 201 E. 50th Street, New York, NY 10022.

Highlights '94 and Fodor's Choice

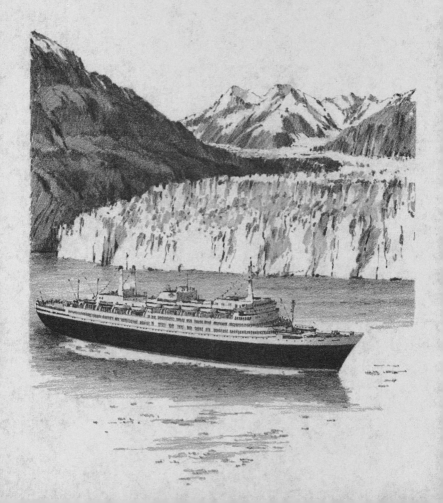

Highlights '94

With nearly 5 million passengers expected to take to the high seas in 1994—doubling 1986's tally—the cruise industry appears impervious to every obstacle today's volatile world throws before it. Through summer 1993, the number of bookings has risen roughly 10% since 1990. Nine of every 10 cruise cabins are occupied, itineraries continue to expand rapidly, the '93–'94 cruise seasons will see nearly 20 new ships plying the waters, and discounts range from 10% to 60% on every type of cruise imaginable.

Rampant discounting may taper off in the coming years. Rising airfare costs will force cruise lines to cut back or eliminate free flights, and many cruise destinations, especially those in the Caribbean, have begun raising port taxes—a cost that's passed directly to passengers. Fuel costs, too, are slowly creeping up. The one hope for consumers is that the cruise industry should eventually reach a saturation point, with so many ships debuting during the next few years. It's still a terribly competitive market, and early-booking discounts are now offered by nearly every cruise line.

Regardless of how many ships sail the seven seas in 1994, the cruise industry will always have plenty of customers. Consider the recent study conducted by the Cruise Line International Association. Among descriptions passengers selected to summarize their cruise experiences, "Pampered by the staff," "Fun," and "Well organized" top the list. "Relaxing," "Safe," "Good value," and "Hassle-free" are not far behind. Overall, 85% of all passengers were "extremely/very satisfied" with their vacations. More than 90% of them plan on cruising again. Today's passengers younger, more budget-conscious, and more diverse than ever, and the variety of cruises available in 1994 is limitless—so you're almost guaranteed to find the ship that's tailored to your needs.

What's Hot Lower-Caribbean loop cruises out of San Juan are grabbing a nice share of the market, along with similar loops out of Aruba. Theme cruises continue to be popular; one cruise-only travel agency, Landry and Kling, now sponsors everything from chocolate voyages to Scottish heritage cruises.

With the average vacation time of the American worker having dropped to under four nights, an increasing number of three- and four-night loop cruises are available. Popular short-cruise destinations are Nassau–Freeport/Lucaya–Key West cruises out of Miami or Fort Lauderdale and Ensenada and Catalina Island cruises out of Los Angeles.

Airport Aggravation Overcrowding, overbooking, and delays at major U.S. airports may force cruise companies to book flights a day ahead of cruise departures. One cruise line has already begun its own charter airline. Others will flee to less congested gateways such as Palm Beach and Fort Lauderdale's Port Everglades. And in Port of Miami, the notoriously maddening experience of getting to and from the pier has been greatly relieved by the recent opening of a $52 million fixed-span bridge that connects the mainland to downtown Miami.

New Ships on the Horizon One ship that sunk beneath the horizon in 1993 was **Ocean Cruise Lines'** *Ocean Princess*, a 460-passenger ship that ran aground during an Amazon River cruise in April. The ship itself was the only casualty, and Ocean is currently shopping around for a new ship, hoping to unveil it by early to mid-1994.

Celebrity recently announced plans to build three 1,740-passenger luxury vessels between 1995 and 1997. The first of these 70,000-ton megaships will sail year-round out of Fort Lauderdale through the Caribbean. Accommodations will be opulent: Many suites will have verandas, marble baths, and whirlpool tubs.

A new cruise line, **Silversea Cruises,** also plans to unveil two chic ships meant to compete directly with such small splendors as **Seabourn's** *Spirit* and **Cunard's** *Sea Goddesses.* The 13,000-ton *Silver Cloud* will set sail in spring 1994; it will share the seas with a sister-ship, the *Silver Wind,* the following season. With about a dozen luxury ships charging staggering fares, Silversea is banking on the questionable belief that the pockets of cruise passengers run very deep. Time will determine which cruise lines remain solvent.

In 1993, **Carnival** became the first mainstream cruise line to target the Latin market, launching a new division, **FiestaMarina Cruises.** Its first ship, the *Carnivale,* which sailed previously under the parent company, serves up the best of Cuban, Spanish, South American, and Mexican cuisine; sails from San Juan to Caracas, with calls at St. Thomas and Santo Domingo (Dominican Republic); and presents Latin-flavor entertainment and facilities. On-board communication is in Spanish.

In 1996, Carnival will introduce a mammoth 95,000-ton megaship, expected to be the largest cruise ship ever built. This on the heels of three-year project that will have seen the issue of three identical 2,600-passenger ships, the *Sensation, Fascination,* and *Imagination.* Carnival, which owns **Holland America Line, Windstar Cruises,** and **Seabourn Cruise Line,** is poised to remain the world's largest cruise line for many years to come.

Princess is adding a gargantuan ship of its own, the *Sun Princess,* which is due to enter service in fall 1995. This $300 million, 1,950-passenger vessel will stretch about three football fields in length and feature a high-tech fitness center, two main show lounges, and a cobblestone-floor pizza parlor.

The **Delta Steamboat Company's** two riverboats, the *Delta Queen* and the *Mississippi Queen,* were reviewed in this book for the first time in 1994. And already, we're planning to expand our coverage in next year's edition: Delta's new *Belle of America,* a 420-passenger replica of a mid-19th-century riverboat, will be plying the Mississippi River by July 1994.

Child's Play When Bruce Nierenberg left family-oriented **Premier Cruise Lines** in 1991 to take the helm of **Costa Cruise Lines,** industry experts wondered how the change would affect Costa's then-limited hold of the traveling-with-kids market. Sure enough, a new cruise line, **American Family Cruises,** was developed in 1993 by Nierenberg as a joint venture between Costa and its parent company, **Costa Crociere.** Two old Costa ships, the *EugenioCosta* and *CostaRiviera* have been refitted and renamed as the *American Adventure* and *American Pioneer,* respectively. The *Adventure* debuted late in 1993 and will sail the Caribbean; the *Pioneer* will follow in 1994, sailing Alaska's Inside Passage. Both ships offer nonstop children's activities that address four distinct age groups, a trained staff to supervise the kids, and shore excursions geared specifically toward families.

Cargo Cruising A cruising craze of late is sharing your trip with a few hundred tons of coffee, nuts, and honey. You wouldn't think many passengers would *choose* to sail from New York to Buenos Aires aboard a fully working cargo ship, but **Ivaran Lines'** *Americana* draws as many as 85 passengers during its regular round-trip voyages between North and South America. Accommodations are surprisingly plush, and per diems are quite reasonable. For information, see the South America section of Chapter 4 or call 201/798–5656.

Green Ships The ecotourism, or "green", travel market is due for its own global warming. These small, floating classrooms are staffed with top scientists and researchers. They often lack white-glove service and luxury cuisine; what they don't lack is luxury fares and passengers willing to pay them. Why so high? The remote itineraries—including the Northwest Passage, Siberia, Antarctica, and the Amazon River region.

There Goes the Neighborhood? With the increase in traffic comes concerns about the effects on the environment. The cruise industry has worked hard to show itself in an environmentally sensitive light—installing state-of-the-art waste and sewage management systems, appointing environmental experts to their staffs—but for now, most older ships continue their old, not-so-sensitive practices. Furthermore, the number of ships exploring unchartered waters and calling at uninhabited ports, such as Antarctica, is rising. If the *QE2* grounded off Martha's Vineyard in 1992, and the *Ocean Princess* sank in the Amazon River in 1993, can a serious environmental cruise-ship disaster be far behind? Preservation, safety, and profit are conflicting imperatives, and it remains to be seen how cruise lines will resolve this problem.

Fodor's Choice

No two people agree on what makes a perfect cruise, but it's fun and helpful to know what others think. We hope you'll have a chance to experience some of Fodor's Choices while on your cruise. For detailed information about each entry, refer to the appropriate chapter in this guidebook.

Special Moments

On Board   Breakfast on your cabin's veranda while transiting the Panama Canal aboard the *Royal Princess*

Listening to the crackle of glacial ice in Alaska's Inside Passage

Following a pod of whales in rubber Zodiac boats launched from the *Polaris*

The *Wind Star* under full sail

Sailing under the Verrazano Bridge as you approach New York City

Approaching Rio de Janeiro

Ashore   Riding a moped along the Railway Trail in Bermuda

Tea at the Empress Hotel in Victoria, British Columbia

Swimming with the dolphins in Freeport, Bahamas

Meeting the green monkeys at the Wildlife Reserve on Barbados

In Antarctica, meeting a chinstrap penguin face-to-face

Scuba diving at Sting Ray City, Grand Cayman Island

Charter-boat fishing out of Sitka, Alaska

Hiking on the Kenai Peninsula, Alaska

Watching the Acapulco cliff divers at night

Shore Excursions

Alaska   Gold Creek Salmon Bake, Juneau

Mendenhall Glacier Float Trip, Juneau

Mendenhall Glacier Helicopter Ride, Juneau

Misty Fjords Flightseeing, Ketchikan

Kenai River Float Trip and Salmon Bake, Seward

Bahamas   Coral World, Nassau

Beach Barbecue on a private Bahamian island

Caribbean   Any Caribbean submarine tour

Angel Falls and Canaima Lagoon, Caracas, Venezuela

Chichén Itzá Mayan ruins, Cozumel, Mexico

Dunn's River Falls, Ocho Rios, Jamaica

Island Tour, Martinique

La Soufrière and the Pitons, St. Lucia

Sailing and Snorkeling Tour, St. John

El Yunque Rain Forest, San Juan, Puerto Rico

Nightlife Tour, San Juan, Puerto Rico

Mexican Riviera Sierra Madre Tour, Mazatlán

Beach Tour, Zihuatanejo/Ixtápa

South America The private Carnival celebration in the tiny Amazon village of Parantins

Entertainment

Any theme cruise

High-stakes "horse racing" extravaganzas on the *Royal Princess*

Carnival Cruises' high-energy shows

The classical music ensembles and piano soloists on the *Sovereign of the Seas*

The harpist on the *Crystal Harmony*

The revues on the *Norway*

Dining

The pasta made fresh at the table on Princess Cruises' ships

Self-serve ice cream/yogurt bars and taco stands on all Holland America ships

The Princess Grill on the *Queen Elizabeth 2*

The Lido luncheon buffet on the *Sagafjord*

The sumptuous luncheon buffets on the *Seabourn Pride*

The superb Japanese cuisine on the *Crystal Harmony*'s Kyoto restaurant

Facilities

The atrium and the shopping arcade on the *Sovereign of the Seas*

The extensive art collections aboard Holland's *Statendam* and *Maasdam*

The theater on the *Rotterdam*

The huge sun deck on the *Oceanic*

The sun-filled Vista Lounge on the *Crystal Harmony*

The promenade deck on the *Norway*

Cabins

The cabins/suites on the *Sea Goddess* and the *Seabourn Pride*

The cabins with private verandas on the *Crown Princess*

The Penthouse suites on the *Queen Elizabeth 2*

The Owner's Suite, furnished with Louis XVI antiques, on the *Sea Cloud*

Shopping

Early morning in Charlotte Amalie, St. Thomas

St. George's, Bermuda

Acapulco's Mercado Municipal

Front Street in Philipsburg, St. Martin

Bagshaw Studios, St. Lucia

Beaches

Playa del Amor, Cabo San Lucas, Mexico

Playa Isla de los Venados, Mazatlán, Mexico

Hawksnest, St. John, U.S. Virgin Islands

Grand Anse, Grenada

Seven Mile Beach, Grand Cayman

Most of Antigua's 365 beaches

Bermuda's south shore

Scenic Views

Calving icebergs in Glacier Bay, Alaska

Kenai Peninsula, Alaska

Prince William Sound, Alaska

Grand Etang, Grenada

El Yunque Rain Forest, Puerto Rico

The Pitons (Petit and Gros), St. Lucia

Los Arcos, Cabo San Lucas, Mexico

The lights of Acapulco, Mexico

The waterways in Belize, overgrown with mangrove trees.

The ocean during a storm

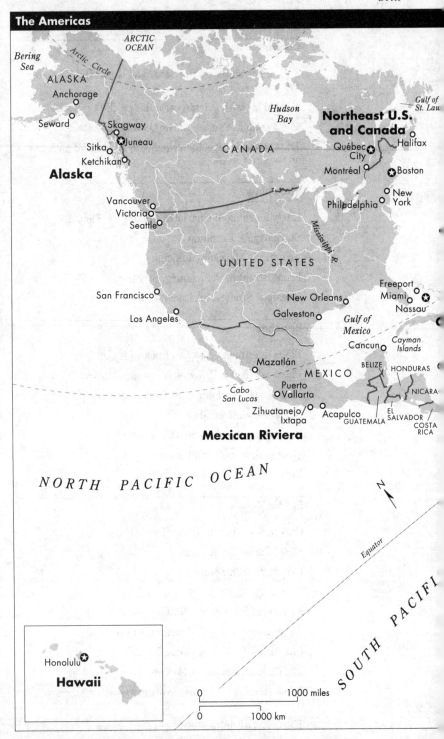

The Americas

ARCTIC OCEAN

Bering Sea

Arctic Circle

ALASKA
Anchorage

Seward

Skagway

Sitka
Juneau

Ketchikan

Alaska

Hudson Bay

CANADA

Gulf of St. Lau

Northeast U.S. and Canada

Québec City

Halifax

Montréal

Boston

Vancouver
Victoria
Seattle

New York

Philadelphia

UNITED STATES

Mississippi R.

San Francisco

New Orleans

Freeport
Miami
Nassau

Los Angeles

Galveston

Gulf of Mexico

Cayman Islands

Cancun

Mazatlán

MEXICO

BELIZE

HONDURAS

NICARA

Cabo San Lucas

Puerto Vallarta

GUATEMALA

EL SALVADOR

COSTA RICA

Zihuatanejo/ Ixtapa

Acapulco

Mexican Riviera

NORTH PACIFIC OCEAN

N

Equator

Honolulu

Hawaii

SOUTH PACIFI

0   1000 miles

0   1000 km

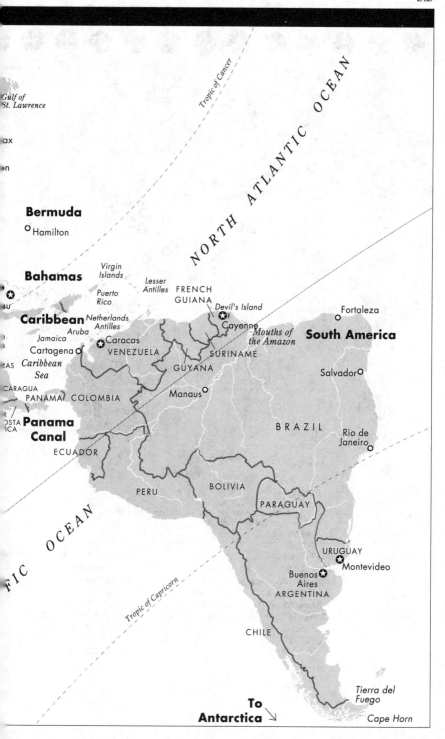

World Time Zones

Numbers below vertical bands relate each zone to Greenwich Mean Time (0 hrs.).
Local times frequently differ from these general indications,
as indicated by light-face numbers on map.

Algiers, **29**
Anchorage, **3**
Athens, **41**
Auckland, **1**
Baghdad, **46**
Bangkok, **50**
Beijing, **54**

Berlin, **34**
Bogotá, **19**
Budapest, **37**
Buenos Aires, **24**
Caracas, **22**
Chicago, **9**
Copenhagen, **33**
Dallas, **10**

Delhi, **48**
Denver, **8**
Djakarta, **53**
Dublin, **26**
Edmonton, **7**
Hong Kong, **56**
Honolulu, **2**

Istanbul, **40**
Jerusalem, **42**
Johannesburg, **44**
Lima, **20**
Lisbon, **28**
London (Greenwich), **27**
Los Angeles, **6**
Madrid, **38**
Manila, **57**

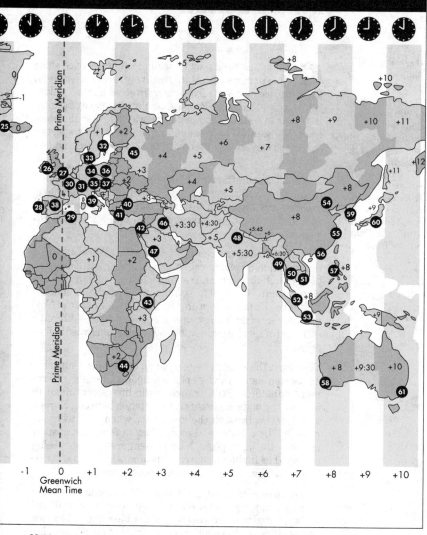

Introduction

*By Daniel and
Sally Grotta*

*Daniel and Sally
Grotta's work has
appeared in many
national magazines
and newspapers,
including
American Heritage,
Reader's Digest,
Islands, and the
Boston Globe. They
are the authors of
The Green Travel
Source Book.*

Sailing has been part of the human experience since time immemorial. Until relatively recently, however, an ocean voyage frequently involved hardship, danger, and great expense. People took ships primarily because they had to — there was no other way to cross the seas. Even the wealthiest passengers had to endure spartan shipboard conditions, often with spoiled food and cramped cabins.

It wasn't until after the Canadian Sir Samuel Cunard founded his famous steamship company in 1840 that naval architects finally began designing and building vessels that specifically featured passenger amenities and conveniences.

From the turn of the century to the eve of World War II a fierce national rivalry raged among the great European powers to build and sail the finest, fastest, and most luxurious ocean liners. These monarchs of the oceans — Britain's *Mauritania* and *Queen Mary,* France's *Normandie,* Germany's *Imperator,* and Italy's *Rex* — offered a standard of service and opulence on a scale unrivaled before or since.

The Great Depression helped put an end to these superliners, which had always depended upon generous government subsidies. Still, transatlantic liners continued to provide the main means of transportation between Europe and America through the mid-1960s, when they were superseded by a faster and more efficient form of transportation — the jet airplane. Most passenger ships faced being scrapped or finding a source of income other than transatlantic sailings. Thus, the cruise industry was born.

The simplest definition of a cruise is a vacation at sea during which all major services, such as meals, entertainment, and accommodations, are covered in the base price. Modern cruise ships are the nautical equivalents of good resort hotels. Most cruises travel in a loop, or circle, originating and terminating at the same port. During a cruise, most ships stop briefly at various ports, so passengers can sightsee, shop, and play. Today the prime sailing regions in the Americas are the Caribbean and the Bahamas, Alaska, and the Mexican Riviera, but increasing numbers of ships are visiting South America and Antarctica. Although not many ships pass through the Hawaiian Islands, American Hawaii Cruises gives passengers the opportunity to cruise among four major islands. Even the northeastern United States and Canada are benefiting from the surge in the popularity of cruises.

Wherever you're headed, a cruise might be the perfect opportunity for you to curl up in a deck chair to read the latest best-seller. If you're looking for action, however, the large majority of cruise ships provide a panoply of organized activities — dance classes, trivia contests, bridge tournaments, scavenger hunts, and so on. Facilities such as swimming pools, saunas, fitness centers, movie theaters, discos, and gift shops are also commonly featured.

Today's composite cruise passenger is a far cry from her more staid counterpart of just a few years past. She (a substantial majority of cruise passengers are female) is younger, more athletically inclined, and enjoys traveling with her spouse and children. She spends relatively little time in her cabin, enthusiastically participates in a variety of shipboard activities, and enjoys shopping in foreign ports. At night she drops between $200 and $400 in the casino and on bingo, and stays up late for the shows and to dance. Unfortunately she also gains four pounds on average during a one-week cruise.

But for every stereotype, there are a thousand other kinds of passengers, and today's cruises cater to many of them. Whether they are party ships in the Caribbean or adventure ships navigating ice-choked channels in Antarctica, cruises have become as diverse as the ports at which they call.

1 Essential Information

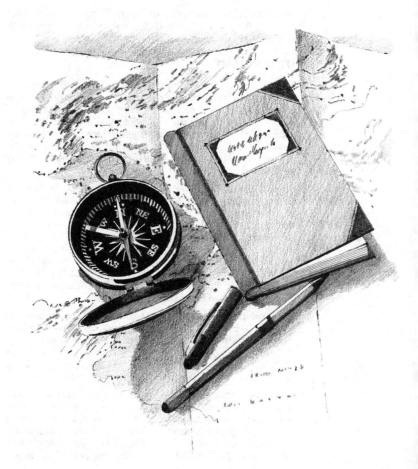

Choosing Your Cruise

Cruise Information

Magazines
Cruises & Tours profiles new ships and covers ports and itineraries; $11.80 per year for four issues (Vacation Publications, 1502 Augusta St., Suite 415, Houston, TX 77057, tel. 713/974–6903).

Cruise Travel Magazine has photos and features on ships and ports of call; $9.97 per year for six issues (Box 342, Mt. Morris, IL 61054, tel. 815/734–4151 or 800/877–5893).

Newsletters
Cruise Digest Reports has detailed ship reports, evaluations and ratings, and cruise industry news; $35 per year for six issues (1521 Alton Rd., Suite 350, Miami Beach, FL 33139, tel. 305/374–2224).

The Millegram is a newsletter with information on new ships, shipbuilding contracts, and changes in itineraries; $10 per year for four issues (Bill Miller Cruises Everywhere, Box 1463, Secaucus, NJ 07096, tel. 201/348–9390).

Ocean & Cruise News reviews a different ship each month; $28 per year for 12 issues (World Ocean & Cruise Liner Society, Box 92, Stamford, CT 06901, tel. 203/329–2787).

Types of Ships

The bigger the ship, the more it can offer: a greater number of activities, public rooms, and dining options; a broader range of entertainment; and, of course, more passengers—a boon if you're gregarious, a burden if you're not. Rates on large ships can be slightly lower; the newer megaships are significantly less expensive per passenger to operate. Some ships, though, are too unwieldy to dock in smaller ports, and passengers may be shuttled to shore in a tender (a small boat).

Smaller cruise ships offer intimacy; the crew may be more informal, the level of activity less intense. Small ships can often slip into tiny, shallow harbors, cruise narrow waterways, and dock right at quayside. Small ships come in two versions: simple excursion vessels and ultraluxurious ships. The excursion vessels usually don't have such amenities as pools, theaters, casinos, or libraries, and cabins are almost always closetlike. Small luxury ships, which usually carry up to 200 passengers, have all the big-ship amenities, all-outside suites, and an exacting level of personalized service.

In considering size, don't forget to factor in other variables. In Chapter 3, individual ship reviews show the passenger/crew ratio (or service ratio), which indicates how many passengers each crew member must serve. A ratio of 2:1 indicates that there's a crew member for every two passengers. All things being equal, choose the ship with the lower service ratio.

Space ratio, which indicates the relative size of cabins and public areas, is also important. Divide a ship's gross tonnage by its passenger capacity to find this. A 25,000-ton vessel carrying 1,000 passengers will have a 25:1 ratio. By industry standards, a ratio of 45:1 or above is considered spacious. Vessels with ratios under 25:1 can feel a bit like floating cans of sardines.

Also study carefully a ship's on-board facilities. Is there a pool? How many entertainment lounges and movie theaters? How well equipped is the library or the health club? Facilities vary greatly.

Mainstream Ships These ships carry between 700 and 2,000 passengers and are similar to self-contained, all-inclusive resorts. You'll find pools, spas and saunas, movie theaters, exercise rooms, Las Vegas–style entertainment, a casino, and shore excursions, not to mention plenty of planned group activities.

The per diem is the daily rate, per passenger, when two persons share a cabin. Differences in ships, cabin categories, itineraries, and discounts, however, can skew that figure.

Within the mainstream cruise ship category, there are several subcategories: standard, premium, and luxury. The per diem listed with each one is based on a standard outside cabin in peak season—this being any ship's middle-of-the-road accommodation. Inside cabins have lower fares; fancy suites, with verandas or VCRs, cost more.

Luxury Here you'll savor the finest cuisine afloat, dining at single seatings and by special order, and unusually large cabins. Most cabins are outside; some have verandas. These ships have high service and space ratios and extremely personalized service. Passengers are experienced and sophisticated cruisers. Evenings are dressy, with some formal occasions. You'll find fewer families and more seniors. **Per diem:** $300–$800.

Premium Most ships fall into this category. They are run by highly experienced cruise lines, and you can expect competent, consistently professional service and entertainment and above-average itineraries. Waiters are apt to be of one nationality, adding a distinctive flair to the dining room. Hours and room service selection are better, the menu choice and quality of food higher, than those of the standard class. Featured dishes may be prepared tableside, and you're often able, with advance notice, to place special orders. Evenings are dressier, and the ambience similar to that of a good restaurant. There are usually a couple of formal nights. **Per diem:** $260–$590.

Standard Menus are probably not extensive, and the food good but not extraordinary. Dress is more casual. Some of these ships are older, refitted vessels lacking modern amenities and state-of-the-art facilities. Others are gleaming new 60,000-ton megaships, carrying more than 2,000 passengers, that have been patterned after all-inclusive resorts where everything, from staff members to cabins to public spaces, seem rather impersonal. **Per diem:** $200–$410.

Yachtlike Ships These ships carry an average of 50–200 passengers.

Ultraluxurious These have the optimum level of personalized service, fine dining, and cushy amenities, including top-of-the-line health centers, pools, whirlpools, casinos, and entertainment. The cabins, all outside suites, are spacious and equipped with every comfort to pamper passengers. The itineraries are an incredible roll call of the world's most exotic ports. **Per diem:** $700–$900.

Upscale Though not as elegant as ultraluxurious vessels, these also offer good service and unusual itineraries. There are few planned shipboard activities beyond impromptu Scrabble games or music provided by local entertainers. **Per diem: $200–$300.**

Excursion   These vessels have been designed specifically to visit out-of-the-way destinations where larger ships can't go. The trade-off is usually modest accommodations, small public rooms, informal service, and casual, family- style dining. **Per diem: $100–$200.**

Ships in the latter two categories sail mostly along the U.S. eastern seaboard, the Pacific Northwest, the Caribbean, and Central America.

Specialty Ships   Designed for a particular type of cruise—such as a hybrid vessel powered by both sails and turbine engines. They vary widely in price and quality. **Per diem: $125–$675.**

Adventure Ships   These small ships, carrying from 50 to 400 passengers, sail almost anywhere in the world, from Antarctica to the Amazon. They usually have tiny, spartan cabins, few traditional onboard activities, and informal service. Food quality varies from ship to ship; meals are usually open seating. Lecturers on the wildlife or culture of the region visited sail on every cruise. Newer ships have better amenities, the philosophy these days being that adventure cruising need not mean roughing it. **Per diem: $250–$700.**

Types of Cruises

Cost, destination, and cruise duration determine whether a ship will be oriented toward older or younger passengers. On some ships, the average age is over 60 and the number of children can be counted on one hand. Without exception, such cruises are 10 or more days in duration, have a significantly higher per diem charge, and visit unusual or out-of-the-way ports. Ships offering voyages of three or four days and modest rates attract the younger set. On these cruises kids are common, especially during school holidays.

Traditional Cruises   On a mainstream ship, these combine a standard set of onboard amenities and services with a sprinkling of brief stopovers at mainstream ports. Captain's parties, get-togethers, costume parties, bingo, and specific activities for newlyweds, singles, senior citizens, teenagers, and other special groups are typical.

Those catering to younger passengers add lively, even rowdy activities such as beer chugalug contests, greased-pole pillow fights, and singles' mingles.

Theme Cruises   Special lectures, demonstrations, or seminars—in addition to normal activities—are what set theme cruises apart from mainstream cruises. Most cruise ships offer these special trips at slack times throughout the year. Sports personalities, Hollywood actors, best-selling authors, and even high-powered Ivy League professors perform or lecture on board. Recent cruises have been organized around such themes as classical music, wine-tasting, and computers. One unusual theme cruise involves a murder mystery, with the passengers playing detective. Country-and-western cruises and '50s and '60s cruises often feature appropriate celebrity performers who entertain and mingle with guests. There is no extra charge for most theme cruises, although a handful, such as wine-tasting cruises, carry premiums for those who participate. Some special programs and theme cruises are advertised many months ahead. Others are not announced to the public; you can learn about them by contacting your travel agent or the cruise line directly.

A recent trend is booking an elaborate theme cruise through an outside agency. For example, an agency might work with a cruise line to design a special cruise for tennis enthusiasts, arranging all details for the participant. Schedules on such cruises are packed with private parties and lectures and may include casual interaction with celebrities or excursions to exotic locales. The voyages are more intimate, because usually only a portion of the ship is set aside for theme-package participants. **Landry and Kling's Themes at Sea** (Gables Waterway 1, 1390 S. Dixie Hwy., Suite 1207, Coral Gables, FL 33146, tel. 800/223-2026) caters to a variety of special-interest groups, from chocolate lovers to ham radio operators.

Excursion Cruises Small vessels that emphasize unusual ports over shipboard entertainment are gaining in popularity. These cruises are highly unstructured, leaving passengers to their own devices: Sunbathing, card games, and reading are major pastimes. Ships often tie up at a small island or village pier for the night, allowing passengers to take part in the local nightlife. Excursion cruises are available in all price ranges.

Cultural or Adventure Cruises These voyages may feature seminars by college professors or distinguished government officials, or they may be organized around a special activity such as whale-watching, retracing the routes of the early explorers, or photographing a rare mid-ocean solar eclipse. Other cultural cruises are centered on exotic destinations, such as the Amazon River, Antarctica, or the Galápagos Islands. Per diems are often higher, and itineraries often span more than two weeks, therefore attracting older, more affluent passengers. These cruises are often offered in conjunction with pre- or post-cruise supplemental travel packages. Because most cultural cruises are on small or specialty ships, amenities and services may be limited.

Windjammer Cruises Unfurling their sails for part of each day and night (motor-powered the rest of the time), windjammers are not your traditional cruise ships. In this class are schooners, topsail schooners, barquentines, sailing yachts, and barques—all carrying an aura of adventure and romance. Evenings are peaceful; conversation and stargazing may be the main entertainment. By day, life aboard is totally casual and unstructured, with few scheduled group activities. Instead, guests enjoy sea breezes and the simple life; many windjammer lines encourage passengers to help with the sails, even offering informal sailing classes.

Clothing is casual—on some ships shoes are seldom donned. Your windjammer cruise wardrobe can easily fit into a duffel bag. Windjammers vary in size, accommodation, and degree of luxury. They carry from 18 to more than 100 passengers, and fares start at $100 per diem. Cabins range in size from small to moderate. The most basic have upper and lower bunks, cold-water basins, and shared hand-pumped cool water showers; others may have double beds and/or tiny private showers and toilets. Food is hearty and simple. Beach picnics are features of the Caribbean experience, and lobster bakes are the highlight of New England cruises.

Most windjammers sailing the New England coast are restored wooden-hull schooners. The Caribbean has some larger steel-hulled vessels, some restored beauties formerly owned by millionaires. The most luxurious is the 75-passenger *Sea Cloud*, built in 1931 as private yacht for Marjorie Merriweather Post (*see* Special Expeditions, in Chapter 3). Some even have air-conditioning and lounges with TVS and VCRs.

New England, especially Long Island Sound and coastal Maine, is a popular windjammer area. The main bases for the fleets are Camden and Rockland, Maine, and Mystic, Connecticut. The Caribbean fleet has home ports and itineraries throughout the islands.

Ports tend to be off the beaten track—smaller, less spoiled ones rarely, if ever, visited by the large cruise ships. Most anchor off isolated beaches for beachcombing and sunning; there's little organized sightseeing. The more ambitious operators offer plenty of swimming, snorkeling, scuba diving, windsurfing, and small-boat sailing. Poking through villages and whale-watching are part of the New England experience.

Windjammer cruises appeal to nature lovers, photographers, sailors, and those who just want to get away from it all. As with the cruise ship fleet, sailing styles vary—some are family oriented, others designed for adults only—so check with the operator to find your perfect match.

Below are some of the major windjammer operators:
Maine Windjammer Association (Box 317P, Rockport, ME 04856, tel. 800/624–6380), with 13 vessels based in Camden, Rockport, and Rockland.
Tall Ship Adventures (1010 S. Joliet St., Suite 200, Aurora, CO 80012, tel. 303/341–0335 or 800/662–0090), offering three- to seven-day Caribbean cruises on the *Sir Francis Drake*.
Windjammer Barefoot Cruises (1759 Bay Rd., Box 120, Miami Beach, FL 33119, tel. 305/534–7447 or 800/327–2601), with six vessels plying the Caribbean.

Ship Itineraries

Note: Itineraries listed in Chapter 3 are for the late 1993–mid-1994 cruise season but are subject to change. Contact your travel agent or the cruise line directly for up-to-the-minute itineraries.

A cruise's itinerary is an important consideration in determining the best ship for you. Many ships visit three or four ports a week, stopping for a morning or a day at each. This style of cruise is not as exhausting as a comparable land-based tour, because your ship acts as a floating hotel that moves you from one locale to the next without a worry. Passports, paperwork, and other details are attended to when you first board the ship, and you can generally book a shore excursion that will pick you up dockside. So brief a taste of a port's culture can be frustrating, however. Also remember that the more ports scheduled per week, the fewer days you will spend at sea.

Loop cruises start and end at the same port; **one-way cruises** start at one port and end at another. Typically, one-way cruises travel farther than loop cruises, spend fewer days at sea, and cover more ground. Alaska cruises that start and end in Vancouver sail over the same area twice, offering passengers less time in Alaska than those cruises that sail one-way. One-way Alaska cruises also give passengers the option of spending more time in Alaska before or after the cruise. Loop cruises out of San Juan, Puerto Rico, can visit up to six ports on a seven-day cruise. Loop cruises out of Florida can reach up to four ports in seven days; it will take one day to reach the first port.

Many ships sailing the Caribbean or the Mexican Riviera in winter and spring move to Alaska or New England in summer and fall. Other ships spend part of the year in the Caribbean, part outside the Western Hemisphere. When a ship moves from one cruising area to another, it offers a **repositioning cruise,** which typically stops at infrequently visited ports and attracts fewer passengers. It often has a lower per diem.

A handful of ships offer an annual one- to two-month **cruise around South America** or a three- to four-month **around-the-world cruise,** stopping at dozens of fabulous ports. This continent-straddling itinerary typically costs from $7,000 per person for a small inside cabin to tens of thousands of dollars for a suite; partial segments, usually of 14 to 21 days, are also available.

There are two basic loop itineraries for **cruises to Antarctica.** The most common route starts from the tip of South America and sails to the Antarctic Peninsula. The other itinerary starts in New Zealand or Australia and runs to the Ross Sea. The latter covers much longer distances, so more time is spent at sea and less on shore—though it does include a stop at the explorers' historic huts.

There's been a boom lately in **three- and four-day cruises.** Many first-timers take them to test their sea legs, before investing more vacation time and money on a longer cruise; others just prefer short getaways. Once the exclusive province of old, out-of-style ships, the short-cruise market is now serviced by sleek new vessels, some built exclusively for these runs. The short cruises operate out of Florida to the Bahamas and out of Los Angeles to both Mexico and the southern Californian coast and islands.

Cost

For one all-inclusive price (plus tips, shopping, bar bills, and other incidentals), you can have what many have called the trip of a lifetime. The axiom "the more you pay, the more you get" doesn't always hold true: Most mainstream ships are one-class vessels on which the passenger in the cheapest inside cabin eats the same food, sees the same shows, and share the same amenities as one paying more than $1,000 per day for the top suite. (A notable exception is the *Queen Elizabeth 2*, where your dining-room assignment is based on your per diem.) To some, a larger cabin—used principally for sleeping, showering, and changing clothes—is not worth the extra money. Where price does make a difference is in the choice of ship.

A handy way to compare costs is to look at the per diem cost—the price of a cruise on a daily basis for each passenger, when two people occupy one cabin. If a seven-day cruise costs $700 per person, the per diem is $100.

Consider using the following checklist to help figure roughly what your costs will total. The goal is to match your individual per diem budget—the bottom line on your worksheet—to the per diem price of a cabin aboard a ship in Chapter 3 that interests you.

Note: Per diem prices quoted in Chapter 3 are for the late 1993–mid-1994 cruise season but are subject to change. Contact your travel agent or cruise specialist for up-to-the-minute fares.

Cruise Budget Worksheet

1/	*Total budget for you and your companions (what you can afford to pay for the entire vacation)*	$
2/	*Pre- or post-cruise arrangements*	$
3/	*Airfare, airport taxes, etc.*	$
4/	*Transfer to and from airport*	$
5/	*Transfer to and from ship*	$
6/	*Pre-trip incidentals*	$
7/	*Shore excursions*	$
8/	*Casino, bingo, etc.*	$
9/	*Shopping*	$
10/	*On-board incidentals for you and your companions for the entire cruise*	$
11/	*Subtotal (add lines 2–10)*	$
12/	*Net working budget (subtract line 11 from line 1)*	$
13/	*Number of travelers in your party*	
14/	*Individual budget (divide line 12 by line 13)*	$
15/	*Number of days in cruise*	
16/	*Individual per diem budget (divide line 14 by line 15)*	$

Pre- and post-cruise arrangements: If you plan to arrive a day or two early at the port of embarkation, or linger a few days for sightseeing afterward, estimate the cost of your hotel, meals, car rental, sightseeing, and other expenditures. Cruise lines sell packages for pre- and post-cruise stays that can include hotel accommodations, transportation, tours, extras such as car rentals, and some meals. These packages can cost less than similar stays you arrange on your own, but comparison shopping may reveal that you can do better on your own.

Airfare: Airfare and transfers are often included in the basic cruise fare; however, the cruise line chooses your airline and flight. Lines give an air transportation credit of $200–$400 for passengers who make their own air arrangements. You may find a better airfare or more convenient routing, or use frequent-flyer miles.

Pretrip incidentals: These may include trip or flight insurance, the cost of boarding your pets, airport or port parking, departure tax, visas, long- distance calls home, clothing, film or videotape, and other miscellaneous expenses.

Shore excursions/expenses: Estimate an average of $70–$140 per passenger on a seven-day cruise.

Amusement and gambling allowance: Losses at bingo, in the casino, or in other forms of gambling, plus the cost of video games, can set you back a bundle. Of course, this is an entirely avoidable expense, but if you plan to bet, plan to lose. You must be over 18 to gamble on a cruise ship.

Shopping: Include what you expect to spend for both inexpensive souvenirs and major duty-free purchases.

On-board incidentals: According to CLIA (Cruise Lines International Association), passengers can expect to tip an average of $7–$11 per day. Daily on-board expenditures—bar tabs, wine with meals, laundry, beauty parlor services, gift shop purchases—vary widely from person to person.

Accommodations

Where you sleep matters only if you enjoy extra creature comforts and are willing to pay for them; on most of today's one-class cruise ships no particular status or stigma is attached to your choice of cabin. Having said that, there's certainly an advantage to personally selecting the best cabin within your budget, rather than having your travel agent or cruise line representative simply book you into the next available accommodation. Also, the earlier you book, the better the selection.

Cabin Size The term "stateroom," used on some ships, is usually interchangeable with "cabin." Price is directly proportional to size and location, and the overwhelming majority are tiny.

Suites are the roomiest and best-equipped accommodations; even on one ship, they may differ in size, facilities, and price. Steward service may be more attentive (top suites on some ships are even assigned private butlers). Most have a sitting area with a sofa and chairs; some have two bathrooms, occasionally with a whirlpool bath. The most expensive suites may be priced without regard to the number of passengers occupying them.

Furnishings Almost all modern cabins are equipped with individually controlled air-conditioning and a private bathroom—usually closet-size, with a toilet, small shower, and washbasin. More expensive cabins, especially on newer ships, may have a bathtub. Most cabins also have limited closet space, a small desk or dresser, a reading light, and, on many ships, a phone and TV, sometimes even a VCR.

Selecting a Cabin*

Luxury Suite/Apartment

The largest accommodations on board, luxury suites have sitting areas, queen-size beds, vanity desks, and walk-in closets (with safes).

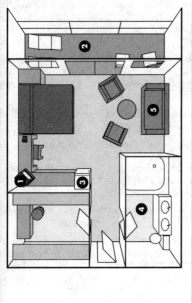
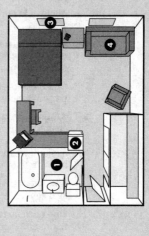

❶ Although televisions are common, luxury suites often have VCRs (and access to a video library) and stereos as well.

❷ Private verandas, connected by sliding doors, are on some ships.

❸ Most luxury suites have refrigerators, often with stocked bars. Butler service is provided on some ships.

❹ Twin sinks and Jacuzzi bathtubs (with shower) are typical.

❺ The sofa can usually unfold into a bed for additional passengers.

Suite

Though much more expensive than regular cabins, suites are also larger, featuring double beds, sitting areas, televisions, and comparatively large closets.

❶ Bathrooms are likely to have single sinks and bathtubs (with showers).

❷ Refrigerators are often included, although alcoholic beverages may not be complimentary.

❸ Suites, which tend to be on upper decks, usually have large picture windows.

❹ The sofa can be converted into a bed.

11

Outside Cabin

Outside cabins have showers rather than bathtubs and seldom have refrigerators. Most cabins have phones, and many have televisions.

❶ Many cabins, especially those on lower decks, have portholes instead of picture windows. Cabins on newer ships, however, often have large windows.

❷ Twin beds are common, although many ships now offer a double bed. Upper berths for additional passengers fold into the wall.

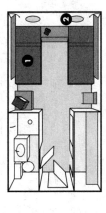

Inside Cabin

The least expensive accommodations, inside cabins have no portholes, tend to be tiny and oddly configured, have miniscule clothes closets, and bathrooms with showers only.

❶ Almost all cabins have phones, but few have televisions.

❷ Many inside cabins have upper and lower berths; the upper berth folds into the wall during the day, and the lower berth is made a couch.

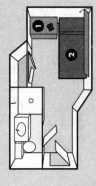

* Cruise lines offer a wide range of cabins, with a variety of names. This chart is intended as a general guide only.

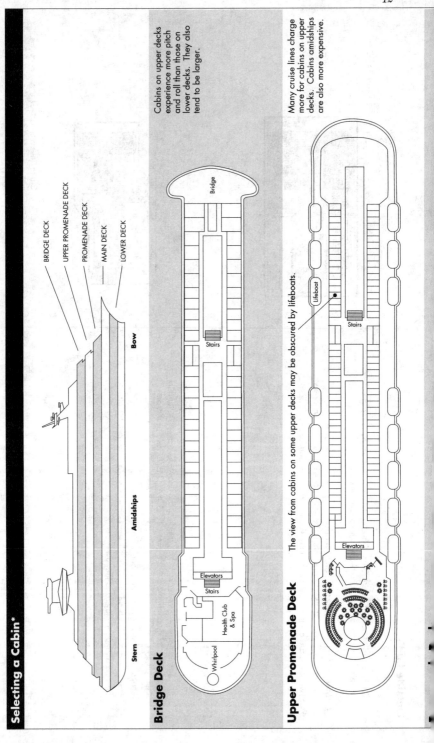

12

Selecting a Cabin*

Stern   Amidships   Bow

BRIDGE DECK
UPPER PROMENADE DECK
PROMENADE DECK
MAIN DECK
LOWER DECK

Cabins on upper decks experience more pitch and roll than those on lower decks. They also tend to be larger.

Many cruise lines charge more for cabins on upper decks. Cabins amidships are also more expensive.

Bridge Deck

Bridge

Stairs

Elevators
Stairs

Health Club & Spa

Whirlpool

Upper Promenade Deck

The view from cabins on some upper decks may be obscured by lifeboats.

Lifeboat

Stairs

Elevators

13

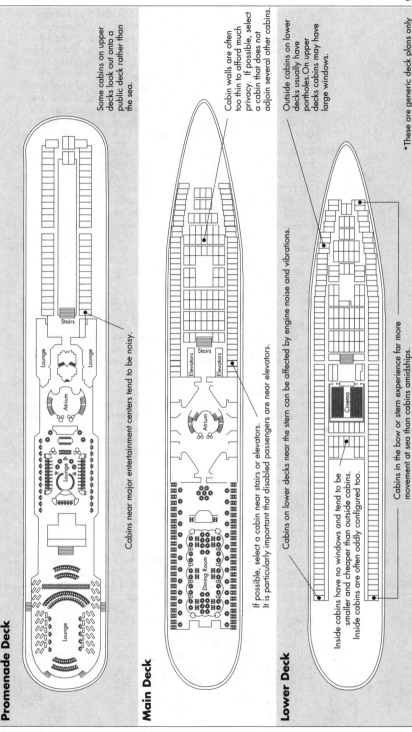

Promenade Deck

Some cabins on upper decks look out onto a public deck rather than the sea.

Cabins near major entertainment centers tend to be noisy.

Main Deck

Cabin walls are often too thin to afford much privacy. If possible, select a cabin that does not adjoin several other cabins.

If possible, select a cabin near stairs or elevators. It is particularly important that disabled passengers are near elevators.

Lower Deck

Outside cabins on lower decks usually have portholes. On upper decks cabins may have large windows.

Cabins on lower decks near the stern can be affected by engine noise and vibrations.

Cabins in the bow or stern experience far more movement at sea than cabins amidships.

Inside cabins have no windows and tend to be smaller and cheaper than outside cabins. Inside cabins are often oddly configured too.

*These are generic deck plans only

Depending upon the ship and category, a cabin may have beds or berths. The beds may be twins, either side-by-side or at right angles. On many new ships, twin beds convert into a double. Lower-price cabins and cabins on smaller or older ships may have upper and lower bunks, or berths, especially when three or four people share the same accommodation. To provide more living space in the daytime, the room steward folds the berths into the wall and may convert single beds into couches. More and more ships are reconfiguring cabins to offer double beds; if you require this, get an assurance in writing that you have been assigned a cabin with a double bed.

Sharing Most cabins are designed for two people. If more than two people share a cabin, a substantial discount to the third and fourth persons is usually offered; therefore, the per-person price for the room for all three or four passengers is lower. An additional discount is often offered for children sharing a cabin with their parents. Smaller, one-person cabins usually carry a premium price. When no single cabins are available, passengers traveling on their own must pay a single supplement, which usually ranges from 125% to 200% of the double-occupancy per-person rate. On request, however, many cruise lines will match up two strangers of the same sex in a cabin at the double-occupancy rate.

Location On all ships, regardless of size or design, the bow (front) and stern (back) bounce up and down on the waves far more than amidships (middle). Similarly, the closer your deck is to the true center of the ship—about halfway between the bottom of the hull and the highest deck—the less you will feel the ship's movement. Some cruise lines charge more for cabins amidships; most charge more for the higher decks.

Outside cabins have portholes or windows (which cannot be opened); on the upper decks, the view from outside cabins may be partially obstructed by lifeboats or overlook a public deck. Because outside cabins are more desirable, many newer upscale and luxury ships are configured with outside cabins only. On a few ships more expensive outside cabins have a private veranda that opens onto the sea.

Inside cabins on older vessels are often smaller and oddly shaped in order to fit around the ship's particular configuration. On newer ships, the floor plans of inside cabins are virtually identical to those of outside cabins. Providing windowless inside cabins don't make you feel claustrophobic, they're a great way to save money.

Cruise brochures show the ship's layout deck by deck and the approximate location and shape of every cabin and suite. Study the deck plan to make sure the cabin you pick is not near the noise of public rooms or the ship's engine, and make sure that you are near stairs or an elevator. If detailed layouts of typical cabins are printed, you can determine what kind of beds the cabin has, if it has a window or a porthole, and what furnishings are provided. In Chapter 3 we have tried to indicate those outside-cabin locations that may be partially obstructed by lifeboats or that overlook a public deck. Be aware that configurations within each category can differ.

When to Go

Although the cruise industry is booming year-round, there are definite cruise seasons, and the most desirable times command the highest prices. Here are the most popular seasons:

- November–April in the Caribbean
- Mid-June–Labor Day in the Caribbean for families
- Late April–early October in Bermuda
- October–mid-May along the Mexican Riviera
- Early December–early March around South America
- Holidays, such as Christmas, Easter, and, in South America, Carnival time
- September–October, December–March, and May for the Panama Canal
- June–August and holidays in Hawaii
- Mid-May–mid-September in Alaska
- June–mid-October in Canada and the northeastern U.S. seacoast
- December–February for Antarctica

While the weather might be marginally cooler or drier during high season in the Caribbean and Mexican Riviera, there is no reason not to go to these areas during the low and shoulder seasons, when both ships and ports are less crowded and fares are often lower. The one exception to this rule is that fall Caribbean cruises risk an encounter with a tropical storm or hurricane. Alaska cruises run in summer only, and Antarctic cruises have an even shorter season because of extreme weather conditions.

Booking Your Cruise

Most cruise ships sail at or near capacity, especially during high season, so consider making reservations six months to a year ahead. On the other hand, you may be able to save a bundle by booking close to the sailing date, especially if you go through a cruise specialist or a discounter.

Getting the Best Cruise for Your Dollar

It used to be an article of faith that one travel agent would give you cruise rates identical to those offered by any other. In fact, until airline deregulation in 1978, it was illegal for travel agents to discount the set price for airline tickets. And by custom, most other bookings—from cruise ships to hotels to car rentals—were also sold at the same price, regardless of the agency. The rare discount or rebate was kept discreetly under the table. In recent years, however, this practice among travel agencies has declined—and cruise travelers benefit.

Like everything in retail, each cruise has a list price. However, the actual selling price can vary tremendously: These days, if you ask any 10 passengers on almost any given ship what they're paying per diem, they'll give you 10 sharply different answers. Discounts on the same accommodation can range from 5% on a single fare to 50% on the second fare in a cabin. The deepest discounts are in the Caribbean. Top-of-the line cruises may not be discounted. However, added-values, such as free business-class air transportation, may be dangled before you to promote certain sailings of certain ships.

Approach deep discounts with skepticism. Fewer than a dozen cabins may be offered at the discounted price, they may be inside cabins, and the fare may not include air transportation or transfer.

Though a single, sure-fire path to whopping savings may not exist, you can maximize your chances in several ways:

Full-Service Travel Agents Consider booking with a full-service travel agent. He or she can make your arrangements and deal directly with airlines, cruise companies, car-rental agencies, hotels, and resorts. You won't be charged a service fee—agents make money on commissions from the cruise lines and other suppliers—and you'll eliminate such expenses as long-distance phone calls and postage. Some agents even throw in complimentary flight bags and champagne.

However, you may not wish to rely solely on your agent when selecting your ship and itinerary. Since most travel agencies book everything from cruises to business flights to theme-park vacations, your local agent may not possess a full knowledge of the cruise industry. Agents may have sailed on some of the ships and seen some ports, but most have acquired their knowledge of competing cruise lines from the same booklets and brochures available to the public. Because agents work on commission, there is some potential conflict of interest. Fortunately, disreputable agents remain relatively scarce.

Cruise-Only Travel Agents "Cruise-only" travel agencies constitute one of the fastest-growing segments of the travel industry, and most major towns and cities have at least one. Their knowledgeable employees may have sailed on many of these ships themselves. But that's only one of their strengths. Working in conjunction with specific cruise lines, cruise-only agencies obtain significant discounts by agreeing to sell large blocs of tickets. To make their quotas, they pass along savings to their clients. The discount you get depends upon agency, cruise line, popularity of the ship, season, and current demand.

Cruise Travel Clubs Some cruise-only agencies are run as private clubs, and for an annual fee of $25 to $50 offer members a newsletter, flight bags or other free gifts, special benefits to repeat clients, and sometimes, if the agency negotiates a group price with the cruise line, better rates.

Haggling Shopping around may or may not get you a better deal. Some cruise-only travel agencies discount every cruise they sell—one agency may sell at fixed prices, while another may charge whatever supply and demand will allow. Even when an agent quotes a particular price, go ahead and politely try for a further discount. You have absolutely nothing to lose. If you don't *ask* for the lowest price, you're probably not going to get it. On the other hand, this ploy is best used by experienced cruisers who know what they're looking for. Beginners may find it's worth paying a little more for the sound advice an experienced agent may offer.

Last-Minute Booking When cruise companies have cancellations or unsold cabins, they use cruise-only agencies and cruise specialists to recoup revenue. The closer it is to the sailing date, the bigger the savings. Typically, this type of discount is upward of 25%. You can't book very far in advance—usually only from two weeks to a month. To obtain the best discount, you have to be flexible, and ideally be prepared to leave on as little as 24 hours' notice. You might end up spending your vacation at home, or you might luck into the travel bargain of a lifetime.

A caveat: Cabin choice is limited, air transportation may not be included, and you may not get the meal seating you prefer. Also, think about why those cabins haven't been sold. Do you want to sail for less on the leftovers, or pay more to sail on a ship that is consistently full because it is consistently good?

Early-Booking Discounts Several cruise lines have recently begun offering discounts to customers who book early. In addition to the discount, an early booking gives you a better choice of cabin and sailing date. Some lines guarantee that passengers who book early will receive any lower rate that the line subsequently posts on that particular cruise. Some lines offer an additional discount for paying the full fare in advance.

Spotting Swindlers Always be on the lookout for a scam. Although reputable agencies far outnumber crooks, a handful of marketeers use deceptive and unethical tactics. The best way to avoid being fleeced is to deal with an agency that has been in business for at least five years. If you have any doubts about its credibility, consult your Better Business Bureau or consumer protection agency—*before* you mail in any deposits. Or call the cruise line to verify the agent's reliability. Be wary of bait-and-switch tactics: If you're told that an advertised bargain cruise is sold out, do not be persuaded to book a more expensive substitute. Also, if you're told that your cruise reservation was canceled because of overbooking and that you must pay extra for a confirmed rescheduled sailing, demand a full refund. Finally, if ever you fail to receive a voucher or ticket on the promised date, place an inquiry immediately.

Choosing the Right Agency or Club How do you find an honest, competent travel agent? Word of mouth is always a safe bet—get recommendations from friends, family, and colleagues, especially those who have cruised before. Or look in the Yellow Pages for agents identified as members of CLIA (Cruise Lines International Association) or ASTA (American Society of Travel Agents). CLIA agents have had extensive training, have cruised on several ships and inspected others, and have the background and resources to match carefully prospective passengers with the appropriate cruise line. Agents who are CLIA Accredited Cruise Counsellors or Master Cruise Counsellors are most knowledgeable. There are 20,000 CLIA affiliates nationwide. Larger, well-established agencies are more likely to employ experienced cruisers, but smaller agencies may give you more personal attention. Check around and weigh your options carefully. Then phone for an appointment to interview a few prospects.

Keep one crucial point in mind: To have a wonderful cruise, you need to pick the right ship. Bon vivants will find long cruises on certain upscale ships boring; foodies and highbrows will be miserable on mass-market Caribbean cruises. A romantic getaway cannot be had in the company of families with howling young children. Thus, an agent's first step should be to ask *you* questions about *your* lifestyle, vacation preferences, and expectations. If an agent places promotion of a specific ship or cruise line over consideration of your particular needs, move on.

Here are a few of the better agencies handling cruises; some are full- service, others cruise-only. Publications such as *Cruise Travel Magazine* and *Cruises & Tours* (*see* Choosing Your Cruise, *above*) also list agencies.

Ambassador Tours, Inc. (165 Post St., 2nd floor, San Francisco, CA 94108, tel. 415/981–5678 or 800/989–9000).

Cruise Fairs of America (2029 Century Park E, Los Angeles, CA 90067, tel. 310/556–2925 or 800/456–4386).

Cruise Headquarters (4225 Executive Sq. #1200, La Jolla, CA 92037, tel. 619/453–1201 or 800/424–6111).

Cruise Holidays International (9665 Chesapeake Dr., Suite 401, San Diego, CA 92123, tel. 619/279–4780 or 800/866–7245).

The Cruise Line, Inc. (4770 Biscayne Blvd., Penthouse 1, Miami, FL 33137, tel. 800/777–0707).

Cruise Pro (99 Long Ct., Suite 200, Thousand Oaks, CA 91360, tel. 800/222–7447, 800/258–7447 in CA, or 800/433–8747 in Canada).

Cruise Quarters of America (1241 E. Dyer Rd., Suite 110, Santa Ana, CA 92705, tel. 714/549–3445 or 800/648–2444).

Crui$e Value (c/o Golden Bear Travel, 16 Digital Dr., Suite 100, Box 6115, Novato, CA 94948, tel. 415/382–8900 or 800/551–1000 outside CA).

CruiseMasters (3415 Sepulveda Blvd., Suite 645, Los Angeles, CA 90034, tel. 310/397–7175, 800/242–9444, or 800/242–9000 in CA).

Cruises of Distinction (460 Bloomfield Ave., Montclair, NJ 07042, tel. 201/744–1331 or 800/634–3445).

Don Ton Cruise Tours (3151 Airway Ave., E–1, Costa Mesa, CA 92626, tel. 800/688–4785).

Kelly Cruises (2001 Midwest Rd., Suite 108, Oak Park, IL 60521, tel. 708/932–8300 or 800/837–7447 outside IL).

Landry and Kling East, Inc. Cruise Specialists (Gables Waterway 1, 1390 S. Dixie Hwy., Suite 1207, Coral Gables, FL 33146, tel. 800/223–2026).

MVP Cruise Club ($30 annual membership; 917 N. Broadway, North Massapequa, NY 11758, tel. 516/541–7782 or 800/253–4242 outside NY).

South Florida Cruises (5352 N.W. 53rd Ave., Fort Lauderdale, FL 33309, tel. 305/739–7447 or 800/327–7447).

Time to Travel (582 Market St., San Francisco, CA 94104, tel. 415/421–3333 or 800/524–3300).

The Travel Company (El Camino Real, Suite 250, Dept. CT, Atherton, CA 94027, tel. 415/367–6000 or 800/367–6090).

Trips 'n Travel (9592 Harding Ave., Surfside, FL 33154, tel. 305/864–2222 or 800/331–2745 outside FL).

Vacations at Sea (4919 Canal St., New Orleans, LA 70119, tel. 504/482–1572 or 800/749–4950 outside LA).

White Travel Service, Inc. (127 Park Rd., West Hartford, CT 06119, tel. 203/233–2648 or 800/547–4790).

Videotapes

Most travel agencies have a library of travel tapes, including some on specific cruise ships; usually you can also borrow, rent, or buy tapes directly from the cruise line. As you view the tape, keep in mind that the cruise company produced it to show its ship in the best light. Still, you will get a visual idea of the size and shape of the cabins, dining room, swimming pool, and public rooms; the kinds of attractions, amenities, and entertainment on board; and the ports and islands at which you'll stop.

You can also obtain VHS or Beta videos about many cruises and cruise ships at about $20 each from **Vacations on Video** (1309 E. Northern St., Phoenix, AZ 85020, tel. 602/483–1551). **Vacations Ashore & All the Ships at Sea** (173 Minuteman Causeway, Cocoa Beach, FL 32931, tel. 407/868–2131), a bimonthly video magazine, reviews five ships per issue ($90 per year or $25 per issue).

Cruise Brochures

Although a brochure is as promotional as a videotape, it can provide valuable information about a ship and what it has to offer. Make sure the brochures you select are the most recent versions: Schedules, itineraries, and prices change constantly. Study the maps of the decks and cabin layouts, and be sure to read the fine print to find out just what you'll be getting for your money. Check out the details on fly/cruise programs; optional pre- and post-cruise packages; the ship's credit-card and check-cashing policy; embarkation and debarkation procedures; and legal matters of payment, cancellation, insurance, and liability.

Payment

Deposit Most cruises must be reserved with a refundable deposit of $200–$500 per person, depending upon how expensive the cruise is; the balance is due one to two months before you sail. Don't let a travel agent pressure you into paying a larger deposit or paying the balance earlier. If the cruise is less than a month away, however, it may be legitimate for the agency to require the entire amount immediately.

If possible, pay your deposit and balance with a credit card. This gives you some recourse if you need to cancel, and you can ask the credit-card company to intercede on your behalf in case of problems. Don't forget to get a receipt.

Handing money over to your travel agent constitutes a contract, so before you pay your deposit, study the cruise brochure to find out the provisions of the cruise contract. What is the payment schedule and cancellation policy? Will there be any additional charges before you can board your ship, such as transfers, port fees, or local taxes? If your air connection requires you to spend an evening in a hotel near the port before or after the cruise, is there an extra cost?

Cancellation If you cancel your reservation 45–60 days prior to your scheduled cruise (the grace period varies from line to line), you may receive your entire deposit or payment back. You will forfeit some or even all of your deposit if you cancel any later. In rare cases, however, if your reason for canceling is unavoidable, the cruise line may decide, at its discretion, to waive some or all of the forfeiture. An average cancellation charge is $100 one month before sailing, $100 plus 50% of the ticket price 15–30 days before sailing, and $100 plus 75% of the ticket price between 14 days and 24 hours before sailing. If you simply fail to show up when the ship sails, you will lose the entire amount. Many travel agents also assess a small cancellation fee. Check their policy.

Insurance Cruise lines sell cancellation insurance for about $65 for a seven-day cruise. The amount varies according to the line, the number of days in the cruise, and the price you paid for the ticket. Such insurance protects you against cancellation fees; it may also reimburse you, on a deductible basis, if your luggage is lost or damaged. Note, however, that there are usually some restrictions. For instance, the policy may insure that you receive a full refund *only* if you cancel and notify the cruise line no fewer than 72 hours in advance. Some travel agencies and cruise clubs give customers free trip insurance; be sure to ask when booking your cruise.

Before You Go

Tickets, Vouchers, and Other Travel Documents

Cruise lines give you your cruise ticket and transfer vouchers (which will get you from the airport to the ship and vice versa) after you make the final payment to your travel agent. Depending upon the airline, and whether or not you have purchased a fly/cruise package, you may receive your plane tickets or charter flight vouchers at the same time; you may also receive vouchers for any shore excursions, although most cruise lines prefer to hand those over when you board your ship. Should your travel documents not arrive when promised, contact your travel agent or call the cruise line directly. Occasionally tickets are delivered directly to the ship for those who book late.

Once you board your ship, you may be asked to turn over your passport for group immigration clearance (*see* Passports, *below*; Embarkation in Arriving and Departing, *below*) or to turn over your return plane ticket so the ship's staff may reconfirm your flight home. Otherwise, keep travel documents in a safe place, such as a shipboard safe-deposit box.

Passports

U.S. Citizens If you are traveling to Canada, Mexico, or Bermuda, your birth certificate, baptismal certificate, or even driver's license may be sufficient identification. But the surest bet is a passport.

Passport Renewals You may renew your passport by mail. Send a completed renewal form (DSP–82), plus two recent, identical passport photographs; your current passport, providing it's less than 12 years old and was issued after your 18th birthday; and a check or money order for $55 to the National Passport Center (Box 371971, Pittsburgh, PA 15250). Newly created, this center supersedes passport-agency addresses on older renewal forms that may still be in use.

New Passports You must appear in person at any of the 13 U.S. Passport Agency offices or at post offices and courthouses accepting applications. Bring the completed application form (DSP–11) plus proof of U.S. citizenship, such as a certified copy of your birth certificate or a certificate of naturalization; proof of identity, such as a valid driver's license, military ID, student ID, or other unexpired document with your signature and photo; two passport photographs; and either cash, check or money order made out to Passport Services in the amount of the fee ($65 for 10-year passports, issued to those 18 and older, or $40 for five-year passports, issued only to those under 18). Although passports are usually mailed within two weeks of your application's receipt, it's best to allow three weeks for delivery in low season, five weeks or more from April through summer.

General You can pick up new and renewal application forms at any of
Information the 13 U.S. Passport Agency offices and at some post offices and courthouses. All photographs must be recent, identical, and 2 inches square; black-and-white and color photos are acceptable. Call the Department of State Office of Passport Services' information line (1425 K St. NW, Washington, DC 20522, tel. 202/647–0518) for details.

If your passport is lost or stolen abroad, report it immediately to the nearest embassy or consulate and to the local police. If you can provide the consular officer with the information contained in the passport, they will usually be able to issue you a new passport. For this reason, it is a good idea to keep a copy of the data page of your passport in a separate place, or to leave the passport number, date, and place of issuance with a relative or friend at home.

Non-U.S. Citizens If you plan to cruise from an American gateway, such as Miami or Los Angeles, and return to the United States at the end of the trip, you may need a passport from your own country, along with a B-2 visa, which allows multiple entries into the United States.

Canadians An identity card will be sufficient for entry and reentry into the United States.

Passport application forms are available at 23 regional passport offices as well as post offices and travel agencies. Whether applying for a first or subsequent passport, you must apply in person. You'll need the completed application plus the originals of documents confirming your Canadian citizenship (birth certificate, certificate of Canadian citizenship, or, if born in Québec, a record of birth issued by a provincial religious, municipal, or judicial authority); two identical photographs, preferably black-and-white, measuring no more than 2″ by 2¾″; the $35 passport fee, payable by money order, certified check, bank draft made out to the Receiver General for Canada, or in cash; and any passport or other travel document issued within the last five years. In addition, your application and one of the photographs must be signed by an eligible guarantor—that is, a Canadian citizen who is a doctor, dentist, minister, bank officer, or notary public who has known you for at least two years. Children under 16 may be included on a parent's passport but must have their own passport to travel alone. Passports are valid for five years and are usually mailed within two weeks of an application's receipt. For more information in English or French, call the passport office (tel. 514/283–2152).

U.K. Citizens Applications for new and renewal passports are available from main post offices as well as at the six passport offices, located in Belfast, Glasgow, Liverpool, London, Newport, and Peterborough. You may apply in person at all passport offices, or by mail to all except the London office; Londoners should mail applications to the Glasgow office (3 Northgate, 96 Milton St.,

Cowcaddens, Glasgow G4 0BT, tel. 041/332–0271). For your first passport, you must submit the completed form plus the original of your birth or adoption certificate; two recent, identical photographs measuring 45 millimeters by 35 millimeters; and, if you're a married or divorced woman, the original of your marriage certificate or divorce documents. The form and one of the photographs must be countersigned by a Commonwealth citizen who has known you personally for at least two years and is a minister, judge, doctor, lawyer, teacher, civil servant, member of parliament, police officer, or person of similar standing. For a renewal passport, you may submit the renewal application along with your old passport and new photos; the application and photographs must be countersigned as above only if your appearance has changed so much that you no longer look like the same person. The fee is £18 for a 32-page passport, £27 for a 48-page document. If applying by mail, send a postal order or check made out to "Passport Office," crossed "Account Payee," and with your name and address written on the back; if applying in person, you must pay cash or support the check with a bank card. Children under 16 may travel on a parent's passport when accompanying them. All passports are valid for 10 years. Allow a month for processing.

A British Visitor's Passport is valid for holidays and some business trips of up to three months to Bermuda as well as various European countries. It can include both partners of a married couple. You must apply in person at a main post office and present your uncanceled British passport (or the original of your birth or adoption certificate, an uncanceled British visitor's passport, a U.K. passport in which you were included as a child, your naturalization certificate, or your pension book or card, plus your NHS medical card, driver's license, valid check or credit card, your child- benefit book, or a recent gas, phone, or electricity bill). In addition, you need two recent, identical photographs 35 millimeters by 45 millimeters and the fee (£12, or £18 if your spouse is included on the document). A British visitor's passport is valid for one year and will be issued on the same day that you apply.

Visas

Information about visa requirements for various cruise destinations may be found in Chapter 4. Some destinations require a tourist card—a kind of ad hoc visa—which often can be filled out at your travel agent's office or during the plane ride to your ship. Most nations simply stamp an entry and exit visa when you come in and leave the country. (Many do not even bother with the stamp, so if you want a page of colorful stamps as a souvenir of your voyage, ask immigration officials specifically to stamp your passport.)

Many ships that ply Central and South American ports have the local immigration officials inspect and stamp all the passengers' passports at the same time, so the boarding card issued to each passenger is the only document you'll need to get on or off the ship. But there are some countries, especially in South America, from which you must obtain a visa stamp in advance. Your travel agent should inform you if you need a visa and should even help you obtain it, by mail or directly from the consulate or embassy. (There may be a charge of up to $25 for this service, added to the nominal visa charge of about $5.)

Vaccinations and Inoculations

Unless you plan to cruise to exotic or out-of-the-way destinations, you probably will not need any shots before you leave. However, if you are in a high-risk category (middle-age, overweight, high blood pressure, diabetes), your doctor may wish to prescribe certain inoculations (such as a flu shot) not normally recommended for otherwise healthy people.

If you intend to visit some of the more remote Central or South American jungles, you may have to take antimalaria pills (begin taking them three weeks in advance of your trip to build immunity). Hepatitis, once rare, now crops up periodically throughout the Americas; check with your doctor about whether or not to have a gamma-globulin shot. Cruise ships regularly avoid regions that have typhoid, typhus, and cholera. If it's been years or decades since you received a polio vaccination, and you're headed for South America, it's advisable to take a booster dose. It's also a good idea to have a tetanus shot if you haven't had one within the past five years or so. Visit your doctor for shots three or four weeks before your trip since some vaccinations must be given in a series of shots.

Certain rarely given inoculations, such as that for yellow fever (if you are going into the Amazon), are administered, at a nominal cost, only by U.S. Health Department clinics. Your physician or the local hospital can give you the address and hours of the nearest facility. After getting such a shot, you will be given an International Certificate of Vaccination, which should be carried with your passport.

Traveling with Children

Many ships provide fare breaks, special facilities, and programs for parents taking a cruise with their children. A few lines allow children under 12 staying in the same cabin with two adults to travel free, while others offer rates that range between half-price and $30 per diem per child. Airfare for children to and from the port of departure is frequently discounted, as are many shore excursions and museum admission charges, especially on Alaska cruises. Fares for children vary widely from line to line and often change according to the season.

At least during summer vacation and holiday periods, many ships now have supervised play areas for children and teenagers. Programs include arts and crafts, computer instruction, games and quizzes, kids' movies, swimming pool parties, scavenger hunts, ship tours, magic shows, snorkeling lessons, kite-flying, cooking classes, and teaching sessions on the history of the ports to be visited. Premier, the official cruise line of Walt Disney World, has children's breakfasts with costumed Disney characters. Find out in advance whether there are special programs for your child's specific age group, how many hours a day are scheduled, whether meals are included, and what the counselor-to-child ratio is.

Some ships provide day care and baby-sitting for younger children at no extra charge, while others charge a nominal hourly rate. On many ships, baby-sitting is by private arrangement (at a negotiated price). If you plan to bring an infant or toddler, be sure to request a crib, high chair, or booster seat in advance and bring plenty of diapers and formula.

Ships with two dinner seatings routinely assign passengers with children to the earlier seating; some lines will not permit children to eat in the dining room on their own. If your kids are picky eaters, check ahead to see if special children's menus are offered.

Publications Several excellent sources on family traveling exist. But above all, call the line and ask if it is attuned to traveling with children, and talk it over with your travel agent.

The most comprehensive guide on cruising with children is *Cruising with Children,* which contains the nitty-gritty details—from pricing to kids' programs to crib availability—on 30 cruise lines. It is available from **Travel With Your Children** (TWYCH, 45 W. 18th St., 7th floor Tower, New York, NY 10011, tel. 212/206–0688; $20 plus $3 postage). TWYCH's newsletter *Family Travel Times,* issued 10 times year (annual subscription $55), features a column on cruising. **Premier Cruise Lines'** complimentary brochure "Pack Up the Kids" is full of helpful hints (400 Challenger Rd., Cape Canaveral, FL 32920, tel. 800/473–3262).

Hints for Older Passengers

For the older traveler, cruise vacations strike an excellent balance: They offer a tremendous variety of activities and itineraries but require only moderate investment of energy, planning time, and money. You can do as much or as little as you want, meet new people, see new places, enjoy shows and bingo, learn to play bridge, or take up needlepoint—all within a very safe, familiar environment. Cruises are *not* a good idea for those who are bedridden, have a serious medical condition that is likely to flare up on board, or are prone to periods of confusion or severe memory loss.

No particular rules apply to senior citizens on cruises, except to exercise caution and common sense. Those who want a leisurely, relaxed pace will probably be happiest on ships that attract a higher percentage of older passengers: upscale vessels, small specialty cruises, and voyages of longer than seven days. Passengers who are less than spry should select a cabin near an elevator or stairway amidships, on the deck nearest the main public rooms. Do not book a cabin with upper and lower berths.

Only a couple of cruise lines, notably Premier, have reduced senior-citizen rates, but senior citizens may be able to take advantage of local discounts at ports. Showing proof of age often ensures reduced admissions, half-fares on public transportation, and special dining rates.

Organizations The **American Association of Retired Persons** (AARP, 601 E St. NW, Washington, DC 20049, tel. 202/434–2277) has several programs, including the Purchase Privilege Program (which offers discounts on hotels, car rentals, and sightseeing) and the AARP Travel Experience from American Express (400 Pinnacle Way, Suite 450, Norcross, GA 30071, tel. 800/745–4567 for cruises, 800/927–0111 for other arrangements). AARP membership is open to those 50 and over; annual dues are $8 per person or couple.

Two other membership organizations offer discounts on lodgings, car rentals, and other travel products, along with such nontravel perks as magazines and newsletters. The **National Council of Senior Citizens** (1331 F St. NW, Washington, DC 20004, tel. 202/347–8800) is a nonprofit advocacy group with some 5,000 local clubs across the United States; membership costs $12 per person or couple annually. **Mature Outlook** (6001 N. Clark St., Chicago, IL 60660, tel. 800/336–6330), a Sears Roebuck & Co. subsidiary with 800,000 members, charges $9.95 for an annual membership.

Note: If you use any senior-citizen identification card for reduced hotel rates before or after your cruise, mention it when booking, not when checking out. At restaurants, show your card before you're seated; discounts may be limited to certain menus, days, or hours. If you need to rent a car, ask about promotional rates that might improve on your senior-citizen discount.

Tour Operators **Saga International Holidays** (222 Berkeley St., Boston, MA 02116, tel. 800/343–0273), which specializes in group travel for people over 60, offers a selection of variously priced cruises as well as tours.

Publications ***The International Health Guide for Senior Citizen Travelers,*** by W. Robert Lange MD ($4.95 plus $1.50 for shipping; Pilot Books, 103 Cooper St., Babylon, NY 11702, tel. 516/422–2225), advises on pretrip planning and on traveling with specific medical conditions. It includes a list of what to pack in a basic medical travel kit and a chart showing how to adjust insulin dosages when flying across multiple time zones. ***Get Up and Go*** ($10.95 plus $1.75 postage; Gem Publishing Group, Box 50820, Reno, NV 89513, tel. 702/786–7419) is a 325-page handbook of travel tips and deals for Americans over 49; the same organization publishes the monthly ***Mature Traveler*** newsletter ($24.50 annually), covering travel bargains and programs for senior citizens.

Hints for Passengers with Disabilities

Unfortunately, some cruise lines make things difficult for travelers with disabilities. Disclaimers on every cruise brochure allow ships to refuse passage to anyone whose disability might endanger others. Most ships require that you travel with a full-fare companion if you have severe disabilities or even if you use a wheelchair.

If you have a mobility impairment, even though you do not use a wheelchair, tell your travel agent. Follow up by making sure that the cruise line is fully informed of your disabilities and special needs. Get written confirmation of any promises of a special cabin and provisions for transfer to and from the airport. The line may request a letter from your doctor stating that you need neither a wheelchair nor a companion, or that you will not require special medical attention on board.

If you have a chronic problem that may require medical attention, notify the ship's doctor soon after you board so that he or she will be able to recognize the symptoms—and be prepared to treat you as needed.

Passengers in Many modern cruise ships have modified a small number cab-
Wheelchairs ins by enlarging the bathroom, mounting handrails on the beds

and grab bars by the toilets, and clearing the floor of obstructions. If you need such a cabin, book as far in advance as possible. On several ships—mostly new ones, but some refitted older ones as well—corridors and promenades are wider, ramps have been installed where necessary, elevator buttons are at chest level, and the like. If you book a cabin that is supposed to be navigable by someone in a wheelchair, ask specifically how it is equipped. Is the entrance level or ramped? Are all doorways at least 30″ (wider if your wheelchair is not standard-size)? Are pathways to beds, closets, and bathrooms at least 36″ wide, and unobstructed? In the bathroom, is there 42″ of clear space in front of the toilet, grab bars behind and on one side of it and in the bathtub or shower? Ask whether there is a three-prong outlet in the cabin, and whether the bathroom has a hand-held showerhead, a bath bench, roll-in shower or shower stall with fold-down seat, if you need them.

The best cruise ship for passengers who use wheelchairs is one that ties up right at the dock at every port, at which time a ramp or even an elevator is always made available. Unfortunately, it's hard to ascertain this in advance, for a ship may dock at a particular port on one voyage and anchor in the harbor on the next. Ask your travel agent to find out which ships are scheduled to dock on which cruises. If a tender is used, some ships will have crew members carry the wheelchair and passenger from the ship to the tender. Unfortunately, other ships point-blank refuse to take wheelchairs on tenders, especially if the water is choppy.

Visually Impaired Passengers Some ships allow guide dogs to accompany blind passengers; however, if your cruise is scheduled to visit foreign ports (as most do), you won't be able to take a guide dog ashore in most countries without later subjecting your animal to a two- to six-month quarantine upon return to the United States. There are a few exceptions, including Bermuda, so check with your travel agent before booking.

Pregnant Women Advanced pregnancy is considered a disability, and a pregnant woman may be refused passage. Check with the cruise line about its definition of "advanced," but it usually refers to any time during the third trimester.

Organizations The **Information Center for Individuals with Disabilities** (Fort Point Pl., 27–43 Wormwood St., Boston, MA 02210, tel. 617/727–5540 or 800/462–5015 in MA between 11 and 4, or leave message; TDD/TTY tel. 617/345–9743) helps with problem-solving and publishes a monthly newsletter and numerous fact sheets, including the 10-page "Tips for Planning a Vacation" (with airlines' toll-free TDD numbers and sections on auto and van, bus, train, ship, and plane travel) and the state-by-state list of "Tour Operators, Travel Agencies, and Travel Resources for People with Disabilities" (23 pages at present). On out-of-state orders, enclose $2 per sheet for postage. **Mobility International USA** (Box 3551, Eugene, OR 97403, voice and TDD tel. 503/343–1284) is the U.S. branch of an international organization based in Britain (*see below*) and present in 30 countries. It coordinates exchange programs for disabled people, especially programs with an educational, work, or community-service component; provides travel information; and publishes and sells *A World of Options for the '90s*, a guide to travel for people with disabilities ($16). Annual membership costs $20 and includes a quarterly newsletter and access to a referral service.

MossRehab Hospital Travel Information Service (1200 W. Tabor Rd., Philadelphia, PA 19141, tel. 215/456–9603, TDD tel. 215/456–9602) tries to get people started with their travel plans; for a nominal postage and handling fee, it will send information on tourist sights, transportation, and accommodations in destinations around the world. The **Society for the Advancement of Travel for the Handicapped** (SATH, 347 5th Ave., Suite 610, New York, NY 10016, tel. 212/447–7284, fax 212/725–8253) provides lists of tour operators specializing in travel for the disabled, information sheets on traveling with specific disabilities and to specific countries, and a quarterly newsletter. Annual membership is $45, $25 for students and senior citizens. Nonmembers may send $3 and a self-addressed, stamped envelope for information on specific destinations. **Travel Industry and Disabled Exchange** (TIDE, 5435 Donna Ave., Tarzana, CA 91356, tel. 818/368–5648) supplies travel information and publishes a quarterly newsletter. Annual membership is $15; most members are travel suppliers (travel agents, cruise lines, etc.), but consumers are welcome. **Travelin' Talk** (Box 3534, Clarksville, TN 37043, tel. 615/552–6670) is a network of disabled people worldwide ready to provide the lowdown on accessibility in their area. To join, there is a onetime registration fee (on a sliding scale of $1–$10 for individuals, $15–$50 for organizations) that also entitles you to a quarterly newsletter.

In the United Kingdom Main sources include the **Royal Association for Disability and Rehabilitation** (RADAR, 25 Mortimer St., London W1N 8AB, tel. 071/637–5400), which publishes travel information for the disabled in Britain, and **Mobility International** (228 Borough High St., London SE1 1JX, tel. 071/403–5688), the headquarters of an international membership organization that serves as a clearinghouse of travel information for people with disabilities.

Travel Agencies and Tour Operators **Directions Unlimited** (720 N. Bedford Rd., Bedford Hills, NY 10507, tel. 914/241–1700), a travel agency, has expertise in tours and cruises for the disabled. **Evergreen Travel Service** (4114 198th St. SW, Suite 13, Lynnwood, WA 98036, tel. 206/776–1184 or 800/435–2288) operates Wings on Wheels Tours for those in wheelchairs, White Cane Tours for the blind, and tours for the deaf and makes group and independent arrangements for travelers with any disability. **Flying Wheels Travel** (143 W. Bridge St., Box 382, Owatonna, MN 55060, tel. 800/535–6790 or 800/722–9351 in MN), a tour operator and travel agency, arranges international tours, cruises, and independent travel itineraries for people with mobility disabilities. **Nautilus,** at the same address as TIDE (*see above*), packages tours for the disabled internationally.

Publications In addition to the fact sheets, newsletters, and books mentioned above are several free publications available from the Consumer Information Center (Pueblo, CO 81009): "New Horizons for the Air Traveler with a Disability," a U.S. Department of Transportation booklet describing changes resulting from the 1986 Air Carrier Access Act and those still to come from the 1990 Americans with Disabilities Act (include Department 608Y in the address), and the Airport Operators Council's "Access Travel: Airports" (Dept. 5804), which describes facilities and services for the disabled at more than 500 airports worldwide.

Twin Peaks Press (Box 129, Vancouver, WA 98666, tel. 206/694–2462 or 800/637–2256) publishes the *Directory of Travel Agencies for the Disabled* ($19.95), listing more than 370 agencies worldwide; *Travel for the Disabled* ($19.95), listing some 500 access guides and accessible places worldwide; the *Directory of Accessible Van Rentals* ($9.95) for campers and RV travelers worldwide; and *Wheelchair Vagabond* ($14.95), a collection of personal travel tips. Add $2 per book for shipping.

What to Pack

Some cruise passengers like to bring a huge wardrobe so they can parade in their finest clothes as part of the cruise fantasy; others prefer to travel light, reasoning that they have no need to impress fellow travelers whom they will never see again. In general, anything goes, because most cruise ships today are far less formal than their ocean-liner predecessors—although upscale and luxury vessels are more formal than regular mainstream and small, budget ships. When in doubt, bring less, not more, because cabin closets are small. You really don't need more than one outfit for every two to two-and-a-half days of travel, especially if you coordinate an interchangeable wardrobe. Ships often have convenient laundry facilities as well (*see* Shipboard Services in On Board, *below*). And don't overload your luggage with extra toiletries and sundry items; they are easily available in port and in the ship's gift shop (though usually at a premium price).

You will naturally pack differently for the tropics than for an Alaskan cruise, but even if you're heading for the warmer climes, bring along a sweater in case of cool evening ocean breezes or overactive air-conditioning. (To find out what to pack for cruises to Antarctica, *see* Chapter 4.) Make sure you bring at least one pair of comfortable walking shoes for exploring port towns. Shorts or slacks are convenient for shore excursions, but remember that in Latin America women are expected to dress modestly and men to wear slacks. In Chapter 3 we indicate how many formal evenings each ship has during a typical cruise—usually two per seven-day cruise. Men should pack a dark suit, a tuxedo, or a white dinner jacket. Women should pack one long or cocktail dress for every two or three formal evenings on board. Most ships have semiformal evenings, when men should wear a jacket and tie. On a few upscale ships, men should wear a jacket and tie every evening. A few lines have no dress codes or guidelines.

Health

Sanitation All passenger ships sailing from American ports to foreign ports are inspected at least twice a year by the Centers for Disease Control (CDC) Vessel Sanitation Program. (Since American Hawaii Cruises' ships do not leave American waters, they are not subject to inspection.) Those that are rated as unsatisfactory—about 10% of them—are still permitted to sail, as, according to the CDC, "a low score does not necessarily imply an imminent risk of an outbreak of gastrointestinal disease." The CDC rates cruise ships on the following: water; food preparation and handling; potential contamination of food; and general cleanliness, storage, and repair. For a free copy of the latest sanitation inspection report, write: Chief, Vessel Program, Center for Environmental Health and Injury Control (1015 North America Way, Room 107, Miami, FL 33132).

Medical Care If you have a preexisting condition or a chronic disease, it's a good idea to let your steward know, because he or she can help you if you run into trouble. And if you have any dietary needs, let the cruise line know in advance so they tailor your meals to you diet.

All but the tiniest ships carry at least one doctor, and larger ones have fully equipped infirmaries, staffed with doctors and nurses, most of whom have emergency-room experience and who are prepared to handle medical emergencies. Doctors have office hours and make cabin calls if you are bedridden. Fees for medical services are usually nominal—$10–$25 for a consultation, including any medicine you may need—but not always: The charge can run into the hundreds of dollars for broken bones or emergency surgery, for which you must pay cash, by check, or with a credit card; you may then apply for reimbursement from your insurance company when you get home. In addition, most ships carry small quantities of the most frequently dispensed prescription drugs, from insulin to hypertension pills.

If you become seriously ill or injured and happen to be near a modern major city, it will be a relatively routine matter for a ship's captain to have you taken ashore. But if you're farther afield, you may have to be airlifted off the ship by helicopter and flown either to the nearest American territory or to an airport where you can be Medivaced by charter jet to the United States. If you have any reason to feel that you could have a medical emergency, ask your travel agent about buying trip insurance (*see* Insurance, *below*).

If you take medication regularly, visit your pharmacist and obtain a larger-than-usual supply of your particular prescription. Also, be sure to pack an extra pair of your prescription glasses. Keep all your medicine in a purse or a carry-on bag; don't pack it in luggage that must be checked through.

Seasickness Modern cruise ships, unlike their earlier transatlantic predecessors, are relatively motion-free vessels with computer-controlled stabilizers, and they usually sail in comparatively calm waters. According to many experts, antimotion medicine just isn't necessary for most people on most cruises. It's best to get treatment *before* you begin to feel ill, however. The easiest, most painless method is to ask your doctor or the ship's doctor to prescribe a Transderm patch, good for about 72 hours, which tapes behind your ear; the medicine, contained in a semipermeable membrane, is automatically absorbed through the skin into your bloodstream. Side effects can be strong and may include blurred vision and a dulled sense of taste. Two other antimotion drugs of preference are Bonine and Dramamine, both sold over the counter (in fact, many cruise ships hand out free packets of Dramamine at the purser's office or in the dining room); their one undesirable side effect is drowsiness. Some swear by wristbands (with an embedded plastic button) that employ acupressure to ward off seasickness; they're sold through travel-supplies catalogues, at some travel agencies, and in some ships' shops. If you do feel seasick, don't talk about it; stay away from anybody complaining about seasickness, and go out on deck. Breathe in the fresh air. Look at the horizon rather than the waves. Get involved in fun activities. This is one problem that, when ignored, will often go away. Typically, seasickness does not last longer than three to ten hours. In an emergency, ships' doctors can administer a shot that quickly relieves all symptoms of seasickness.

Potable Water Water and food on board any ship listed in this book is as safe as at any stateside restaurant. Canada, Bermuda, Puerto Rico, the Virgin Islands, and a handful of other well-developed countries and islands are quite safe in terms of sanitation, but at many other ports, precautions are in order. Local water may taste good, but it can contain bacteria to which locals are immune but visitors are susceptible. Diarrhea and intestinal disorders can result.

In such situations, drink only water that has been boiled for at least fifteen minutes. Unless you are sure that the ice in your drink comes from a pure source, avoid ice, which is often made from straight tap water; it may be fine in luxury hotels, which usually have their own distillation units. Because the glass you use may have been washed in suspect water, drink beer or soda straight from the can or bottle. In tropical climates, stay away from fruits or raw vegetables that you don't peel yourself.

Swimming Water While swimming in the sea or salt water doesn't present any health hazard (unless the area is polluted, as in Acapulco), swimming in rivers, freshwater lakes, and streams in undeveloped countries may expose you to harmful microorganisms or aquatic parasites. So, unless you are on a ship-sponsored shore excursion or have been specifically told by the cruise director that the local creeks and lakes are safe, stick with the ocean or chlorinated swimming pools.

Insurance

For U.S. Residents Most tour operators, travel agents, and insurance agents sell specialized health-and-accident, flight, trip-cancellation, and luggage insurance as well as comprehensive policies with some or all of these features. But before you make any purchase, review your existing health and homeowner policies to find out whether they cover expenses incurred while traveling.

Health-and-Accident Insurance Supplemental health-and-accident insurance for travelers is usually a part of comprehensive policies. Specific policy provisions vary, but they tend to address three general areas, beginning with reimbursement for medical expenses caused by illness or an accident during a trip. Such policies may reimburse anywhere from $1,000 to $150,000 worth of medical expenses; dental benefits may also be included. A second common feature is the personal-accident, or death-and-dismemberment, provision, which pays a lump sum to your beneficiaries if your die or to you if you lose one or both limbs or your eyesight. This is similar to the flight insurance described below, although it is not necessarily limited to accidents involving airplanes or even other "common carriers" (buses, trains, and ships) and can be in effect 24 hours a day. The lump sum awarded can range from $15,000 to $500,000. A third area generally addressed by these policies is medical assistance (referrals, evacuation, or repatriation and other services). Some policies reimburse travelers for the cost of such services; others may automatically enroll you as a member of a particular medical-assistance company.

Flight Insurance This insurance, often bought as a last-minute impulse at the airport, pays a lump sum to a beneficiary when a plane crashes and the insured dies (and sometimes to a surviving passenger who loses eyesight or a limb); thus it supplements the airlines' own coverage as described in the limits-of- liability paragraphs on your ticket (up to $75,000 on international flights, $20,000 on domestic ones—and that is generally subject to litigation). Charging an airline ticket to a major credit card often automatically signs you up for flight insurance; in this case, the coverage may also embrace travel by bus, train, and ship.

Baggage Insurance In the event of loss, damage, or theft on international flights, airlines limit their liability to $20 per kilogram for checked baggage (roughly about $640 per 70-pound bag) and $400 per passenger for unchecked baggage. On domestic flights, the ceiling is $1,250 per passenger. Excess-valuation insurance can be bought directly from the airline at check-in but leaves your bags vulnerable on the ground.

Trip Insurance There are two sides to this coin. **Trip-cancellation-and-interruption insurance** protects you in the event you are unable to undertake or finish your trip. **Default** or **bankruptcy insurance** protects you against a supplier's failure to deliver. Consider the former if your airline ticket, cruise, or package tour does not allow changes or cancellations. The amount of coverage to buy should equal the cost of your trip should you, a traveling companion, or a family member get sick, forcing you to stay home, plus the nondiscounted one-way airline ticket you would need to buy if you had to return home early. Read the fine print carefully; pay attention to sections defining "family member" and "preexisting medical conditions." A characteristic quirk of default policies is that they often do not cover default by travel agencies or default by a tour operator, airline, or cruise line if you bought your tour and the coverage directly from the firm in question. To reduce your need for default insurance, give preference to tours packaged by members of the United States Tour Operators Association (USTOA), which maintains a fund to reimburse clients in the event of member defaults. Even better, pay for travel arrangements with a major credit card, so you can refuse to pay the bill if services have not been rendered—and let the card company fight your battles.

Comprehensive Policies Companies supplying comprehensive policies with some or all of the above features include **Access America, Inc.,** underwritten by BCS Insurance Company (Box 11188, Richmond, VA 23230, tel. 800/284–8300); **Carefree Travel Insurance,** underwritten by The Hartford (Box 310, 120 Mineola Blvd., Mineola, NY 11501, tel. 516/294–0220 or 800/323–3149); **Tele-Trip** (Mutual of Omaha Plaza, Box 31762, Omaha, NE 68131, tel. 800/228–9792), a subsidiary of Mutual of Omaha; **The Travelers Companies** (1 Tower Sq., Hartford, CT 06183, tel. 203/277–0111 or 800/243–3174); **Travel Guard International,** underwritten by Transamerica Occidental Life Companies (1145 Clark St., Stevens Point, WI 54481, tel. 715/345–0505 or 800/782–5151); and **Wallach and Company, Inc.** (107 W. Federal St., Box 480, Middleburg, VA 22117, tel. 703/687–3166 or 800/237–6615), underwritten by Lloyds, London. These companies may also offer the above types of insurance separately.

U.K. Residents Most tour operators, travel agents, and insurance agents sell specialized policies covering accident, medical expenses, personal liability, trip cancellation, and loss or theft of personal

property. Some policies include coverage for delayed departure and legal expenses, winter-sports, accidents, or motoring
abroad. You can also purchase an annual travel- insurance policy valid for every trip you make during the year in which it's
purchased (usually only trips of less than 90 days). Before you
leave, make sure you will be covered if you have a preexisting
medical condition or are pregnant; your insurers may not pay
for routine or continuing treatment, or may require a note from
your doctor certifying your fitness to travel.

The Association of British Insurers, a trade association representing 450 insurance companies, advises extra medical coverage for visitors to the United States.

For advice by phone or a free booklet, "Holiday Insurance,"
that sets out what to expect from a holiday-insurance policy
and gives price guidelines, contact the Association of British
Insurers (51 Gresham St., London EC2V 7HQ, tel. 071/600–
3333; 30 Gordon St., Glasgow G1 3PU, tel. 041/226–3905; Scottish Provincial Bldg., Donegal Sq. W, Belfast BT1 6JE, tel.
0232/249176; call for other locations).

Getting Money

Some ships will not cash personal checks or take certain credit
cards. However, the purser's office usually cashes traveler's
checks, and on some ships, you can even open an account there
and get cash when you need it; it will be added to your bill along
with on-board purchases, and you pay at the end of the cruise.
Cashiers of on-board casinos also cash traveler's checks and
dispense cash advances on your credit card, even to those who
don't intend to gamble.

Traveler's Checks The most widely recognized are **American Express, Barclay's,
Thomas Cook,** and those issued by major commercial banks
such as **Citibank** and **Bank of America.** American Express also
issues *Traveler's Cheques for Two,* which can be signed and used
by you or your traveling companion. Some checks are free; usually the issuing company or the bank at which you make your
purchase charges 1% of the checks' face value as a fee. Be sure
to buy a few checks in small denominations to cash toward the
end of your trip, when you don't want to be left with more foreign currency than you can spend. Always record the numbers
of checks as you spend them, and keep this list separate from
the checks.

Cash Machines While there are many itineraries that never get near a port
with automated- teller machines, ATMs are proliferating and
can be found in most major tourist areas as well as aboard some
ships; many are tied to international networks such as **Cirrus**
and **Plus.** You can use your bank card at ATMs away from home
to withdraw money from your checking account and get cash
advances on a credit-card account (providing your card has
been programmed with a personal identification number, or
PIN). Check in advance on limits on withdrawals and cash advances within specified periods. Ask whether your bank-card
or credit-card PIN number will need to be reprogrammed for
use in the area you'll be visiting—a possibility if the number
has more than four digits. Remember that finance charges
apply on credit-card cash advances from ATMs as well as on
those from tellers. And note that, although transaction fees for
ATM withdrawals abroad will probably be higher than fees for

withdrawals at home, Cirrus and Plus exchange rates tend to be good.

Be sure to plan ahead: Obtain ATM locations and the names of affiliated cash-machine networks before departure. For specific foreign Cirrus locations, call 800/4–CIRRUS; for foreign Plus locations, consult the Plus directory at your local bank.

American Express Cardholder Services The company's **Express Cash** system lets you withdraw cash and/or traveler's checks from a worldwide network of 57,000 American Express dispensers and participating bank ATMs. You must *enroll first* (call 800/CASH–NOW for a form and allow two weeks for processing). Withdrawals are charged not to your card but to a designated bank account. You can withdraw up to $1,000 per seven-day period on the basic card, more if your card is gold or platinum. There is a 2% fee (minimum $2.50, maximum $10) for each cash transaction, and a 1% fee for traveler's checks (except for the platinum card), which are available only from American Express dispensers.

At AmEx offices, cardholders can also cash personal checks for up to $1,000 in any seven-day period (21 days abroad); of this $200 can be in cash, more if available, with the balance paid in traveler's checks, for which all but platinum cardholders pay a 1% fee. Higher limits apply to the gold and platinum cards.

Currency

U.S. dollars, traveler's checks, and credit cards are accepted in almost every port frequented by cruise ships. Many local businesses and vendors actually prefer receiving U.S. dollars.

But there are always times when foreign currency will come in handy—for museum and theater admissions, public buses, telephones, vending machines, and small tips. When you change money, change just as much as you need (since it can be difficult to reconvert it to U.S. dollars), and do it at a bank or money-exchange booth, where you will probably get better rates than at hotels, restaurants, shops, or the ship's purser's office. If you do change too much, look for the box that several cruise keep somewhere near the purser's office or reception desk, where passengers' leftover local bills and coins go to local charities or UNICEF.

Photography

Bring with you all the film, tapes, and batteries that you need. Such items are more expensive abroad or in the ship's commissary, and often the particular brand or size you want is not available.

Many long-distance shots cannot be captured with a normal lens, so bring a telephoto if possible. An ultraviolet or haze filter will remove excess blues that predominate at sea level and will protect your lens against sand and salt spray. Polarizing filters enhance bright skies and seas.

If you intend to charge videocamera batteries aboard ship, make certain that the ship supplies 110V–120V current, or that you use the proper converter. Don't attempt to attach your camcorder to the television in your cabin in order to play back tapes—many ships' televisions use European broadcast standards, making them incompatible with U.S.-made video equipment.

Further Reading

Those who wish to learn about the modern sailing era should read *Great Cruise Ships and Ocean Liners from 1954 to 1986*, by William H. Miller, Jr. Miller has assembled a marvelous collection of rare black-and-white photographs of many of history's greatest superliners, accompanied by a wealth of history and anecdotes that make wonderful shipboard reading.

Peter Freuchen's *Book of the Seven Seas* is an ambitious novel incorporating all that's best from the mythology, history, and exploration of the world's oceans. John Maxtone-Graham's three books, *The Only Way to Cross, Liners to the Sun*, and *Crossing & Cruising*, chronicle the growth of shipping from a mode of travel to a mode of pleasure. David McCullough's *The Path Between the Seas* is a fascinating account of the construction of the Panama Canal, from its ill-fated French origins to the battle against yellow fever and the creation of the country of Panama.

For practical information on cruising, **Cruise Lines International Association** (500 Fifth Ave., Suite 1407, New York, NY 10110; send self- addressed business-size envelope with 52¢ postage) offers a free booklet, "Cruising—Answers to Your Questions."

Arriving and Departing

Getting to the Port

By Plane   Most cruise passengers fly from their home cities on regularly scheduled or chartered flights to the principal ports of embarkation: Miami, Fort Lauderdale, Vancouver, San Francisco, Los Angeles, New York, and a few other coastal cities (*see* Ports of Embarkation in Chapter 4). Many cruise lines offer heavily discounted or even free plane tickets from 30 or more gateway cities in the United States and Canada. One advantage of these package flights is that if the flight is late, the ship may temporarily delay sailing to wait for it, or passengers may be flown to the next port. Most fly/cruise packages include transfers from the airport to the ship but not transportation to and from your home to your local airport.

If you have purchased a fly/cruise package, you will be met by a cruise company representative when your plane lands at the port city and then shuttled directly to the ship in buses or minivans. Some cruise lines arrange to transport your luggage between airport and ship—you don't have to hassle with baggage claim at the start of your cruise or with baggage check-in at the end. If you decide not to buy the fly/cruise package but still plan to fly, ask your travel agent if you can use the ship's transfer bus anyway. Some ships require you to purchase a round-trip transfer voucher ($5–$20) for this service.

By Bus   Round-trip bus connections are sometimes arranged by local travel agents or cruise brokers who book large numbers of cruise passengers from a nearby town or city. Ask your travel agent for information or call the cruise line directly. A number of local bus lines that serve major port cities such as New York or San Francisco offer occasional charters or extensions of their normal runs directly to the dock.

By Car In most ports, you can drop off your luggage directly in front of the pier, as well as park in protected lots near the ship (at fees of $3–$6 per day). Let a porter carry your bags, rather than doing it yourself, and tip him a dollar or two, even if he takes them only 10 feet or so.

Early Arrivals If your schedule entails arriving a day early, as part of your fly/cruise package you may be given transfer vouchers good from the airport to your hotel. Many hotels used as part of precruise packages provide free or inexpensive transportation to the ship on the day of sailing. If yours doesn't, find out whether it would be more expensive to take a taxi from the hotel to the ship or to return to the airport and wait for the bus to the ship.

Luggage

Allowances Because closet space is so limited, many cruise ships ask that
On Board Ship each passenger bring no more than two suitcases weighing under 70 pounds total. Because luggage is often tossed about and stacked as it is moved between ship and airport, bring suitcases that can take abuse.

Inflight Free baggage allowances on an airline depend on the airline, the route, and the class of your ticket. In general, on domestic flights and on international flights between the United States and foreign destinations, you are entitled to check two bags— neither exceeding 62 inches, or 158 centimeters (length + width + height), or weighing more than 70 pounds (32 kilograms). A third piece may be brought aboard as a carryon; its total dimensions are generally limited to less than 45 inches (114 centimeters), so it will fit easily under the seat in front of you or in the overhead compartment. There are variations, so ask in advance. The only rule, a Federal Aviation Administration safety regulation that pertains to carry-on baggage on U.S. airlines, requires only that carryons be properly stowed and allows the airline to limit allowances and tailor them to different aircraft and operational conditions. Charges for excess, oversize, or overweight pieces vary, so inquire before you pack.

Safeguarding Your Before leaving home, itemize your bags' contents and their
Luggage worth; this list will help you estimate the extent of your loss if your bags go astray. To minimize that risk, tag them inside and out with your name, address, and phone number. (If you use your home address, cover it so that potential thieves can't see it.) When you check in for your pre- or post-cruise flight, make sure that the tag attached by baggage handlers bears the correct three-letter code for your destination; and if your bags do not arrive with you, or if you detect damage, do not leave the airport until you've filed a written report with the airline.

Embarkation

Check-in On arrival at the dock, you must check in before boarding your ship. (A handful of smaller cruise ships handle check-in at the airport.) An officer will collect or stamp your ticket, inspect or even retain your passport or other official identification, ask you to fill out a tourist card, check that you have the correct visas, and collect any unpaid port or departure tax. Seating assignments for the dining room are often handed out at this time, too. You may also register your credit card to open a shipboard account, although that may be done later at the purser's office.

After this you may be required to go through a security check and to pass your hand baggage through an X-ray inspection. To be safe, never put film through an X-ray machine—such machines have been known to fog photosensitive materials—but, rather, request a hand-inspection.

Although check-in takes only five or 10 minutes per family, lines are often long, so aim for a off-peak time. The worst time tends to be immediately after the ship begins boarding; the later it is, the less crowded check-in counters tend to be. For example, if boarding begins at 2 PM and continues until 4:30, try to arrive after 3:30.

Boarding the Ship Before you walk up the gangway, the ship's photographer will probably take your picture; there's no charge unless you buy the picture. On board, stewards may serve welcome drinks in souvenir glasses—for which you're usually charged $3–$5 cash.

You will either be escorted to your cabin by a steward or, on a smaller ship, given your key by a ship's officer and directed to your cabin. Some elevators are unavailable to passengers during boarding, since they are used to transport luggage. You may arrive to find your luggage outside your stateroom or just inside the door; if it doesn't arrive within a half-hour before sailing, contact the purser. If you are among the unlucky few whose luggage doesn't make it to the ship in time, the purser will trace it and arrange to have it flown to the next port.

Visitors' Passes Some cruise ships permit passengers' guests on board prior to sailing, although an increasing number of cruise lines prohibit all but paying passengers for reasons of security and insurance liability. Cruise companies that allow visitors on board usually require that you obtain passes several weeks in advance; call the companies for policies and procedures.

Most ships do not allow visitors on board while docked in a port of call. If you meet a friend on shore, you won't be able to invite him or her back to your stateroom.

Disembarkation

The last night of your cruise is full of business. On most ships you must place everything except your hand luggage outside your cabin door, ready to be picked up by midnight. Your shipboard bill is left in your room during the last day; to pay the bill (if you haven't already put it on your credit card) or to settle any questions, you must stand in line at the purser's office. Tips to the cabin steward and dining staff are distributed on the last night.

The next morning, in-room breakfast service is usually not available because stewards are too busy. Most passengers clear out of their cabins as soon as possible, gather their hand luggage, and stake out a chair in one of the public lounges to await the ship's clearance through customs. Be patient—it takes a long time to unload and sort thousands of pieces of luggage. Passengers are disembarked by groups; those with the earliest flights get off first. If you have a tight connection for a flight, notify the purser before the last day, and he or she may be able to arrange faster preclearing and disembarkation for you.

Customs and Duties

On Departure If you plan to take more than $10,000 in cash, traveler's checks, or other negotiable instruments (such as bearer bonds or money orders) in or out of the United States, you must file Customs Form 4790 before you leave. U.S. residents bringing any foreign-made equipment from home, such as cameras, are wise to carry the original receipts with them or to register the items with U.S. Customs before leaving home (Form 4457). Otherwise, you may end up paying duty on your return.

Returning Home To ease customs clearance at the end of your cruise, keep a detailed record of your purchases, save all receipts, and pack your overseas purchases on top of all your other belongings, in case the customs officer wishes to inspect them.

U.S. Customs Before your ship lands, each individual or family must fill out a customs declaration, regardless of whether anything was purchased abroad. If you have fewer than $1,400 worth of goods, you will not need to itemize individual purchases. Be prepared to pay whatever duties are owed directly to the customs inspector, with cash or check.

U.S. Customs now preclears a number of ships sailing in and out of Miami and other ports—it's done on the ship before you disembark. In other ports you must collect your luggage from the dock, then stand in line to pass through the inspection point. This can take up to an hour.

Allowances: Provided you've been out of the country for at least 48 hours and haven't already used the exemption, or any part of it, in the past 30 days, you may bring $400 worth of goods home duty-free from *most* countries. A more generous amount, $600, applies to two dozen Caribbean Basin Initiative beneficiary countries. If you're returning from the U.S. Virgin Islands, the duty-free allowance is even higher—$1,200. A flat 10% duty applies to the next $1,000 of goods; above that, the rate varies with the merchandise. These exemptions may be pooled among family members, regardless of age, so one may bring in more if another brings in less. If the 48-hour or 30-day limits apply, your duty-free allowance drops to $25, which may *not* be pooled. Some wrinkles to the above: If you are visiting more than one island, say the U.S. Virgins and the Dominican Republic (a beneficiary country), you may bring in a total of $1,200 duty-free, of which no more than $600 may be from the Dominican Republic. If you visit a beneficiary country and an excluded one, such as Martinique, you may bring in a total of $600 goods duty-free, of which no more than $400 may be from Martinique.

In addition, the Generalized System of Preferences, aimed at helping developing countries improve their economies through trade, exempts certain items from the same beneficiary countries from duty entirely, meaning that they do not count toward the duty-free total at all. At press time, however, the future of GSP beyond its July 4, 1994, expiration date was unknown.

Alcohol and Tobacco: Travelers 21 or older may bring back one liter of alcohol duty-free from most countries (two liters from most Caribbean countries), provided the beverage laws of the state through which they reenter the U.S. allow it. In the case of the U.S. Virgin Islands, five liters are allowed. If you are visiting a beneficiary country and an excluded one, no more than one of the two liters allowed may be from the excluded country; if you are visiting the U.S. Virgin Islands and a beneficiary country, no more than two liters of the five allowed may be from the beneficiary country. Regardless of your age, you may bring 100 non-Cuban cigars and 200 cigarettes back to the U.S. From the U.S. Virgin Islands, 1,000 cigarettes are allowed, but only 200 of them may have been acquired elsewhere.

Gifts: Gifts under $50 may be mailed duty-free to stateside friends and relatives, with a limit of one package per day per addressee (do not send alcohol or tobacco products, nor perfume valued at over $5). These gifts do not count as part of your exemption, although if you bring them home with you, they do. Mark the package "Unsolicited Gift" and include the nature of the gift and its retail value.

Restrictions: Certain goods require a special license to be imported into the United States, and others cannot be brought in at all. These include products made from endangered species such as turtles and coral; any fruits, vegetables, or meats; and any controlled substances, such as cocaine, heroin, or marijuana. Also banned are firearms, explosives, Cuban cigars, liquor-filled candies, pre-Columbian art, obscene material or publications violating U.S. copyright law, switchblades, restricted trademarked goods like certain cameras and watches, and even foreign lottery tickets. Live animals will be subjected to a two-month quarantine (six months in Hawaii).

For More Information: The free brochure "Know Before You Go" lists all Caribbean Basin Initiative beneficiary countries, and details what you may and may not bring back to this country, rates of duty, and other pointers; to obtain it, contact the U.S. Customs Service (Box 7407, Washington, DC 20044, tel. 202/927–6724). A copy of "GSP and the Traveler" is available from the same source.

Canadian Customs **Allowances:** Once per calendar year, when you've been out of Canada for at least seven days, you may bring in $300 worth of goods duty-free. If you've been away less than seven days but more than 48 hours, the duty-free exemption drops to $100 but can be claimed any number of times (as can a $20 duty-free exemption for absences of 24 hours or more). You cannot combine the yearly and 48-hour exemptions, use the $300 exemption only partially (to save the balance for a later trip), or pool exemptions with family members. Goods claimed under the $300 exemption may follow you by mail; those claimed under the lesser exemptions must accompany you on your return.

Alcohol and Tobacco: Alcohol and tobacco products may be included in the yearly and 48-hour exemptions but not in the 24-hour exemption. If you meet the age requirements of the province through which you reenter Canada, you may bring in, duty-free, 1.14 liters (40 imperial ounces) of wine or liquor *or* two dozen 12-ounce cans or bottles of beer or ale. If you are 16 or older, you may bring in, duty-free, 200 cigarettes, 50 cigars or cigarillos, and 400 tobacco sticks or 400 grams of manufactured tobacco. Alcohol and tobacco must accompany you on your return.

Gifts: Gifts may be mailed to friends in Canada duty-free. These do not count as part of your exemption. Each gift may be worth up to of $60—label the package "Unsolicited Gift— Value under $60." There are no limits on the number of gifts that may be sent per day or per addressee, but you can't mail alcohol or tobacco.

For More Information: For details, including specifics of duties on items that exceed your duty-free limit, ask the Revenue Canada Customs and Excise Department (Connaught Bldg., MacKenzie Ave., Ottawa, Ont., K1A OL5, tel. 613/957–0275) for a copy of the free brochure "I Declare/Je Déclare."

U.K. Customs **Allowances:** If your journey was wholly within EC countries, you no longer need to pass through customs when you return to the United Kingdom. According to EC guidelines, you may bring in 800 cigarettes, 400 cigarillos, 200 cigars, and 1 kilogram of smoking tobacco, plus 10 liters of spirits, 20 liters of fortified wine, 90 liters of wine, and 110 liters of beer. If you exceed these limits, you may be required to prove that the goods are for your personal use or are gifts.

From countries outside the EC, you may import duty-free 200 cigarettes, 100 cigarillos, 50 cigars or 250 grams of tobacco; 1 liter of spirits or 2 liters of fortified or sparkling wine; 2 liters of still table wine; 60 milliliters of perfume; 250 milliliters of toilet water; plus £36 worth of other goods, including gifts and souvenirs.

For More Information: "A Guide for Travellers" details standard customs procedures as well as what you may bring into the United Kingdom from abroad; to obtain a copy or for other information, contact HM Customs and Excise (New King's Beam House, 22 Upper Ground, London SE1 9PJ, tel. 071/620–1313).

U.S. Customs for If you hold a foreign passport and will be returning home
Foreigners within 48 hours of docking, you may be exempt from all U.S. Customs duties. Everything you bring into the United States must leave with you when you return home. When you reach your own country you will have to pay appropriate duties there.

On Board

Checking Out Your Cabin

The first thing you should do upon arriving at your cabin or suite is ensure that everything is in working order. Is the cabin clean and orderly, with fresh linens on the bed and toiletries in the bathroom? Do you have enough blankets and pillows? Do the toilet, shower, and faucets work satisfactorily? Are there sufficient towels? If you have a bathtub, does it have a stopper? Check the telephone, television, radio, lights, and all locks and keys. Are there enough clothes hangers? Are there an ice bucket and drinking glasses? Your dining time and seating assignment card may be in your cabin; now is the time to check it and immediately request any changes. Since your cabin is your home away from home for a few days or weeks, everything should be to your satisfaction. If not, ask your room steward to make whatever corrections are necessary *before* the ship disembarks.

If there are any serious problems, such as two twin beds instead of the expected double bed, ask to be moved. Unless the ship is full, you can usually persuade the chief housekeeper or hotel manager to allow you to change cabins. It is customary to tip the stewards who assist you in moving to another cabin.

The Crew

Cruise ships carry a full complement of crew (the people who actually sail the ship) and staff (the employees who feed, serve, and entertain you while you are on board). It's highly unlikely that you will see or meet the great majority of the ship's employees, since most work behind the scenes in the engine room, galleys, and other areas that are off-limits to passengers. Here are some with whom you will come in contact:

Captains have many years of experience at sea and are officially certified and licensed as master mariners by their governments. On cruise ships the captain is responsible not only for sailing the ship and ensuring its safety, but also for setting the tenor of the cruise. Most are charming, sophisticated diplomats who act as troubleshooters for almost any on-board problem. The **staff captain,** who is second-in-command to the captain, also holds master mariner papers and is fully qualified to take over should the captain become incapacitated. Usually, the staff captain oversees the day-to-day operations of the crew in matters of navigation and seamanship. Smaller ships may not carry a staff captain, in which case the second-in-command is the **first mate.**

The **chief purser** is the ship's accountant, responsible for a number of services, such as check cashing, money changing, account payments, safe-deposit boxes, customs, and daily schedules. The shipboard **hotel manager** serves much the same function as a land-based hotel manager: supervising all housekeeping and dining-room staff. The hotel manager is the final authority on any problems you may have with your cabin, the food, or any other aspect of the ship. Small and medium-size ships that do not have a hotel manager split these responsibilities between the staff captain and the chief purser.

The **cruise director**—usually dressed in a brightly colored blazer rather than a uniform—is probably the most visible person on the ship. Besides planning, scheduling, and directing all shipboard social activities, the cruise director acts as an ombudsman and troubleshooter. The **entertainment director** oversees entertainment activities, from lounge music to guest lecturers. The **shore excursion director** sells tour tickets, gives an informative talk on each port before docking, and arranges almost everything on land—including tour buses, guides, and admissions to attractions. On smaller ships, the cruise director may take on the duties of one or both of the latter positions.

The **chief steward** oversees the dining room, the galley, the Lido, and the pantry, and supervises all waiters, busboys, and maître d's. Talk to the chief steward first if you have any complaints about the food or the service; if you don't get satisfaction, see the hotel manager. On some ships the title of chief steward is used for the officer in charge of the room stewards, in which case the duties described above are often assumed by the maître d' or dining room manager. Talk to the **maître d'** if you have any dietary preferences, wish to change tables, or want a picnic lunch packed for a trek ashore.

The **room steward/stewardess** or **cabin steward/stewardess** cleans and tidies your cabin throughout the voyage and also usually delivers any food or drink ordered through room service. Depending upon the ship, your steward may be visible enough that you become quite friendly, or you may seldom see him or her until the last evening, when tips traditionally are distributed. If there are any maintenance problems with your cabin or if you have special requests, such as extra pillows, first talk to your steward. If necessary, your next recourse is the **chief housekeeper,** who supervises the small army of stewards and cleaning and laundry personnel.

Tipping

For better or worse, tipping is an integral part of the cruise experience. Most companies pay their cruise staff nominal wages and expect tips to make up the difference. A number of European ships have replaced "voluntary" tipping with a mandatory 15% service charge, which is then divided among the crew. On most small adventure ships, a collection box is placed in the dining room or lounge on the last full day of the cruise, and passengers are encouraged to contribute anonymously. Several upscale companies have a "tips optional" policy that takes the pressure off both crew and passengers; surprisingly, it's reported that the level of tipping on board these ships is almost exactly the same as on those where tipping is a fact of life. A handful of luxury lines have eliminated tipping altogether, and any employee caught accepting a gratuity is reprimanded.

Tips are certainly a major motivation for some crews, but the level of service on no-tip and tips-optional ships is generally as high as, or even higher than, on ships that encourage tipping. On some ships the pressure to tip is heavy-handed: Stewards may actually stand and wait in the doorway with their palms upturned after performing some regular service (most ships' rules prohibit them from actually *asking* for a tip).

Lines that encourage tipping advertise a recommended tipping policy in their brochures and even on information sheets left on your pillow (along with envelopes addressed to Steward, Waiter, Busboy, and so on). These are guidelines only; you may tip as little or as much as you wish. On most cruise ships it is customary to tip on the last night at sea. Always tip in cash, preferably in U.S. dollars. Generally, tip your regular waiter and cabin steward. On some ships you should also tip the busboy, but on others the waiter shares his tips with the busboy. If the maître d' provides any special services, such as moving you to another table, he should be tipped a nominal amount, usually between $5 and $15. If you order wine with your meals, the wine steward should be tipped 15% of the total bill, unless a service charge is added automatically. Do not tip any of the officers, the entertainers, or the cruise staff. On some ships bartenders and bar stewards are tipped when the drinks are served, but on others a 15% service charge is added to your account. Each cruise line's current recommendations for tipping are listed in Chapter 3.

Dining

Restaurants The chief meals of the day are served in the dining room. Most ships' dining rooms and kitchens are too small to serve all passengers simultaneously, so there are usually two mealtimes—early (or main) and late (or second) seatings—usually about 1½ hours apart.

Most cruise ships have a Lido deck, adjacent to the swimming pool, where fast food and snacks are served cafeteria-style. Entrées available in the regular dining room may also be served here. Most Lidos have restricted hours—sunrise coffee, breakfast, morning snacks, lunch, and afternoon tea. Many ships provide self-serve coffee or tea around the clock at a table on the Lido.

A handful of ships have recently introduced alternative restaurants providing superior dining, sometimes at an additional charge. A growing trend is to offer specialty outlets—pizzerias, ice-cream parlors, coffee shops—where food may be available for free or at extra cost.

Meals Traditional cruise ships offer at least five meals a day: breakfast, lunch, afternoon tea, dinner, and midnight buffet. There may be up to four breakfast options: early morning coffee and pastries on deck, breakfast in bed via room service, buffet-style breakfast on the Lido, and breakfast in the dining room. There may also be two or three choices for lunch, and late-night snacks and buffets to complement dinner. You can eat whatever is on the menu, in any quantity, at as many of these meals as you wish. Room service is traditionally, but not always, free (*see* Shipboard Services, *below*).

Seatings When it comes to your dining table assignment, you should have options on four important points: early or late seating; smoking or no-smoking section; a table for two, four, six, or eight; and special dietary needs. If you like staying up into the night or remaining late in port, choose the late seating; if you like to get to bed early or plan on leaving the ship as soon as possible when it hits port in the evening, then select an early seating. To disembark as early as possible in the morning, either order breakfast in bed or grab a bite at the Lido Deck buffet.

Several cruise lines preassign seatings, either through the travel agent or at the time of check-in; make your preferences clear to your agent when you book, and get a confirmation in writing. Other ships do not hand out assignments until after the vessel sails—usually an announcement over the PA system tells where and when such assignments are made. The lines may be long, but get there early to assure your preferred selection.

Not all ships follow seating assignments strictly. Several have open seating for breakfast or lunch, which means you may sit anywhere at any time. Smaller or more luxurious ships offer open seating for all meals.

Changing Tables Dining is a focal point of the cruise experience, and your companions at meals may become your best friends on the cruise.

On some ships the maître d' actually tries to match people with similar interests and personalities, but there's always the chance that you won't enjoy the company. The maître d' can usually move you to another table if the dining room isn't completely full—a tip helps. He will probably be reluctant to comply with your request after the first full day at sea, however, because the waiters, busboys, and wine steward who have been serving you up to that point won't receive their tips at the end of the cruise. Be persistent if you are truly unhappy.

Cuisine Some passengers actually select a ship according to the variety of cuisine it offers. Most ships sailing in the Western Hemisphere serve food geared to the American palate, but theme dinners are often scheduled, featuring the cuisine of a particular country. Some European ships, especially smaller vessels, may specialize in one particular cuisine throughout the cruise—Scandinavian, German, Italian, or Greek, perhaps-depending on the ship's or the crew's nationality. The quality of the food on board is uniformly high, since provisions are usually purchased in the United States and shipped in containerized cargo holds directly to the vessel, wherever it is. Such foodstuffs as Kansas City steaks, Alaskan king crabs, Maine lobsters, Idaho potatoes, Texas shrimp, Florida fruits, Cape Cod fish, California vegetables, and other regional specialties are brought fresh to the ship. The quality of the cooking is generally good but certainly not memorable, for even a skilled chef is hard-put to serve 500 or more extraordinary dinners per hour. On the other hand, the presentation is often spectacular, especially at gala midnight buffets.

There is a direct relationship between the cost of a cruise and the quality and sophistication of its cuisine. Some (mostly upscale) vessels specialize in gourmet food, among them the *Sea Goddess I*, *The Royal Viking Queen*, the *Seabourn Pride* and *Seabourn Spirit*, the *Crystal Harmony*, and (in its Queen's Grill and Princess Grill) the *Queen Elizabeth 2*.

Special Diets With notification well in advance, most ships can provide a special menu (kosher, vegetarian, sugar-free) for those who need it. However, there's always a chance that the wrong dish will somehow be handed to you. Check especially on soups and desserts.

An increasing number of cruise ships offer an alternative "light" or "spa" menu based upon American Heart Association guidelines, using less fat, leaner cuts of meat, low-cholesterol or low-sodium preparations, smaller portions, and plenty of healthy garnishes, salads, and fresh-fruit desserts. Some smaller ships may not be able to prepare separate food or accommodate special diets. Vegetarians generally have no trouble finding appropriate selections on ship menus.

Wine Most ships charge for wine at meals. The tariffs for popular wines and vintages are comparable to typical restaurant prices and are charged to your shipboard account. Some ships, however (especially some Italian, French, and Greek vessels), include *vin ordinaire* (table wine) with meals. A handful of luxury vessels throw in all the wine and liquor you want.

The Captain's Table It is both a privilege and a marvelous experience to be invited to dine one evening at the captain's table. Although some seats are given to celebrities, repeat passengers, and passengers in the most expensive suites, other invitations are given at random to ordinary passengers. Cruise passengers can actually request an invitation from the chief steward or the hotel manager, although there is no guarantee you will be accommodated. The captain's guests always wear a suit and tie or a dress, even if the dress code for that evening is casual. On many ships, passengers may also be invited to dine at the other officers' special tables, or officers may visit a different passenger table each evening.

Bars

Ship's bars, whether adjacent to the pool or attached to one of the lounges, tend to be the social center of a ship. Except for a handful of luxury-class ships where everything is included in the ticket price, on-board bars operate on a pay-as-it's-poured basis. Rather than demand cash after every round, however, most ships allow passengers to charge drinks to their accounts. There was a time when ships charged a pittance for bar drinks, but nowadays expect resort prices.

In international waters there are, technically, no laws against teenage drinking, but almost all ships require passengers to be over 18 or 21. Many cruise ships have chapters of Alcoholics Anonymous (aka "Friends of Bill W") or will organize meetings on request.

Entertainment

Lounges and Nightclubs
Many ships—specifically mainstream vessels—offer organized entertainment from morning to late night, starting with a steel band by the pool during the day, continuing with before-dinner music in the lounges or bars, and featuring two major shows each night—one each for the early and late-dinner seatings. From the end of the main show until the wee hours of the morning there may be disco, a dance band, and/or a piano bar.

Generally the quality of the entertainment on board is good but not up to New York, London, or Las Vegas standards. Many performers are on short-term contracts in between road tours or while waiting for a part in a Broadway play. On smaller ships entertainers may be hired less for their singing and dancing skills than for their willingness to do double duty in the off-hours—a ballroom dancer may teach aerobics, or a singer may be tapped to accompany shore excursions.

The main entertainment lounge, which may also be called a theater or showroom, offers everything from Vegas-style revues to production shows. Generally, the larger the ship, the bigger and more elaborate the productions. During the rest of the day the room is used for group activities, such as shore-excursion talks or bingo games.

Many larger ships have a second lounge, sometimes used for bingo or trivia contests while the main show is under way elsewhere. This lounge often features entertainers and ballroom dancing late into the night. Elsewhere you may find a disco, nightclub, or cabaret, usually built around a bar and a dance floor. Music is provided by a piano player, disc jockey, or small performing ensembles such as country-and-western duos or jazz combos.

On smaller ships the entertainment options are more limited, sometimes consisting of no more than a piano around which passengers gather. Whereas party ships emphasize social activities, cultural adventure cruises place the accent on lectures and more sedate forms of entertainment.

Library Most cruise ships have a library with anywhere from 500 to 1,500 volumes, including everything from the latest bestsellers to reference works on whales, flora, fauna, and other cruise-related topics. Party ships may have no library, or just one or two shelves of paperbacks. Increasingly, ship libraries require a substantial deposit to check out a book.

Movie Theaters Most vessels (other than the smallest) have at least one movie theater. The films are frequently one or two months past their first release but not yet available on videotape or cable TV. Films rated "R" are edited to tone down sex and violence. A weeklong voyage may feature a dozen different films, repeated at various showings throughout the day. Theaters are also used for lectures, religious services, and private meetings.

A number of ships now have TVs in some or all of the cabins, offering movies (some newer ships show movies continuously), closed-circuit showings of shipboard activities, and satellite reception of regular programs. Ships with VCRs in the cabins usually provide a selection of movies on cassette at no charge (a deposit is usually required).

Casinos Once a ship is 12 miles off American shores, it is in international waters and gambling is permitted. (Some "cruises to nowhere," in fact, are little more than sailing casinos.) All mainstream, as well as many smaller or specialty ships, have casinos. On larger vessels, they usually have poker, baccarat, blackjack, roulette, craps, and slot machines. House stakes are much more modest than those at Las Vegas or Atlantic City—usually $100 tables are tops—and payouts on the slot machines (some of which take as little as a nickel) are generally much lower. Credit is never extended, but many casinos have handy credit-card machines that dispense cash for a hefty fee. An exception is the *Cyrstal Harmony:* The ship's Caesar's Palace at Sea Casino, regulated by the Nevada Gaming Commission, offers the same gambling limits as in Las Vegas and, by prior arrangement, will extend credit.

Children are officially barred from the casinos, but it's common to see them playing the slots rather than the adjacent video machines. Most ships offer free individual instruction and even gambling classes in the off-hours. Casinos are usually open from early morning to late night, although you may find only unattended slot machines before evening. In adherence to local laws, casinos are always closed while in port.

Game Rooms Most ships have a game or card room with card tables and board games. These rooms are for serious players and are often the site of friendly round-robin competitions and tournaments. Most ships furnish everything for free (cards, chips, games, etc.), but a few charge $1 or more for each deck of cards. Be aware that professional cardsharps and hustlers have been fleecing ship passengers almost as long as there have been ships.

Most medium and large ships have small video arcades. A few also feature a room with personal computers equipped with games and popular business programs such as WordPerfect and Lotus 1-2-3, all available at no charge.

Bingo and Other Games The daily high-stakes bingo games are even more popular than the casinos. You can play for as little as a dollar a card. Most ships have a snowball bingo game with a jackpot that grows throughout the cruise into hundreds or even thousands of dollars. These crowded games have become big moneymakers for the cruise lines.

Even more competitive are the so-called "horse races": Eight fictional horses are auctioned off, usually for about $50 or $60, then "run" according to dice throws or computer-generated random numbers. The audience bets on their favorites.

Sports and Fitness

Swimming Pools All but the smallest ships have at least one pool, some of them elaborate affairs with water slides or retractable roofs; hot tubs and whirlpools are quite common. Ship's pools are filled with salt water (to conserve fresh water) and are often emptied or covered with canvas while in port or during rough weather. Many are too narrow or short to allow swimmers more than a few strokes in any direction; none have diving boards; some are not heated. Simple wading pools are sometimes provided for small children.

Sun Deck The top deck is usually called the Sun Deck or Sports Deck. On some ships this is where you'll find the pool or whirlpool; on others it is dedicated to volleyball, table tennis, shuffleboard, and other such sports. A number of ships have paddle-tennis courts, and a few have golf driving ranges. (Skeet shooting is usually offered at the stern of a lower deck.) Often, at twilight or after the sun goes down, the Sun Deck is used for dancing, barbecues, limbo contests, or other social activities.

Exercise and Fitness Rooms Most newer ships and some older ones have well-equipped fitness centers, many with massage, sauna, and whirlpools. An upper-deck fitness center often has an airy and sunny view of the sea; an inside, lower-deck health club is often dark and small, except those that have indoor pools or beauty salons. Many ships feature full-service exercise rooms with bodybuilding equipment, stationary bicycles, rowing machines, treadmills, aerobics classes, and personal fitness instruction. Some ships even have structured cruise-length physical fitness programs, which may include lectures on weight loss or nutrition. Beauty salons adjacent to the health club may offer spa treatments such as facials and mud wraps. The more extensive programs are often sold on a daily or weekly basis.

Promenade Deck Many vessels designate certain decks for fitness walks and may post the number of laps per mile. Fitness instructors may lead daily walks around the Promenade Deck. A number of ships discourage jogging and running on the decks or ask that no one take fitness walks before 8 AM or after 10 PM, so as not to disturb passengers in cabins.

Shipboard Services

Charge Account Although your cruise ticket entitles you to an inclusive package of services and facilities, there are always purchases to make on board—shore excursions, massages, hair styling, drinks, souvenir photographs, wine with dinner, laundry, dry cleaning, and items from the gift shop. On some ships you may sign for everything, settling your account on the last day of the cruise with a credit card, traveler's checks, or cash. Other ships—typically during three- or four-day cruises—allow you to sign only for bar purchases and require cash on the spot for everything else. In either case you can usually open a shipboard account with the purser's office by presenting your credit card. You will receive an accounting of charges at the end of the cruise.

Room Service A small number of ships have no room service at all, except when the ship's doctor orders it for an ill passenger. Many offer only breakfast (Continental on some, full on others), while others provide no more than a limited menu at certain hours of the day. Most, however, have certain selections that you can order at any time. Some upscale ships have unlimited round-the-clock room service. There may or may not be a charge for room service (other than for drinks). Check before you order.

Minibars An increasing number of ships equip higher-price cabins with small refrigerators or minibars stocked with various snacks, soft drinks, and liquors, which may or may not be free.

Laundry and Dry Cleaning All but the smallest ships and shortest cruises offer laundry services—valet, self-service, or both. Use of machines is generally free; some ships charge for washing supplies. Valet laundry service includes cabin pickup and delivery and usually takes 24 hours. Most ships also offer dry-cleaning services.

Hairdressers Even the smallest ships have a hairdresser on staff. Larger ships have complete beauty parlors, and some have barber shops. Book hairdressers well in advance, especially before such popular events as the farewell dinner.

Film Processing Many cruise ships have color-film processing and printing equipment to develop film overnight. It's expensive but convenient.

Photographer The staff photographer, a near-universal fixture on cruise ships, records every memorable, photogenic moment. The thousands of photos snapped over the course of a cruise are displayed publicly in special cases every morning and are offered for sale, usually for $6 for a 5″ × 7″ color print. If you want a special photo or a portrait, the photographer is usually happy to oblige.

Office/Meeting Facilities Few cruise ships currently provide the kind of business services often found in large hotels, but some larger vessels have installed computer rooms equipped with PCs, and some have faxing and secretarial services. If you bring your own equipment, make certain you have the right connectors and transformer. Most cruise ships use U.S.-type 110V, 60-cycle electricity and grounded plugs, but others feature 220V, 50-cycle current and are fitted with European- or English-type outlets. (*See* Chapter 3 for information on the kind of electricity each ship uses.) Generally it is difficult, if not impossible, to use a computer modem or portable fax through most ships' phone systems.

Some ships, such as the *Crystal Harmony*, *CostaClassica*, and *Royal Viking Sun*, have meeting rooms that can be used for conferences. The *Radisson Diamond*, built specifically for conference and incentive groups, has a large ballroom and plenty of versatile meeting space.

Religious Services   Most ships provide nondenominational religious services on Sundays and religious holidays, and a number offer daily Catholic masses and Friday-evening Jewish services. The kind of service held depends upon the clergy the cruise line invites on board. Usually religious services are held in the library, the theater, or one of the private lounges, although a few ships have actual chapels.

Communications   Most cabins have loudspeakers and telephones. Generally, the
Shipboard   loudspeakers cannot be switched off because they are needed to broadcast important notices. Telephones are used to call fellow passengers, order room service, summon a doctor, leave a wake-up call, or speak with any of the ship's officers or departments. On most ships, cabin telephones connect directly to the radio room or satellite for calls to shore.

Ship to Shore   Satellite facilities make it possible to call anywhere in the world from most ships. Most are also equipped with telex and fax machines, and some provide credit card phones. It may take as long as a half-hour to make a connection, but unless a storm is raging outside, conversation is clear and easy. On smaller ships, voice calls must be put through on short-wave wireless or via the one phone in the radio room. Be warned: The cost of sending any message, regardless of the method, can be quite expensive—at least $15 per minute. Faxing is more economical.

Lifeboats

By international law all ships must be equipped with lifeboats, and according to Coast Guard regulations and the SOLAS (Safety Of Life At Sea) convention, every cruise ship must conduct at least one lifeboat drill, mandatory for all passengers, early in the voyage. Every passenger must correctly don a life preserver, which is usually found in the cabin under the bed or in the closet. On the back of the cabin door or nearby on the wall will be an instruction chart and possibly a map indicating how to get to your lifeboat mustering station. At the signal for abandoning ship—six long blasts of the ship's horn, followed by six short blasts—every passenger must proceed to a mustering station. All ships follow this drill with at least one full-fledged crew practice (usually while most passengers are ashore at one of the ports of call), and some ships have additional emergency drills during the cruise.

For safety's sake make certain that the ship's purser knows if you or your spouse has some physical infirmity that may hamper a speedy exit from your cabin. In case of a real emergency, the purser can quickly dispatch a crew member to assist you. If you are traveling with children, be sure child-size life jackets are placed in your cabin.

2 Portraits of Cruising

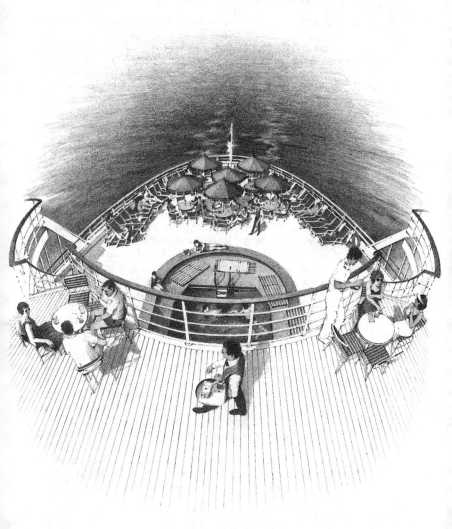

At One with the Sea

By John
Maxtone-Graham

A marine
historian, John
Maxtone-Graham
is the author of
The Only Way to
Cross, liners to
the Sun, Cunard:
150 Glorious
Years, and
Crossing &
Cruising.

I have a picture of my American grandfather taken on the deck of an unnamed ship in the early 1920s. It was probably the *Adriatic,* for she was his favorite among the White Star Line's fleet. The photograph was taken the morning of arrival in New York; he is dressed for city rather than ship, in waistcoat, overcoat and Homburg, and his expression combines anxiety and regret. It is a portrait of a passenger half-impatient to reach his Manhattan office yet half-reluctant to quit the vessel on which (during that crossing and many others) he so enjoyed himself. It is a disembarkation angst I myself know well.

I must have inherited his and my mother's devotion to shipboard. I am in love no less with days at sea than with the very logistics of ocean travel—the challenge of luggage, even the ordeal of transfer to ship from plane, car or train. Indeed, the boat-train might have been made especially for me: for so many years that anticipatory rail journey before embarkation served as the ideal overture to the voyage, wherein, at the pier terminus, funnel smoke from locomotive and steamer intermingled evocatively, an acrid yet haunting travel essence.

I am absolutely besotted with ships. Neither yachtsman nor sailor, my preoccupation remains firmly with passenger vessels, steam or diesel. Every one of them provides architectural and decorative delights, good companionship, splendid service, civilized comfort and, perhaps most compelling of all, indescribable peace. Familiar shipboard sights, sounds and smells remain fresh in my sense memory. After a half-century of ship travel, I have reached the startling conclusion that, whether old or new, wood or Formica-paneled, ritzy or glitzy, crossing or cruising, the spirit on all ships is essentially the same; so, not surprisingly, is the spirit among their passengers who, though differing ashore, on board are mantled immediately in universal passengerhood.

Since I have family on both sides of the Atlantic, ocean passage between England and the United States dominated my early life. I am often asked how many times I have sailed; quite honestly, I've never counted. I do know that when I was six months old I made my first eastbound Atlantic crossing from New York to Tilbury, on the long-departed *Minnewaska.* My transatlantic sailings continued, except during the war, at the rate of at least one each year. Predictably, when I had children of my own, they joined me on summer crossings to Europe throughout the last years of what we used to call the Atlantic Ferry. Nowadays, I spend about a third of each year afloat, lecturing to passengers about ships and researching new books.

I came to cruising—as opposed to crossing—two decades ago. One Christmas season in the late Sixties, just as the appeal of shipboard life was starting its epic renaissance, I sailed on the *France* (now the *Norway*) from New York to the Caribbean. Not surprisingly, I enjoyed it immensely. The *Normandie* had been my all-time favorite, but since her tragic demise denied me the chance to book on her, I was delighted to be able to sail on the *France*, her obvious successor. For the first time, I remained on board the same vessel for a fortnight, five days longer than my previous record, a nine-day westbound crossing on the *Franconia* in 1956.

It was, admittedly, a radically different on-board regimen, combining as it did days at sea with days in port. Transatlantic passengers see nothing between New York and Southampton but gray ocean and the occasional freighter. But on that novel *France* cruise, there was always something on the horizon. Every other dawn, we dropped anchor off an island. The ports were agreeable but of less interest to me than our arrival in them and—even more pleasurable—our departure from them. For, however vaunted a landscape might be, the seascape always beckoned more compellingly. I found myself, then as now, invariably impatient to sail. Perhaps the same could be said of a moored or anchored vessel: whether hawsered to a pier or swinging at anchor, ships appear restless, their departure imminent. They seem immobilized against their will, merely awaiting their dilatory human cargo.

It was on that initial cruise that I experienced the shiphound's chronic dichotomy, brought on by proximity to land: Was it more intriguing to stand on deck looking at the land or to go ashore and have the vision of the ship anchored at sea? Wherever I was, I longed to enjoy, vicariously, the opposing vantage point, to be—momentarily—pierside spectator instead of shipboard passenger. Also, on that long-ago *France* cruise, I was more seasick during the northbound passage to New York than I've ever been since. We ran into a fearsome January gale off Cape Hatteras, and it was then I discovered the utter folly of packing during rough weather: bending over a drawer or suitcase compounds the discomfort. With the memory of that final violent sea day still fresh in my inner ear, I appreciate the present-day wisdom of embarking at Miami rather than New York for winter cruises.

During the Sixties, historically a decade of protest, I protested the layup, disappearance, and loss of so many old Atlantic ships. Something infinitely more precious than the time saved by transatlantic flight was being thoughtlessly discarded. One by one, the great liners vanished until only *Queen Elizabeth 2* was left in undisputed sway on the North

Atlantic. But in warmer waters, a new shipboard lifestyle began to thrive. Cruising, that maritime adventure for inquisitive Victorians and Edwardians, reemerged as a vital modern-day passion. Prevented from crossing, Americans—always the most numerous and enthusiastic passengers—have flocked in record numbers to board cruise ships.

What changes await them! Benign seas and relaxed itineraries have engendered completely different hulls. Liberated from a prudence of design dictated by harsh transatlantic weather and schedules, naval architects glory in delicate soaring prows, towering superstructures and futuristic deckscapes. Contemporary passenger ships have become glistening white fantasies, seemingly styled rather than wrought. More passengers are accommodated on board. Cabin size has decreased, deck space proliferated. Enclosed promenades have been supplanted by pools and open decks, as a predominantly indoor Atlantic experience has become, in sun-burnished waters, overwhelmingly outdoor. Portholes are sealed against humidity no less than seas, as air conditioning, paradoxically, isolates these new "outdoor" ships' interiors from balmy weather.

But familiar traditions remain: Once the last port and/or the sun disappears beneath the horizon, evenings are festive and elegant. The Atlantic ritual of dressing for dinner survives intact on many well-run cruise ships.

The most significant (and delightful) characteristic of a cruise, however, is its aimlessness. Passengers usually embark and disembark at the same place; they might call at a succession of intervening ports, but they achieve no geographical objective. Rather than persevere across a hostile ocean, cruise ships dabble along the fringes of benign seas. This navigational insouciance, the absolute unessentiality of the voyage, is mirrored on board among amiable passengers embarked exclusively for pleasure. No other conveyance offers the same grand specific: whereas passengers in trains, planes, buses or automobiles are bound on errands of compulsion, cruise-ship passengers embrace indolence, eschew haste and laze in a pleasant nautical limbo that *Punch*, the British humor magazine, once characterized as "a menace to activity."

Of course, for those who are interested, there are still crossings available. In addition to the *QE2*'s scheduled sailings, repositioning cruises are offered by several lines as they move ships from one seasonal market to another. The parade of ships through the Panama Canal, for instance, in spring and fall, en route to or from Alaska's summer season, offers a wealth of crossing experiences every bit as pleasing as those on conventional but rarer ocean voyages. Most crossings are treated like cruises. Vessels spanning the Atlantic, for instance, will often stop for an unnecessary day in Bermuda or Iceland, a way of breaking the voyage for those passengers who find interminable sea days intolerable. I am *not* among them—for me, the ship at sea is in her element, with passengers and crew united within a miraculous symbiosis. And the attendant blessing of every sea voyage, whether crossing or cruising, is detachment not only from land but also the day-to-day cares or responsibilities that surround us ashore. Escapist? Indubitably.

Given this blessed shipboard idleness, it seems curious that cruise lines go to such extraordinary lengths to vitiate the very peace they have marketed! In the *Great Cruise Manual in the Sky*, it has apparently been written that ships' passengers require continuous diversion. Unstructured moments are discouraged. As a result, many cruise ships become indoor-outdoor arenas of endeavor. On most cruise ships, more than one activity is planned for the same time, partly because there is seldom room for all the passengers to attend any one and partly because the company feels obliged to cater to a bewildering variety of tastes.

Does this nearly universal anomaly—busy passengers on indolent vessels—in fact illustrate and confirm the apparent contradiction in those curious buzzwords "leisure industry"? Does a Protestant work ethic obtrude, as though the prospect of unalloyed idleness afloat would somehow subvert the passenger psyche? Those who book long cruises thrive on lectures and seminars, perhaps in an attempt to allay hedonism's persistent guilt.

For my part, I shun most shipboard scheduling, playing socio-recreational hooky that, thankfully, ships are large enough to indulge. The shipboard experience, for my taste, is inextricably linked to deck chair and book, and a quiet stretch of sheltered deck is my preferred objective. The view of sea over railing, a soft breeze, the whispering glissando of hull through water and, once daily, a breathtaking sunset, fulfill to perfection my cruise expectation. Of course, I am only one passenger among many and do not mean to discourage my fellows from enjoying a strenuous cruise; but I sometimes feel that hyperactivity obscures the essential seagoing experience.

Years ago, in *Mirror of the Sea*, Joseph Conrad wrote: "It needed a few days after the taking of your departure for a ship's company to shake down into their places, and for the soothing deep-water ship routine to establish its beneficent sway." His words underscore a remarkable shipboard continuum. Indeed, "shaking down" today's passengers is actually accelerated by an apparent digression, the initial excursion ashore. Paradoxically, that first day on land bonds passengers even more potently than uninterrupted days at sea. I think this hastened camaraderie results from an underlying threat of displacement. Passengers cherish their vessel and cherish their comfortable life on board; relinquishing either, even for a day, is somehow unsettling. So, comparative strangers from the ship when encountered ashore become instant friends, co-ship conspirators, if you will, among an alien populace. Wherever they meet, all are inevitably linked within that sublime, unquestioned assemblage called fellow passengers. In fact, an unmistakable smugness characterizes all of us shiphounds enduring the rigors of going ashore. There, we are outsiders; back on board, we belong.

A word about service. Neglected (and exasperated) at a table in a Barbadian hotel, my twin brother was once offered this puzzling rebuke by his waiter: "If you want good service in the Caribbean, you've got to wait." However dicey service might be on an island, on board ship it must be close to perfection. Good service is the lubricant of shipboard life, and without it, the cruise momentum grinds to a sticky halt. The largest crew contingent on board any vessel, outnumbering deck and engine departments combined, is the hotel staff, numbering dozens of stewards.

In late-20th-century self-help America, most passengers are unused to servants and are unsure how to treat the staff members anxious to help them on board. Establishing a good rapport is a vital task, well worth accomplishing, because stewards are every ship's greatest hidden asset and their ministrations, whether in cabin, dining room, lounge or on deck, are the very essence of life at sea.

Too often stewards are abused. I talked recently with the maître d'hôtel of a ship's dining room who had risen through the ranks from steward to captain to his present rank. He is Italian, a skillful and deft company stalwart who remembers being cautioned, when he first boarded, with the same words that he still uses to caution his subordinates today: "Americans are seldom as polite as Europeans." It seems an abrupt though, I must agree, sometimes inescapable verdict.

I once sat at a large table for lunch (it was a port day, when passengers are seated indiscriminately at anonymous tables with anonymous stewards) and was appalled to note that not one of my fellow passengers said "please" or "thank you" to the stewards throughout the meal. Small wonder that some tend toward indifference; yet—Catch 22—they must be civil, regardless, since the bulk of their livelihood depends on it. One sure way to correct this courtesy imbalance is to keep in mind the inversion of a familiar credo, to wit: the passenger is often wrong. Treat all shipboard staff with consideration and the same courtesy you expect in return. In fact, the returns are remarkable.

One supposed peril of the ship's dining room is the possibility of uncongenial tablemates. Some companies have suggested avoiding this potential difficulty by having passengers sit at different tables at every meal. I dislike the idea, for it vitiates one of shipboard dining's perennial delights, the subtle passenger-steward relationship. A steward is far more than a restaurant waiter officiating over dinner: he is a knowledgeable, cheerful and resourceful factotum for at least a score of meals. You will get to know him and, far more important, he will get to know you and what you like and do not like. By the cruise's end, he can almost order for you. He is no less your steward than you are his passenger—exquisitely interdependent.

The task of selecting or assigning table companions is not easy. A maître d'hôtel told me once that he used to station two clever stewards near the door as newly embarked passengers came in to book seats. Although they never knew it, the passengers were being screened at once, ushered discreetly into one line or the other depending on their age. Younger couples arrived at one seating plan, older ones at another. There, once again, they were grouped by equally clever captains. But seldom is everyone happy. One man on a long Royal Viking cruise did not get his requested window table and refused to speak to the maître d'hôtel for the entire three-week voyage; thank heaven, that kind of rudeness is the exception.

Indeed, the reverse usually obtains. Recently, on another ship, I sat next to a table of eight. They had been selected by computer in the sales department long before they reached the pier, and I can only marvel at whatever electronic wizardry had masterminded the job: it was absolutely on target. All four couples were enjoying their first cruise, all were in their thirties, and the obvious rightness of the combination was apparent from the first evening. Moreover, their salubrious dining-room experience initiated an ensuing network of liaisons in the lounge, on deck and ashore.

Of course, one foolproof way of ensuring a congenial table is to book a cruise with friends from home. I know one man who must have set some kind of record by arranging for not less than 45 members of his extended family to come together on a Panama Canal cruise. But however the tables are stacked, it is obvious that the choice of meal companions is no less pivotal than the meal itself; successful tables make for contented dining rooms. It is a curious thing about which I have remarked before: the vigor of conversational hum in a ship's dining room increases each successive evening of a cruise as Conrad's "shake down" works immutably.

I have saved for last that paradigmatic perquisite, the cabin. They come in every configuration but, almost without exception, share a unique and cozy ingenuity lacking in even the most palatial accommodation ashore. When we book a room in a hotel, we take what we are given; on board ship, we have the privilege of preliminary selection. Hence, a cabin is not only a passenger's ultimate on-board retreat, it is also chosen space, selected carefully after sober evaluation of checkbook and deck plan. What delectable promise those brochure symbols and photographs hold, and how often we envision the layout and design of our cabin-to-come: berth and bureau, closet and shelf, shower and sink, porthole and chair mean something special to every passenger.

Sadly, tighter confinement has meant the gradual disappearance of tubs from many cabin bathrooms, and their replacement by the space-economical shower. And that vanishing tub (increasingly a feature of only the most expensive cabins) reflects ruthless design choices forced on naval architects by owners and builders anxious to squeeze in as many passengers as possible. Cabin planners are awarded a crucial square-footage figure, within which they must apportion living, sleeping and bathing space. At stake is not only a large measure of future passenger contentment but, inevitably, an assignment of space priorities that will probably remain unchanged for the life of the vessel.

Additional closets, shelves or even drawers are as unlikely to be added to a cabin as the wall dividing bedroom from bathroom is to be redeployed. To my mind, the best cabins, of the most generous nautical design, are those on older ships that were built for the Atlantic.

But, regardless of occasional shortcomings, the cabin mystique persists. I am convinced that for every passenger, the most pervasive cruise recollection will not concern the dining table, the swimming pool or deck chairs, nor the ship's profile or ports of call but, inevitably, the cabin. In my travel diary, I list every voyage and record the name of every steward and stewardess, every master and hotel manager, every chief steward, maître d'hôtel and cruise director; but first, at the top of each ship's roster, is the number of my cabin. I recall with delight each of the dozens of cabins I have occupied over years of sailing. Some were larger than others; some admitted too many inadvertent confidences from next door; some had inadequate curtains to keep out early light; some seemed, at first glance, impossibly cramped. But after things are unpacked, suitcases stowed beneath berths, belongings put in place, and, most evocatively, beds turned down by the steward, every cabin becomes, without fail, an ideal seagoing home away from home.

Those reassuring interior pleasures, juxtaposed with each day's novel exterior scenes through the porthole, are the stuff of shipboard dreams. And the saddest view through that same porthole is the sight of tugs shepherding the ship to the final pier. How neatly that image brings us, by the great circle route, back to my grandfather's photographed distress on leaving the *Adriatic*. My wife, Mary, and I have a fixed strategy to combat that worrisome separation anxiety: We never disembark from one cruise without having booked another. Short of staying on board forever, it is the best antidote I know.

How to Talk Like an Old Salt—or a Salt Substitute

By Henry Beard

Henry Beard is the author of Sailing: A Sailor's Dictionary.

Abbreviations: Size and means of propulsion are designated by a pair of letters that precede a cruise ship's name, for example, M.V. (Motor Vessel), S.S. (Steam Ship), T.S.S. (Turbine Steam Ship), M.S. (Motor Ship), and so on. As a rule, do not book passage on ships with the following designations: T.T. (Tub Toy), P.P.S. (Passenger Powered Ship), M.V.R.S. (Motor Vessel in Receivership), V.D.C. (Vessel Driven by a Curse) and T.G.B. (Towed Garbage Barge).

Aboard: On a ship, as opposed to Ashore. Toward the rear of a ship is Aft or Abaft; behind the rear of a ship is Astern. Anything overhead is Aloft, and something off to one side is Abeam. Someone leaning over the side in heavy weather is Awhoops or Afish. A passenger at the bar is Aswig, people in the buffet line are Agrub or Anosh, a person skeet-shooting off the stern is Ablam and anyone playing the slot machine is Abilk. Someone who cuts in front of you in the line for the tender is Abum. And a less-than-exciting person next to you at dinner is a pain in the Aft.

Ballast: Weight placed in the hold of a vessel to keep her on an even keel. On most cruise ships, the ballast is a single 900,000-gallon container of potato salad.

Bells: Thirty-minute nautical time units. The 24-hour day on most ships is measured in six "watches" of four hours each, marked by one to eight bells rung at half-hour intervals. But on cruise ships it is divided into six meals of four courses each, separated by eight snacks at half-hour intervals.

Bermuda Triangle: Awkward cruise-ship romance involving three people.

Bingo: See "Rain."

Bridge: Where you find the captain and the ship's wheel. On the bridge, look for the immense foam-rubber dice that seafaring superstition dictates be hung in front of the windshield.

Captain: Although the master of a ship on the high seas has considerable power, passengers should be advised that the captain cannot renew driver's licenses, postpone overdue mortgage payments, approve expense vouchers, issue college acceptances or authorize substitutions in diets.

Captain's Table: Odd tradition on oceangoing vessels by which rich and well connected individuals who wouldn't be caught dead eating with their chauffeurs fight to have dinner with the guy who drives the ship.

Companionway: A narrow interior stairway on shipboard. Its name derives from the fact that trying to pass another person while climbing up or going down one is the quickest way for two passengers to become close companions.

Crew: The employees of a ship are referred to as "hands" for reasons that become clear as the cruise draws to a close and all hands are out, palms upward.

Crow's Nest: 1. Lookout platform on the top of a ship's mast. 2. A woman's hairdo as it appears in a candid snapshot taken on deck by the ship's photographer.

Cruise Director: Individual whose responsibility it is to see that even if there is a mutiny, the crew members involved in the uprising won't interfere with the volleyball tournament on the afterdeck; that passengers get a chance to bet on which officer is forced to walk the plank first; and that the mutineers dress up like pirates for a formal Captain Kidd Cocktail Party and Buccaneer Dinner Gala.

Debark: 1. To leave a ship in port. 2. The sound a dog makes in Jamaica or Barbados.

Deck: The floor of a ship. The ceiling is known as the Overhead, walls are called Bulkheads, doorways are Bangheads and deck plans are Scratchheads or Shakeheads.

Deck Chair: Adjustable lounging chair with two basic seating positions: Ogle and Snooze.

Fly-Cruise Package: Prearranged travel option that permits an individual to be airsick and seasick on the same vacation.

Free Port: Duty-free shopping area where, because there are no import taxes or other fees, prices are usually no more than half of twice what they should be.

Head: Salty nautical term for a shipboard toilet. Some passengers properly object to this usage, but attempts to make it more delicate while retaining its maritime flavor are hopeless, since crew members will almost certainly react with bafflement to a request to be directed to the nearest temple, pate, brow, dome, cranium, sconce or noodle.

Hotel Manager: Shipboard officer who on most cruise vessels has supplanted the Purser as the individual responsible for all passenger comforts. He performs the same role as his counterpart on land, though it should be said that the manager of a Sheraton does not have to worry about his establishment colliding with a Hyatt across the street, or being in the wrong city when his guests arrive or having to arrange an air drop if he runs out of olives.

Inside Cabin: A cabin from which it's impossible to tell that it's too dark, too foggy or too rainy outside. See "Outside Cabin."

Jacob's Ladder: Somewhat unsafe rope ladder with wooden rungs once used to get from a moored ship to a tender, now replaced by more substantial folding metal stairs—thanks to a couple of lawsuits won by Jacob's Lawyer.

Knots: Speed as calculated in nautical miles (1 = about 1.15 statute miles, or 6,000 feet) per hour. Other maritime measurements that differ from those on land include: cabin size (1 nautical foot = 3.4 inches), cabin temperature (70 nautical degrees = 87 degrees Fahrenheit), time spent waiting for the tender (1 nautical minute = 357 seconds), closet capacity (1 nautical closet = .63 suitcase), price of items in shops (1 nautical dollar = 47 cents), liquid measure (1 nautical concoction = 2.6 drinks) and weight (100 pounds before embarking = 147 pounds on arrival).

Lifeboat Drill: Shipboard evacuation exercise during which passengers find out if the potential disaster of a shipwreck is going to be compounded by assignment to a lifeboat filled with boring, un-fun people.

Maître d': Hardworking, scrupulously fair individual whose job it is to see that all passengers are equally unhappy with their seating arrangements.

Nowhere: The "destination" of very short cruises of two or three days that remain at sea the whole time. Although Nowhere doesn't photograph very well for cruise-ship brochures, it remains a very popular port of call because there are absolutely no sights to miss, no amazing bargains to overlook, no cheap and charming restaurants to walk right by without even noticing, no fabulous beach to run out of time to swim at, no spectacular view to have no film left to photograph and no tender to wait for when it's time to leave.

Outside Cabin: A cabin into which the sun shines directly at 7 AM regardless of the ship's position, course or destination.

Pier Group: Passengers waiting on shore for a tender.

Pier Pressure: Force exerted by passengers on one another as they push forward toward an arriving tender.

Pitch and Roll: Two of the 19 separate motions a ship makes in moderate-to-heavy seas. The others are: wallow, lurch, quiver, shudder, plunge, reel, rock, sway, swing, heave, pound, yaw, yeow, damn, yuck, ohno and aaaaaaaag.

Port: On board ship, left is Port and right is Starboard. The way to remember this is to recall the handy mnemonic phrases: "The Port we Left was a dump" and "During the entertainment, the Star Bored me Right from the start."

Port of Call: Exotic, fascinating place where life is cheap, but *Time* and *Newsweek* cost $3 each; where fortunes change hands at the closing of a taxi door; where natives in crowded marketplaces sell precious goods from the fabled islands of Taiwan, Hong Kong and Singapore and strange articles of clothing in a single size that mysteriously fits all; where the drinks taste like lollipops but pack the wallop of a rocket; where danger is spelled Special Fish of the Day, and there is no word for Rest Room.

Purser: The ship's officer in charge of finances, information, public relations and day-to-day ship's business. He is thus the individual whose responsibility it is—if the ship starts to sink—to report in the ship's newspaper that new saltwater swimming pools are now open in the ship's hold; that passengers with outside cabins on the lower decks will now find free aquariums where their portholes used to be; and, if necessary, that there will be a Lifejacket Fashion Show on the Promenade Deck followed by a free but mandatory Lifeboat Excursion to Nowhere.

Quay: A dock. You'd think it would be pronounced "kway," but sailors pronounce it "key." Here are some other words with nautical pronunciations: When you ask your dining-room steward how a particular dish is, he might say it's "crummy," which is pronounced "yummy"; if you ask the purser when the next tender will arrive to take you ashore, he might say "I don't know," which is pronounced, "Oh, in 10 minutes"; and when a female passenger who's been having a fling with a ship's officer asks him if he'll call her when he's in port next, he might answer "no," which is pronounced "yes."

Rain: See "Bingo."

Running Lights: Small red and green flashlights worn in the left and right ears, respectively, by joggers on deck after dusk or in a fog so that strolling passengers can avoid being trampled.

Skipper: Slang term for Captain. The Radio Officer is "Sparks," the Ship's Doctor is "Bones," the Ship's Photographer is "Snaps," the Ship's Barber is "Clips," the Ship's Masseur is "Slaps" or "Chops," the Ship's Croupier is "Chips" and the Ship's Passengers are "Tips."

Tender: Motorboat transport used to separate the passengers of a cruise ship moored in a shallow harbor into two groups: those who wish they'd stayed on board, and those who wish they'd gone ashore.

Tipping: Nothing causes more needless worry on the last day of a cruise than deciding how much to tip the cabin and dining-room stewards. In fact, the calculations are perfectly straightforward. Cabin stewards: Number of days you were seasick times $20, plus number of mornings you didn't remember returning to your cabin the night before times $10. Dining-room stewards: $20 per pound gained for each week of the cruise. (Note to exercise nuts: if you actually lost weight on the voyage, give the dining-room steward $4 per day and tip the ship's athletic director $500.)

Weigh Anchor: To raise the anchor prior to sailing. The huge iron mooring devices on the prow of the ship aren't actually "weighed" when cruise ships leave the harbor at the end of a voyage, but crew members taking an inventory of the missing silverware and stolen ashtrays do generally check to make sure that the ship still has its anchors, hatches, rudder, propeller and funnels.

What to Read at Sea—If Anything

By Robert
Benchley

*Until his death in
1945, Robert
Benchley led a
distinguished
career as an
actor, a humorist,
and an author. He
was editor of Life
magazine in the
1920s and won an
Academy Award
for his role in
How to Sleep.
Among his many
books the
best-known are
20,000 Leagues
under the Sea,
or, David
Copperfield and
My Ten Years in
a Quandary and
How It Grew.*

The choice of books for whiling away the time on an ocean voyage is a question to which considerable thought should be given. One shouldn't rush off with the first three books that happen to be lying on the library-table as one leaves for the boat, neither should one rely on the generosity of friends to supply one with reading matter for the trip across. For no matter how many people send books to the boat, you are quite sure to find, on settling down to read the next day, that they are all copies of the same one. I think that book-store clerks do it on purpose.

An ocean voyage is a good time not only to get in a little light reading but to catch up with some of the books you never have quite got around to wading through on shore. So I would recommend, in addition to the current fiction success and the latest humorous "steamer-book," of which you will have five copies each given to you, taking a copy of "The Life of Lord Morley" or "Aspects of International Diplomacy" or something good and meaty to give balance to your mental diet. You *might* read a couple of pages in one of them, who can tell?

On the first day out you will appear with three books under your arm and settle down in your chair. You bring three in case you finish one quickly. It would be a nuisance to have to keep running to your cabin for fresh books as fast as you finish one. You wouldn't be surprised if you finished all three before lunch. So you begin on the popular fiction work.

The first page is easy-going and in no time you are on page 2. Then something happens. You take a look at the ocean as you turn the page. It is a funny thing about the ocean. Nobody ever took a quick look at it and turned right away again. You always look a little longer than you intended to. It isn't that you *see* anything. The waves all look alike and follow each other with considerable regularity. But they have a hypnotic quality which makes it possible to look at them for hours at a time without any good excuse. It is maybe five minutes before you get back to page 2 again.

Page 2 suddenly presents tremendous difficulties. You can't seem to get into it. There is too much type, in the first place, and somehow the author doesn't seem to have caught the knack of holding your attention. Before you know it your eyes are back on the ocean again, watching with fascination a slight dipping of the horizon along the top of the rail. It's a funny thing, the ocean. All that water.

But come, come! This isn't reading! Let's skip page 2 and get over on to page 3. That's better. A lot of conversation. Not very good conversation though. Let's see. "'I am glad that you told me this before I had a chance to fall in love with you,' said Eunice, holding her spoon gingerly poised above her cup." Who was that who just walked past on the deck? You look up to see, although you are sure it was no one you know, and on the way back to page 3 your eyes get caught in the ocean again. Five more minutes out.

"The Life of Lord Morley" has slipped off your lap onto the deck, but somehow that doesn't make much difference. The current fiction success has your forefinger inserted between pages 2 and 3, but otherwise your contact with it has been broken. You have frankly given yourself over to an intense contemplation of the sea and a half-hearted examination of everyone that walks past. You will do this for ten more minutes, you say to yourself, and then go back to your book. Perhaps "The Life of Lord Morley" would be good for a change. This fiction thing seems to be rather footless.

But before you have got around to opening "The Life of Lord Morley" the stewards have come around with bouillon and some of those hearty German sandwiches and there isn't much else to do but stack your three books up very neatly beside your chair and give yourself over to nourishment. A man has got to look out for his health, after all. And then, after eating, he certainly ought to take a turn around the deck or perhaps play a game of deck-tennis. He can't sit in his chair *all* day.

And here is where the books really fulfill their purpose. As they lie on the empty chair, waiting for their owner to come back to read them, they are the object of curious scrutiny by people walking by and those in neighboring chairs. There is always a great interest displayed by passengers in what their fellows are reading—or leaving lying around on their chairs. People in the next chairs will walk past, tipping their heads to one side to see what the title of the book is, and, if they are sure that the owner is on another deck, will even take the book up and thumb its pages. And from these books they judge the occupant of the chair.

Now, since it is pretty well understood that, so long as the ocean presents its distractions and so long as people keep walking past, you are not going to get much further than page 4 in any book you may take out on deck, you might as well get credit among your neighbors for being an important person mentally. Don't leave a paper-covered copy of an Edgar Wallace book lying about. Pick a good one that will look impressive. I used a copy of *The Masters of Modern French Criticism* on my last trip and got quite a name for myself with it. I got about two pages read, but all the people on my side of the ship had me sized up as a serious thinker. Everything went all right until one night a man came up to me and said "I see you are reading Professor Babbitt's book on French Criticism. I would be interested to know what you think of it. I wrote a review of it for the *Nation* when it came out and I wonder if you find the same fault with it that I do." So I had to say that I really had just begun it (he must have seen it lying around for five days) and that I hadn't really formed any opinion on it yet. Eventually, I had to read the book in my berth at night, for he wouldn't let me go.

So it would be well to pick even more esoteric works than that, in order not to get caught by someone who has already read them. The main point is, in all ocean reading, to take books which you don't have to read yourself.

3 Cruise Lines and Ships

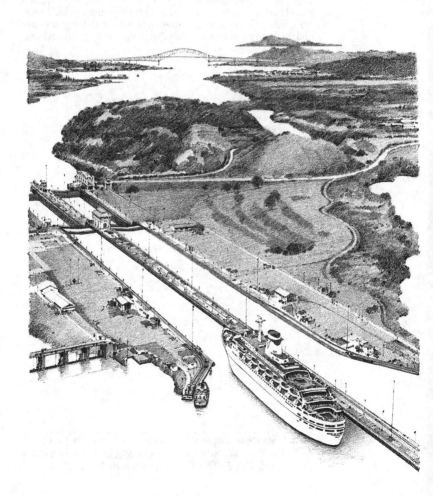

This chapter provides detailed reviews of the major cruise lines and ships that sail the Western Hemisphere. Not included are small European lines whose ships only occasionally sail in American waters.

The cruise industry is in a remarkable state of flux. Several new ships that were still under construction when this book went to press are now cruising American waters. Lines and ships reviewed here may have altered itineraries, prices, and even the amenities offered. For this reason, readers are urged to check with their travel agent or the cruise lines to confirm all details of the cruises that interest them.

No system for rating ships, such as the awarding of stars or points, has been used in this guide. Such ratings can be misleading, because people's preferences in elements of the cruise experience vary enormously. Cunard's *Sagafjord*, for example, is almost always rated five stars in appreciation of its luxurious trappings and superb service; young singles looking for round-the-clock action, however, would probably find the ship too bland for their tastes and too rich for their pocketbooks. Therefore, this guide relies on written evaluations and comparative charts to give readers an idea of what each cruise line and ship has to offer them.

Chart Symbols. *The following symbols are used in the Cruise Facilities chart.* ●: *The ship has this facility;* ○: *The ship does not have this facility;* ◐: *This facility/service is limited on the ship.*

Abercrombie & Kent

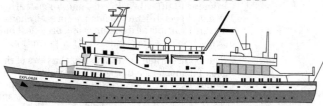

Ship MS *Explorer*

Evaluation **Abercrombie & Kent** (A&K)—established in 1962 as a luxury safari operation and today a world-renowned adventure-touring outfit—bought the *Explorer* (formerly the *Lindblad Explorer* and later the *Society Explorer*) in 1992. One of the industry's foremost advocates of environmentally responsible travel, or ecotourism, A&K captured the prestigious ASTA/Smithsonian Magazine Environmental Award in 1993.

Every aspect of A&K's operations is carefully overseen by its owners, the Kents. (There never was a Mr. Abercrombie—the name was appropriated from the former safari provisioner Abercrombie & Fitch.) While A&K's land tours to exotic locales cater to a decidedly upscale crowd, prices for its cruises are quite competitive. A&K ships spend most of the year outside the Western Hemisphere, but the *Explorer* covers Antarctica in winter, as she has done since she first pioneered cruising this destination rapidly growing in popularity.

Activities As with other adventure cruise ships, daytime activities are outside the mold of traditional cruising. A typical day at sea might start at dawn with an announcement that whales have been sighted off the starboard bow—whereupon most passengers pile enthusiastically out of bed to join the naturalists on deck or in the navigation bridge. When conditions allow, Zodiacs are lowered to follow the whales through the floating ice. During the morning, you might hear a lecture on some aspect of Antarctica or a description of an upcoming landing, perhaps at a penguin rookerie or a research station. The day is punctuated with these sightings, lectures, and landings, as well as films and Zodiac tours. Passengers might engage in card games or Scrabble, but there are no organized activities. In 1993, A&K introduced an intensive massage-therapy program.

Dining Meals are served at a single seating in a rather diminutive dining room; dinner is at roughly 7:30. With no formal seating arrangements, you can pop around from meal to meal, mingling with fellow travelers. This is no glamour cruise: The two semiformal evenings are frequently attended by casually dressed passengers who have wisely junked fancier duds to economize

---

Chart Symbols. *The following symbols are used in the cabin charts that accompany each ship's evaluation.* **D:** *Double bed;* **K:** *King-size bed;* **Q:** *Queen-size bed;* **T:** *Twin bed;* **U/L:** *Upper and lower berths;* ●: *All cabins have this facility;* ○: *No cabins have this facility;* ◐: *Some cabins have this facility*

on packing space. Food is of the hearty Northern European variety—not bad, not gourmet. You'll find heavy meat dishes, standard buffet breakfasts, and a smattering of American dishes. Special dietary needs are not easily handled. Coffee and tea are available all day. Lunch and breakfast buffets are sometimes presented deckside, weather permitting.

Entertainment The lecturers and naturalists are the stars of this cruise. Don't look for much else in the way of traditional shipboard entertainment. Otherwise, passengers may group around the piano for an impromptu sing-along or enjoy movies and nature documentaries on the lecture hall's VCR, which may also be used to screen passengers' camcorder tapes.

Service and Tipping Service is competent and friendly. A service charge is included in the fare, and tipping is not accepted.

For More Information Abercrombie & Kent (1520 Kensington Rd., Oak Brook, IL 60521, tel. 708/954–2944 or 800/323–7308).

MS Explorer

Specifications *Type of ship:* Specialty
Type of cruise: Adventure

Size: Small (2,398 tons)
Number of cabins: 51
Outside cabins: 100%

Passengers: 96
Crew: 67 (European and Filipino)
Officers: West German
Passenger/crew ratio: 1.4 to 1
Year built: 1969

Itinerary **Fall:** Outside the Western Hemisphere. **Winter:** Fifteen- to 22-day Antarctica cruises leave Ushuaiya (Argentina), calling at a research station, along the Beagle Channel (Chile/Argentina), and at Deception Island (U.K./Antarctica); or at the Falkland Islands or South Georgia Island. Local weather and ice conditions and the discretion of research stations may force unexpected changes in itinerary. Twelve-day Chilean Fjords cruises leave from Puerto Montt, calling at Chiloe Island, Puerto Natales, Glacier Passage, and Puerto Williams. The two itineraries may be combined.

Port tax: None in Antarctica.

Overview After a five-month, $1 million refurbishment, completed in 1993, the *Explorer* has retained its title as the grand dame of adventure cruising. It was the first to feature an ice-hardened hull, a relatively shallow draft, a small profile for entering otherwise inaccessible coves and harbors, and a fleet of Zodiacs. Recently, the waste containment and treatment system was completely revamped to minimize the ship's environmental impact on these remote regions. Compared with the new better-equipped, bigger adventure vessels, the *Explorer* is a bit spartan. The design is strictly utilitarian, with narrow decks, exposed pipes, and cramped quarters with no frills. Instead of deferential white-glove service, you'll find naturalists and lecturers eating and moving about among the passengers, avoiding a them-and-us mentality. The feeling is intimate, as if one were a valued guest on a private working operation. Despite the *Explorer*'s age and size, its red hull continues to be a beacon to adventure cruisers, some of whom would never dream of sailing to Antarctica on any other ship.

Cabins and Rates

	Beds	Phone	TV	Sitting Area	Fridge	Tub	Per Diem
Category 5	T	○	○	●	●	○	$471–$733
Category 4	T	○	○	○	○	○	$382–$599
Category 3	T	○	○	○	○	○	$331–$526
Category 2	T	○	○	○	○	○	$312–$495
Category 1	T	○	○	○	○	○	$268–$436

Cabins are tiny; all have hair dryers. In the daytime, beds are converted into side-by-side sofas. Closet space is extremely limited. Cabins on the Boat Deck look onto the public promenade, but all have outside views.

Outlet voltage: 220 AC.

Single supplement: 140%–170% of double-occupancy rate.

Discounts: A third passenger in a cabin pays half the double-occupancy rate; no cabins accommodate four passengers. Airfare is not included in rates.

Sports and Fitness **Health club:** Reclining bike, ski machines, free weights, sauna.

Other sports: The tiny pool is not filled on Antarctic cruises.

Facilities **Public rooms:** Dining room, lecture hall, lounge; access to navigation bridge.

Shops: Small gift shop, hairdresser.

Health care: Doctor on call.

Child care: None.

Services: Laundry.

Other: Purser's safe.

Access for the Disabled No elevator. Not recommended for those using wheelchairs.

Cruise Facilities

Ship	Cruise Line	Principle Cruising Regions	Size (in tons)	Type of Ship	Type of Cruise	Per Diem Rates	Length of Cruise	Number of Passengers
Amerikanis	Fantasy	Caribbean	20,000	Mainstream	Party	$85-$221	7-day	617
Aurora I	Classical	Mexico	2,928	Specialty	Cultural Excursion	$250-$550	18,20 day	80
Britanis	Fantasy	Caribbean/ South America	26,000	Mainstream	Party	$80-$220	3,4,5, 7-day	922
Caribbean Prince	Amer. Canadian Caribbean	Caribbean/N.E. U.S. & Canada	89.5	Specialty	Excursion Senior	$135-$192	12,15- day	80
Caribe I	Commodore	Caribbean	23,000	Economy mainstream	Party	$142-$206	7-day	875
Carnivale	Carnival/ FiestaMarina	Caribbean	27,250	Specialty	Party	$144-$297	3,4- 7-day	950
Celebration	Carnival Cruise	Caribbean	48,000	Mainstream	Party	$164-$354	7-day	1486
Club Med I	Club Med	Caribbean	14,000	Specialty	Sail-power Excursion	$250-$555	7-day	386
Columbus Caravelle	Marquest	S. America/ Carib./N.E.U.S.	7,560	Specialty	Adventure	$124-$301	12,15- 16-day	250
Constitution	American Hawaii	Hawaii	30,090	Mainstream	Traditional	$204-$585	3,4- 7-day	798
CostaAllegra	Costa	Caribbean	30,000	Mainstream	Traditional	$192-$599	7-day	800
CostaClassica	Costa	Caribbean	50,000	Mainstream	Traditional	$192-$599	7,10- 11-day	1300
CostaRomantica	Costa	Caribbean	50,000	Mainstream	Traditional	$192-$599	7,10- day	1300
Crown Dynasty	Cunard	Caribbean Alaska	20,000	Upscale mainstream	Traditional	$178-$389	7-day	820
Crown Jewel	Cunard	Caribbean	20,000	Upscale mainstream	Traditional	$178-$389	7-day	820
Crown Odyssey	Royal	Worldwide	34,250	Luxury mainstream	Traditional Senior	$156-$879	varies	1052
Crown Princess	Princess	Caribbean/ Alaska	70,000	Mainstream megaship	Traditional	$199-$463	11- day	1590
Cunard Countess	Cunard	Caribbean	17,593	Economy mainstream	Traditional	$156-$382	7,14- day	796
Crystal Harmony	Crystal	Caribbean/ Panama	49,400	Luxury mainstream	Traditional	$243-$1101	10,17- day	960
Delta Queen	Delta Queen Steamboat	Mississippi River	1,650	Paddlewheel steamboat	Upscale Excursion/ Theme	$243-$565	2-12- day	182

Passenger/Crew Ratio	Sanitation Rating*	Disabled Access	Special Dietary Options	Gymnasium	Walking/Jogging Circuit	Swimming Pool	Whirlpool	Sauna/Massage	Deck Sports	Casino	Disco	Cinema/Theater	Library	Boutiques/Gift shops	Video Arcade	Child Care
1.5:1	97	○	●	◐	●	2	○	●	●	●	●	●	●	●	●	●	●
1.6:1	N/A	◐	◐	●	●	1	○	○	○	○	○	◐	●	○	○	○
1.7:1	91	○	●	◐	●	1	○	◐	●	●	●	●	●	●	●	○	◐
4.7:1	79	○	●	○	●		○	○	○	○	○	○	○	○	○	○
2.5:1	87	◐	◐	●	○	1	●	○	●	●	●	●	●	●	○	●	◐
1.7:1	91	○	◐	●	○	4	○	●	●	●	●	●	●	●	●	●	●
2.2:1	86	○	◐	●	●	2	●	◐	●	●	●	●	○	●	●	●	●
2.1:1	92	○	◐	●	●	2	○	●	●	●	●	◐	●	●	●	○	○
2:1	N/A	◐	●	◐	○	1	●	◐	◐	○	○	○	●	●	◐	○	◐
2.5:1	N/A	○	◐	●	◐	2	○	●	●	○	●	◐	○	●	●	○	◐
2:1	90	●	●	●	●	1	●	●	●	●	●	●	○	●	●	○	●
2:1	86	●	●	◐	●	2	○	●	●	●	●	●	●	●	●	●	●
2:1	N/A	●	●	●	●	2	●	●	●	●	●	●	○	●	●	●	●
2.75:1	N/A	◐	◐	●	●	1	●	●	○	●	●	●	●	●	●	○	○
2.75:1	91	◐	◐	●	●	1	●	●	○	●	●	●	●	●	●	○	◐
2.2:1	89	●	●	●	●	2	●	●	●	●	●	●	●	●	●	○	○
2.2:1	83	●	●	◐	●	2	●	●	●	●	●	●	●	●	●	○	◐
2.3:1	94	◐	●	●	◐	1	●	●	●	●	●	●	●	●	●	●	◐
1.76:1	95	●	●	●	●	2	●	●	●	●	●	●	○	●	●	●	◐
2.4:1	N/A	○	◐	◐	●		○	○	○	○	○	○	○	◐	○	○

Ship	Cruise Line	Principle Cruising Regions	Size (in tons)	Type of Ship	Type of Cruise	Per Diem Rates	Length of Cruise	Number of Passengers
Dolphin IV	Dolphin/Majesty	Bahamas	13,007	Economy mainstream	Traditional Theme	$141-$156	3, 4-day	588
Dreamward	Norwegian	Caribbean/Bermuda	41,000	Mainstream	Traditional	$182-$427	7-day	1246
Ecstasy	Carnival	Bahamas	70,367	Mainstream megaship	Party	$149-$334	3,4-day	2040
Enchanted Isle/Enchanted Seas	Commodore	Caribbean/Mexico	23,395	Economy mainstream	Traditional	$88-$271	7-day	731
Explorer	Abercrombie & Kent	South America	2,398	Specialty	Adventure	$268-$733	15, 22-day	96
Fair Princess	Princess	Mex. Riviera/Alaska/Hawaii	25,000	Upscale mainstream	Traditional Senior	$128-$501	7, 9-day	890
Fantasy	Carnival	Bahamas	70,367	Mainstream megaship	Party	$149-$334	3,4-day	2044
Festivale	Carnival	Caribbean	38,275	Mainstream	Party	$164-$354	7-day	1146
Golden Odyssey	Royal	Panama/Alaska Carib./N.E.U.S.	10,500	Luxury mainstream	Traditional Senior	$197-$814	7-day	460
Golden Princess	Princess	Mexico/Hawaii	28,000	Upscale mainstream	Traditional Senior	$174-$708	7, 10-day	830
Holiday	Carnival	Caribbean	46,052	Mainstream	Party	$164-$354	7-day	1452
Horizon	Celebrity	Caribbean/Bermuda	46,000	Upscale mainstream	Traditional	$171-$439	7-day	1354
Independence	American Hawaii	Hawaii	30,090	Mainstream	Traditional	$195-$614	3, 4-7-day	798
Island Princess	Princess	South America/Caribbean	20,000	Upscale mainstream	Traditional	$206-$726	7, 11-14-day	610
Jubilee	Carnival	Mexico	48,000	Mainstream	Party	$164-$354	7-day	1486
Maasdam	Holland America	Caribbean/Alaska	52,000	Upscale mainstream	Traditional	$243-$795	7, 10-day	1266
Majesty of the Seas	Royal Caribbean	Caribbean	73,941	Mainstream megaship	Party	$177-$513	7-day	2766
Mayan Prince	Amer. Canadian Caribbean	Caribbean/Canada/N.E.U.S.	92	Specialty	Excursion Senior	$141-$200	12-day	96
Meridian	Celebrity	Caribbean/Bermuda	30,440	Upscale mainstream	Traditional	$160-$410	7,10-11-day	1106
Mississippi Queen	Delta Queen Steamboat	Mississippi River	3,364	Paddlewheel steamboat	Upscale Excursion/Theme	$243-$565	2–12-day	436

Passenger/Crew Ratio	Sanitation Rating*	Disabled Access	Special Dietary Options	Gymnasium	Walking/Jogging Circuit	Swimming Pool	Whirlpool	Sauna/Massage	Deck Sports	Casino	Disco	Cinema/Theater	Library	Boutiques/Gift shops	Video Arcade	Child Care
2.1:1	92	◐	●	○	●	1	○	○	●	●	●	○	●	●	●	◐
2.5:1	89	●	●	●	●	2	●	●	●	●	●	●	●	●	●	●
2.2:1	87	○	◐	●	●	2	●	●	●	●	●	○	●	●	●	●
2.1:1	89/92	◐	●	◐	○	1	○	◐	●	●	●	●	●	●	●	◐
1.4:1	N/A	○	○	●	○		○	◐	○	○	○	○	○	○	○	○
2:1	88	◐	●	●	◐	3	○	●	●	●	●	●	●	●	●	◐
2.2:1	86	○	◐	●	●	2	●	●	●	●	●	○	●	●	●	●
1.9:1	92	○	◐	●	●	2	○	●	●	●	●	●	●	●	●	●
2.3:1	89	◐	●	●	●	1	○	◐	●	●	●	●	●	●	○	○
2:1	N/A	○	●	●	●	2	●	●	●	●	●	○	●	●	○	◐
2.2:1	86	○	◐	●	●	2	○	●	●	●	●	○	●	●	●	●
2.1:1	90	●	●	●	●	2	●	●	●	●	●	○	●	●	●	●
2.5:1	N/A	○	◐	●	◐	2	○	●	●	○	●	●	○	●	●	◐
1.7:1	89	○	◐	●	◐	2	○	●	●	○	●	●	○	●	●	◐
2.2:1	95	○	◐	●	●	2	●	●	●	●	●	○	●	●	●	●
2.2:1	N/A	●	●	●	●	2	●	●	●	●	●	●	●	●	●	●
2.8:1	97	●	●	●	●	2	●	●	●	●	●	●	●	●	●	●
4.7:1	N/A	○	●	○	●		○	○	○	○	○	○	○	○	○	○
1.7:1	89	◐	●	●	●	2	●	●	●	●	●	●	●	●	●	●
2.6:1	N/A	◐	◐	●	●		●	●	○	○	○	◐	●	●	○	○

4

Ship	Cruise Line	Principle Cruising Regions	Size (in tons)	Type of Ship	Type of Cruise	Per Diem Rates	Length of Cruise	Number of Passengers
Monarch of the Seas	Royal Caribbean	Caribbean	73,941	Mainstream megaship	Party	$177-$513	7-day	2354
Nantucket/ Yorktown Clipper	Clipper	Caribbean/N.E. U.S./Panama/Mex	98	Upscale yacht-like	Excursion Senior	$183-$360	8-day	102
New Shoreham II	Amer. Canadian Caribbean	Caribbean/N.E. U.S. & Canada	89	Specialty	Excursion Senior	$99-$175	12-day	76
Nieuw Amsterdam	Holland America	Alaska/Caribbean	33,930	Upscale mainstream	Traditional	$163-$471	7,10-day	1214
Noordam	Holland American	Alaska/Caribbean	33,930	Upscale mainstream	Traditional	$163-$471	7,10-day	1214
Nordic Empress	Royal Caribbean	Bahamas	48,563	Mainstream	Party	$121-$386	3,4-day	1600
Nordic Prince	Royal Caribbean	Mexico/Alaska	23,000	Mainstream	Traditional Party	$163-$389	7-day	1012
Norway	Norwegian	Caribbean	76,000	Mainstream liner	Traditional Theme	$208-$806	7-day	2044
Oceanbreeze	Dolphin/Majesty	Caribbean	21,486	Mainstream	Traditional	$164-$349	7-day	776
Pacific Princess	Princess	Panama Canal	20,000	Upscale mainstream	Traditional	$206-$726	14-day	610
Polaris	Special Expeditions	Worldwide	2,214	Adventure	Cultural	$318-$583	10,12-14-day	84
Queen Elizabeth 2	Cunard	Worldwide	67,139	Luxury mainstream	Traditional	$202-$4155	varies	1864
Radisson Diamond	Diamond	Caribbean/Mediterranean	20,000	Luxury	Traditional	$600-$900	3,4 7-day	354
Regal Princess	Princess	Caribbean/Alaska	70,000	Upscale mainstream	Traditional	$199-$463	10,11-day	1590
Regent Rainbow	Regency	Caribbean	25,000	Mainstream	Traditional Budget	$98-$218	2-5-day	960
Regent Sea	Regency	Caribbean/Haw./S.Amer./Alaska	22,000	Mainstream	Traditional Budget	$169-$419	7,10-day	729
Regent Star	Regency	Panama Canal/Carib./Alaska	24,500	Mainstream	Traditional Budget	$176-$464	7-day	950
Regent Sun	Regency	Carib./New England/Canada	25,500	Mainstream	Traditional Budget	$176-$354	7-day	836
Renaissance III,VI	Renaissance	Caribbean	4,500	Luxury yacht-like	Cultural	$249-$499	8-day	114
Rotterdam	Holland America	Worldwide	38,000	Upscale mainstream	Traditional	$130-$493	7,10-day	1114

Passenger/Crew Ratio	Sanitation Rating*	Disabled Access	Special Dietary Options	Gymnasium	Walking/Jogging Circuit	Swimming Pool	Whirlpool	Sauna/Massage	Deck Sports	Casino	Disco	Cinema/Theater	Library	Boutiques/Gift shops	Video Arcade	Child Care
2.8:1	93	●	●	●	●	2	●	●	●	●	●	●	●	●	●	●
3.6:1	70/92	○	◐	○	●		○	○	○	○	○	◐	○	○	○	○
4.7:1	95	○	●	○	●		○	○	○	○	○	○	○	○	○	○
2.2:1	93	●	●	●	●	2	●	●	●	●	●	●	●	●	●	◐
2.2:1	96	●	●	●	●	2	●	●	●	●	●	●	●	●	●	◐
2.3:1	98	●	●	●	●	1	●	●	●	●	●	○	○	●	●	◐
2.4:1	89	◐	●	●	●	1	○	●	●	●	●	○	○	●	○	◐
2.3:1	87	◐	●	●	●	3	●	●	●	●	●	●	●	●	●	●
2.5:1	N/A	◐	●	●	●	1	●	●	◐	●	●	●	◐	◐	○	●
1.7:1	91	●	●	●	●	2	○	●	●	●	●	●	●	●	●	◐
1.9:1	76	○	◐	○	○		○	◐	○	○	○	○	●	●	○	○
1.8:1	88	◐	●	●	●	4	●	●	●	●	●	●	●	●	●	●
1.8:1	92	●	●	●	●	1	●	●	●	●	●	○	●	●	○	○
2.2:1	96	●	●	●	●	2	●	●	●	●	●	●	●	●	○	◐
2.3:1	90	●	●	◐	●	2	○	●	◐	●	●	○	●	●	○	●
2:1	89	●	●	●	●	1	●	●	●	●	●	●	●	●	○	◐
2:1	97	◐	●	●	◐	1	●	●	●	●	●	●	●	●	○	◐
2.1:1	90	◐	●	●	○	1	○	●	●	●	●	●	●	●	○	◐
1.6:1	67-86	○	●	○	●	1	●	●	◐	◐	○	○	●	●	○	○
1.9:1	94	●	●	●	●	2	○	◐	●	●	●	●	●	●	●	◐

Ship	Cruise Line	Principle Cruising Regions	Size (in tons)	Type of Ship	Type of Cruise	Per Diem Rates	Length of Cruise	Number of Passengers
Royal Majesty	Dolphin/Majesty	Bahamas/Caribbean	32,400	Mainstream	Traditional	$149-$530	3,4-day	1056
Royal Princess	Princess	Panama Canal/Caribbean	45,000	Luxury mainstream	Traditional	$265-$865	10,11-day	1200
Royal Viking Sun	Royal Viking	Worldwide	38,000	Luxury mainstream	Traditional Senior	$336-$1252	Varies	740
Sagafjord	Cunard	Carib./N.E.U.S.& Can./Panama	24,474	Luxury mainstream	Traditional	$216-$1252	10,11-14-day	618
Sea Bird	Special Expeditions	Alaska/Mex. Riviera/Oregon	99.7	Adventure	Cultural	$173-$423	10,14-day	70
Sea Cloud	Special Expeditions	Caribbean	2,323	Sailing yacht	Cultural Adventure	$495-$871	12-day	70
Sea Goddess I	Cunard	Caribbean	4,250	Luxury, yacht-like	Traditional	$600-$900	7-day	116
Sea Lion	Special Expeditions	Alaska/Mex. Riviera/Oregon	99.7	Adventure	Cultural	$173-$423	10,14-day	70
Seabourn Pride	Seabourn	Carib./S. Amer./N.E.U.S.&Canada	10,000	Luxury, yacht-like	Traditional	$510-$1465	7,14-21-day	212
SeaBreeze	Dolphin/Majesty	Caribbean	21,000	Economy mainstream	Traditional Theme	$158-$265	7-day	842
Seaward	Norwegian	Caribbean/Bahamas	42,276	Mainstream	Traditional	$178-$383	7-day	1798
Seawind Crown	Seawind	Caribbean	24,000	Economy mainstream	Traditional	$128-$385	7-day	624
Sky Princess	Princess	Caribbean/Alaska	46,000	Upscale mainstream	Traditional	$171-$631	7,11-day	1200
Song of America	Royal Caribbean	Caribbean/Bermuda	37,584	Mainstream	Traditional Party	$177-$435	10,11-day	1402
Song of Norway	Royal Caribbean	Panama Canal	23,000	Mainstream	Traditional Party	$163-$389	11-day	1022
Southward	Norwegian	West Coast U.S.	16,607	Mainstream	Party	$134-$299	3,4-day	754
Sovereign of the Seas	Royal Caribbean	Caribbean	73,192	Mainstream megaship	Party	$177-$513	7-day	2278
Star Princess	Princess	Caribbean	63,500	Upscale mainstream	Traditional	$171-$669	7-day	1494
Star/Ship Atlantic	Premier	Bahamas	36,500	Mainstream	Traditional Family	$148-$385	3,4-day	1769
Star/Ship Majestic	Premier	Bahamas/Key West	17,750	Mainstream	Traditional Family	$148-$351	3,4-day	759

Passenger/Crew Ratio	Sanitation Rating*	Disabled Access	Special Dietary Options	Gymnasium	Walking/Jogging Circuit	Swimming Pool	Whirlpool	Sauna/Massage	Deck Sports	Casino	Disco	Cinema/Theater	Library	Boutiques/Gift shops	Video Arcade	Child Care
2.1:1	N/A	●	●	●	●	1	●	○	○	●	●	○	●	●	○	◐
2.4:1	93	●	●	●	●	4	●	●	●	●	●	●	●	●	●	◐
1.6:1	92	●	●	●	●	2	●	●	●	●	●	●	●	●	○	◐
1.9:1	93	●	●	●	●	2	●	●	●	●	○	●	●	●	○	◐
3.3:1	95	○	○	○	○		○	○	○	○	○	◐	○	◐	○	○
1:1	N/A	○	○	○	●		○	○	○	○	○	○	●	○	○	○
1.3:1	95	○	●	●	●	1	○	●	●	●	○	○	●	●	○	◐
3.3:1	93	○	○	○	○		○	○	○	○	○	◐	○	◐	○	○
1.5:1	89	●	●	●	●	3	●	●	●	●	○	○	●	●	○	◐
2.1:1	86	◐	●	●	●	1	●	◐	●	●	●	●	○	●	●	◐
2.9:1	86	●	●	●	●	2	●	●	●	●	●	○	○	●	○	●
2.1:1	N/A	●	●	●	●	2	○	●	●	●	●	●	●	○	○	●
2.2:1	86	●	●	●	●	3	●	●	●	●	●	●	●	●	●	●
2.6:1	86	○	●	●	●	2	○	●	●	●	●	●	○	●	○	◐
2.4:1	86	○	●	●	●	1	○	◐	●	●	●	○	○	●	○	◐
2.4:1	86	○	●	●	●	1	○	●	●	●	●	●	●	●	●	●
2.8:1	90	●	●	●	●	2	●	●	●	●	●	●	●	●	●	●
2.5:1	91	●	●	●	●	3	●	●	●	●	●	●	●	●	●	●
3.2:1	89	◐	●	●	●	3	●	◐	●	●	●	●	●	●	●	●
2.7:1	90	○	●	●	○	1	○	◐	●	●	○	●	○	●	●	●

Ship	Cruise Line	Principle Cruising Regions	Size (in tons)	Type of Ship	Type of Cruise	Per Diem Rates	Length of Cruise	Number of Passengers
Star/Ship Oceanic	Premier	Bahamas	40,000	Mainstream	Traditional Family	$148-$385	3,4-day	1180
Starward	Norwegian	Mexico	16,107	Mainstream	Party	$161-$321	7-day	758
Statendam	Holland America	Caribbean	52,000	Upscale mainstream	Traditional	$243-$795	10,12-day	1266
Stella Solaris	Sun Line	Caribbean/Panama Canal	18,000	Mainstream	Traditional Senior	$138-$519	10,14-16-day	620
Sun Viking	Royal Caribbean	Caribbean	18,559	Mainstream	Traditional	$180-$423	7-day	714
Tropicale	Carnival	Caribbean	36,674	Mainstream	Party	$164-$354	7-day	1022
Universe	World Explorer	Alaska	18,100	Specialty	Cultural	$193-$285	14-day	500
Viking Serenade	Royal Caribbean	Ensenada/Los Angeles	40,132	Mainstream	Traditional Party	$143-$461	3,4-day	1,512
Vistafjord	Cunard	Caribbean	24,492	Luxury mainstream	Traditional	$242-$1252	14,16-day	749
Westerdam	Holland America	Caribbean/Alaska/Panama	53,872	Upscale mainstream	Traditional	$142-$536	7,14-day	1494
Westward	Norwegian	Bahamas	28,000	Mainstream	Traditional	$179-$442	7-day	829
Wind Spirit/Wind Star	Windstar	Caribbean	5,350	Luxury specialty	Sail-power Excursion	$368-$410	7-day	148
Windward	Norwegian	Caribbean	41,000	Mainstream	Traditional	$182-$427	7-day	1246
World Discoverer	Clipper	Alaska/South America	3,153	Adventure	Cultural	$282-$605	15,30-day	138
Zenith	Celebrity	Caribbean	47,000	Upscale mainstream	Traditional	$171-$439	7-day	1374

Passenger/Crew Ratio	Sanitation Rating*	Disabled Access	Special Dietary Options	Gymnasium	Walking/Jogging Circuit	Swimming Pool	Whirlpool	Sauna/Massage	Deck Sports	Casino	Disco	Cinema/Theater	Library	Boutiques/Gift shops	Video Arcade	Child Care
3:1	93	○	●	●	●	2	●	◑	●	●	●	●	○	●	●	●
2.4:1	92	◑	●	●	●	2	○	●	●	●	●	●	●	●	○	◑
2.2:1	83	●	●	●	●	2	●	●	●	●	●	●	●	●	●	●
2:1	80	●	●	●	●	1	○	●	●	◑	●	●	●	●	○	◑
2.3:1	96	○	●	●	●	1	○	◑	●	◑	●	○	○	●	○	◑
1.9:1	94	○	◑	●	●	2	○	●	●	●	●	○	●	●	●	●
2.3:1	91	◑	◑	●	●		○	◑	●	○	○	●	●	●	○	◑
2.4:1	86	●	●	●	●	1	●	●	●	●	●	○	●	●	●	●
1.9:1	93	●	●	●	●	2	●	●	●	●	○	●	●	●	○	◑
2.4:1	91	●	●	●	●	2	●	●	●	●	○	●	●	●	○	◑
2.5:1	83	◑	●	●	○		○	●	●	●	●	●	●	●	●	●
1.6:1	93	○	●	●	◑	1	○	●	●	◑	●	○	●	●	○	○
2.5:1	N/A	●	●	●	●	2	●	●	●	●	●	●	●	●	●	●
1.8:1	N/A	○	◑	◑	○	1	○	◑	●	○	○	●	●	●	○	○
2.1:1	90	●	●	●	●	2	●	●	●	●	●	○	●	●	●	●

*Sanitation ratings are provided by the Vessel Sanitation Program, Center for Environmental Health and Injury Control. Ships are rated on water, food preparation and holding, potential contamination of food, and general cleanliness, storage, and repair. A score of 86 or higher indicates an acceptable level of sanitation. According to the center, "a low score does not necessarily imply an imminent outbreak of gastrointestinal disease." Chart ratings come from the center's April 23, 1993, report. Not all ships are covered.

American Canadian Caribbean Line

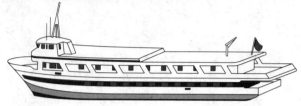

Caribbean Prince

Ships *Caribbean Prince*
Mayan Prince
New Shoreham II

Evaluation American Canadian Caribbean Line's (ACCL) three yacht-sized ships sail to spots that larger cruise ships can't visit, making for some unusual itineraries. With their shallow drafts and bow ramps, the ships can reach isolated beaches and let passengers walk directly ashore. The ships' small size and low rates mean that ACCL offers few traditional services and facilities—it's even suggested that you pack your own beach towel. These no-frills cruises are an excellent value, nevertheless. Everything is included in the base price except tips and shore excursions. No alcohol is sold on board, although passengers are free to bring their own. Mixers and other nonalcoholic drinks are available free from the bar at all hours.

An ACCL cruise will not appeal to those seeking the glamour and pampering of luxury liners; these elements are cheerfully replaced, however, with down-home charm and personal service. Passengers find themselves on easy terms with one another as well as with the crew. ACCL cruisers tend to be educated and older (63 on average), and children under 14 are not permitted. On some Caribbean cruises you can board a day early and use the ship as a floating hotel for $75 per passenger, $100 per couple. A new ACCL ship, the *Niagara*, may be plying the seas as early as mid-1994—it's currently under construction.

Activities Life on board is laid-back, with almost no organized activities. In the Caribbean the focus is on beachcombing and water sports. Two Sailfish, snorkeling equipment, and a 21-seat glass-bottom boat are available free to passengers; you can swim or sail from the stern platform. Fishing from ship or beach is encouraged; bring your own tackle. Shore excursions tend to be informative and extremely worthwhile; if the local tour guides don't meet ACCL standards, the ship supplies a guide. The

Chart Symbols. *The following symbols are used in the cabin charts that accompany each ship's evaluation.* **D:** *Double bed;* **K:** *King-size bed;* **Q:** *Queen-size bed;* **T:** *Twin bed;* **U/L:** *Upper and lower berths;* ●: *All cabins have this facility;* ○: *No cabins have this facility;* ◐: *Some cabins have this facility*

average price for shore excursions is only $12; the most expensive (in Belize) costs $17.

Dining Meals are served family-style at a single, open seating. Breakfast is a Continental-style buffet. The cuisine is basic American, with an emphasis on fresh seafood. Special diets, including low-fat, kosher, sugar-free, and low-salt, must be requested at least two weeks before departure. Passengers can help themselves any time to tea, coffee, lemonade, and snacks. There are no formal nights.

Entertainment Though there is no organized entertainment, a number of innovative programs are devised by the exceptionally creative cruise directors. Most passengers pass the time playing cards or reading.

Service and Tipping Service is quite casual. Tips are given via anonymous envelopes that you place in a basket in the lounge (tip $7 per diem per passenger); the total is pooled among the crew.

For More Information American Canadian Caribbean Line (Box 368, Warren, RI 02885, tel. 401/247–0955 or 800/556–7450).

Caribbean Prince

Specifications *Type of ship:* Specialty *Passengers:* 80
Type of cruise: Excursion/Senior *Crew:* 17 (American)
Size: Very small (89.5 tons) *Officers:* American
Number of cabins: 38 *Passenger/crew ratio:* 4.7 to 1
Outside cabins: 84% *Year built:* 1983

Itinerary **Fall:** Twelve-day cruises sail between Warren (RI) and Québec City, visiting Narragansett Bay, New York Harbor, the Hudson River Valley, West Point, Kingston, Troy, Little Falls, Erie Canal Village, Sylvan Beach, Oswego, the Thousand Islands, Clayton, Upper Canada Village, and Montréal. A 15-day repositioning cruise between Warren and Palm Beach Garden visits New York Harbor, Baltimore, Crisfield (MD), Norfolk (VA), Beaufort (NC), Wrightsville Beach (NC), Georgetown (SC), Charleston, Beaufort (SC), Savannah, St. Simons Island (GA), and, in Florida, St. Augustine, Titusville, and through Hobe Sound. **Winter:** Twelve-day loop cruises leave Belize City, calling at isolated islands and coves along the coasts of Guatemala and Belize, the exquisite barrier reef, and along the Rio Dulce. **Spring–Summer:** Same as Fall.

Port tax: $50–$100 per passenger.

Overview The *Caribbean Prince*, built in 1983, is one of the smallest cruise ships afloat, looking like a cross between an oversize yacht and a little ferry. Its unique bow lowers to offload passengers directly to shore, and small sailboats and other water-sports equipment are launched from the stern. There are only two public rooms. The dining room, furnished with mahogany cabinets, tables for six, and pink- and blue-flowered curtains, doubles by day as a recreation room and lobby. In the cozy forward lounge, the bartender dispenses nonalcoholic drinks or will mix whatever concoctions you wish from liquor you bring aboard. The pilothouse retracts so the ship can pass under low bridges along the Erie Canal and other narrow waterways.

Cabins and Rates

	Beds	Phone	TV	Sitting Area	Fridge	Tub	Per Diem
Cabins 50–59	T/D	○	○	○	○	○	$188–$192
Cabins 40–46	T/D	○	○	○	○	○	$171–$175
Cabins 20–22	T	○	○	○	○	○	$135–$139

The more expensive cabins have picture windows, a lounge chair, and, on request, a small table; other outside cabins have portholes. Some Sun Deck cabins have partially obstructed views. Cabins 20–22 are for nonsmokers.

Outlet voltage: 110 AC.

Single supplement: 175% of double-occupancy rate (cabins 20–22 only).

Discounts: 15% per passenger when three passengers share a cabin. You get a 10% discount when booking consecutive cruises. Airfare is not included in rates.

Sports and Fitness **Walking/jogging:** Unobstructed circuit on Sun Deck (11 laps = 1 mile).

Other sports: Early-morning exercises, fishing, snorkeling, sailing.

Access for the Disabled None.

Mayan Prince

Specifications *Type of ship:* Specialty
Type of cruise: Excursion/senior
Size: Very small (92 tons)
Number of cabins: 45
Outside cabins: 87%

Passengers: 92
Crew: 18 (American)
Officers: American
Passenger/crew ratio: 4.7 to 1
Year built: 1992

Itinerary The *Mayan Prince*'s itinerary changes throughout the year, allowing for a variety of repositioning cruises. **Fall:** Same as *Caribbean Prince*. **Winter:** Twelve-day cruises between Antigua and Grenada call at Guadeloupe, Dominica, Martinique, St. Lucia, St. Vincent, and the Grenadines' Bequia, Canouan, Mayreau, and Carriacou. Twelve-day cruises sail around the southern Caribbean, including calls at Aruba, Bonaire, and Curaçao. Twelve-day cruises through the Panama Canal call at Caldera (Costa Rica), the San Blas Islands, and a number of smaller ports. **Spring–Summer:** Same as Fall.

Port tax: $60–$120 per passenger.

Overview The *Mayan Prince* was built in 1992 at ACCL's Blount Shipyard in Warren, Rhode Island, inspired by feedback from questionnaires collected from passengers on the *Caribbean Prince* and *New Shoreham II*. Well designed and modern in both layout and convenience, the new ship features an efficient electrical generator positioned outside the stern, resulting in an unusually quiet vessel. A new type of ductless air-conditioning lets passengers individually control cabin temperature. The new ship also features 20% more deck space than its fellows. The decor reflects the art of the Mayans, indigenous to many areas visited by the ship, as well as teak railings and enclosed staircases. A retractable pilothouse allows the boat to travel under 22-foot-high bridges frequently encountered on cruises along the Erie Canal or the Saguenay Fjord. And because it draws just 6 feet of water and is equipped with a 40-foot bow ramp that allows dry descent to spectacularly remote beaches, the *Mayan Prince* is able to call at some relatively unspoiled Caribbean islands. Carried on board are a glass-bottom boat, two dinghies, and a 25-passenger tender.

Cabins and Rates

	Beds	Phone	TV	Sitting Area	Fridge	Tub	Per Diem
Cabins 60–63	T/D	○	○	●	○	○	$175–$200
Cabins 50–58	T/D	○	○	●	○	○	$173–$198
Cabins 40–47	T/D	○	○	○	○	○	$163–$176
Cabins 20–22	T	○	○	○	○	○	$135–$141

All cabins except 20–22 have picture windows and twin beds that can be converted to doubles on request. There's ample storage space and hanging closets. Bathrooms have a state-of-the-art silent commode—not the roaring vacuum-type systems found on other ships.

Outlet voltage: 110 AC.

Single supplement: 175% of double-occupancy rate (cabins 20–22 only).

Discounts: 15% per passenger when three passengers share a cabin. You get a 10% discount when booking consecutive cruises. Airfare is not included in rates.

Sports and Fitness **Sports:** Informal workouts, fishing, snorkeling.

Access for the Disabled None.

New Shoreham II

Specifications

Type of ship: Specialty
Type of cruise: Excursion/senior
Size: Very small (89 tons)
Number of cabins: 36
Outside cabins: 50%

Passengers: 76
Crew: 16 (American)
Officers: American
Passenger/crew ratio: 4.7 to 1
Year built: 1979

Itinerary **Fall:** Same as *Caribbean Prince*. **Winter:** Not in service. **Spring:** Twelve-day cruises in and around a number of small Bahamian islands, including Nassau, Exuma, and Eleuthera. Eight- to 15-day cruises sail from West Palm Beach to New Orleans, New Orleans to Natchez (MS), New Orleans to Chicago, and Chicago to Warren (RI); ports include Houma, Morgan City, and Baton Rouge (LA); Biloxi and Columbus (MS); Peoria and Joliet (IL); St. Louis; Mobile; Nashville; Mackinaw City and Detroit (MI); Lake Erie; and Lake Ontario. **Summer:** Several six- to 15-day cruises explore New England's coast, including calls at Cape Cod, Bar Harbor, and Block Island.

Port tax: $50–$120 per passenger.

Overview As with its companion ships, everything about the *New Shore-ham II* is Lilliputian. Separated by a pair of cabins are the two intimate public rooms, the lounge (with liquorless bar) and the dining room, both with frilly curtains and antique-style lamps. The ship has a Sun Deck, a Promenade Deck, and a swimming platform that folds down from the stern. A bow ramp, which can be raised and lowered, allows passengers to disembark directly onto beaches. The pilothouse retracts to allow the ship to pass under the low bridges along the Erie Canal.

Cabins and Rates

	Beds	Phone	TV	Sitting Area	Fridge	Tub	Per Diem
Cabins 91–92	T	○	○	○	○	○	$175–$188
Cabins 81–82	T	○	○	○	○	○	$169–$182
Cabins 42–59	T	○	○	○	○	○	$165–$179
Cabins 31–34	U/L	○	○	○	○	○	$99
Cabins 14–28	T or U/L	○	○	○	○	○	$116–$128

More expensive cabins have picture windows, a lounge chair, and, on request, a small table; other outside cabins have port-holes. The view from some cabins on the Sun Deck is partially obstructed. Cabins 42–59 can accommodate a third passenger in a portable berth; in cabins 14–28 two passengers can squeeze into the wide twin bed, freeing the other bed for a third passenger. Stateroom A, not available on northern cruises, has no private bathroom facilities.

Outlet voltage: 110 AC.

Single supplement: 175% of double-occupancy rate.

Discounts: 15% per passenger when three passengers share a cabin. You get a 10% discount when booking consecutive cruises. Airfare is not included in rates.

Sports and Fitness **Walking/jogging:** Unobstructed circuit on Sun Deck (12 laps = 1 mile).

Other sports: Informal workouts, fishing, snorkeling, sailing.

Access for the Disabled None.

American Hawaii Cruises

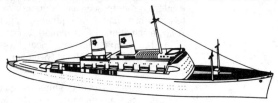

Ships SS *Constitution*
SS *Independence*

Evaluation Built in 1951, these were the first modern liners to sail between New York and the Mediterranean. In 1956 the *Constitution* brought Grace Kelly and her wedding party to Monaco for her marriage to Prince Rainier. Since American Hawaii Cruises bought them in 1980, both ships have continued to play host to the stars, including Rex Reed, June Allyson, and various San Francisco Forty-Niners. But these mainstream cruises also attract honeymooners, families, and older passengers—or anyone wishing to avoid the round of hotels and interisland airports usually involved in visiting the major islands. Many passengers take comfort in the fact that the ship is never more than 2 miles from land. Singles, however, will probably feel left out.

The staff is friendly and accommodating, and the public areas are in good condition, having undergone a $40 million refurbishment between 1988 and 1992. There's plenty of room to relax on deck and in public rooms, and numerous scheduled activities are gently offered. The main attractions, however, are the islands themselves; passengers choose from 45 shore excursions on the four islands. Only one day is spent at sea, as the ships sail between ports at night. Options include three-, four-, and seven- day cruises or a seven-day Cruise/Resort Vacation combining a three- or four-day cruise with hotel stays. Several theme cruises are held each year; 1994's lineup includes "Save the Humpback Whales" (late March), three "Health and Fitness" cruises (June, July, August), "Aloha Festival" (mid-September), and "1940s Remembered" (early May and early December).

Activities Passengers who stay aboard find plenty to do, from the usual cruise activities to ukulele, hula, lei-making, palm-weaving, and Hawaiian-language lessons. Popular shore excursions include flightseeing by helicopter over an active volcano, bicycling down the slopes of a dormant volcano, or visiting Volcano National Park—you should be detecting a theme here. Also big are whale watching, snorkeling, and kayaking.

Chart Symbols. *The following symbols are used in the cabin charts that accompany each ship's evaluation.* **D:** *Double bed;* **K:** *King-size bed;* **Q:** *Queen-size bed;* **T:** *Twin bed;* **U/L:** *Upper and lower berths;* **●**: *All cabins have this facility;* ○: *No cabins have this facility;* **◑**: *Some cabins have this facility*

Dining The food is average, though service is efficient and friendly. American, Continental, and Polynesian dishes incorporate local ingredients, such as mahimahi, *lomi lomi* salmon, Manoa lettuce, macadamia nuts, pineapple, papaya, and Kona coffee. A large selection of Californian, French, and German wines is offered to complement your meal. Passengers may sign on to the Pu'uwai (Healthy Heart) program, which guarantees them a low-fat, low- cholesterol entrée at every meal.

The dining rooms on both ships are spacious and quiet. On the *Constitution,* you can choose between two restaurants, Bird of Paradise or Hibiscus. The *Independence* offers the Palms, an elegant room with etched glass dividers. Passengers are assigned tables at one of two seatings, at 6 and 8:15. The first evening, dinner is a grand buffet. Sunday is the one semiformal evening; a jacket and tie or a simple dress will easily suffice. Other nights, attire is always casual, except for the Polynesian dinner, at which Hawaiian dress is expected.

Coffee is served on the Upper and Sun Decks from 6:30 to 10 AM for early risers. A breakfast buffet and lunch are served on the Upper Deck or in the dining rooms at open seating (the buffet is recommended to those planning shore excursions, since breakfast service in the dining room can be slow). Sherbet is offered mid-morning, tea and a hamburger-and-hot-dog cookout are held mid-afternoon, and midnight snacks round out the day. A limited menu of beverages and snacks are available 24 hours a day from room service.

Entertainment Evening entertainment is family oriented and includes traditional Broadway-style revues, comedy nights, magic shows, big-band and swing music, and dance orchestras. Participatory activities include talent shows, pajama parties, and '50s sock hops. The Hawaiian entertainers are particularly enjoyable, with favorite local stars, such as the Naluai Brothers and the Johnny Lum Ho troupe, performing island music. Both ships have both a movie theater and a disco.

Service and Tipping The American crew are personable and enthusiastic, but room service can be slow. Recommended tips per passenger per diem: dining room waiter, $3; assistant waiter, $1.50; cabin steward, $3. A 15% gratuity is automatically added to bar and wine service.

For More Information American Hawaii Cruises and Land Vacations (550 Kearny St., San Francisco, CA 94108, tel. 415/392–9400 or 800/765–7000).

SS Constitution and SS Independence

Specifications *Type of ship:* Mainstream *Passengers:* 798
Type of cruise: Traditional *Crew:* 320 (American)
Size: Medium (30,090 tons) *Officers:* American
Number of cabins: 383 *Passenger/crew ratio:* 2.5 to 1
Outside cabins: 44%/43% *Year built:* 1950

Itinerary **Year-round:** Seven-day loops leave Honolulu Saturdays, calling
Constitution at Kahului (Maui), Hilo and Kona (Big Island), and Nawiliwili (Kauai).

Port tax: $58 per passenger.

Independence **Year-round:** Seven-day loops reversing the *Constitution*'s route leave Honolulu Saturdays, with an overnight at Kahului.

Port tax: $58 per passenger.

Overview   The *Constitution* and the *Independence*—the only cruise ships sailing under the American flag—combine modern features with the traditional designs of transatlantic liners. Each sleek white ship, funnels emblazoned with the line's red hibiscus flower logo—contains 23,000 square feet of open deck and roomy staterooms. The delightful main lounges provide ample room for relaxing, reading, and playing cards and board games. Each ship also has a writing room in soothing pastels, for catching up on correspondence, and a Whale Gallery, with photographs of and information on endangered humpbacks—spottings of which are a rare treat in these waters.

On the Sun Deck the casual Beachcomber Bar (*Constitution*) and Barefoot Bar (*Independence*) are located poolside and incorporate tropical mosaics by Hawaiian artist Martin Charlot. The somewhat more elegant Tradewinds Terrace (*Constitution*) and Commodore's Terrace (*Independence*) are popular for predinner drinks and musical entertainment. The Upper Deck's Lahaina Landing (*Constitution*) and Latitude 20 (*Independence*) are located near the buffet/cookout areas and feature nighttime dancing and entertainment. On both ships the Showplace areas, with recently upgraded sound systems, can become crowded at night; you need to arrive early to find good seats. The pools are freshwater. A sleekly designed fitness center offers up-to-date equipment and good views.

Cabins and Rates

	Beds	Phone	TV	Sitting Area	Fridge	Tub	Per Diem*
Owner's Suite	T, K	●	●	●	●	●	$585
Deluxe Suite	T, K	●	○	◐	●	●	$556
Outside Suite	T, K	●	○	◐	●	◐	$356
Outside Stateroom	T	●	○	○	○	○	$307
Inside Stateroom	T, D, or U/L	●	○	○	○	○	$263
Outside Cabin	T, D, or U/L	●	○	○	○	○	$280
Economy Inside Cabin	T, D, or K	●	○	○	○	○	$225
Budget Inside Cabin	T, D	●	○	○	○	○	$204

Rates are for seven-day cruises. Not all categories are listed.

Between 1988 and 1992, staterooms were redecorated with new fabrics and carpeting in tropical colors; the rest retain older furnishings that show their age. Tropical plants and Polynesian-theme art by Luigi Fumagalli and Hawaiian artist Pegge Hopper brighten the cabins. Views from some Sun Deck cabins are partially obstructed by lifeboat stations. The Owner's Suite pampers splurgers with a king-size bed in the master bedroom; a marble-tile master bath; a sitting room with TV, VCR, bar, refrigerator, and two daybeds; and a second bath.

Outlet voltage: 110 AC.

Single supplement: 200% of double-occupancy rate for suites, 160% for other categories. Some cabins available as singles at no extra charge.

Discounts: A third or fourth passenger in a cabin pays about $650 per cruise. Children under 17 traveling with two full-fare adults in select cabin categories sail free, except on certain summer dates. Airfare is not included in rates.

Sports and Fitness   **Health club:** Recently refurbished top-deck gym, with large windows, Life Cycles, Stairmasters, free weights, rowing machines, multistation Polaris exercise machines, men's and women's saunas, massage (extra charge).

Walking/jogging: Boat Deck circuit (9 laps = 1 mile).

Other sports: Aerobics, yoga, dancercise, and stretch-and-tone classes; two freshwater pools.

Facilities   **Public rooms:** Three bars, lounge, show/conference room, writing room, Whale Gallery, disco, cinema, game room, photo gallery.

Shops: Shopping arcade, beauty parlor/barber.

Health care: Doctor and nurse on call.

Child care: Supervised activities for children 5–16 summer and holidays, youth recreation center, baby-sitting arranged privately with staff member.

Services: Laundromat, irons and ironing boards, dry cleaning arranged off ship, photo lab on *Independence.*

Other: Safe-deposit boxes, religious services on weekends, Alcoholics Anonymous (occasionally); shipboard purchases, including bar tabs, can be signed for against a credit card.

Access for the Disabled   Although the ships do not have designated cabins for passengers with wheelchairs, the line makes an effort to assign disabled passengers to larger cabins off a main hallway on the Main Deck or on the decks above. Elevators are accessible for slim, folding wheelchairs. Disabled passengers must be accompanied by an able-bodied individual.

Carnival Cruise Lines/FiestaMarina Cruises

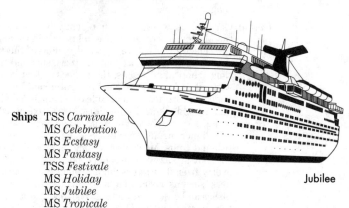

Jubilee

Ships   TSS *Carnivale*
MS *Celebration*
MS *Ecstasy*
MS *Fantasy*
TSS *Festivale*
MS *Holiday*
MS *Jubilee*
MS *Tropicale*

Evaluation   For better or worse, Carnival is the standard by which all lower-priced cruise lines are measured. Advertising hype aside, not even its critics can deny that the line delivers all it promises: Activities and entertainment are nonstop, food is plentiful, and cabins are spacious and comfortable. Though there's nothing exotic about it, and it has none of the gentility or grace of some other lines, brash and sometimes crass Carnival does throw a great party. Passengers are young, or at least young at heart (though those under 18 must be accompanied by an adult 21 or older, and infants under four months are not allowed). More singles cruise on Carnival than on any other line. Sure to contribute to the carefree atmosphere is the line's recent adoption of a "Sail and Sign" card allowing passengers to go about cashless, charging drinks and other purchases to their cabin.

In October 1993, Carnival introduced a subsidiary cruise line, FiestaMarina Cruises, geared specifically toward the Latin American market. For now, its only ship is the *Carnivale*, which offers a variety of cruises out of San Juan and La Guaira, Venezuela—the port of Caracas.

Carnival pioneered the fly/cruise program, which offers free or greatly reduced airfares from major cities to Miami or Los Angeles, though not for lower-fare cabins on three- and four-cruises—be sure to check when booking. Carnival also offers

Chart Symbols. *The following symbols are used in the cabin charts that accompany each ship's evaluation.* **D:** *Double bed;* **K:** *King-size bed;* **Q:** *Queen-size bed;* **T:** *Twin bed;* **U/L:** *Upper and lower berths;* ●: *All cabins have this facility;* ○: *No cabins have this facility;* ◐: *Some cabins have this facility*

a variety of packages combining a cruise with a stay at Walt Disney World.

Activities   Carnival vessels offer every activity that a cruise ship could have, including beer-drinking contests, greased-pole pillow fights, bingo, masquerade parties, pool games, water-balloon tosses, and trivia contests. No one can do it all, but many passengers try.

Dining   Carnival has worked hard in recent years to shed its image as the McDonald's of the cruise industry, and though in the past the selection gravitated toward middle-of-the-road Italian-American fare, such as pastas, pizzas, surf-and-turf combinations, chops, and roasts, the majority of current dishes are seafood and poultry served in lighter and healthier sauces. Vegetarian dishes are available on all lunch and dinner menus, and the odd ethnic dish—fajitas, blackened swordfish—is featured, too. All ships have quiche-and-salad bars. Kids' lunch and dinner menus offer basics like raviolis, hamburgers, and fish-and-chips. Meals are nothing less than feasts, with oversize but attractively arranged portions, noisy conversation, overly friendly waiters, and strolling musicians. Theme dinners, such as French night or Spanish night, feature special dishes and costumed waiters. The food quality is average, but the quantity and hoopla associated with its presentation make it seem better than it is.

The dining room has two seatings per meal, at 7 and 9:30, tables are assigned, though you may ask to be placed at a table of your peers, or with families traveling with children. Requests for special diets should be made two weeks in advance. Kosher food is not available.

Breakfast and lunch buffets are also served on the Lido, as are mid-morning snacks and afternoon tea. Coffee is on 24 hours a day; specialty coffees are available (at extra cost) on the new ships, *Celebration, Ecstasy, Fantasy, Holiday,* and *Jubilee.* Every night there's a midnight buffet; some ships even offer a still- later buffet for those who party into the wee hours. All ships feature 24-hour room service from a limited menu. Two formal evenings are held on cruises of four days or longer, one on three-day cruises.

Entertainment   It would be nearly impossible to be bored on a Carnival cruise. The action begins just after sunrise and continues well into the night. Movies run nonstop from morning until past midnight, and disco music begins throbbing by mid-afternoon. At any given time you can choose from an abundance of contests, parties, classes, games, bar and lounge entertainers, and bands.

Carnival apportions a significant part of its operating budget to entertainment, so it attracts better-than-average musicians, magicians, dancers, comedians, jugglers, and other specialty acts. On the larger ships it's not unusual to have a country-and-western duo, a full-size dance band, a rock 'n' roll group, a '40s swing band, a song stylist, a cocktail pianist, *and* a classical-music quartet, all performing simultaneously—in addition to the offerings from the disco and the teenage dance club. Even the smaller Carnival ships have more entertainment options than most cruise lines' largest.

Carnival's casinos are the largest afloat, and heavy emphasis is placed on gambling. The line also owns a casino/resort at

Cable Beach, which is featured in its Nassau shore excursions. The year-round children's programs include "Coketail" parties, kite-flying contests, arts and crafts, bridge tours, and bingo. Baby-sitting is available in the playroom for a nominal charge. The *Ecstasy* and *Fantasy* have teen clubs with video games and music.

Service and Tipping The pressure to tip on a Carnival cruise is palpable. You may be forced to endure the life story of your waiter or steward, complete with tales of poverty (and the threat of dismissal they're under, unless they receive the highest rating on the review sheets passengers fill out). If you tip well, however, you can be assured of snappy service. Tip the room steward and the waiter $3 each per passenger per diem, the busboy $1.50. Bar waiters, bellboys, deck stewards, and room-service waiters expect to be tipped at the time of service; 15% is customary. Tip the maître d' and the head waiter at your own discretion and whenever you request a special service, such as a change in your table assignment.

For More Information Carnival Cruise Lines (Carnival Pl., 3655 NW 87 Ave., Miami, FL 33178, tel. 800/327-7373). 205-599-2600

TSS Carnivale

Specifications

Type of ship: Mainstream	*Passengers:* 950
Type of cruise: Specialty	*Crew:* 550 (international)
Size: Medium (27,250 tons)	*Officers:* Italian
Number of cabins: 482	*Passenger/crew ratio:* 1.7 to 1
Outside cabins: 45%	*Year built:* 1956

Itinerary Year-round, three-, four-, and seven-day loops out of both La Guaira (Venezuela) and San Juan call at St. Thomas/St. John, either San Juan or Caracas/La Guaira (Venezuela), and Santo Domingo (Dominican Republic).

Port tax: $69 per passenger.

Overview Now run by Carnival's Latin American subsidiary, FiestaMarina Cruises, the *Carnivale* offers food, activities, and entertainment with Latin appeal. All onboard communication is in Spanish; cuisine is heavily Cuban, Mexican, South American, and Spanish; and a salsa dance club offers music and fun until dawn.

The *Carnivale*, built in 1956 as the ocean liner *Empress of Britain*, was purchased in 1976 by Carnival to join its sister ship, the *Mardi Gras*, which is now stationed in Europe. Despite a $10 million refurbishment in 1991, the *Carnivale*, which is the oldest ship in the line, retains much of its traditional appearance. Instead of the ubiquitous steel, fabric, and plastic found in most modern ships, here you'll find interiors enriched by wood paneling, columns, and trim. The *Carnivale* is decorated in the art deco style. Perhaps the two most popular gathering spots are the ornate, oversize casino and the three swimming pools and wading pool on the Sun and Sports Deck.

Cabins and Rates

	Beds	Phone	TV	Sitting Area	Fridge	Tub	Per Diem
Veranda Suite	T	○	○	●	○	●	$274–$297
Outside	D, T	○	○	○	○	◐	$164–$262
Inside	D, T, or U/L	○	○	○	○	◐	$144–$242

Cabins are larger than average, especially in the upper categories; some cabins even have queen- and king-size beds. There are more inside cabins than on other Carnival vessels. Bathrooms are tiny.

Outlet voltage: 110 AC.

Single supplement: 150%–200% of double-occupancy rate. Carnival can match up to four same-sex adults in a cabin at $275 each (three-day), $395 each (four-day), or $650 (seven-day).

Discounts: A third or fourth passenger in a cabin pays $66 per diem. You get a discount of up to $1,000 per cabin for early booking and up to $250 for arranging your own airfare.

Sports and Fitness   **Health club:** Exercise equipment, sauna, indoor pool, facial- and body-treatment center.

Other sports: Exercise classes, shuffleboard, table tennis, trap-shooting, indoor pool, two outdoor pools.

Facilities   **Public rooms:** Five bars, four entertainment lounges, casino, cinema, disco, Lido, tapas bar, library.

Shops: Boutique and gift shop, drugstore, beauty salon/barber.

Health care: Doctor and nurse on call.

Child care: Playroom, supervised youth programs, baby-sitting arranged privately with crew member.

Services: Full-service laundry, ironing room, photographer.

Other: Safe-deposit boxes, electrical converters.

Access for the Disabled   None.

MS Celebration and MS Jubilee

Specifications   *Type of ship:* Mainstream
Type of cruise: Party
Size: Large (48,000 tons)
Number of cabins: 743
Outside cabins: 61%

Passengers: 1,486
Crew: 670 (international)
Officers: Italian
Passenger/crew ratio: 2.2 to 1
Year built: 1987/1986

Itinerary
Celebration   **Year-round:** Seven-day loops leave Miami Saturdays, calling at San Juan, St. Thomas/St. John, and St. Maarten/St. Martin.

Port tax: $69 per passenger.

Jubilee   **Year-round:** Seven-day loops leave Los Angeles Sundays, calling at Puerto Vallarta, Cabo San Lucas (if tidal conditions favorable), and Mazatlán.

Port tax: $69 per passenger.

Overview Showy, brassy art, brightly colored walls, neon lights, spectacularly lighted ceilings and floors—when it comes to design and decor, there is nothing subtle about these vessels. Just about every decorative material imaginable—wrought iron, stained glass, wood paneling, padded leather, Plexiglas—has been used, to startling effect. Scattered throughout the two ships are a trolley car, a Wizard of Oz–theme disco, a '20s Speakeasy Café, and other imaginative touches. The result is overwhelming and is guaranteed to keep your adrenaline flowing from the moment you get up until you collapse into bed. Both ships have an arcade of lounges and bars, each with its own motif, several dance floors, and a number of small nooks. The large bars are awfully rowdy. The main entertainment lounges are spacious steel-and-marble extravaganzas, as flashy and tacky as anything aglow in Las Vegas. Discos on both ships have a futuristic, sci-fi look.

Cabins and Rates

	Beds	Phone	TV	Sitting Area	Fridge	Tub	Per Diem
Veranda Suite	T/K	●	●	●	●	●	$332–$354
Outside Twin/King	T/K	●	●	○	●	○	$254–$275
Outside Upper/Lower	U/L	●	●	○	●	○	$194–$215
Inside Twin/King	T/K	●	●	○	●	○	$207–$267
Inside Upper/Lower	U/L	●	●	○	●	○	$164–$207

Cabins are of similar size, shape, and appearance. The Veranda Suite, however, has a whirlpool and a veranda. Closed-circuit TV plays films all day and most of the night.

Outlet voltage: 110 AC.

Single supplement: 150%–200% of double-occupancy rate. Carnival can match up to four same-sex adults in a cabin for $650 each.

Discounts: A third or fourth passenger in a cabin pays $57 per diem. You get a discount of up to $1,000 for booking early, and up to $250 for arranging your own airfare.

Sports and Fitness **Health club:** Gym with exercise equipment; men's and women's spas with whirlpools, saunas, facial- and body-treatment center.

Walking/jogging: Unobstructed circuit on Lido Deck.

Other sports: Aerobics classes, shuffleboard, table tennis, trapshooting, two pools, children's wading pool.

Facilities **Public rooms:** Seven bars, six entertainment lounges, card area, casino, disco, indoor Lido cafeteria, library, piano bar, specialty coffee café, video-game room.

Shops: Gift shops, beauty salon/barber.

Health care: Doctor and nurse on call.

Child care: Playroom, youth programs run by counselors, baby-sitting arranged privately with crew member.

Services: Full-service laundry, laundromat, photographer.

Access for the Disabled None.

MS Ecstasy and MS Fantasy

Specifications
Type of ship: Mainstream
Type of cruise: Party
Size: Megaship (70,367 tons)
Number of cabins: 1,020/1,022
Outside cabins: 60.7%

Passengers: 2,040/2,044
Crew: 920 (international)
Officers: Italian
Passenger/crew ratio: 2.2 to 1
Year built: 1990/1991

Itinerary
Fantasy **Year-round:** From Port Canaveral (FL), three-day loops leave Thursdays for Nassau, four-day loops leave Sundays for Nassau and Freeport/Lucaya.

Port tax: $49 per passenger.

Ecstasy **Year-round:** From Miami, three-day loops leave Fridays for Nassau, four-day loops leave Mondays for Nassau and Freeport/Lucaya.

Port tax: $49 per passenger.

Overview These two $225-million ships, the newest in the Carnival fleet, appeal to a younger set, the kind of crowd that loves Atlantic City and Las Vegas. They are identical in all but decor, though on both, marble, brass, mirrors, and electric lights throughout heighten Carnival's now-notorious hyperactivity. In addition to Olympic-size pools, the ships also have unique banked and padded jogging tracks with a special surface; their casinos and fitness centers are the largest afloat.

Big, bright, bold, and brassy, the *Fantasy* lives up to its name, resembling a series of fantastic Hollywood sets rather than a cruise ship. Fifteen miles of bright neon tubing snake through the ship. The public rooms are lavishly decorated in elaborate motifs; the Cats Lounge, for example, was inspired by the famous musical, and Cleopatra's Bar re-creates the interior of an Egyptian tomb. The six-story Grand Spectrum atrium, with its glass-enclosed elevators, amazing skylight, white-marble staircase, and brilliant neon trim, is straight out of science fiction.

The *Ecstasy* is less futuristic and more elegant, with a cityscape theme. The centerpiece is the seven-deck-high Grand Atrium and City Lights Boulevard, evoking a city street scene. The other public rooms capture a variety of city moods: The Rolls Royce Café is built around an antique Rolls, the Metropolis Bar is home to a skyscraperlike neon sculpture, and the entrance to the Chinatown lounge is guarded by twin lion-head Foo dog sculptures reminiscent of ancient China.

Cabins and Rates

	Beds	Phone	TV	Sitting Area	Fridge	Tub	Per Diem
Veranda Suite	T/K	●	●	●	●	●	$309–$334
Demi Suite	Q	●	●	●	●	○	$284–$309
Outside	T/K	●	●	○	○	○	$237–$279

Inside	T/K or U/L	●	●	○	○	○	$149– $267

Cabins are quite spacious, with closed-circuit TV and private safes. Veranda Suites and Demi Suites have private verandas, wet bars, and VCRs. Veranda Suites have tubs with whirlpool jets. Some outside cabins on the Veranda Deck have partially obstructed views.

Outlet voltage: 110 AC.

Single supplement: 150%–200% of double-occupancy rate. Carnival can match up to four same-sex adults in a cabin for $275 (three-day cruises) or $395 (four-day cruises) each.

Discounts: A third or fourth passenger in a cabin pays $66 per diem (three-day) or $49 per diem (four-day). You get a discount of up to $400 for early booking and up to $100 for arranging your own airfare.

Sports and Fitness **Health club:** Gym, aerobics room, massage room, women's and men's locker rooms with steam rooms and saunas, fitness machines, two whirlpools, facial and body treatments.

Walking/jogging: Banked jogging track on Sun Deck (11 laps=1 mile).

Other sports: Aerobics classes, shuffleboard, table tennis, trapshooting, two outdoor pools (one with slide), children's wading pool, four outdoor whirlpools.

Facilities **Public rooms:** Six bars, four entertainment lounges, card room, casino, disco, indoor Lido bar/grill, outdoor snack bar, library, specialty coffee café (extra charge).

Shops: Boutiques, drugstore, beauty salon/barber.

Health care: Doctor and nurse on call.

Child care: Playroom, teen center (with video games), youth programs run by counselors, baby-sitting arranged privately with crew member.

Services: Full-service laundry, laundromat, photographer.

Access for the Disabled None.

TSS Festivale

Specifications *Type of ship:* Mainstream
Type of cruise: Party
Size: Large (38,275 tons)
Number of cabins: 580
Outside cabins: 47%

Passengers: 1,146
Crew: 580 (international)
Officers: Italian
Passenger/crew ratio: 1.9 to 1
Year built: 1961

Itinerary **Year-round:** Seven-day loops leave San Juan Sundays, calling at St. Thomas/St. John, St. Maarten/St. Martin, Barbados, and Martinique.

Port tax: $69 per passenger.

Overview Carnival purchased this vessel, built in 1961 as the *Transvaal Castle*, in 1978 and refurbished it in 1986. Although the ship now conforms to Carnival's cruising specifications, its age and original design are still apparent. Many of the cabins are roomy, but original fixtures are often chipped, cracked, or corroded.

This ship does not offer the glitz and glitter some Carnival passengers desire, but its classic lines, winged bridge, and single smokestack make it one of the best-looking ships in the fleet. The public areas, too, retain much of the original wood paneling and have polished brass railings and doors. The decor is conservative by Carnival standards, with muted colors, classic etched glass, and a fabulous art deco steel stairway. The Tradewinds and Copa Cabana lounges are reminiscent of 1930s film sets. The Gaslight Café looks like a mishmash of every B movie ever made, mixing teak paneling with a mirrored ceiling, petite pink tables, and overstuffed purple chairs.

Cabins and Rates

	Beds	Phone	TV	Sitting Area	Fridge	Tub	Per Diem
Veranda Suite	T	○	○	●	○	●	$332–$354
Demi Suite	T	○	○	○	○	◑	$289–$311
Outside Cabin	Q, T or U/L	○	○	○	○	●	$185–$297
Inside Cabin	Q, T or U/L	○	○	○	○	○	$164–$261

Recalling the ship's heyday as an ocean liner, some suites have wooden headboards, full-length mirrors, and separate sitting rooms. Demi Suite V55 does not have a bathtub. Some outside cabins on the Veranda Deck have partially obstructed views.

Outlet voltage: 110 AC.

Single supplement: 150%–200% of double-occupancy rate. Carnival can match up to four same-sex adults in a cabin for $650 each.

Discounts: A third or fourth passenger in a cabin pays $57 per diem. You get a discount of up to $1,000 for booking early and up to $250 for arranging your own airfare.

Sports and Fitness **Health club:** Exercise equipment, sauna, massage room, facial- and body-treatment center.

Walking/jogging: Walking circuit (7.5 laps=1 mile).

Other sports: Aerobics classes, shuffleboard, table tennis, trapshooting, two pools, wading pool.

Facilities **Public rooms:** Five bars, four entertainment lounges, casino, cinema, disco, library, Lido, video games.

Shops: Boutique, gift shop, liquor/sundries shop, beauty salon/barber.

Health care: Doctor and nurse on call.

Child care: Playroom, play deck, youth programs with counselors, baby-sitting arranged privately with crew member.

Services: Full-service laundry, photographer.

Other: Safe-deposit boxes.

Access for the Disabled None.

MS Holiday

Specifications *Type of ship:* Mainstream *Passengers:* 1,452
Type of cruise: Party *Crew:* 660 (international)
Size: Large (46,052 tons) *Officers:* Italian
Number of cabins: 726 *Passenger/crew ratio:* 2.2 to 1
Outside cabins: 61.5% *Year built:* 1985

Itinerary **Year-round:** Seven-day loops leave Miami Saturdays, calling at Cozumel/Playa del Carmen (Mexico), Grand Cayman, and Ocho Rios (Jamaica).

Port tax: $69 per passenger.

Overview One of the first generation of "superliners" built for Carnival, the *Holiday* is a bulky, ungainly ship from the outside. Inside, however, it's a spacious, fantasy-filled palace—not unlike a Disney theme park. A bar called The Bus Stop has red-top luncheonette stools, traffic signs, and an actual red-and-white bus from the 1930s. Another bar, Carnegie's, has the luxurious look of a private club, with overstuffed leather chairs and sofas, and glass-door library shelves. Rick's American Café is straight from *Casablanca.* An unusual design feature is the extra-wide, enclosed walkway that runs along the port side of the Promenade Deck. The teak passageway called Broadway connects the casino and all the bars and lounges on the deck. The main entertainment lounge, the Americana, is a six-level, curved room that accommodates more than 900 passengers. The Gaming Club Casino has more than 100 slot machines and 250 seats.

Cabins and Rates

	Beds	Phone	TV	Sitting Area	Fridge	Tub	Per Diem
Veranda Suite	T/K	●	●	●	●	●	$332–$354
Outside Twin/King	T/K	●	●	○	○	○	$231–$275
Outside Upper/Lower	U/L	●	●	○	○	○	$185–$215
Inside Twin/King	T/K	●	●	○	○	○	$207–$261
Inside Upper/Lower	U/L	●	●	○	○	○	$164–$215

Cabins are slightly larger than average. The Veranda Suites have a sitting room, private veranda, and whirlpool. All cabins have wall safes.

Outlet voltage: 110 AC.

Single supplement: 150%–200% of double-occupancy rate. Carnival can match up to four same-sex adults in a cabin for $650 each.

Discounts: A third or fourth passenger in a cabin pays $57 per diem. You get a discount of up to $1,000 for booking early and up to $250 for arranging your own airfare.

Sports and Fitness   **Health club:** Exercise equipment, spas with whirlpools, sauna, massage room, facial- and body-treatment center.

Walking/jogging: Unobstructed fitness-walk circuit on Lido Deck.

Other sports: Aerobics, golf driving, shuffleboard, table tennis, trapshooting, two outdoor pools, wading pool.

Facilities   **Public rooms:** Seven bars, four entertainment lounges, casino, disco, library, enclosed Lido cafeteria, piano bar, specialty- coffee café (extra charge), video-game room.

Shops: Boutique, gift shop, beauty salon/barber.

Health care: Doctor and nurse on call.

Child care: Playroom, youth programs run by counselors, baby-sitting arranged privately with crew member.

Services: Full-service laundry, laundromat, photographer.

Access for the Disabled   None.

MS Tropicale

Specifications   *Type of ship:* Mainstream   *Passengers:* 1,022
Type of cruise: Party   *Crew:* 550 (international)
Size: Large (36,674 tons)   *Officers:* Italian
Number of cabins: 511   *Passenger/crew ratio:* 1.9 to 1
Outside cabins: 63%   *Year built:* 1981

Itinerary   **Year-round:** Seven-day loops leave San Juan Saturdays, calling at St. Thomas/St. John, Guadeloupe, Grenada, Caracas/La Guaira, and Aruba.

Port tax: $69 per passenger.

Overview   The *Tropicale* is the model for most new cruise ships. Passenger polls encouraged Carnival to build a large ship filled with open spaces; a good choice of bars, lounges, and play arenas; and a spectacular swimming pool. However, the *Tropicale* has been criticized for its impersonal staff and disorganization— those used to the red carpet may be disappointed.

Although its design has been imitated many times since it was launched, the *Tropicale* is still recognizable by its clean lines, sloping superstructure, oversize portholes, and the raked, single smokestack near the stern. The interior is ultramodern and utilizes the entire spectrum of colors. The Exta-Z Disco's dance floor, for instance, is alive with red and yellow lights, the elaborate ceiling with blue, green, and red neon lights. Indirect lighting sets a more appetizing mood in the Riviera Restaurant, which, with its rattan furniture, resembles a tropical grand hotel.

Cabins and Rates

	Beds	Phone	TV	Sitting Area	Fridge	Tub	Per Diem
Veranda Suite	T/K	●	●	●	●	●	$332–$354
Outside Twin/King	T/K	●	●	○	○	○	$231–$275

Outside Upper/Lower	U/L	●	●	○	○	○	$185–$207
Inside Twin/King	T/K	●	●	○	○	○	$207–$261
Inside Upper/Lower	U/L	●	●	○	○	○	$164–$215

Cabins are of similar size and appearance, comfortable and larger than average; the majority have twin beds that can be made into a king. Veranda Suites have balconies. Most outside cabins have large square windows rather than portholes.

Outlet voltage: 110 AC.

Single supplement: 150%–200% of double-occupancy rate. Carnival can match up to four same-sex adults in a cabin for $650 each.

Discounts: A third or fourth passenger in a cabin pays $57 per diem. You get a discount of up to $1,000 for booking early and up to $250 for arranging your own airfare.

Sports and Fitness **Health club:** Exercise equipment, men's and women's saunas and massage rooms, facial- and body-treatment center.

Walking/jogging: Small, unobstructed circuit on Sports Deck.

Other sports: Aerobics classes, shuffleboard, table tennis, trap-shooting, two pools, wading pool.

Facilities **Public rooms:** Five bars, four entertainment lounges, card room, casino, disco, library, enclosed Lido, video-game room.

Shops: Gift shops, beauty salon/barber.

Health care: Doctor and nurse on call.

Child care: Playroom, youth programs run by counselors, baby-sitting arranged privately with crew member.

Services: Full-service laundry, laundromat, photographer.

Other: Safe-deposit boxes.

Access for the Disabled None.

Celebrity Cruises

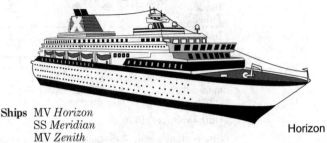

Horizon

Ships MV *Horizon*
SS *Meridian*
MV *Zenith*

Evaluation Introduced in 1990, Chandris's Celebrity Cruises provides a more elegant—and expensive—alternative to its sister line, Fantasy Cruises, including roomier accommodations, slightly more personalized service, and more amenities. All three ships feature similar tasteful and attractive furnishings, fixtures, and artwork, but ambience and level of service differ. The *Horizon* and *Zenith* are new ships, with modern amenities and a practical design. The *Meridian* is a vintage transatlantic liner that was stretched and redesigned in 1990 during a $55-million renovation. Celebrity delivers above-average cuisine, friendly and enthusiastic service, and generally good value—plus special programs for children during holiday sailings. The median age is about 50 on Celebrity cruises, the less expensive spring and fall repositioning cruises, offered on the *Horizon* and the *Meridian*, usually attract a younger crowd.

Activities Though not party ships, Celebrity packs plenty of fun into its cruises. Activities include pool and card games, shuffleboard, snorkeling instruction, "horse racing," skeet shooting, and golf putting. Passengers are not pressured, and many choose to read or relax on their own in a lounge chair.

Dining Celebrity has risen nicely above typical cruise cuisine by hiring Chef Michel Roux, proprietor of two of Britain's finest restaurants, as a consultant. Roux's experience in creating and cooking for large numbers of discriminating diners has been put to wonderful use. Food is truly outstanding, both familiar and exotic dishes have been customized to appeal to the mellow palate of American cruisers. To keep things fresh, the menu rotates constantly. At least one "lean and light" entrée is offered at every meal, and special diets, such as kosher or salt-free, can be catered to when booked in advance or with the maître d' on the day of sailing.

Outside the dining rooms, options include an enormous café on the Marina Deck, which is open for breakfast, lunch, and afternoon tea. Dinner is at two assigned seatings, at 6:15 and 8:30.

Chart Symbols. *The following symbols are used in the cabin charts that accompany each ship's evaluation.* **D:** *Double bed;* **K:** *King-size bed;* **Q:** *Queen-size bed;* **T:** *Twin bed;* **U/L:** *Upper and lower berths;* ●: *All cabins have this facility;* ○: *No cabins have this facility;* ◑: *Some cabins have this facility*

Room service is available 24 hours. Two formal evenings are held each cruise. Passengers can sign for drinks.

Entertainment All three ships present lavish, if predictable, variety shows, enlivened by the occasional surprise guest (e.g., performers from a Russian circus). Smaller lounges offer low-key jazz and big-band music. Kareoke parties are popular, and the Marina Disco rocks until 3 AM.

Service and Tipping Service is friendly and first class—rapid and accurate in the dining room, slower and uneven in the bars. Waiters, stewards, and bartenders are enthusiastic, take pride in their work, and try to please—though not all have full command of English. Tip your room steward and your waiter $3 each per passenger per diem, the busboy and the assistant steward $1.50 each; the maître d' gets $5 per passenger per cruise. Bar stewards should be tipped 15% of the bill at the time of service.

For More Information Celebrity Cruises (5200 Blue Lagoon Dr., Miami, FL 33126, tel. 800/437–3111).

MV Horizon and MV Zenith

Specifications *Type of ship:* Upscale mainstream   *Passengers:* 1,354/1,374
Type of cruise: Traditional (international)   Crew: 642/657
Officers: Greek
Size: Large (46,811/47,811 tons)   Passenger/crew ratio: 2.1 to 1
Number of cabins: 677/687   *Year built:* 1990/1992
Outside cabins: 84%

Itinerary
Horizon **Early Fall:** Seven-night cruises leave New York Saturdays for Bermuda, with two nights each at Hamilton and St. George's. **Late Fall–Winter:** Seven-night loops leave San Juan Saturdays, calling at Martinique, Barbados, St. Lucia, Antigua, and St. Thomas/St. John. **Spring–Summer:** Same as Fall.

Port tax: $87 (Bermuda) or $67 (Caribbean) per passenger.

Zenith **Year-round:** Seven-day western and eastern Caribbean loops leave Fort Lauderdale alternate Saturdays. Eastern loops call at San Juan, St. Thomas/St. John, St. Maarten/St. Martin, and Nassau; Western loops, at Cozumel/Playa del Carmen (Mexico), Grand Cayman, Montego Bay (Jamaica), and Key West.

Port tax: $67 per passenger.

Overview As with many huge modern cruise ships, the exterior looks ungainly—here primarily because of the long rows of large windows and portholes, the squared-off stern, and the boxy smokestack (which, like all Fantasy and Celebrity ships, is marked with a large, distinctive *X*). However, the interior is surprisingly gracious, airy, and comfortable. Because there is no central architectural focus (such as an atrium), the ships seem more intimate than other 1,300-passenger ships. The design makes the most of natural light through strategically placed oversize windows. The nine passenger decks sport several bars, entertainment lounges, and ample deck space. Wide corridors, broad staircases, seven elevators, and well-placed signs make it easy to get around. Decor is contemporary and attractive, the artwork pleasant rather than memorable. The *Zenith* is has a slightly different lay-out than its sister ship: There are two fewer bars—though others have been enlarged, more suites, a larger health club, more deck space, and a meeting room.

Cabins and Rates

	Beds*	Phone	TV	Sitting Area	Fridge	Tub	Per Diem
Deluxe Suites	D	●	●	●	○	●	$367–$439
Deluxe Cabins	D or T/K	●	●	●	○	○	$296–$310
Outside	D or T/K	●	●	○	○	○	$240–$293
Inside	D or T/K	●	●	○	○	○	$171–$239

* Twins convert to king-size beds on only the Zenith.

The cabins are modern and quite roomy. Suites come with butler service. A number of upper-priced cabins have tubs with whirlpool jets. The view from many outside cabins on the Bermuda Deck is partially obstructed by lifeboats.

Outlet voltage: 110/220 AC.

Single supplement: 150%–200% of double-occupancy rate.

Discounts: A third or fourth passenger in a cabin pays $121. Children 2–12 traveling with two full-paying adults pay $56 (Bermuda) or $99 (Caribbean) per diem. Children under 2 travel free. Airfare is not included in the rates.

Sports and Fitness **Health club:** Bright, sunny upper-deck spa with sauna, massage, weight machines, stationary bicycles, rowing machine, treadmill, separate mirrored aerobics area, massage, facial/body treatments.

Walking/jogging: Marina Deck (5 laps=1 mile).

Other sports: Exercise classes, putting green, shuffleboard, snorkeling, trapshooting, ping-pong, two pools, three whirlpools.

Facilities **Public rooms:** Eight bars (*Horizon*) and 6 bars (*Zenith*), three showrooms, disco, teen room, casino, 2 restaurant, library/reading room, card room, video arcade.

Shops: Gift shop, boutique, perfume shop, cigarette/liquor store, photo shop.

Health care: Hospital staffed by doctor and nurse, limited dispensary for prescriptions.

Child care: Playroom, teen room on Sun Deck, preteen and teen youth programs supervised by counselors, baby-sitting arranged with crew member.

Services: Photographer, valet laundry, beauty shop/barber.

Other: Safe-deposit boxes.

Access for the Disabled Four cabins with 39½-inch doorways are wheelchair- accessible. Specially equipped public elevators are 35½" wide. Certain areas may not be wide enough for wheelchairs. The captain cannot guarantee that passengers in wheelchairs will be accommodated at every port. Disabled passengers must provide their own small collapsible wheelchairs and travel with an able-bodied passenger.

SS Meridian

Specifications *Type of ship:* Upscale mainstream   *Passengers:* 1,106
Type of cruise: Traditional   *Crew:* 580 (international)
Size: Large (30,440 tons)   *Officers:* Greek
Number of cabins: 553   *Passenger/crew ratio:* 1.7 to 1
Outside cabins: 54%   *Year built:* 1967 (rebuilt 1990)

Itinerary **Fall:** Seven-day loops leave New York (or, occasionally, Baltimore, Boston, Charleston, Philadelphia, or Fort Lauderdale) for Somerset, Bermuda. **Winter:** Out of San Juan, 10-day cruises call at Aruba, Caracas/La Guaira, Grenada, Barbados, St. Lucia, Martinique, St. Maarten/St. Martin, and St. Thomas/St. John; and 11-day cruises call at Montego Bay (Jamaica), Aruba, Caracas/La Guaira, Grenada, Barbados, Martinique, Virgin Gorda, and Tortola (British Virgin Islands), and St. Thomas/St. John. **Spring–Summer:** Same as Fall.

Port tax: $92 (Caribbean) per passenger.

Overview Originally the *Galileo*, this former transatlantic liner was stretched and totally refurbished before reemerging as the *Meridian.* It now possesses a relaxed, personable charm—it's like staying in someone's home. The beige tile that borders the pool is pretty and unpretentious, and the Zodiac Club's simple terra-cotta theme is cozy. Most of the public rooms are on the same deck, allowing easy access.

Cabins and Rates

	Beds	Phone	TV	Sitting Area	Fridge	Tub	Per Diem
Presidential Suite	T	●	●	●	○	●	$395–$410
Starlight Suite	T	●	●	●	○	●	$370–$385
Deluxe Suite	D	●	●	●	○	●	$335–$350
Deluxe Cabin	T or D	●	○	●	○	○	$275–$305
Outside	T or D	●	○	○	○	○	$235–$285
Inside	T, D, or U/L	●	○	○	○	○	$160–$247

Bathtubs in the Presidential, Starlight, and Deluxe suites have whirlpool jets. Outside cabins on the Horizon Deck have floor-to-ceiling windows. Many outside cabins on the Atlantic Deck have obstructed or partially obstructed views.

Outlet voltage: 110/220 AC.

Single supplement: 150%–200% double-occupancy rate.

Discounts: A third or fourth passenger in a cabin pays $99 (Caribbean) per diem. Children 2–12 sharing a cabin with two full-paying adults pay $35–$99 per diem. Children under 2 travel free. Airfare is not included in the rates.

Sports and Fitness **Health club:** Stationary bikes, weight machines, treadmill, rowing machines, sauna, massage, facial/body treatment.

Walking/jogging: Jogging track on Captain Deck (8 laps=1 mile).

Other sports: Exercise classes, putting green, golf driving, shuffleboard, snorkeling, trapshooting, ping-pong, pool, children's pool, three outdoor whirlpools.

Facilities **Public rooms:** Seven bars, four entertainment lounges (including main showroom), card room/library, casino, chapel/synagogue, cinema, dining room, disco, Lido, video arcade.

Shops: Boutique, perfumerie, drug store, photo shop, beauty salon/barber.

Health care: Doctor on call.

Child care: Playroom with large windows, patio, and wading pool; youth programs with counselors when needed; baby-sitting arranged privately with crew member.

Services: Photographer, valet laundry, beauty shop/barber.

Other: Safe-deposit boxes.

Access for the Disabled Two cabins have wheelchair access. Celebrity demands that passengers in wheelchairs travel with an able-bodied adult who will take full responsibility in case of emergency.

Classical Cruises

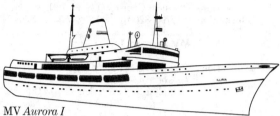

Ships MV *Aurora I*

Evaluation Classical shies away from just about everything a traditional cruise ship offers. Bingo and skeet shooting have been replaced with animated, engaging lectures and discussions, led by experts, about the extremely varied destinations. The *Aurora I*, built in 1991 in Lübeck, Germany, is intimate and luxurious; its sister, *the Aurora II*, sails outside the Western Hemisphere. Classical is the retail arm of Travel Dynamics, the tour operator that designs cruises for such special-interest groups as the American Museum of Natural History and the Smithsonian. Many of these itineraries are available to the general public.

Life on board is gracious but informal. Passengers are usually involved, well-educated, in their mid-fifties, and well-traveled, with the time and money to continue learning. Fares are higher than on mainstream ships but competitive with other adventure-cruise lines of this caliber.

Activities Shipboard activities focus on learning about the ports of call. Lectures and slide shows on the local culture, wildlife, and history are well attended, and the libraries are packed with reference works and information. Noted guest lecturers give in-depth presentations on an assortment of fascinating topics. There are no other organized activities; some passengers play cards or join in ad hoc after-dinner piano sing-alongs.

Dining Meals, featuring American and Continental cuisine, are served at a single open seating. At breakfast and lunch, you usually have a buffet option. Other food options include full breakfast, afternoon tea, and late-night snacks.

Entertainment A piano player provides evening entertainment, and there's a TV and VCR in the library, where at least one movie is aired daily. A state-of-the-art sound system pipes music through the ships. Each cabin is equipped with a TV and VCR, allowing passengers to view arrivals into each port through outdoor video cameras.

Service and Tipping Service is competent and unobtrusive, though Classical's staff won't wow you with personality or impeccable service. Tips are given anonymously and pooled among the staff (tip $10 per pas-

Chart Symbols. *The following symbols are used in the cabin charts that accompany each ship's evaluation.* **D:** *Double bed;* **K:** *King-size bed;* **Q:** *Queen-size bed;* **T:** *Twin bed;* **U/L:** *Upper and lower berths;* ●: *All cabins have this facility;* ○: *No cabins have this facility;* ◐: *Some cabins have this facility*

senger per diem); the company discourages tipping individuals.

For More Information   Classical Cruises (132 E. 70th St., New York, NY 10021, tel. 212/794–3200 or 800/252–7745 outside NY).

MV Aurora I

Specifications	*Type of ship:* Specialty	*Passengers:* 80
	Type of cruise: Cultural/ natural-history excursion	*Crew:* 55 (Greek and Filipino)
		Officers: Greek
	Size: Small (2,928 tons)	*Passenger/crew ratio:* 1.6 to 1
	Number of cabins: 44	*Year built:* 1991
	Outside cabins: 100%	

Itinerary   **Year-round:** Outside the Western Hemisphere, except in **March,** when a series of eight-day cruises are offered around Baja California, the Sea of Cortés, and the Copper Canyon (Mexico).

Port tax: Included in fare.

Overview   The small, *Aurora* features all outside staterooms, furnished in the style of a gracious private yacht. The restaurant is quite spacious, and a generously apportioned lounge beckon after dinner. The ship meets the latest environmental and safety standards as well as those of the U.S. Coast Guard and the U.S. Department of Health. Retractable fin stabilizers provide maximum comfort even in rough waters. Super-launches and Zodiacs give access to small or inaccessible ports.

Cabins and Rates

	Beds	Phone	TV	Sitting Area	Fridge	Tub	Per Diem
Outside	T	●	●	●	●	●	$250–$550

Cabins measure 250 square feet, comparable in size to suites on other small ships. They are furnished with writing desks, two picture windows, and an oversize bathroom. Single cabins have portholes and a bathroom with shower. All rooms have individual climate control and ample storage space. The Aurora Suite is twice the size of a double cabin.

Outlet voltage: 110 AC.

Single supplement: 200% of double-occupancy rate.

Discounts: Airfare is not included in rates.

Sports and Fitness   **Health club:** Computerized stationary bicycle, Stairmaster, other small fitness machines.

Walking/jogging: Unobstructed circuit on Sun Deck.

Other sports: Aerobics, pool.

Facilities   **Public rooms:** Two bars, game room, deck buffet, dining room, lecture hall, library, lounge, IBM-compatible computer, reception area.

Shops: Boutique, hair salon.

Health care: Hospital with doctor on call.

Child care: None; children under 12 discouraged.

Access for the Disabled None.

Clipper Cruise Line

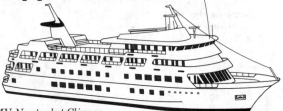

Ships MV *Nantucket Clipper*
MS *World Discoverer*   **Yorktown Clipper**
MV *Yorktown Clipper*

Evaluation Clipper Cruise Line offers two distinct styles of cruising: Clipper Classic and Clipper Adventure. On the famous *World Discoverer* adventure cruises, Zodiacs ferry passengers to remote beaches, pristine forests, small villages, and wildlife refuges; a team of naturalists and lecturers conduct seminars on board and unusual walking tours ashore.

Clipper Classic cruises, available on the *Nantucket Clipper* and the *Yorktown Clipper,* offer upscale vacations with a relaxed, country-club ambience. With fewer than 140 passengers aboard, the ships don't disrupt the lifestyles of the small islands they visit. The ships' size allows docking at marinas or at town piers, eliminating the need for tenders or taxis. Aboard ship, passengers entertain themselves, most preferring Clipper's emphasis on beachcombing over bingo and reading over roulette. Compared with other small vessels, the Clipper Classic ships are more sophisticated and service-oriented than those of American Canadian Caribbean Line but nowhere near as elegant or expensive as Cunard's *Sea Goddess*es.

Clipper Cruises subscribes to guidelines for environmentally responsible travel. There is no question that the adventure style has influenced the traditional country-club "Classic" style and vice versa. Passengers are older (typically in their mid-sixties), wealthier, and better-educated than the average cruise passenger.

Activities Apart from occasional lectures, organized activities are few. Board games and card games are popular, but reading and socializing are the main on-board activities.

Dining Clipper's cuisine is simply prepared and plainly served. Selections are quite limited and portions rather small, although passengers can always order more. Dinner, at 7:30, is served at one assigned seating. Special dietary requests should be made in writing three weeks before departure; no kosher meals are available. There are two "dressy" evenings per cruise, but for-

---

Chart Symbols. *The following symbols are used in the cabin charts that accompany each ship's evaluation.* **D:** *Double bed;* **K:** *King-size bed;* **Q:** *Queen-size bed;* **T:** *Twin bed;* **U/L:** *Upper and lower berths;* ●: *All cabins have this facility;* ○: *No cabins have this facility;* ◐: *Some cabins have this facility*

mal attire is not necessary. An alternate Continental breakfast is served in the Observation Lounge, and fresh chocolate-chip cookies are available in the afternoon. Coffee and tea can be had at any time, but there is no room service.

Entertainment Though local entertainers sometimes perform on board and movies may be shown, evenings are low-key; socializing in the lounge over drinks is about as rowdy as this crowd usually gets. Many passengers venture ashore to enjoy the nightlife or take evening strolls.

Service and Tipping Though small, the staff is young, energetic, and capable, working nicely together to provide good service without lobbying for tips. On the last evening passengers are asked to leave tips in an envelope on the purser's desk (tip $8 per passenger per diem); these are pooled and distributed.

For More Information Clipper Cruise Line (7711 Bonhomme Ave., St. Louis, MO 63105, tel. 800/325–0010).

MV Nantucket Clipper and MV Yorktown Clipper

Specifications *Type of ship:* Upscale, yachtlike
Type of cruise: Excursion/senior
Size: Very small (99.5 tons)
Number of cabins: 51/69
Outside cabins: 100%

Passengers: 102/138
Crew: 28/37 (American)
Officers: American
Passenger/crew ratio: 3.6 to 1
Year built: 1984/1988

Itinerary *Nantucket Clipper* **Fall:** A variety of seven- to 14-day cruises sail along the eastern seaboard, calling at Boston, Gloucester (MA), Rockport (ME), Nantucket, Newport (RI), New York City, Philadelphia, Baltimore, Annapolis, Washington (DC), Alexandria and Norfolk (VA), Beaufort and Wilmington (NC), Charleston, Savannah, St. Simons Island (GA), and Jacksonville. Northeastern Canada cruises call at Charlottetown (Prince Edward Island), Caraquet (New Brunswick), Percé (Québec), along the Saguenay Fjord, Québec City, Montréal, Prescott (Ontario), the Thousand Islands, and Rochester. **Winter:** Eight-day loops leave St. Thomas, calling at various Virgin Islands, including St. John, Tortola, Norman Island, Virgin Gorda, Soper's Hole, and Jost Van Dyke. **Spring:** A variety of seven- to 14-day cruises sail along the eastern seaboard (same as Fall). Also, a variety of cruises sail along the Gulf of Mexico, leaving Miami and calling at the Florida ports of Key West, Dry Tortugas, Sanibel Island, Captiva Island, Tampa, Panama City, and Pensacola, plus Mobile, Biloxi, and New Orleans. **Summer:** Same as Fall.

Port tax: $65–$90 per passenger.

Yorktown Clipper **Fall:** Various cruises sail throughout the Pacific Northwest, calling in British Columbia and along the Columbia River. Northern California cruises call at Redwood City, Sausalito, Stockton, Sacramento, and Napa Valley. Mexican Riviera cruises call at Acapulco, Zihuatanejo/Ixtapa, Puerto Vallarta, the San Blas Islands, Mazatlán, Isla San Francisco, Isla San José (Panama), Isla Santa Catalina, Los Islotes, Isla Espiritu Santo, Cabo San Lucas, and San Diego. Panama Canal Transits call at the Panamanian ports of Panama City, Colón, Portobelo, the San Blas Islands, Isla Cebaco, Marenco, Manuel Antonio Park, and Punta Leonara, and at Puerto Caldera and San José in Costa Rica. **Winter:** Various Caribbean cruises call at An-

tigua, Anguilla, Saba, St. Maarten/St. Martin, St. Kitts, Iles
des Saintes (Guadeloupe), Dominica, St. Lucia, Bequia and
Union Island (Grenadines), and Grenada; or Trinidad, Ciudad
Guayana/Angel Falls and along the Orinoco River (Venezuela),
Tobago, Isla Chimana Grande, Bonaire, and Curaçao. **Spring:**
Same as Fall. **Summer:** Northern California and Pacific North-
west cruises (same as in Fall). Also, various Alaska cruises call
at Juneau, along the Tracy Arm Fjord, Sawyer Glacier, at The
Brothers, Baranof Island, Sitka, Glacier Bay National Park,
Haines, and Skagway.

Port taxes: $40–$95 per passenger.

Overview The *Clippers* look more like yachts than cruise ships. The
trademark design, dominated by a large bridge and large picture windows that ensure bright interior public spaces, is sleek
and attractive. There are only a few public rooms, and deck
space is limited. The glass-walled Observation Lounge is small
enough to foster conversation that can be heard anywhere in
the room, so it's usually quite friendly. The ships' coziness can
engender camaraderie or claustrophobia, but generally passengers are made to feel like invited guests. A knowledgeable
crew offers advice as to what and what not to see in port. And
day or night, you're usually welcome to stop by the bridge for
a cup of coffee with the captain and crew.

Cabins and Rates

	Beds	Phone	TV	Sitting Area	Fridge	Tub	Per Diem
Category 5	T	○	○	○	○	○	$313–$360
Category 4	T	○	○	○	○	○	$275–$323
Category 3	T	○	○	○	○	○	$250–$293
Category 2	T	○	○	○	○	○	$217–$267
Category 1	T	○	○	○	○	○	$183–$297

Cabins are all small. How the designers stuffed two beds, a
dresser, a desk, a bathroom, and a closet into such a tiny space
is a great mystery. Category 2 cabins open onto the public
promenade.

Outlet voltage: 110 AC.

Single supplement: 108%–170% of double-occupancy rate.

Discounts: A third passenger in a cabin pays $800–$2,050 per
cruise, depending upon the itinerary. Airfare is not included in
the rates.

Sports and Fitness **Walking/jogging:** Unobstructed circuit on Promenade Deck.

Other sports: Snorkeling equipment and instruction; no organized deck sports or facilities.

Facilities **Public rooms:** Small lounge serves as living room, bar, card
room, and entertainment center; TVs in dining room and
lounge.

Shops: None, but souvenir items available.

Health care: None, but the ship seldom strays far from land.

Access for the Disabled None.

MS World Discoverer

Specifications

Type of ship: Adventure
Type of cruise: Cultural
Size: Very small (3,153 tons)
Number of cabins: 71
Outside cabins: 100%

Passengers: 138
Crew: 75 (international)
Officers: West German
Passenger/crew ratio: 1.8 to 1
Year built: 1974

Itinerary **Fall:** Alaska Inside Passage cruises leave Kodiak, calling at Katmai Peninsula, Geographic Harbor, Semidi Islands, Shumagin Islands, Dutch Harbor, Aleutian Islands, Pribilof Islands, St. Matthew Island, St. Lawrence Island, Provideniye, Novoye Chaplino, Russia Far East, Arakamchechen Archipelago, and Nome. Consecutive cruises run south along the west coast of the United States to the Gulf of California, the coast of Costa Rica, the Panama Canal, and western South America. **Winter:** Cruises to Antarctica and through the Chilean Fjords call at a variety of small islands and research stations. **Spring–Summer:** Same as Fall. Cruises also call throughout the Aleutian Islands and Siberia.

Port tax: $85–$90 per passenger; no port tax on Antarctica cruises.

Overview The *World Discoverer* conforms to exacting standards for adventure cruises, including the useful feature of a hardened hull to plow through ice-choked channels. Originally built for Society Expeditions, the ship in 1985 made the first Northwest Passage crossing by a passenger ship, making an unscheduled excursion across the Bering Strait during an Alaskan cruise. The U.S. government fined the line for this historic bold stroke; these days, crossing to the Russian Far East is an accepted itinerary.

The ship is not luxurious, but it is comfortable. Instead of casinos, theaters, and mega-fitness centers, you get such utilitarian amenities as a well-stocked library, easy-access gangways, sturdy Zodiacs, and top-notch safety and navigational equipment.

Cabins and Rates

	Beds	Phone	TV	Sitting Area	Fridge	Tub	Per Diem
Suite	T	●	○	●	○	●	$482–$605
Category 6	T or U/L	●	○	○	○	○	$404–$532
Category 5	T or U/L	●	○	○	○	○	$382–$512
Category 4	T	●	○	○	○	○	$350–$465
Category 3	T	●	○	○	○	○	$325–$432

Category 2	T	●	○	○	○	○	$304 $402
Category 1	T or U/L	●	○	○	○	○	$282– $371

Cabins are small but more than adequate for the typical adventure passenger, who tends to be active and use the cabin for little besides sleep.

Outlet voltage: 220 AC.

Single supplement: 150% of double-occupancy rates; however, five single outside cabins with phone are available at $423–$562 per cruise.

Discounts: A third or fourth passenger in a cabin pays $1,750–$3,450 per cruise, depending upon the itinerary. Airfare is not included in the rates.

Sports and Fitness   **Health club:** Tiny gym, sauna, solarium, massage (sometimes).

Other sports: Pool; equipment for diving, fishing, snorkeling, waterskiing, windsurfing.

Facilities   **Public rooms:** Three bars, two lounges, observation lounge, cinema/lecture hall, library/card room; navigation bridge open to passengers.

Shops: Gift shop, beauty salon/barber.

Health care: Doctor on call.

Other: Safe-deposit boxes.

Access for the Disabled   None.

Club Med

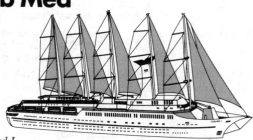

Ship *Club Med I*

Evaluation Club Med's reputation for relaxed, activity-oriented vacations extends to one of its latest additions: its first cruise ship, introduced in 1990. Built by the French shipyard that produced the graceful Windstar ships, the *Club Med I* is a distinctive, sleek white vessel that combines ancient sail power with cutting-edge technology. It is also one of the largest passenger sailing ships afloat. Excursions focus on the seldom-seen side of the Caribbean. Like the Club Med vacation villages scattered throughout the world, the ship attracts an active, convivial crowd, including many couples. Its sister ship, the *Club Med II*, debuted in October 1992, and sails the seas of New Caledonia.

Activities *Club Med I*'s daytime activities center on island exploration and water sports. Tenders transport passengers to nearby islands for tours, or to a deserted beach. A large platform built into the stern lowers to water level when the ship is anchored, and passengers are given free use of all sailing, scuba diving, and snorkeling equipment. Calisthenics and aerobics are offered on deck and in the pool. Club Med's social staff, the *gentils organisateurs*, or G.O.'s, supervise all shipboard activities, including such traditional offerings as bridge lessons and classical-music concerts.

Dining Cuisine is mainly French and Continental. Seating is open in both dining rooms for all meals, though passengers can request table size (single to 10-person). The more formal dining room, La Louisiane, offers lunch and dinner. The informal Odyssey has both indoor and outdoor seating, and the buffet dinner is usually prepared around a theme, such as Italian or seafood. Beer and Club Med's private-label red, white, rosé, and Bordeaux wines are complimentary; other wines may be ordered at an additional charge. Early birds can partake of Continental breakfast on the top deck from 5 to 7 AM, and afternoon tea is served. Except for complimentary Continental breakfast in the cabin, there is a charge for 24-hour room service.

Chart Symbols. *The following symbols are used in the cabin charts that accompany each ship's evaluation.* **D:** *Double bed;* **K:** *King-size bed;* **Q:** *Queen-size bed;* **T:** *Twin bed;* **U/L:** *Upper and lower berths;* ●: *All cabins have this facility;* ○: *No cabins have this facility;* ◖: *Some cabins have this facility*

Entertainment	A piano bar, a disco, and a cabaret lounge with performances by G.O.'s and local bands constitute the entertainment. Don't look for the Vegas-style shows you see on some ships.
Service and Tipping	The G.O.'s are neither servile nor condescending. The friendly and informal staff seem genuinely enthused and eager to help passengers, and most are bilingual. No tips are accepted.
For More Information	Club Med (40 W. 57th St., New York, NY 10019, tel. 800/CLUB–MED).

Club Med I

Specifications	*Type of ship:* Specialty
	Type of cruise: Sail-powered/excursion
	Size: Medium (14,000 tons)
	Number of cabins: 193
	Outside cabins: 100%

Passengers: 386
Crew: 188 (international)
Officers: French
Passenger/crew ratio: 2.1 to 1
Year built: 1990

Itinerary **Fall:** Seven-day alternating loops leave Martinique Saturdays, calling at various Virgin Islands including Les Saintes, Virgin Gorda, Jost Van Dyke, and St. Thomas/St. John, as well as St. Barts and St. Kitts; or St. Lucia, Barbados, Tobago Cays (British Virgin Islands), and Bequia, Mayreau, and Carriacou in the Grenadines; or Marie Galante (near Guadaloupe), Nevis, Virgin Gorda, St. Maarten/St. Martin, Tintamarre (near St. Martin), and Dominica. **Winter–early Spring:** Same as Fall. **Late Spring–Summer:** Transatlantic and Mediterranean cruises.

Port tax: Included in fare.

Overview There's no mistaking the *Club Med I* when all seven white sails are unfurled. It is a vessel of beauty and grace, reminiscent of great clipper ships of old. Its main power source is the wind, augmented by nonpolluting electric diesel engines, all controlled by a state-of-the-art computer. A draft of only 15 feet allows the ship to sail safely into small, off-the-beaten-track harbors.

Eschewing the chrome, neon, and plastic decor of glitzy megacruise ships plying the seas today, Club Med wisely opted instead for a yachtlike ambience achieved through rich teak and mahogany decks and paneling. The public rooms, designed by Albert Pinto, one of Europe's best-known interior designers, are furnished in an art deco style, with muted blue and beige fabrics, and are wrapped in large windows that make you feel very much at one with the sea.

Cabins and Rates

	Beds	Phone	TV	Sitting Area	Fridge	Tub	Per Diem
Suite	T/K	●	●	●	●	○	$396–$555
Da Balaia Deck	T or D	●	●	●	●	○	$278–$384
Cancun Deck	T or D	●	●	●	●	○	$264–$370
Bali Deck	T or D	●	●	●	●	○	$250–$355

Passengers are required to join Club Med by paying a $30 initiation fee and an annual membership fee of $50. Cabins are outside and have twin portholes, local and closed-circuit TV, a telephone, a radio, an honor bar, two mini-safes, a hair dryer, and a terry robe. The two suites (which look onto the sea) are 321 square feet, cabins 188 square feet—not huge, but roomy enough for most cruisers.

Outlet voltage: 110/220 AC.

Single supplement: 150% of double-occupancy rates.

Discounts: A third passenger in a cabin ups the double-occupancy rate by 120%. Airfare is not included in rates.

Sports and Fitness   **Health club:** Spacious top-deck fitness center with sea-view windows and modern weight-training machines, stationary bikes, rowing machines, and treadmill; massage, tanning, sauna.

Walking/jogging: Two unobstructed circuits.

Other sports: Aerobics and other exercise classes, Windsurfers, Sunfish sailboats, scuba equipment (for certified divers), waterskiing off swimming platform, two pools, two Zodiac dive boats.

Facilities   **Public rooms:** Five bars, disco, casino, multipurpose theater, two dining rooms, piano bar.

Shops: Gift shop, beauty salon.

Health care: Doctor on call.

Child care: None; children under 12 not allowed.

Services: Bank, laundry, pressing service.

Access for the Disabled   None.

Commodore Cruise Line

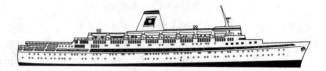

Ships   MS *Caribe I*
SS *Enchanted Isle*
SS *Enchanted Seas*

Evaluation   Commodore is one of the best values afloat. Low prices and an unusually pleasant staff, rather than luxury or extensive amenities, are the major draws. The acquisition of the Bermuda Star Line added two like vessels to its fleet, the *Enchanted Isle* and the *Enchanted Seas*. Commodore's ships were all originally built in the 1950s as transatlantic liners. They have been completely refurbished but show signs of aging: corroded brass, thick layers of paint, scarred and pitted wood. Facilities commonly found on more modern cruise ships are also lacking. Families with children will appreciate being able to fit three, four, or five passengers in many of the staterooms at greatly reduced rates—Commodore is most popular among younger (mid-forties) professionals.

Activities   Commodore bills its vessels as the "Happy Ships," and activities are geared to ensure their claim. All the activities expected on a mainstream cruise ship—bingo, scavenger hunts, wine-and-cheese tastings, food-carving demonstrations, poolside games—are offered, though at a pace somewhat less frenetic than on party ships.

Dining   Commodore's food preparation and quality are above average, but the strictly American fare (what one would expect from an economy cruise line) is sometimes served lukewarm. Some tables are so large that it's difficult to carry on a conversation across them. Although the cruise line officially designates smoking and nonsmoking sections in the dining room, the maître d' may not always seat passengers according to their preferences. Meals are served at two seatings (6 and 8:15) with tables assigned, except at two open- seating lunches. Champagne is included in the Captain's Gala Dinner and at holiday dinners. Low-fat, no-sugar, low-salt, vegetarian, and low-calorie diets are available, but kosher meals are not. There are two formal evenings. A buffet breakfast and lunch are available on the Lido, as are ice cream, cakes, and cookies at teatime. Pizza

---

Chart Symbols. *The following symbols are used in the cabin charts that accompany each ship's evaluation.* **D:** *Double bed;* **K:** *King-size bed;* **Q:** *Queen-size bed;* **T:** *Twin bed;* **U/L:** *Upper and lower berths;* ●: *All cabins have this facility;* ○: *No cabins have this facility;* ◑: *Some cabins have this facility*

and other hot snacks are served in some lounges and bars after 11 PM. Room service from a limited menu is available 24 hours.

Entertainment Commodore is currently revamping its onboard programs, and the catchphrase these days is "party, party, party." The push toward a highly charged good-time attitude is reflected primarily in the revitalized entertainment. Shows may take a destination as a theme, and the general shipboard atmosphere reflects the ports, too: Embarkation staff, waiters, and bartenders wear colorful uniforms—Mexican sombreros, Caribbean tropical wear, or perhaps Dixieland jazz tuxedos, depending upon the ship's itinerary. In the fall, there's an Oktoberfest cruise. Other onboard pastimes include dancing, music, and movies—shown in the two-tiered theaters (which double as late-night discos) on a large-screen TV projector that can be hard to see.

Service and Tipping Tip the room steward and waiter $2.50 each per passenger per diem, the busboy $1.50. A 15% service charge is automatically added to beverage purchases.

For More Commodore Cruise Lines (800 Douglas Rd., Suite 700, Coral **Information** Gables, FL 33134, tel. 800/237–5361).

MS Caribe I

Specifications | *Type of ship:* Economy mainstream | *Passengers:* 875 |
| --- | --- |
| *Type of cruise:* Party | *Crew:* 350 (international) |
| *Size:* Medium (23,000 tons) | *Officers:* International |
| *Number of cabins:* 440 | (mostly northern European) |
| *Outside cabins:* 47% | *Passenger/crew ratio:* 2.5 to 1 |
| | *Year built:* 1953 |

Itinerary **Year-round:** Alternating seven-day loops leave Miami Saturdays, calling at Puerto Plata (Dominican Republic), San Juan, and St. Thomas/St. John; or at Ocho Rios and Montego Bay (Jamaica), Grand Cayman, and Nassau and Blue Lagoon Island (the Bahamas).

Port tax: $68 per passenger.

Overview This former transatlantic ocean liner is one of the most graceful afloat. The interior is no less attractive, with its handsome hardwood paneling, highly polished brass fixtures, and etched glass. Unfortunately, most of the public rooms are small and claustrophobic, especially the Grand Lounge, which may be the most cramped main lounge of any major cruise ship. The glass-enclosed library, however, is wonderful, filled with leatherbound volumes, leather chairs, and walnut-paneled bookshelves. Popular are the modern, airy Mermaid Lounge and Tradewinds Bar; cold and seldom used is the highly touted, two-tiered disco/theater.

The crew is quite spirited, and a typical cruise features a variety of shows and activities, such as Broadway or '50s- and '60s-style, high-energy revues or a Carnival/Mardi Gras celebration.

Cabins and Rates

	Beds	Phone	TV	Sitting Area	Fridge	Tub	Per Diem
Outside Deluxe Suite	T or T/D	●	●	●	●	○	$185–$206
Deluxe Cabin	T/D	●	○	●	●	○	$178–$192
Outside Stateroom	D, T, or U/L	●	○	○	○	○	$106–$185
Inside Stateroom	T or U/L	●	○	○	○	○	$85–$146
Outside Single	T	●	○	○	○	○	$171–$185
Inside Single	T	●	○	○	○	○	$142–$156

Suites are unusually spacious, retaining much from the ship's days as a transatlantic liner, but the lower-category cabins are small and cramped. The Honeymoon Suite is a Deluxe Suite with a double bed.

Outlet voltage: 110 AC.

Single supplement: 150%–200% the double-occupancy rate. Commodore will match two same-sex adults in a cabin at the double-occupancy rate.

Discounts: A third, fourth, or fifth passenger in a cabin pays $52–$66 per diem. A child under 17 sharing with two adults pays $39–$42 per diem. You get a $300 discount for arranging your own airfare.

Sports and Fitness **Health club:** Small exercise room with Life Cycle, rower, Universal gym, two whirlpools.

Walking/jogging: Partially enclosed, air-conditioned Promenade Deck (6 laps=1 mile).

Other sports: Exercise classes, golf driving, table tennis, scuba-diving and snorkeling lessons, shuffleboard, skeet shooting, pool.

Facilities **Public rooms:** Six bars, four lounges, casino, disco, video arcade, library, theater.

Health care: Doctor on call.

Child care: Playroom, youth programs.

Services: Full-service laundry, dry-cleaning.

Shops: Gift shop, beauty salon/barber.

Other: Alcoholics Anonymous.

Access for the Disabled Some public areas are inaccessible to wheelchairs; there is a 2- to 12-inch step to cabin bathrooms, and public lavatories are not equipped for wheelchairs. Despite these severe limitations, disabled passengers are welcome; 22.5″ wheelchairs are provided free.

SS Enchanted Isle and SS Enchanted Seas

Specifications *Type of ship:* Economy mainstream
Type of cruise: Traditional
Size: Medium (23,395/ 23,500 tons)
Number of cabins: 358
Outside cabins: 80%

Passengers: 731/736
Crew: 350 (international)
Officers: European and American
Passenger/crew ratio: 2.1 to 1
Year built: 1957

Itinerary
Enchanted Isle **Year-round:** Seven-day loops leave San Diego Saturdays, calling at Cabo San Lucas, Mazatlán, and Puerto Vallarta.

Port tax: $58 per passenger.

Enchanted Seas **Year-round:** Seven-day loops leave New Orleans Saturdays, calling at Montego Bay (Jamaica), Grand Cayman, Cozumel/Playa del Carmen (Mexico), and Key West.

Port tax: $55 per passenger.

Overview The *Enchanted Seas,* formerly the *Queen of Bermuda,* and the *Enchanted Isle,* formerly the *Bermuda Star* and built in 1957 as the *Argentina,* are virtually identical, though minor structural differences exist—the *Enchanted Seas* is 100 tons heavier, for example. Both ships have long and illustrious histories, and both were recently refurbished.

Despite new paint and paneling, there's no disguising the fact that these ships don't cater to the luxury market. But cruises are reasonably priced, and passengers definitely get what they pay for. The irregular and fairly small design of public rooms, narrow corridors, and lack of light, open spaces can be vexing at times, and some of the facilities—the gym, for example—look like afterthoughts. The minuses are balanced, however, by the fact that the passenger capacity is relatively low and cabins are quite large. Oddly, cabins on the upper decks cost less than those on the lower ones.

Cabins and Rates

	Beds	Phone	TV	Sitting Area	Fridge	Tub	Per Diem
Superior Deluxe Outside Stateroom	D or T	●	●	●	○	●	$157–$271
Superior Outside Stateroom	T	●	○	●	○	●	$146–$256
Deluxe Outside Stateroom	D or T	●	○	●	○	●	$135–$242
Outside Stateroom	D or T	●	○	○	○	○	$123–$235
Outside Cabin	D, T or U/L	●	○	○	○	○	$123–$235
Deluxe Inside Cabin	D or T	●	○	○	○	○	$105–$199

Economy	D, T	◖	○	○	○	○	$88–
Inside	or U/L						$174

Though large, cabins have tiny closets barely adequate for two people, and some cabins have neither a desk nor a sitting area. Recent redecoration helped spruce things up, but many cabins still look cheap and dreary. The view from outside cabins on the Sun Deck, except 222–224, is partially obstructed, and lifeboats block the view of all outside cabins on the Navigation Deck except those looking forward. Outside cabins on the Boat Deck look onto a public promenade.

Outlet voltage: 110 AC.

Single supplement: 135%–200% of double-occupancy rate. Commodore will match two same-sex adults in a cabin at the double-occupancy rate.

Discounts: A third or fourth passenger in a cabin pays $50 per diem. A child under 17 sharing with two adults pays $39–$42. You get a $300 discount for arranging your own airfare.

Sports and Fitness   **Health club:** Small, inside exercise room, sauna.

Other sports: Aerobics, golf driving, table tennis, shuffleboard, skeet shooting, pool.

Facilities   **Public rooms:** Four bars, two entertainment lounges, card/writing room, casino, cinema, disco, indoor Lido, library, piano bar, video-game room.

Shops: Boutique, sundries shop, beauty salon/barber.

Health care: Doctor on call.

Child care: Playroom, baby-sitting, youth programs run by counselors during holidays and in summer.

Services: Full-service laundry, laundromat, photographer, film processing.

Other: Safe-deposit boxes, Alcoholics Anonymous.

Access for the Disabled   Elevators are wheelchair-accessible, and public doorways with ledges are fitted with ramps. However, cabin bathrooms have a step-up ledge with which most passengers in wheelchairs require assistance. Disabled passengers are welcome, however, and the crew makes an effort to help.

Costa Cruises

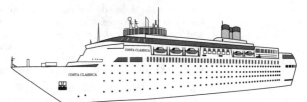

Costa Classica

Ships MS *CostaAllegra*
MS *CostaClassica*
MS *CostaRomantica*

Evaluation By the end of 1993, when the *CostaRomantica* has joined the *Classica* and the *Allegra*, Costa Cruise Lines will have completely revamped itself, operating no ship in the Western Hemisphere older than two. When the *Classica* was introduced in January 1992, the plan was to move away from the cruise line's established lively Italian style and toward a more refined elegance. But, in response to passenger pleas to the contrary, Costa has reintroduced its famed Italian sass. On the *Classica*, and likely on its twin, the *Romantica*, the result is like having a festival in a stately European hotel. The ships themselves are elegant and sleek, but the mood onboard is distinctly jovial—such as singing waiters who prepare specialty dishes at your table and a toga party the last night of the cruise. Overall, the *Allegra* has a more informal attitude, design, and decor.

Passengers use a Costa "credit card" to pay for shore excursions and onboard expenses. Major credit cards, traveler's checks, and cash are accepted; personal checks are not.

Activities Costa offers the usual bag of merriments—bingo, skeet shooting, and myriad get-togethers—along with more unusual offerings, such as Italian language lessons and lectures on such topics as wine, astrology, and Italian history. In keeping with the Italian flair for romance, Costa's captains invite married couples to renew their vows in a special ceremony—after which they'll happily sell you champagne. Recently, Costa began conducting a snorkeling school on its Caribbean sailings.

Dining With the introduction of the three new ships, Costa has revamped its gastronomic experience, keeping old favorites and introducing some delightful alternatives. In the main dining room you'll find the usual lavish fare, with rich but unadventurous pasta dishes as well as beef and fresh fish. Throughout the ship at different times of day and night are a variety of speciality foods; a poolside gelati stand and, on the *Classica* and *Romantica*, a Viennese-style patisserie and a café serving individual gourmet pizzas. At least three times per cruise, chefs

---

Chart Symbols. *The following symbols are used in the cabin charts that accompany each ship's evaluation.* **D:***Double bed;* **K:***King-size bed;* **Q:***Queen-size bed;* **T:***Twin bed;* **U/L:** *Upper and lower berths;* ●: *All cabins have this facility;* ○: *No cabins have this facility;* ◐: *Some cabins have this facility*

set up a pasta buffet poolside—cooking several different dishes on the spot.

On all the ships, the dining room offers two assigned seatings per meal, though open seating sometimes obtains at breakfast and lunch when the ship is in port. Low-calorie SpaCosta meals are available, but special dietary requests, as well as arrangements for birthday and anniversary celebrations, should be made in writing at least four weeks in advance.

On the Lido Deck, you can help yourself to early-morning coffee with juice and pastries, a full buffet breakfast and lunch, and afternoon tea and snacks. Room service is available 24 hours but is limited to sandwiches and Continental breakfast. Other options include a formal afternoon tea and a midnight buffet. Also, each cruise has one pizza/focaccia poolside party, an outdoor barbecue, and a buffet/galley tour. Night owls munch on Italian pastries at 2 AM. Noteworthy on the older ships are the free pizzerias and gelaterias, open daily with limited hours.

Entertainment Each event has a theme; most popular are the Italian *festa* and the Roman Bacchanalia, for which passengers fashion togas out of bedsheets. Otherwise, entertainment is fairly typical, from cabaret shows to dancing to shows in the piano bar. Bingo is held late afternoon or early evening, sometimes pushing back the second seating's main show until around 11 PM. Nonbingo fans can get a little testy about this.

Service and Tipping The current level of service and attention to detail are greatly improved. A 24-hour Concierge Desk handles special requests, and the crew tends to its passengers with traditional European deference. Tip the room steward and waiter $3 each per passenger per diem, the head waiter $1, the busboy $1.50.

For More Information Costa Cruises (World Trade Center, 80 S.W. 8th St., Miami, FL 33130, tel. 800/462–6782).

MS CostaAllegra

Specifications

Type of ship: Mainstream	*Passengers:* 800
Type of cruise: Traditional	*Crew:* 400 (International)
Size: Medium (30,000 tons)	*Officers:* Italian
Number of cabins: 405	*Passenger/crew ratio:* 2 to 1
Outside cabins: 60%	*Year built:* 1992

Itinerary **Fall:** In the Mediterranean. **Winter–Spring:** Seven-day loops leave San Juan, calling at St. Maarten/St. Maarten, St. Lucia, Barbados, Serena Cay (Costa's private island), Casa de Campo (Dominican Republic), and St. Thomas/St. John. **Summer:** Same as Fall.

Port tax: $79 per passenger.

Overview With a more low-slung profile than its sister ship, the *Allegra* also has an unpretentious atmosphere that attracts an older, less affluent and less active crowd. The ship is comfortable and easy to get around, with all the public rooms on one deck, including a descending staircase into the main dining room. The designers also made wonderful use of the sunlight and sea in the public areas: A stunning plant-filled atrium caps the health club, and the boxy aft of the ship allows high windows in the dining room, with a splendid view of the ocean. Public areas have the feel of being underwater because of a series of skylit water-filled compartments overhead and large portholes peering into the main swimming pool above. Extensive use of Italian architectural detailing is made throughout the ship, such as an intricate mosaic bordering the entrance to the dining room and many hand-painted murals.

Cuisine is good, basic international fare, with excellent pasta but rather unimaginative desserts. Although the service in the dining room is fair to good, you won't find the attention to detail found on the *Classica*. Some special buffets are lavish, but in general the lunch and midnight buffets offer only the basics. The pasta dishes are consistently yummy.

Cabins and Rates

	Beds	Phone Area	TV Diem	Sitting	Fridge	Tub	Per
Grand Suite	Q, T	●	●	●	●	●	$570–$599
Suite	Q, T	●	●	●	●	●	$485–$513
Outside	Q, T	●	●	○	○	○	$256–$327
Inside	U/L	●	●	○	○	○	$192–$263

Inside and outside cabins are equally spacious, all decorated with spare Italian furnishings using burnished wood and woven fabrics. Some cabins have twins that convert to a queen and all have built-in hair dryers and safes. The Grand Suite, on the bow, has large windows on two sides but no balcony. Like the Grand Suite, regular suites have whirlpool bathtubs and walk-in closets, but they have private balconies. Suites receive flowers, fruit, and pastry and candy baskets replenished daily.

Outlet voltage: 110/220 AC.

Single supplement: 200% of double occupancy rate for suites, 150% for other cabins.

Other discounts: A third or fourth passenger in a cabin pays $113–$127 per diem. You get a discount for arranging your own airfare.

Sports and Fitness **Health club:** Stair climbers, Lifecycles, treadmills, free weights, aerobics and stretch classes, massage and facial-treatment center.

Walking/jogging: Unobstructed jogging track on top deck.

Other sports: Pool, three jacuzzis.

Facilities: **Public rooms:** Two restaurants, four bars, two entertainment lounges, disco, casino, library, card room, meeting room, chapel.

Shops: Boutique, perfume and jewelry shop, photo shop, beauty salon/barber.

Health care: Doctor on call.

Child care: Supervised childrens center, baby-sitting.

Services: Full-service laundry, photographer.

Other: Safe-deposit boxes.

Access for the Elevators and public lavatories are wheelchair-accessible, as
Disabled are six cabins.

MS CostaClassica and MS CostaRomantica

Specifications *Type of ship:* Mainstream   *Passengers:* 1,300
Type of cruise: Traditional   *Crew:* 650 (international)
Size: Large (53,000 tons)   *Officers:* Italian
Number of cabins: 654   *Passenger/crew ratio:* 2 to 1
Outside cabins: 67%   *Year built:* 1991/1993

Itinerary **Fall:** One transatlantic crossing and a series of Mediterranean
Classica sailings. **Winter:** Alternating seven-day loops leave Miami Sat-
urdays, calling at San Juan, St. Thomas/St. John, and Serena
Cay (Costa's private island), or Ocho Rios (Jamaica), Grand
Cayman, and Cozumel/Playa del Carmen (Mexico). A 10-day
Christmas cruise and 11-day New Year's cruise leave Miami,
calling at St. Maarten/St. Martin, St. Lucia, and Antigua.
Spring–Summer: Same as Fall.

Port tax: $79 per passenger.

Romantica Itinerary and port tax are unannounced at press time (Spring
1993), but the *Romantica* is expected to make several inaugural
Caribbean cruises.

Overview The $325 million *CostaClassica* is one of the world's most ex-
pensively built cruise ships per passenger. It has the regal
bearing of an established European hotel—with plenty of cool
Italian marble and hand-made ceramic tile—but a sassy,
charged Italian spirit. Once past the stark institutional feel of
the hallways, you'll discover utterly charming nooks and cran-
nies: Curl up with a good book in a high-back chair tucked away
in a corner, sip fruit punch at the outdoor café beneath a broad
swath of canvas, or take high tea amid palm fronds in the intimate patisserie. On hot days, you'll want to plant yourself in
one of the blue-and-white-striped lounge chairs by the pool on
the three-tiered teak aft deck.

The main dining room, the Tivoli Restaurant, is spare and elegant, with Louis XIV–style chairs and an Italian marble floor.
It is at once stunning and loud. Unfussy northern Italian food
is the fare of the day, along with a few classic crowd-pleasers,
such as lobster and beef Wellington. Two theme dinners feature
foods of the Renaissance and Roman eras; themes are also reflected in murals on the restaurant's walls. Early breakfasts
and buffet lunches are served at La Trattoria, a contemporary-
style Italian café with hand-painted tiles and marble tables. Its
open-air extension, Café Alfresco, features moss-green wicker
chairs with flowered cushions and marble-top tables. Aug-
menting the luncheon buffet are two refreshing alternatives: a
salad bar and Leonardo's deli, where you build your own sandwich.

Typical Las Vegas–style revues are offered in the Colosseo
Showroom, a faithful reproduction of a Renaissance theater
with tiered seating. The Puccini Ballroom features big-band
music and jazz. The circular Galileo Club and Observatory
perch above the bow of the ship; its floor-to-ceiling windows
allow a 360-degree view.

Cabins and Rates

	Beds	Phone	TV	Sitting Area	Fridge	Tub	Per Diem
Suite	Q	●	●	●	●	●	$422–$446
Outside	Q or T	●	●	●	○	○	$287–$346
Inside	T or U/L	●	●	●	○	○	$170–$299

Staterooms average a roomy 200 square feet, and bathrooms are large, too. Decor is simple and elegant, with cherrywood furniture, designer fabrics, and watercolor prints of European cities on the walls. Light sleepers may grumble, however, about the thin walls. Current movies and CNN news are shown continuously on cabin TVs. Some twins convert to a queen staterooms that accommodate three passengers offer upper and lower berths. Suites sleep up to four, using a twin sofabed and a twin Murphy bed along with the queen-size bed; in addition to a sitting area, the suites have a graceful wood-rimmed balcony large enough to accommodate two chaise longues with room to spare.

Outlet voltage: 110/220 AC

Single supplement: 200% of double-occupancy rate, 150% for other cabins.

Discounts: A third or fourth passenger in a cabin pays $142 per diem. You get a discount for arranging your own airfare.

Sports and Fitness **Health club:** Aerobics studio; exercise room with free weights, Lifecycles, treadmills, stair climbers, circuit weight-training system; whirlpool spas, roman bath, steam and sauna rooms; massage and facial-treatment center; juice bar.

Walking/jogging: Unobstructed jogging track on top deck.

Other sports: Two pools.

Facilities **Public rooms:** Two bars, two entertainment lounges, disco, casino, library, card room, two restaurants, conference center/chapel.

Shops: Boutique, perfume shop, jewelry/gift shop, photo shop, sports-clothing shop, gourmet deli, beauty salon/barber.

Health care: Doctor on call.

Child care: Playroom, supervised youth activity center, babysitting.

Services: Full-service laundry, photographer.

Other: Safe-deposit boxes.

Access for the Disabled Elevators and public lavatories are wheelchair-accessible, as are six cabins.

Crystal Cruises

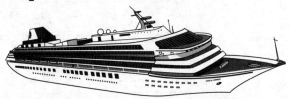

Ship *Crystal Harmony*

Evaluation Japanese-owned Crystal Cruises has "put the luxury back into luxury cruising" in order to lure away high-powered international executives from chartering their own yachts and attract other wealthy passengers who are accustomed to the best. A cruise aboard the $200-million *Crystal Harmony* is not as intimate or unstructured as a *Sea Goddess* cruise, nor as formal or sedentary as one aboard the *Sagafjord*. The *Harmony* is designed for those who love physical activity and fine food and are willing to pay plenty for them.

Crystal combines the best of Japanese industrial know-how with a European flair for service and attention. Engines, radar, and navigational equipment are state-of-the-art. Business services for the hyper executive include audio-visual, translation, and satellite telecommunications equipment, as well as fax machines, computers, and secretarial services. And the fitness center—a 3,000-square-foot space with an ocean view and spa facilities—is arguably the seagoing world's most advanced. White-glove service, stellar cuisine, air-conditioned tenders with toilets, and an exquisite interior complete the effect of total luxury and comfort.

Activities Crystal provides all the mainstream cruise activities: bingo, bridge, a masquerade party, "horse racing," board and card games, dance classes, arts and crafts classes, pool games, table tennis, paddle tennis court, skeet shooting, and shuffleboard. To this it adds high-tech sports facilities, such as a computerized electronic golf course and driving range; high-powered intellectual and cultural debates and destination-oriented lectures by scholars, political figures, and diplomats; a busy fitness center and spa, with lots of pampering; and the first Caesar's-Palace-at-Sea casino.

Dining The Japanese aesthetic is evident in Crystal's lavish, distinctive food presentations. Breaking cruising tradition, the line offers two dinner alternatives to the dining room at no additional charge—Asian cuisine at the superb Kyoto Restaurant and Italian food at Prego. The main dining room has two seatings for breakfast, lunch, and dinner, which is at 6 and 8. Typi-

---

Chart Symbols. *The following symbols are used in the cabin charts that accompany each ship's evaluation.* **D:** *Double bed;* **K:** *King-size bed;* **Q:** *Queen-size bed;* **T:** *Twin bed;* **U/L:** *Upper and lower berths;* **●:** *All cabins have this facility;* **○:** *No cabins have this facility;* **◑:** *Some cabins have this facility*

cally, there are two formal evenings per week. The canopy-covered indoor/outdoor Lido serves breakfast, mid-morning bouillon, and lunch. The swim-up bar in the Neptune Pool serves hot dogs and hamburgers. The Bistro sells specialty coffees and wine and serves international cheeses. 24-hour room service offers a menu including pizza and sandwiches. The ship has an extensive wine cellar.

Entertainment There are pre- and post-dinner cabarets, two nightly reviews in the main lounge, a piano bar, before- and after-dinner dancing, a harpist, a trio (sometimes classical), a sing-along piano bar, and the casino. Local entertainers are sometimes brought on board to entertain during the ship's frequent parties.

Service and Tipping Crystal's staff members are well trained, highly motivated, and thoroughly professional. However, because *Harmony* is the only ship in Crystal's line, crew members are stuck together on the same boat for lengthy periods, and this has been known to cause visible tension. Tip the steward and the waiter $3 each per passenger per diem, the busboy $2. In Prego and Kyoto restaurants, tip $3 per passenger per meal.

For More Information Crystal Cruises (2121 Ave. of the Stars, Los Angeles, CA 90067, tel. 800/446–6645).

Crystal Harmony

Specifications *Type of ship:* Luxury mainstream
Type of cruise: Traditional
Size: Large (49,400 tons)
Number of cabins: 480
Outside cabins: 96%

Passengers: 960
Crew: 545 (European)
Officers: Norwegian and Japanese
Passenger/crew ratio: 1.76 to 1
Year built: 1990

Itinerary **Fall:** Europe and South Pacific. **Winter:** A variety of 10- to 17-day one-way Panama Canal Transits run between Barbados and Acapulco, San Juan and Acapulco, San Juan and Los Angeles, and Fort Lauderdale and Acapulco. Ports may include Aruba, St. Maarten/St. Martin, St. Thomas/St. John, Jamaica, Grand Cayman, Cozumel/Playa del Carmen (Mexico), Key West, Grenada, Puerto Caldera (Costa Rica), Curaçao, Nassau, Puerto Vallarta, and Zihuatanejo/Ixtapa. **Spring–Summer:** Same as Fall.

Port tax: $105–$120 per passenger.

Overview The *Crystal Harmony*, exceptionally sleek and sophisticated, contradicts the conventional wisdom that all new state-of-the-art ships must look like high-rise, barge-bound hotels. Technologically advanced and superbly equipped, it is tastefully decorated as well. Harmonious colors, lots of plants and neoclassical sculptures, and a light-and-airy design give a sense of both luxury and simplicity. At the center is a multilevel atrium, Crystal Plaza—a study in glass stairways and railings, brass fixtures, and dazzling white walls. The Vista Lounge is a beautiful wedding-white room with oversize observation windows. The Lido is covered by a retractable canopy. With one of the highest passenger/space ratios afloat, there's never a feeling of claustrophobia, in either the public rooms or the hallways.

Cabins and Rates

	Beds	Phone	TV	Sitting Area	Fridge	Tub	Per Diem
Crystal Penthouse	T/K	●	●	●	●	●	$1,021–$1,101
Penthouse Suite	T/Q	●	●	●	●	●	$692–$745
Penthouse	T/Q	●	●	●	●	●	$550–$591
Superior	T/Q	●	●	●	●	●	$428–$459
Deluxe Veranda	T/Q	●	●	●	●	●	$371–$415
Deluxe	T/Q	●	●	●	●	●	$259–$352
Inside	T	●	●	●	●	●	$243–$259

Staterooms and cabins are large, beautifully decorated, and equipped with 14-channel TVs (including CNN) and VCRs. Staterooms also have hair dryers and robes. Penthouses have verandas and whirlpools; some deluxe suites have verandas. A butler is available for suites. Some cabins on the Horizon and Promenade decks have obstructed views (Crystal's sales catalog clearly identifies rooms with limited views). Cabins on the Promenade Deck look out onto a public promenade.

Outlet voltage: 110/220 AC.

Single supplement: 160%–200% of double-occupancy rate.

Discounts: A third passenger in a cabin pays the minimum per-person fare for that cruise. Children under 12 with two full-paying adults pay half-fare. You get a $300 discount for arranging your own airfare.

Sports and Fitness **Health club:** Spa with state-of-the-art equipment—stationary bikes, rowing machines, stair climbers—free weights, saunas, steam rooms, massage, exercise classes, weight-reduction regimens, body and facial care, makeup services.

Walking/jogging: Unobstructed circuit on Promenade Deck.

Other sports: Aerobics, jazz-dance, other exercise classes, paddle tennis, shuffleboard, skeet shooting, ping-pong, two pools (one for laps), two whirlpools.

Facilities **Public rooms:** Seven bars, six entertainment lounges, card room, casino, cinema, disco, Lido, library (books, videotapes), piano bar, smoking room, video-game room.

Shops: Shopping arcade of boutiques, beauty salon/barber.

Health care: Doctor on call.

Child care: Youth programs with counselors during holidays or whenever a large number of children are on board, baby-sitting arranged privately with crew member.

Services: Concierge service, full-service laundry and dry cleaning, valet service, self-service laundry room, photographer, video-camera rentals, film processing, secretarial and photocopy services, translation equipment for meetings.

Other: Safe-deposit boxes.

Access for the Disabled   Four cabins have been specially fitted for wheelchair access. Passengers must provide their own small, traveling wheelchairs. All areas are accessible.

Cunard Line Limited

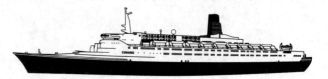

QE 2

Ships MV *Cunard Countess*
SS *Cunard Crown Dynasty*
SS *Cunard Crown Jewel*
RMS *Queen Elizabeth 2*
MS *Sagafjord*
Sea Goddess I
MS *Vistafjord*

Evaluation Cunard offers four distinct styles of cruising. The *Cunard Countess* is one of the most affordable mainstream cruise ships and caters to a relaxed, informal, mostly European crowd. Older passengers are drawn to the tradition and opulence of the *Sagafjord* and *Vistafjord*. The small *Sea Goddess* offers cruises affordable by only a very few; passengers on this ship enjoy the highest standards of luxury and service available. And the *QE2* remains the grande dame of the seas, offering a generous variety of activities and amenities that range from upscale to luxurious, depending on how much you pay for your cabin. In January 1993, Cunard underwent a joint venture with Crown Cruise Line. Cunard now markets its *Countess* and *Princess* (which is stationed in Europe) ships together with Crown's *Monarch* (now stationed in Australia), *Jewel*, and *Dynasty* (which debuted June 1993). Because of the diversity of styles among the Cunard and Cunard Crown ships, information on activities, cuisine, entertainment, and service has been covered in the individual ship evaluations.

For More Information Cunard Line Limited (555 5th Ave., New York, NY 10017, tel. 800/221–4770).

MV Cunard Countess

Specifications *Type of ship:* Economy mainstream
Type of cruise: Traditional
Size: Small (17,593 tons)
Number of cabins: 398
Outside cabins: 66%

Passengers: 790
Crew: 350 (mainly British)
Officers: British
Passenger/crew ratio: 2.3 to 1
Year built: 1976

Chart Symbols. *The following symbols are used in the cabin charts that accompany each ship's evaluation.* **D:** *Double bed;* **K:** *King-size bed;* **Q:** *Queen-size bed;* **T:** *Twin bed;* **U/L:** *Upper and lower berths;* ●: *All cabins have this facility;* ○: *No cabins have this facility;* ◑: *Some cabins have this facility*

Itinerary **Year-round:** Alternating seven-day loops leave San Juan Saturdays, calling at St. Maarten/St. Martin, Guadeloupe, Grenada, St. Lucia, St. Kitts, and St. Thomas/St. John; or Tortola, Antigua, Martinique, Barbados, and St. Thomas/St. John. The itineraries can be combined for 14-day cruises.

Port tax: $80–$95 per passenger.

Overview The *Countess* has all the amenities that a young, budget-oriented clientele might desire, but since these are among the least expensive cruises available, don't mistake the Cunard name for an automatic stamp of luxury. The ship is compact, cabins are small, but public rooms are spacious; the Showtime Lounge, for example, features a 40-square-foot, black marble dance floor. The Starlight Lounge, a card room and entertainment lounge, is one of the ship's highlights; furnished in art-nouveau style, it commands a magnificent view of sea. Public areas and cabins were refurbished in fall 1992—furniture was reupholstered and new navy-and-gold carpeting was installed.

Activities In addition to typical mainstream activities, the ship has a 24-hour health club that offers a wide range of fitness activities. Exercise options continue ashore in the form of hikes, sports programs, and competitive runs—the *Countess* is known for its extensive shore excursion program.

Dining Food is above average, and the service is usually excellent. The dining room has two assigned seatings per meal (at 6:30 and 8:30) and a midnight buffet. A special fitness diet is available, though special dietary requests should be made two weeks before sailing. The Lido serves early morning coffee and pastries, light breakfast, mid-morning bouillon, and light lunch. Self-serve coffee and tea are available all day, and afternoon tea is served; 24-hour room service is available from a limited menu. There are two formal evenings per week.

Entertainment Entertainment is typical of that on other ships. Variety shows are held in the main lounge, and there's an indoor/outdoor nightclub and a piano bar.

Service and Tipping Service is excellent. Tip the room steward and the waiter $3 each per passenger per diem, the busboy $1.50; the wine steward gets 15% of the wine bill.

Cabins and Rates

	Beds	Phone	TV	Sitting Area	Fridge	Tub	Per Diem
Deluxe Outside Double	T	●	●	●	●	●	$320–$382
Outside Double	T	●	○	○	○	○	$268–$310
Inside Double	T	●	○	○	○	○	$186–$270
Double Category H	T or U/L	●	○	○	○	○	$156–$170

Cabins are small but convert into sitting rooms during the day. Recent renovations include thicker mattresses, beds set in an L-shape arrangement, and more luggage space.

Outlet voltage: 110 AC.

Single supplement: 150% of double-occupancy rate; if a confirmed reservation is made at least 30 days prior to sailing, the double-occupancy rate may apply. Cunard will match two same-sex adults in a cabin for the double-occupancy rate.

Discounts: A third or fourth passenger in a cabin pays $127–$142 per diem. You get a discount for arranging your own airfare.

Sports and Fitness   **Health club:** 24-hour gym with free weights, computerized weight machines, rowing machines, stationary bikes, ballet barre, sauna, massage; aerobics, stretch, yoga, and other exercise classes.

Walking/jogging: Boat Deck.

Other sports: Basketball, golf driving, paddle tennis, table tennis, shuffleboard, pool, two outdoor whirlpools.

Facilities   **Public rooms:** Four bars, three entertainment lounges, card room, casino, cinema, disco, library/writing room, Lido, piano bar.

Shops: Small arcade of boutiques and gift shops, beauty salon/barber.

Health care: Doctor on call.

Child care: Wading pool, baby-sitting, youth programs run by counselors during holidays or in summer.

Services: Full-service laundry, photographer.

Other: Safe-deposit boxes.

Access for the Disabled   Not all public areas are wheelchair-accessible, and wheelchairs are not permitted on tenders. Passengers confined to wheelchairs must provide their own small, portable wheelchair.

SS Crown Jewel and SS Crown Dynasty

Specifications

Type of ship: Upscale mainstream	*Passengers:* 820
Type of cruise: Traditional	*Crew:* 300 (Filipino)
Size: Small (20,000 tons)	*Officers:* Northern European
Number of cabins: 410	*Passenger/crew ratio:* 2.75 to 1
Outside cabins: 69.5%	*Year built:* 1992/1993

Itinerary
Cunard Crown Dynasty   **Fall–early Winter:** Ten- and 11-day Panama Canal transits between Acapulco and Fort Lauderdale call at Cozumel/Playa del Carmen (Mexico), along the Canal, Puerto Caldera (Costa Rica), Ocho Rios or Montego Bay (Jamaica), Grand Cayman, and Key West. **Mid-Winter:** Seven-day loops out of Fort Lauderdale call at Puerto Plata (Dominican Republic), St. Thomas/St. John, San Juan, and Nassau. **Late-Winter–early Spring:** Same as fall–early winter. **Late Spring–Summer:** Seven-day cruises between Anchorage/Seward call at Hubbard Glacier, Skagway, Juneau, Petersburg, Ketchikan, Sitka, Tracy Arm Fjord, Misty Fjord, and along the inside passage.

Port tax: $78–$205.

Cunard Crown Jewel   **Year-round:** Alternating seven-day loops out of Fort Lauderdale call at Puerto Plata (Dominican Republic), St. Thomas/St.

John, San Juan, and Nassau; or Ocho Rios (Jamaica), Grand Cayman, and Cozumel/Playa del Carmen.

Port tax: $78 per passenger.

Overview Cunard markets the *Dynasty* and *Jewel* together with its other relatively affordable ships, the *Monarch, Countess,* and *Princess.* The low rates attract a younger, lively crowd looking for Cunard's service on relatively small, casual ships. These identical $100 million ships are stylish and sophisticated, though service has been a little slow on some of the ships' early sailings. The ships have half the passenger capacity of many competitors, thereby offering an intimate voyage replete with personal touches, yet achieving an illusion of spaciousness through clever use of glass. A skylight and three window walls brighten the Bon Vivant dining room, where tiered seating allows unobstructed sea views. In the Crown Plaza atrium, a five-story wall of glass offers a spectacular view as well. A grand staircase and a glass elevator complete the space. At night, you can dance to upbeat videos and music in the lively Chameleon Club or catch a film in the well-appointed cinema, which also serves as a comfortable meeting room.

Activities The ships offer "low density, low impact" activities, such as bingo, pool games, "horse racing," wine tasting, "whodunit" evenings, and crafts classes. The "Seafit" health-and-fitness program combines aerobics, water exercises, walking tours of ports, and low-calorie, low-cholesterol, low-sodium cuisine.

Dining The elaborate, adventurous American and Continental cuisine is presented by a competent, low-key, and cheerful wait-staff. Food, particularly the first courses, is stellar, with only a few exceptions: Pasta is often prepared in a bland, heavy cream sauce. There are always light and healthy offerings, and desserts are good but not excessively rich. Breakfast and lunch in the dining room are open seating. The dining room (capacity 440) utilizes an innovative tiered design, which affords unobstructed sea views from nearly every table. The Palm Court Café, a bright indoor/outdoor facility, serves breakfast, lunch, snacks, and outdoor grill selections. Dinner on both ships is served at two assigned seatings (6 and 8:15). Afternoon tea and midnight buffets are offered. Room service is available 24 hours but is limited to sandwiches and Continental breakfast. Special dietary requests must be made in writing at least two weeks before sailing.

Entertainment Entertainment is not dazzling, and this seems to suit its passengers just fine. Broadway-style shows, cabarets, and dancing take place in the Scheherezade main lounge, with large windows great for sea viewing by day. The aft lounge, Reflections, features jazz combos and dance music, and the Chameleon Club is a popular disco.

Service and Tipping Service has improved tremendously in past years, and the crew takes great pride in the ships. Tip the steward and the waiter $2.50 each per passenger per diem, the busboy $1.50. A 15% service charge is added to bar bills.

Cabins and Rates

	Beds	Phone	TV	Sitting Area	Fridge	Tub	Per Diem
Suites	D	●	●	●	●	○	$232–$389

Outside	T/D	●	●	◑	◑	○	$164–$278
Inside	T/D	●	●	○	○	○	$178–$228

Each stateroom has a private bathroom, two lower beds that convert to a double, remote-control TVs, ample storage, and a safe. Each 350-square-foot Deluxe Suite has a double bed, a sitting area, an extra closet, and a refrigerator. Ten suites have private balconies. All cabins are dressed in a subtle color scheme of mauves, pinks, blues, and greens set against beautiful wood trim. Every passenger is pampered with complimentary fruit, champagne, and other amenities.

Outlet voltage: 110 AC.

Single supplement: No surcharge; however, spaces are limited, and this rate cannot be combined with other offers.

Discounts: A third passenger in a cabin pays $64 per diem, as does a child under 15 sailing with a single parent. You get a discount for arranging your own airfare.

Sports and Fitness **Health club:** Nautilus equipment, aerobics, juice bar, sauna, steam room, massage, facials.

Walking/jogging: Circuit on Promenade Deck.

Facilities **Public rooms:** Library, four lounges, casino, dining room, café, meeting room, cinema, disco.

Shops: Boutiques, beauty salon with manicures and pedicures.

Child care: Teen/youth center.

Access for the Disabled Four cabins (two inside, two outside) and the elevators are wheelchair-accessible. Disabled passengers are welcome, though it is recommended that they travel with an able-bodied companion.

RMS Queen Elizabeth 2

Specifications *Type of ship:* Luxury/ mainstream
Type of cruise: Traditional upscale
Size: Megaship/liner (67,139 tons)
Number of cabins: 957
Outside cabins: 70%

Passengers: 1,800
Crew: 1,025 (international)
Officers: British
Passenger/crew ratio: 1.8 to 1 (varies according to cabin price)
Year built: 1969

Itinerary **Year-round:** Several five-day transatlantic crossings run between New York and Southampton, England. Several loop cruises leave New York for the Caribbean, calling at St. Maarten/St. Martin, Barbados, Martinique, and St. Thomas/St. John. A 100-day circumnavigation of the globe leaves New York, calling at 33 ports on six continents, including Fort Lauderdale, several Caribbean islands, the east and west coasts of South America, Acapulco, Los Angeles, several Hawaiian ports, Auckland, the Australian coast, Bali, Singapore, Bangkok, Hong Kong, other Far East ports, along the Panama Canal, Southampton (UK), and various Mediterranean ports. Several 11- and 13-day Panama Canal Transits leave New York, calling at Fort Lauderdale, St. Thomas/St. John, Cartagena (Colombia), Acapulco, and Los Angeles. Several seven-day cruises sail from New York to Bermuda. Several four-day cruises sail along the Northeastern U.S. and Canadian coast, calling at Bar Harbor, Halifax, and Martha's Vineyard. Itineraries change, often with little notice, from month to month; it's best to check with Cunard for the latest information on the *QE2*'s itineraries.

Port tax: $135–$155 per passenger.

Overview Built in 1969 as the last of the true ocean liners, the *QE2* is both a two-class transatlantic liner and a one-class cruise ship. Even when cruising, however, passengers are assigned (according to their per diem) to one of four restaurants, each offering a different level of quality. Outside the cabin and restaurants, all passengers enjoy the same facilities and amenities.

The ship has undergone numerous refits, including one that transformed it into a military carrier during the Falklands War. Taking the *QE2*'s historic and social position to heart, Cunard continues to invest its flagship with the best, the most, and the largest of whatever can fit into this floating metropolis. An $8 million refurbishment completed in December 1992 saw the redecoration of public rooms and the addition of an art gallery and one of the most comprehensive spas on land or sea.

Thirteen stories high and three football fields long, the *QE2* still possesses the grace that eludes new megaships. High ceilings, wood paneling, and expensive furnishings create the look and ambience of a grand European hotel, and a tony arcade features such posh emporiums as Harrods and Gucci. You'll also find an American Express office, a flower shop, a nursery, and a large, well-equipped Epson computer center. Passengers on the transatlantic run have use of a 30-car garage and a dog kennel.

Close inspection reveals signs of aging. Still, every passenger need has been thought of, and though some passengers find the ship too large, others too stuffy, the wealth of space, impeccable service, and options makes the *QE2* a wonderful, dazzling gem radiating with British elegance and dignity.

Activities Without diverging from the traditional fare of bingo, "horse racing," and similar get-togethers, the *QE2* offers as many activities as any ship afloat, partly because of its size and partly because of Cunard's pride in its flagship. Offerings include numerous lectures and seminars, classical-music concerts, fashion shows, computer courses, and an extensive fitness program. A program designed around the new art gallery includes art-history lectures and workshops and art-museum tours in port.

Dining Your dinner depends on your per diem, and this will always annoy some passengers and please others. The gourmet Queen's Grill and Princess Grill are elegant, single-seating restaurants for occupants of suites and luxury and ultra-deluxe cabins. Offering a virtually limitless menu, both are consistently and justifiably awarded four stars by international food critics. The larger, single-seating Columbia Restaurant serves those in deluxe and higher-priced outside cabins; meals are beautifully prepared and expertly served but fall short of the grills' standards. All other passengers eat at two seatings in the Mauritania Restaurant, which, were it the featured dining room of just about any other ship, would be a stellar restaurant.

On the QE2, it's an admirable fourth-place option. Dinner is assigned, at 6:30 and 8:30.

On transatlantic crossings, a special supervised early dinner for children allows parents to dine on their own. Spa meals are available, but other dietary requests should be made at least three weeks ahead. Two formal evenings are held each week, though dinners in the Queen's Grill and Princess Grill are never casual. The wine cellar stocks more than 20,000 bottles.

The Lido serves early morning coffee and pastries, a buffet breakfast and lunch, plus hamburgers and hot dogs. Health-conscious passengers may opt for the breakfast (and sometimes lunch) spa buffets. International Food Bazaars are sometimes featured in the Mauritania Restaurant. Other food service includes mid-morning bouillon, a traditional high tea, and a midnight buffet; 24-hour room service from a limited menu is available.

Entertainment Nightlife is diverse, including variety shows in the Grand Lounge, cabaret, classical-music concerts, disco parties, and a piano bar. A highlight of *QE2* entertainment is a series of talks given by such celebrities as Jeremy Irons, Meryl Streep, Jason Robards, Art Buchwald, and Barbara Walters. Dance and talent contests and costume parties are also held. The liner has its own 20-station TV network, including CNN, with color sets in every cabin. A daily newspaper is published on board.

Service and Tipping Service in the first-class staterooms and restaurants is impeccable because that's where the most—and the best—staff members work. The service at all levels of the ship, however, is above average. Unfortunately, Cunard suffers from occasional labor problems, and there have been a few incidents of work slowdowns or stoppages. Also, some passengers find the British attitude a bit stuffy and unspontaneous. In the Mauritania Restaurant, tip the cabin steward and waiter $3 each per passenger per diem; in the Columbia Restaurant, $4; in the Queen's and Princess grills, $5. A 10% service charge is added to bar bills.

Cabins and Rates

	Beds	Phone	TV	Sitting Area	Fridge	Tub	Per Diem*
Suite (Queen's Grill)	Q or T/D	●	●	●	●	●	$2,422–$4,155 (per suite)
Luxury (Queen's Grill)	Q or T	●	●	●	●	●	$554–$1,334
Ultra Deluxe (Queen's/ Princess)	T	●	●	●	●	●	$387–$769
Deluxe (Columbia)	T	●	●	○	○	●	$325–$527
Outside (Columbia/ Mauritania)	T	●	●	○	○	◑	$258–$505

Inside	T or	●	●	○	○	○	$202–
(Mauritania)	U/L						$370

*The wide range of rates reflects differences among cabins in the lower-priced categories, as well as differences in itineraries (exotic-destination cruises are most expensive).

Suites accommodate up to four passengers, at no extra charge per passenger, making them more economical for a family of four than two luxury cabins. Penthouse Suites, with verandas and whirlpools, are the largest, most luxurious accommodations afloat; first-class cabins (all with VCRs) compare with those of any luxury ship. Luxury cabins, except No. 8184, have private verandas. Lifeboats partially obstruct the view from some cabins on the Sports Deck, and Boat Deck cabins look onto a public promenade.

Outlet voltage: 110 AC.

Single supplement: 175%–200% of double-occupancy rate; several single cabins are available at $179–$726 a day.

Discounts: A third or fourth passenger in a cabin pays half the minimum fare in the cabin's restaurant grade. Various discounts exist for combining consecutive itineraries, booking and paying early on the World Cruise, and arranging your own airfare.

Sports and Fitness **Health club:** Thalassotherapy pool, inhalation room, French hydrotherapy bath treatment, computerized nutritional and lifestyle evaluation, aerobics and exercise classes, weight machines, Lifecycles, Rowers, Stairmasters, treadmills, sauna, whirlpools, hydrocalisthenics, massage.

Walking/jogging: Jogging track (3.5 laps=1 mile).

Other sports: Putting green, golf driving range, paddle tennis, table tennis, shuffleboard, tetherball, trapshooting, volleyball, two outdoor and two indoor pools, four whirlpools, sports area with separate clubhouses for adults and teens.

Facilities **Public rooms:** Six bars, five entertainment lounges, card room, casino, chapel/synagogue, cinema, art gallery, Epson computer center, disco, executive boardroom, library/reading room, piano bar, video-game room.

Shops: Arcade with men's formal rental shop, Harrods, designer boutiques (Gucci, Christian Dior, Louis Vuitton), florist, beauty center, barbershop.

Health care: Extensive hospital with full staff of doctors and nurses.

Child care: Playroom, wading pool, teen center, baby-sitting, youth programs run by counselors.

Services: Full-service laundry, dry-cleaning, valet service, laundromat, ironing room, photographer, film processing.

Other: American Express foreign exchange and cash center, garage, kennel, safe-deposit boxes, Alcoholics Anonymous.

Access for the Disabled A few cabins have wide doors, low threshold ledges, and specially equipped bathrooms. However, wheelchairs may not be carried aboard tenders, so passengers who use wheelchairs may not have access to every port.

MS Sagafjord and MS Vistafjord

Specifications *Type of ship:* Luxury   *Passengers:* 618/749
mainstream   *Crew:* 320/390 (mainly
Type of cruise: Traditional   Scandinavian)
Size: Medium (24,474/24,492 tons) *Officers:* Norwegian
Number of cabins: 336/404   *Passenger/crew ratio:* 1.9 to 1
Outside cabins: 90%/81%   *Year built:* 1965/1973

Itinerary **Fall:** Fourteen-day cruises between Fort Lauderdale and Mon-
Sagafjord tréal may call at New York, Bermuda, Boston, Newport (RI),
Bar Harbor, Charlottetown (Prince Edward Island), St. John
(New Brunswick), Halifax, along the Saguenay Fjord, Québec
City, and Montréal. Fourteen-day cruises between Fort Lau-
derdale and Rio de Janeiro may call at Devil's Island (off
French Guiana); Fortaleza, Recife, Vitória, Salvador, and
Belém (Brazil); Tobago; and St. Thomas/St. John. Fourteen-
and 16-day loops out of Fort Lauderdale may call at St. Tho-
mas/St. John, St. Maarten/St. Martin, Montserrat, Guadeloupe, Barbados, St. Lucia, Grenada, Caracas/La Guaira,
Curaçao, Grand Cayman, Aruba, St. Barts, and Key West. **Winter–early Spring:** A three-month loop around the Pacific and
the Orient leaves Ft. Lauderdale, calling at St. Thomas; Barbados; Devil's Island; Recife, Salvador, Rio de Janeiro (Brazil);
the South Pacific; the Far East; Hawaii; Los Angeles; Cabo San
Lucas; Acapulco; Puerto Caldera (Costa Rica); along the Panama Canal; and Aruba. **Late Spring–Summer:** Ten- and 11-day
cruises between Vancouver and Anchorage/Seward call at
Ketchikan, Juneau, Skagway, Glacier Bay, Sitka, Valdez, Prince
William Sound, and Homer.

Port tax: $105–$190 per passenger.

Vistafjord **Fall:** Europe. **Winter:** Fourteen- and 16-day Panama Canal
Transits between Fort Lauderdale and Los Angeles may call
at Grand Cayman, Cartagena (Colombia), along the Canal,
Puerto Caldera (Costa Rica), Acapulco, Cabo San Lucas,
Aruba, and Ocho Rios (Jamaica). Eleven- and 13-day Carib-
bean loops out of Fort Lauderdale may call at St. Thomas/St.
John, Antigua, Guadeloupe, Barbados, St. Lucia, St.
Maarten/St. Martin, Grand Cayman, Montego Bay (Jamaica),
Curaçao, Grenada, Martinique, Nevis, St. Kitts, Aruba, and
Tortola. **Spring–Summer:** Europe.

Port tax: $95–$205 per passenger.

Overview Although built eight years later, the *Vistafjord* is the sister ship
of the *Sagafjord* and is operated in much the same way. The
Vistafjord is slightly longer and larger; cabins are the same
size, but the additional 65 staterooms mean more passengers
share the same amount of public space. In all other respects
there is almost no difference between the two ships. Their passengers tend to be older (late fifties and up) and more demand-
ing than those on the *Countess* and prefer the slower pace to
the hustle and bustle of the *QE2*.

The *Sagafjord* and *Vistafjord* add a Scandinavian touch to
Cunard's British demeanor. Both are superb vessels, renowned for their sophistication and elegance. The *Sagafjord*
has captured numerous cruise-industry awards, including Ship
of the Year," and it deserves every accolade: From the white-
glove service to the legendary cuisine, it is superb.

Although the *Sagafjord* and *Vistafjord* are much smaller than the *QE2*, low passenger capacity makes them roomier: Both the dining room and the Grand Ballroom can accommodate all passengers at once. The few public rooms are larger and more attractive than comparable rooms on other ships. Indirect lighting helps to highlight the original artwork and the delicate carvings positioned around the ships. Additional light, softened by the use of rich wood paneling and potted plants, emanates through large picture windows. The stern's elegant tiering of polished woods and white paint resembles a grand staircase.

Activities Activities offered—among them, lectures, dance classes, bridge tours, video golf lessons, and card and board games—reflect the sophisticated tastes of the ships' clientele. Recently, former Jacques Cousteau diver David Brown has begun giving live underwater broadcasts on the *Sagafjord*'s Alaskan cruises.

Dining Menus may be similar to those of other cruise lines, but the food preparation and service are outstanding. Meals are served in a single seating, with a large number of one- and two-person tables. Dinner is served between 7 and 9. Special dietary requests should be made one month in advance, but culinary cravings are accommodated with no fuss. All menus offer a healthy alternative, as well as a dessert suitable for diabetics. Every evening is at least semiformal. Both ships feature an extensive wine collection.

On the Lido Deck, early morning juice and coffee, breakfast and lunch buffets, mid-morning bouillon, and afternoon tea are served. Breakfast in the Lido includes hot entrées cooked to order. The lunch buffet offers great variety, from caviar and smoked salmon at the salad bar to grilled hot dogs and hamburgers. Room service is available at any time.

Entertainment Entertainment is more low-key—with less variety but more sophistication—than most. Instead of the gaudy Las Vegas–style revues of some lines, you're likely to find a jazz band, a concert pianist, or an operatic performer featured. On any given night passengers might watch a light musical revue, dance to two different orchestras, or enjoy cabaret in the charming double-decker Polaris nightclub.

Service and Tipping The staff are highly professional and dignified without being stuffy and are clearly interested in the convenience of the passengers. Tip the room steward $4 per passenger per diem, the waiter $5. A 15% gratuity is recommended for the wine steward.

Cabins and Rates

	Beds	Phone	TV	Sitting Area	Fridge	Tub	Per Diem
Luxury Suite	Q or T/D	●	●	●	●	●	$505–$1,252
Outside Double	Q or T	●	○	●	○	◑	$248–$654
Inside Double	T	●	○	●	○	◑	$216–$330

In keeping with the tone set by the rest of the ship, cabins and staterooms are attractive and spacious; closets and extra cabinets are plentiful. Some staterooms have verandas and even separate sitting rooms; most have large picture windows. Cabins have lockable strongboxes and full-length mirrors. Bathtubs are full-size. Lifeboats partially obstruct the view from some outside cabins on the Sun and Officers decks. Cabins on the Promenade Deck look out onto a public area, and some are actually between decks—with the floor of the upper-level Officers Deck cutting across the window.

Outlet voltage: 110 AC.

Single supplement: 175% of double-occupancy rate; some single rooms are available.

Discounts: A third or fourth passenger in a cabin pays $183–$277 per diem. You get a discount for arranging your own airfare.

Sports and Fitness **Health club:** Excellent below-decks facility, with stationary bikes, rowing machines, free weights, hydrocalisthenics, sauna, massage.

Walking/jogging: Promenade Deck (7 laps=1 mile).

Other sports: Aerobics and other exercise classes, golf driving, shuffleboard, table tennis, trapshooting, whirlpools, indoor pool, outdoor pool.

Facilities **Public rooms:** Four bars, three entertainment lounges, card room, small casino, cinema, library, Lido.

Shops: Gift shop, beauty salon, barbershop.

Health care: Doctor on call.

Child care: Baby-sitting can be arranged.

Services: Full-service laundry, dry-cleaning, valet service, laundromat, ironing room, photographer, film processing.

Other: Safe-deposit boxes, Alcoholics Anonymous.

Access for the Disabled Small travel wheelchairs are required to fit in cabin doorways and rest rooms. If advised in advance, the housekeeper will place a ramp over the ledge at the entrance to cabin bathrooms. However, bathrooms are often too small for wheelchair maneuvering. Elevators are accessible. Disabled passengers are assisted ashore on tenders when seas are calm.

Sea Goddess I

Specifications *Type of ship:* Luxury, yachtlike
Type of cruise: Traditional
Size: Very small (4,250 tons)
Number of cabins: 58
Outside cabins: 100%

Passengers: 116
Crew: 89 (American and European)
Officers: Norwegian
Passenger/crew ratio: 1.3 to 1
Year built: 1984

Itinerary **Fall:** Europe. **Winter:** Fourteen-day loops out of St. Thomas call at Virgin Gorda (British Virgin Islands), St. Maarten/St. Martin, St. Barts, St. Kitts, Martinique, St. Lucia, Mayreau (Grenadines), Barbados, Tobago, Devil's Island (off Guiana Coast), Nevis, Jost Van Dyke (British Virgin Islands), and St. John. There will be a few Amazon River cruises, too. **Spring–Summer:** Europe.

Port tax: $135 per passenger.

Overview *Sea Goddess I* was designed to raise the level of cruise luxury (and prices) to new heights, and largely, it has succeeded. Life aboard ship is unstructured, elegant, and unforgettable. Once you've paid the exorbitant fare, there are no more out-of-pocket expenses—no bar tabs, no bingo games. Like its twin ship *Sea Goddess II* (which doesn't sail in the Western Hemisphere), the *Sea Goddess I* looks like a royal yacht, with dramatic lines, upswept twin funnels, and a distinctive sports platform off the stern. But it is the attention to detail—the marble dance floor in the Main Salon, the lush decor of the Greenhouse, the fine Oriental rugs in the lobby—that really sets this ship apart. Its shallow draft allows it to anchor in out-of-the-way coves and unfrequented ports, where the stern's platform can be lowered for snorkeling, sailing, windsurfing, and swimming. Though small, this intimate, romantic ship offers ample room for 59 couples to enjoy what in many ways remains the trendsetter for luxurious vacations afloat. (The *Sea Goddess I* is also available for charter.)

Activities No structured activities are offered; passengers set their own pace. However, the staff is very accommodating, arranging entry to exclusive on-shore clubs for tennis, golf, gambling, and dancing. Special-interest cruises include lectures and seminars; epicurean cruises, for example, feature guest chefs and talks by California vintners. A Golden Door Spa fitness trainer offers exercise classes and designs personal programs.

Dining In the tradition of the finest restaurants, the kitchen caters to special requests, preparing dishes individually as they are ordered. The quality of the food is excellent but, given the limited kitchen space, not as good as that in the *QE2*'s Queen's Grill. Fine wines and after-dinner drinks are served, and Beluga caviar is dispensed as freely as the champagne. Two formal evenings are held each week, but passengers tend to dress elegantly even on casual nights. The Outdoor Café serves coffee, breakfast, and lunch, but full service is available any time. Room service will provide anything day or night, including full-course meals—all served on china and linen.

Entertainment Entertainment is understated, featuring perhaps a pianist or a dance trio in the piano bar, or local entertainment from the day's port of call. Many passengers visit the casinos or nightclubs in town while in port.

Service and Tipping With one of the best passenger-to-crew ratios, the ship offers attentive and personal service. The aim is to make you feel that all your needs, desires, and perhaps even fantasies will be fulfilled. An elegant black-tie midnight dinner for two on the deck? No problem. Chilled champagne and caviar brought ashore to you while you sunbathe in a quiet white-sand cove? You have but to ask. No tipping is allowed.

Cabins and Rates

	Beds	Phone	TV	Sitting Area	Fridge	Tub	Per Diem*
Suite	Q or T	●	●	●	●	●	$600–$900

Prices differ with itinerary; all cabins cost the same for each trip. Transatlantic cruises are less expensive than these quoted prices.

Cabins on the *Sea Goddess I* set the standard for modern seafaring comfort. Each has an electronic safe, a stereo, a remote-control color TV and VCR, and a minibar. The refrigerator can be stocked with any food from the kitchen or any liquor, wine, or beverage you'd like, at no charge; a personal-preference form is mailed to every passenger before sailing, so the crew can stock the cabin and the kitchen accordingly. A few suites have removable adjoining walls for those who want even more space and a second bathroom; the cost is about 150% of the single-cabin rate. Cabins on Deck Five look onto the Promenade. Cabin 315 is a larger suite that doesn't cost more.

Outlet voltage: 110 AC.

Single supplement: 150%–175% of double-occupancy rate.

Discounts: You get a 50% discount for booking consecutive cruises, a discount for arranging your own airfare.

Sports and Fitness **Health club:** Gym, sauna, massage, showers. Golden Door Spa personnel will develop individualized fitness programs.

Walking/jogging: Unobstructed circuit on open Promenade.

Other sports: Skeet shooting, water sports (windsurfing, snorkeling, sailing, waterskiing off the stern swimming platform), pool.

Facilities **Public rooms:** Three bars, two entertainment lounges, casino, greenhouse, library (including a large selection of VCR tapes), outdoor café (Lido), piano bar.

Shops: Gift shop, beauty salon/barber.

Health care: Doctor on call.

Child care: Baby-sitting can be arranged privately.

Services: Full-service laundry, dry-cleaning.

Access for the Disabled Cabin doorways and rest rooms are not large enough for wheelchairs. Also, passengers in wheelchairs may not be taken on launches at ports where the ship must anchor offshore, thus preventing them from going ashore.

Delta Queen Steamboat Company

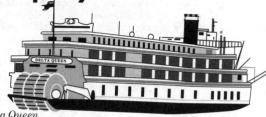

Boats *Delta Queen*
Mississippi Queen

Evaluation: Both boats (they're *not* ships) are authentic steam-driven paddle wheelers that churn along the river at a leisurely 19th-cen-
tury 6 or 7 mph (top speed: 12 mph). They are the only
remaining overnight river boats in the country and have a phe-
nomenal 95–99% occupancy rate. Nostalgia is the name of the
game on both boats, though the *Delta Queen* wins that contest,
hands down. The *DQ* is peaceful and quiet. The younger, glitz-
ier *Mississippi Queen* is sleek, modern, and lively. These floating wedding cakes are both outfitted in Victorian style with
gingerbread trim, Tiffany-type stained glass, polished brass,
crystal chandeliers, plush carpeting, and warm wood paneling.
Public areas have cushy leather wing chairs and handsomely
upholstered Chesterfield sofas. Both boats are fully air-conditioned. On deck, you can watch the country go by from oversize
wooden rocking chairs, old-fashioned porch swings, and white-
iron patio furniture—you can do so while munching freshly
made popcorn or a hot dog. Most passengers are well-heeled
retirees, many of whom return time and again. The Paddlewheel Steamboatin' Society of America Champagne and Punch
Reception for repeat passengers is a special feature. The size
of the two boats governs the scope of the on-board activities
and entertainment; these are covered separately in the individual boat evaluations.

A Riverlorean (the steamboat company's term for river historian) gives lively talks about the river, explains how to find mile
markers and read the river charts, answers questions, lends
books, and provides free binoculars. The captain's lecture is a
not-to-be-missed event. Passengers can try their hands at playing the calliopes. There's little pressure to participate in anything; you can do as little or as much as you like.

Dining Dinner on the *MQ* is a bit dressier than on the *DQ*, but formal
wear is never required. Five meals are served daily, and the
food is good but not outstanding—somewhat surprising since

Chart Symbols. *The following Symbols are used in the cabin
charts that accompany each ship's evaluation.* **D:** *Double bed;*
K: *King-size bed;* **Q:** *Queen-size bed;* **T:** *Twin bed;* **U/L:** *Upper
and lower berths;* ●: *All cabins have this facility;* ○: *No cabins
have this facility;* ◑: *Some cabins have this facility.*

the home port is New Orleans. The menu is more Continental than South Louisiana, and the renditions of regional dishes are on the mild side. Every menu includes at least one "Heart Smart" meal. Passengers with special dietary needs should notify the company a month in advance. "Theme" meals include an old-fashioned family-style picnic, with waiters in jeans passing around huge platters of fried chicken, barbecue ribs, cornbread, corn on the cob, potato salad, and such. Food presentation on the *MQ* is more spectacular than on the *DQ*. Also, the *MQ*'s 200-seat dining room is on the Observation Deck and offers better views; the only good river view in the low-lying *DQ* dining room is from a window seat. Both boats offer two assigned seatings (5:30 and 7) for dinner.

Ports of Call Because the Delta Queen Steamboat Company's ports are not covered in Chapter 4, we've tried to give you a general idea of how time is spent in most river ports on a typical river boat cruise. See individual boat evaluations for full list of ports.

The boats never paddle for more than two days without putting in to port, where they are usually docked for at least a half-day. Things are done at a leisurely pace on the river. Shore excursions are to plantation homes, historic towns and Civil War battlefields, sleepy villages, and major metropolises along the rivers. Tours are either by bus or on foot, and, since there are scores of ports, there is a wide range. The excursions to Houmas House plantation ($5.50 adults, $4 children) and Nottoway Plantation ($8 adults, $3.50 children) involve a stroll at your leisure across the levee and the lawn; tickets can be purchased on board or at the house. A $22, 2½-hour bus tour at Vicksburg is an evening in an antebellum home with dessert and coffee and a performance of John Maxwell's one-man show, "Oh, Mr. Faulkner, Do You Write?". The Battlefield and Siege Tour ($19.50 adults, $15.50 children) is a 3-hour bus tour of the vast Vicksburg National Military Park. In Iowa, gambling is the name of the game on the *Dubuque Casino Belle*, a $9.95, 3½-hour cruise on a four-deck riverboat with slot and poker machines and 26 gaming tables. The most expensive excursion is the Dubuque Victorian House Tour and Progressive Dinner, a 4½-hour bus tour ($45 per person).

In no event is there any pressure to buy a shore excursion, and in some ports the steamboat company provides a free shuttle into town. The latter option is fine if you want to poke around on your own; however, the shore excursions are narrated and take you to plantation homes that you can't always reach on foot. In other ports, you can simply amble down the gangplank and walk into town.

Two special events should be noted: One is the annual Great Steamboat Race, an 11-day cruise from New Orleans to St. Louis that takes place over the Fourth of July. It replicates the famous 19th-century race between the *Natchez* and the *Robert E. Lee*. This is a wildly popular cruise, with the crews competing in various contests and passengers gussied up for the annual Floozy Contest. With their flags flying and calliopes whistling away, the boats race at a dizzying 12 mph or so, while landlubbers line the shore and cheer them on. At Christmas, the Bonfire cruises are also enormously popular. Replicating an age-old Cajun custom (the bonfires light the way for Papa Noel), a huge bonfire is torched, and there is a spectacular fireworks display. Shores and boat decks are lined with folks shouting Christmas greetings back and forth—And Papa Noel does pay a visit.

Service and Tipping The staff and crew are extraordinarily friendly and helpful, not at all intrusive. Dining room service is superb. The night before debarkation, instructions and envelopes for tips are left in each stateroom. Tip waiters, waitresses, and cabin attendants $3.50 per person per night; busboys $2.25 per person per night; maître d's $5 per couple per cruise; porters $1.50 per bag. An automatic 15% is added to wine and bar purchases.

For More Information Delta Queen Steamboat Co. (Robin Street Wharf, New Orleans, LA 70130, tel. 504/586–0631 or 800/543–1949).

Delta Queen

Specifications

Type of boat: Paddle-wheel Steamboat	*Passengers:* 182
Type of cruise: Upscale Excursion/theme	*Crew:* 75 (American)
	Officers: American
Size: Small (1,650 tons)	*Passenger/crew ratio:* 2.4 to 1
Number of cabins: 91	*Year built:* 1926
Outside cabins: 100%	

Itinerary **Year-round:** Three- to 12-day cruises leave New Orleans, Memphis, St. Louis, Louisville, Nashville, Pittsburgh, St. Paul, and Chattanooga, calling at Burnside, White Castle, Baton Rouge and St. Francisville (LA); West Feliciana, Natchez, and Vicksburg (MS); New Madrid (MO); Cairo and Chester (IL); Cape Girardeau, St. Genevieve, and Hannibal (MO); Burlington and Dubuque (IA); Prairie du Chien (WI); Winona and Wabash (MN); Wellsburg and Blennerhasset Island (WV); Marietta and Portsmouth (OH); Maysville, Paducah, and Henderson (KY); Madison (IN); Cave-In-Rock (IL); Dover and Lake Barkley (TN); and Florence and Decatur (AL).

Port tax: $30 per passenger.

Overview If the *Delta Queen* were a song she'd be "Up the Lazy River." This grande dame of America's most famous river first sailed the waters of the Sacramento River and served her country during World War II as a U.S. Navy ferry on San Francisco Bay. She began cruising the Mississippi River System after World War II. In the late '60s, due to federal legislation banning boats with wooden superstructures, she seemed doomed for demolition, but the hue and cry raised by preservationists and nostalgia buffs resulted in a congressional exemption, under which she still sails. The tiny four-decker is a designated National Historic Landmark and is listed on the National Register of Historic Places.

Activities A person can while away a fair amount of time just sitting on deck in a rocking chair or swing. The *DQ* is really not for type A personalities. Bingo and bridge, quilting and hat-making, trivia and kite-flying contests are about as hectic as things get. Free tours are conducted of the Pilot House, and passengers are encouraged to visit the engine room and have a cup of coffee with the crew, who will cheerfully show you how the engines and the 44-ton paddle operate.

Entertainment The boat is so small the dining room has to do extra duty as a lecture and concert hall, a movie theater, and a nightclub. As a result, there is a great deal of moving about chairs and tables between meals and during various functions. The nightly floor shows range from outstanding classical ragtime concerts to corny country hoedowns. Jokes and music are geared toward the older crowd. After the show, the orchestra plays music for dancing, while up in the Texas Lounge a pianist/vocalist entertains with standards and show tunes, mostly from the '40s and '50s, as she does during the cocktail hour. Sing-alongs are also popular, and the Texas Lounge features a great Dixieland band.

Cabins and Rates

	Beds	Phone	TV	Sitting Area	Fridge	Tub	Per Diem
Outside Superior Suite	Q or T	○	○	●	○	●	$565–$570
Outside Luxury Suite Suite	Q	○	○	●	○	○	$480–$485
Outside Superior Stateroom	Q or T	○	○	○	○	○	$408–$410
Outside Deluxe Stateroom	T	○	○	○	○	○	$378–$380
Outside Deluxe Stateroom	T or D	○	○	○	○	○	$344–$345
Outside Stateroom	T	○	○	○	○	○	$283–$285
Outside Stateroom	U/L	○	○	○	○	○	$243–$245

One of the standard jokes aboard the *DQ* is, "You didn't realize that the brochure picture of your cabin was actual size, did you?" They *are* quite tiny (baths are minuscule), but all cabins are outside. A slight disadvantage here is that in order to have any privacy it's necessary to keep your shades or shutters closed; there is a lot of activity on the wraparound decks. Accommodations on the Cabin Deck have inside entrances, while those on the Sun and Texas Decks have outside entrances. All have amenity packages, wall-to-wall carpeting, wood paneling, and limited closet and storage space. Cabins 307 and 308 are up front, on either side of the Pilot House. Cabins 117, 118, 121, and 122 on the Cabin Deck, and 207, 208, 231, and 232 on the Texas Deck have partially obstructed river views. Complimentary Champagne, fresh fruit, and cheese are provided passengers in suites and Superior Staterooms.

Outlet voltage: 110 AC.

Single supplement: 175%–200% of double-occupancy rate.

Other discounts: No cabins accommodate third or fourth passengers. Airfare is not included in rates. There is a discount for booking early.

Sports and Fitness **Health club:** Stationary bike, rowing machine.

Walking/jogging: Three wrap-around decks.

Facilities **Public rooms:** Three lounges, restaurant.

Shops: Gift shop.

Health care: No doctor on board, but the boats are never far from shore.

Child care: Passengers may make private baby-sitting arrangements with a crew member.

Access for Disabled The *Delta Queen* cannot accommodate passengers in wheelchairs. However, disabled passengers can travel aboard the boat provided they can traverse stairways. Every effort is made to assist the physically disabled.

Mississippi Queen

Specifications: *Type of ship:* Paddle wheel steamboat
Type of cruise: Upscale Excursion/theme
Size: Small (3,364 tons)
Number of cabins: 211
Outside cabins: 64%

Passengers: 436
Crew: 160 (American)
Officers: American
Passenger/crew ratio: 2.6 to 1
Year built: 1976

Itinerary Same as *Delta Queen.*

Overview The seven-deck *Mississippi Queen* is the largest steamboat ever built; her huge calliope is the world's largest. She was built in 1976 at a cost of $27 million and refurbished in 1989. There is infinitely more space, in public areas, on decks, and in the cabins. Some passengers debark without ever having completely gotten their bearings. Affluent seniors constitute the majority, but you also see more young people and children here than on the *DQ.*

Activities In addition to bingo, bridge, masquerades, lectures, and contests, the *MQ* offers a gym with exercise machines, Swedish massage, and aerobics classes; a sauna; whirlpool; shuffleboard; full-service beauty shop (perms, cuts, facials, manicures); a first-run movie theater (*Showboat* is frequently screened); a library; and a conference center with audiovisual equipment. As on the *DQ,* tours are conducted of the Pilot House (but not the engine room).

Entertainment The *MQ* is twice the size of the *DQ,* with a separate Grand Saloon for floor shows, and the entertainment is decidedly splashier. There are cabarets with Dixieland bands, ragtime and rinky-dink piano sessions, banjo players, and singers and dancers; the *MQ*'s renditions of the Andrews Sisters, Sophie Tucker, and Al Jolson; Mardi Gras bashes; Broadway-style show revues; and barbershop quartets. The company also follows the current trend of employing "dance hosts", whose job it is to dance with single female passengers. The bars and lounges are large and lively—the Paddlewheel Lounge is a glitzy, two-tier affair on the Observation and Cabin decks.

Cabins and Rates

	Beds	Phone	TV	Sitting Area	Fridge	Tub	Per Diem
Superior Veranda Suite	Q or T	●	○	●	○	●	$565–$570

Luxury Veranda Suite	T	●	○	●	○	●	$480–$485
Deluxe Veranda Suite	T	●	○	●	○	●	$408–$410
Deluxe Veranda Stateroom	T	●	○	●	○	○	$378–$380
Outside Stateroom	T or D	●	○	○	○	○	$344–$345
Inside Stateroom	T or U/L	●	○	○	○	○	$283–$285
Inside Stateroom	U/L	●	○	○	○	○	$243–$245

The *MQ* is not only much larger and more luxurious but also affords more privacy. While none of the staterooms is huge, 94 of them have private verandas, and though some are quite small, they're great places to settle in and contemplate the river in peace and quiet. This boat has much more activity than the *DQ* and can be noisy. Cabins have amenity packages, wall-to-wall carpeting, and wood paneling. Closet and storage space, while not vast, is more generous than on the *DQ*. Inside cabins, however, are not for the claustrophobic. Two suites are adjacent to the Pilot House, with windows facing forward and to the side for a captain's-eye view of the river; two are adjacent to the paddle wheel, with its lulling, sleep-inducing sounds. Cabins 131, 132, 220, 221, 327, and 328 have partially obstructed river views. Some suites have twin beds that can be pushed together to make a king bed as well as sofa beds; others have two single beds and a day-bed, two single beds, additional fold-away upper berths or a lower single bed and a fold-away single upper berth. Complimentary Champagne, fresh fruit, and cheese are provided passengers in suites and Superior Staterooms.

Outlet voltage: 110 AC.

Single supplement: 175%–200% of double-occupancy rate.

Other discounts: A third passenger in a cabin pays $100 per diem. Airfare is not included in rates. You get a discount for booking early.

Sports and Fitness **Health club:** Stationary bike, treadmill, aerobics classes, stairclimber.

Walking/jogging: Unobstructed decks.

Other: Shuffleboard, sauna, whirlpool spa, massage.

Facilities **Public rooms:** Two bars, two lounges, showroom, lecture hall, activity center, game room, library, theater/conference center.

Shops: Gift shop, beauty/barber shop.

Health care: No doctor on board, but the boats are never far from shore.

Child care: Passengers may make private baby-sitting arrangements with a staff or crew member.

Access for Disabled Fold-away wheelchairs are available, and every attempt is made to assist disabled passengers. Elevators and wide hallways accommodate wheelchairs; however, bathroom doors and stateroom doors are only 24 inches wide, have raised thresholds, and will not accommodate wheelchairs. Persons with a physical disability or requiring a wheelchair are advised to travel with a companion who can assist them.

Diamond Cruise Inc.

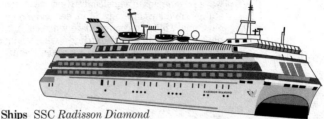

Ships SSC *Radisson Diamond*

Evaluation Diamond Cruise Inc., a Finnish Company, basks in the world-wide reputation of its partner, Radisson Hotels International, which handles all hotel operations and marketing. Impeccable service and attention to detail, along with a private-club ambience, give the *Diamond* the feel of a seagoing Radisson hotel. Although no new Diamond ships are under construction, sister ships are planned over the next few years. Simultaneously, Radisson is developing a new cruise division. Its first ship, the superluxury *Kungsholm*, will debut in 1995.

Activities In keeping with the ship's relaxed mood, there are few onboard organized events. People gather informally around such activities as dancing lessons, card games, backgammon, shuffleboard. The *Diamond* also has an extensive book and videotape library. At least once a cruise, water activities are held off the large marina platform, which is built into the stern of the ship and lowers into the water. Passengers can swim in a small netted swimming pool, ride on a Jet ski, or snorkel. For a fun science fiction–like adventure, the brave should try swimming between the ship's twin hulls.

The *Diamond* offers some interesting alternatives to the usual shore excursions: In St. Maarten you can race on an "America's Cup" 12-meter sailboat. In the *Diamond*'s "Best of the Best" Series, with sports greats, authors, and musicians, focus is on intimate casual discussions with such celebs as James Michner.

Dining Dining aboard the *Diamond* reflects its elegant and exclusive demeanor. Meals are served at one open seating in the Grand Dining Room, so you dine when and with whomever you want. The cuisine is international, taking advantage of each port's fresh foods. There's one formal night per cruise, with relaxed elegant attire the norm other evenings. Breakfast and lunch buffets are served in the Grill, but light à la carte service is also available. At night the Grill is transformed into an intimate gourmet Italian bistro with one seating—run by a couple who came on board to create a small restaurant similar to the one they own in northern Italy, there is a casual congenial atmosphere here. Six wonderful courses are served from a fixed

---

Chart Symbols. *The following symbols are used in the cabin charts that accompany each ship's evaluation.* **D:** *Double bed;* **K:** *King-size bed;* **Q:** *Queen-size bed;* **T:** *Twin bed;* **U/L:** *Upper and lower berths;* ●: *All cabins have this facility;* ○: *No cabins have this facility;* ◑: *Some cabins have this facility*

menu. Reservations should be made as soon as you board, because the restaurant is very popular. Room service is available 24 hours a day from an extensive menu, and you can even order dinner, which arrives complete with linen napery, crystal, china, and flowers. A Continental breakfast buffet is served daily beginning at 6:30 AM, and afternoon tea is served with rich pastries in the Windows Lounge.

Entertainment Evening entertainment is generally mellow and consists of cabaret-style shows, a pianist, a small musical combo, and comedians. Partiers can stay as late as they like in the disco and the casino.

Service and Tipping Diamond Cruise Inc. has a no tipping policy.

For More Information Diamond Cruise Inc. (Concorde Centre, 2875 N.E. 191st St., Suite 304, North Miami Beach, FL 33180, tel. 800/333–3333).

SSC Radisson Diamond

Type of ship: Luxury
Type of cruise: Traditional
Size: Small (20,000 tons)
Number of Cabins: 177
Outside cabins: 100%

Passengers: 354
Crew: 192 (international)
Officers: Finnish
Passenger/Crew Ratio: 1.8 to 1
Year built: 1992

Itinerary **Early Fall:** In the Mediterranean. **Late Fall–Spring:** Three-, four-, and seven-, and ten-night loops out of San Juan call at Key West, Grand Cayman, San Andres Island, Play del Carmen, Cozumel, and Puerto Caldera (Costa Rica).

Port tax: $45–$105 per passenger.

Overview When the 324-passenger *Radisson Diamond* set sail in May 1992, it was the largest twin-hull ship ever constructed specifically for cruising. The futuristic design resembles a spider perched over the sea but actually makes the ship more stable. While you are less likely to get seasick and won't find your legs rubbery when you first step on land, the difference in motion takes some getting used to. During a storm there is none of the normal pitch and roll, but stabilizers cause a very slight side-to-side jerking motion—which only becomes an issue if you are wearing high heels and trying to keep your balance.

The *Diamond* is pure class all the way, catering to the passenger who has seen many ships and has specific demands of a cruise ship. The staff is very flexible and its small-European-hotel ambience is accentuated by a staff of female Austrian, Swiss, and Scandinavian cabin stewardesses. In the dining room, more than 60% of the staff is female. Reflecting its connection with Radisson, the *Diamond* has excellent meeting space and a business center.

Cabins and Rates

	Beds	Phone	TV	Sitting Area	Fridge	Tub	Per Diem
Master Suite	Q or T	●	●	●	●	●	$900
Suite w/balcony	Q or T	●	●	●	●	●	$600
Suite w/window	Q or T	●	●	●	●	●	$600

Cabins are on the outside of the three upper decks and have unobstructed views. Most have a private balcony, others have a large bay window. Soothing mauve or sea-green fabrics are accented by birchwood, and each cabin has a stocked minibar and refrigerator. Bathrooms are spacious, with marble vanities, tubs, and hair driers.

Outlet voltage: 110 AC.

Single supplement: 125% of double-occupancy rate.

Sports and Fitness **Health club:** Aerobics studio, weight room, Lifecycles, Lifesteps, Liferowers, Jacuzzi and body-toning spa with massage and herbal-wrap treatments.

Walking/jogging: Unobstructed track on the top deck.

Other sports: Golf driving range with nets, putting green, mini-golf game, shuffleboard, skeet shooting, and watersports, including snorkeling, windsurfing, jet-skiing, and swimming.

Facilities **Public rooms:** Two restaurants, four bars, entertainment lounge, disco, casino, library, conference center with state-of-the-art video and sound systems.

Shops: Boutique, drug store, beauty salon/barber.

Health care: Doctor on call.

Child care: Though children are not discouraged, no child-care services exist.

Services: Full-service laundry, photographer, film-developing service, and business center with software library, fax, publishing facilities, personal computer hookups.

Other: Safe-deposit boxes.

Access for the Disabled Elevators are accessible to passengers in wheelchairs, and there are two cabins designed to accommodate wheelchairs. Public lavatories are also equipped for wheelchairs.

Dolphin/Majesty Cruise Lines

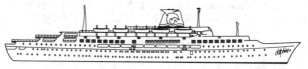

Dolphin IV

Ships SS *Dolphin IV*
SS *Oceanbreeze*
MV *Royal Majesty*
SS *Seabreeze*

Evaluation Because of Dolphin's reputation for offering popular economy cruises, its construction of an upscale luxury liner—the *Royal Majesty*—necessitated the creation of a separate cruise line. Majesty Cruise Line has begun to earn a new place in the luxury market by offering deluxe amenities, oversize cabins, top-quality entertainment, and culinary excellence. While there never has been anything fancy about a Dolphin cruise, passengers get their money's worth, and perhaps a bit more—which keeps a loyal following coming back again and again. Unlike most lower-price cruise lines, Dolphin offers a comprehensive shipboard account system: Passengers sign for all purchases and settle their accounts at the end of the cruise. The tiny island that the *Dolphin IV* visits for its beach party is one of the most picturesque of all those used by cruise lines.

Activities The selection on both lines is typical, including bingo, pool games, grandparents' teas, scavenger hunts, dance classes, and trivia contests.

Dining Menus are extensive and innovative, and food quality is well above average. Buffet breakfast and lunch in the open-air cafés are excellent, by any standard. Waiters hustle and go out of their way to please; what's more, they're genuinely friendly, not just tip-hungry. There are two assigned seatings per meal. A pianist entertains at dinnertime. Make special dietary requests in writing seven days before sailing. Other food service includes 24-hour self-serve coffee and tea, afternoon cookies and cake, a midnight buffet, and 24-hour room service.

Entertainment The usual variety shows, masquerade parties, and dance orchestras are offered. Occasionally, celebrity guests are invited to mingle and perform; such cruises carry a $100 surcharge per passenger.

Chart Symbols. *The following symbols are used in the cabin charts that accompany each ship's evaluation.* **D:** *Double bed;* **K:** *King-size bed;* **Q:** *Queen-size bed;* **T:** *Twin bed;* **U/L:** *Upper and lower berths;* **●:** *All cabins have this facility;* **○:** *No cabins have this facility;* **◑:** *Some cabins have this facility*

Service and Tipping	The staff are energetic, thorough, and unusually personable. Tip the room steward and the waiter each $2.50 per passenger per diem, the busboy $1.25. The maître d' should get $2 per passenger per cruise, the wine steward or bartender 15% of your final tab.
For More Information	Dolphin/Majesty Cruise Lines (901 South America Way, Miami, FL 33132, tel. 800/992–4299).

SS Dolphin IV

Specifications	*Type of ship:* Economy mainstream *Type of cruise:* Traditional *Size:* Small (13,007 tons) *Number of cabins:* 294 *Outside cabins:* 70.4%	*Passengers:* 588 *Crew:* 294 (international) *Officers:* Greek *Passenger/crew ratio:* 2.1 to 1 *Year built:* 1956

Itinerary	**Year-round:** Three- and four-night loops leave Miami Fridays and Mondays, overnighting in Nassau, with a beach party excursion to Blue Lagoon Island (Bahamas), and a stop at Key West on four-night cruises.
	Port tax: $61–$65 per passenger.
Overview	The *Dolphin IV* was the freighter *Ithaca* before Dolphin bought it 10 years ago; it was last renovated in 1990. A masterful conversion enlarged the ship's superstructure and gave the stern a terrace. The ship's design yields more usable space than most other small ships, although it carries a comparatively high number of passengers. The interior combines classic wood paneling and brass trim with bright, upbeat colors and large windows. The Barbizon Restaurant is narrow, with a low ceiling, but mirrors along the walls help create a sense of space and light. The Lido is remarkably well organized, with service divided between a cold buffet and a barbecue; passengers seldom must stand in line. Indeed, for comfort, convenience, and variety, the *Dolphin IV*'s Lido is one of the best. The disco, however, is small and claustrophobic, located on one of the lower decks and accessible only via a flight of steep steps.

Cabins and Rates

	Beds	Phone	TV	Sitting Area	Fridge	Tub	Per Diem*
Junior Suite	D	●	○	●	○	○	$259–$292
Outside	D, T, or U/L	●	○	○	○	○	$188–$249
Inside	D, T, or U/L	●	○	○	○	○	$141–$156

*Prices quoted are for four-night cruises; per diem prices for three-night cruises are usually slightly higher.

Cabins are small but perfectly adequate for short cruises. Views from the outside cabins on the Boat Deck are partially obstructed.

Outlet voltage: 110/220 AC.

Single supplement: 150% of double-occupancy rate.

Discounts: A third or fourth passenger in a cabin pays $445–$505 per cruise. You get a discount of up to $200 per passenger for booking 90 days in advance and a discount of $50–$150 for arranging your own airfare.

Sports and Fitness **Walking/jogging:** Unobstructed circuit on Boat Deck.

Other sports: Aerobics, table tennis, shuffleboard, skeet shooting, pool.

Facilities **Public rooms:** Four bars, two entertainment lounges, card room, casino, disco, small library/movie room, indoor and out-door Lidos, video-game room.

Shops: Gift shop, beauty salon/barber.

Health care: Doctor on call.

Child care: Playroom, baby-sitting, youth programs with counselors during summer and holidays.

Services: Photographer.

Other: Safe-deposit boxes.

Access for the Disabled Elevators and several public areas are not accessible, but public lavatories are equipped for standard-size wheelchairs. Cabins on the Atlantis Deck, the Boat Deck, or the forward Barbizon Deck are recommended for passengers using wheelchairs; they must be accompanied by a an able-bodied companion.

SS Oceanbreeze

Specifications *Type of ship:* Mainstream
Type of cruise: Traditional
Size: Medium (21,486 tons)
Number of cabins: 384
Outside cabins: 61.3%

Passengers: 776
Crew: 310 (international)
Officers: Greek
Passenger/crew ratio: 2.5 to 1
Year built: 1955

Itinerary **Year-round:** Alternating seven-day loops leave Aruba Sundays, calling at Bonaire, Grenada, Barbados, Martinique, and Curaçao; or Cartagena (Colombia), Gatun Lake (along the Panama Canal), the San Blas Islands (near Panama), and Curaçao.

Port tax: $108–$133 per passenger.

Overview The *Oceanbreeze* is the latest addition to Dolphin's fleet, having joined the line in May 1992. It's also one of only two ships based in Aruba. Fans of the now defunct Admiral Cruise Lines may remember the *Oceanbreeze* in its former life as the *Azure Seas.* After extensive renovations, things are a little different on the ship these days. Though it is still no luxury ship, Dolphin has brightened the decor, remodeled cabins, and added a children's room where they and their parents can romp endlessly with Fred Flintstone, Yogi Bear, and other members of the Hanna–Barbera cartoon family. Probably the ship's most stunning feature is the huge two-level casino on the Boat and Promenade decks, where you can chance it on 123 slot machines or try your luck in every other kind of gambling endeavor imaginable.

The atmosphere is decidedly festive and upbeat. Passengers are welcomed aboard with an introductory show and verbal tour of the ship in the Rendezvous Lounge. As is often the case with new ships, the staff, as of early 1993, seemed a bit disoriented and unpolished, though enthusiastic nonetheless. Every so often passengers would show up for an event or movie, only to find that no staff member could be found. If this should happen to you, you might head up to the comfy Mayfair lounge, have a drink, and make the best of it. The evening entertainment is lively and professional; rollicking theme nights include country-and-western and rock 'n' roll parties.

Cabins and Rates

	Beds	Phone	TV	Sitting Area	Fridge	Tub	Per Diem
Penthouse Suite	D	●	●	●	●	●	$328–$349
Outside	D	●	○	○	○	○	$249–$313
Inside Stateroom	D	●	○	○	○	○	$164-$270

Because this is an older vessel, cabins are fairly large. All have a double or two lower beds, plenty of closet and dresser space, and carpeting and are equipped minimally, with climate control and a radio. The new decor is a tasteful array of muted blues, pinks, and greens. The lush Owner's Suite is a two-bedroom pad with all the usual amenities plus a minibar.

Outlet voltage: 110/220 AC.

Single supplement: 150% of double-occupancy rate.

Discounts: A third or fourth passenger in a cabin pays $130–140 per diem. You get a discount of up to $900 per passenger for early booking, and up to $450 for arranging your own airfare.

Sports and Fitness **Health club:** Exercise equipment, whirlpool, sauna.

Other sports: Heated pool.

Facilities **Public rooms:** Three bars, lounges, casino, cinema, two dining rooms, disco, Lido, meeting room, video arcade, card room/library.

Shops: Gift shop, beauty salon/barber.

Health care: Doctor on call.

Child care: Playroom, baby-sitting, youth programs with counselors during holidays or in summer.

Services: Full-service laundry, dry-cleaning, photographer, film processing.

Other: Safe-deposit boxes.

Access for the Disabled Passengers with disabilities must be self-sufficient and travel with an able-bodied adult companion.

MV Royal Majesty

Specifications *Type of ship:* Mainstream
Type of cruise: Traditional
Size: Medium (32,400 tons)
Number of cabins: 544
Outside cabins: 71%

Passengers: 1,056
Crew: 500 (international)
Officers: Greek
Passenger/crew ratio: 2.1 to 1
Year built: 1992

Itinerary **Year-round:** Three-night loops leave Miami, calling at Nassau, with a beach party excursion to Royal Isle. Four-night loops leave Miami, calling at Cozumel/Playa del Carmen (Mexico) and Key West. Occasional seven-night loops combine the two itineraries.

Port tax: $63–$68 per passenger.

Overview With a smoke-free restaurant and a number of smoke-free staterooms, the *Royal Majesty* appeals to a discriminating clientele seeking deluxe pampering on a shorter itinerary. The "royal" theme is carried through the generously proportioned public areas, from the Queen of Hearts Card Room to the House of Lords Executive Conference Room to the Royal Fireworks Lounge. Excellent use of light creates bright, spacious public areas from which passengers can enjoy fine sea views. The Royal Observatory Panorama Bar is a favorite perch from which to watch the ship pull into and out of ports of call.

While other ships slip a daily activities schedule beneath passengers' doors, the *Royal Majesty* presents the days' events via closed-circuit in-cabin TV. In addition to an excellent culinary slate in the main dining room, the outdoor Café Royale serves buffet lunch and breakfast, and the Piazza San Marco pizza and ice cream parlor is great for a late-night snack. Service is good, the staff polite and well-trained. In a push toward environmental consciousness, the ship has its own sewage- and garbage-treatment plants; glass and metal are recycled ashore.

Cabins and Rates

	Beds	Phone	TV	Sitting Area	Fridge	Tub	Per Diem
Royal Suite	D	●	●	●	●	○	$388–$530
Suite	D	●	●	●	●	○	$317–$396
Outside	T/D	●	●	○	○	○	$232–$274
Inside	T/D	●	●	○	○	○	$134–$149

Staterooms have fluffy robes, color TV, five channels of music, direct-dial ship-to-shore telephones, hair dryers, security safes, and ironing boards. Each suite has a minibar, a queen-size bed, and an enormous ocean-view picture window.

Outlet voltage: 110 AC.

Single supplement: 150% of double-occupancy rate.

Discounts: A third or fourth passenger in a cabin pays $150 per diem. You get a discount of up to $100 for arranging your own airfare and a discount of $50 per passenger if you book 100 days in advance.

Sports and Fitness **Health club:** Spa with state-of-the-art workout equipment.

Walking/jogging: Jogging track on Princess Deck.

Other sports: Pool, two whirlpools.

Facilities **Public rooms:** Showroom, dining room, outdoor café, pizza/ice cream parlor, three bars, casino, disco, meeting room, conference room, card room, library.

Shops: Gift shop, beauty salon.

Child care: Playroom, splash pool.

Services: Photographer.

Access for the Disabled:	The ship is fully accessible, including four passenger elevators, rest rooms on various decks, and four specially equipped staterooms.

SS Seabreeze

Specifications	*Type of ship:* Economy mainstream *Type of cruise:* Traditional *Size:* Medium (21,000 tons) *Number of cabins:* 421 *Outside cabins:* 62.5%	*Passengers:* 840 *Crew:* 400 (international) *Officers:* Greek *Passenger/crew ratio:* 2.1 to 1 *Year built:* 1958

Itinerary **Year-round:** Alternating seven-day loops leave Miami Saturdays, calling at Nassau and Blue Lagoon Island (Bahamas), San Juan, and St. Thomas/St. John; or Grand Cayman, Montego Bay (Jamaica), and Cozumel/Playa del Carmen (Mexico).

Port tax: $73–$78 per passenger.

Overview The *Seabreeze* was completely refurbished when it joined the Dolphin fleet in 1989, having previously seen service as Premier's *Royale* and Costa's *Frederico 'C.* The exterior is not beautiful, with twin cargo booms on the fo'c'sle, a bulky superstructure, and a large, squarish stack amidships. But the *Seabreeze* does offer plenty of deck space, easily accommodating the small swimming pool and three honeycomb-shaped whirlpools—maybe the most popular attractions on board. The interior is decorated in electric reds, purples, and oranges. Offsetting these gaudy hues are more traditional naval touches, such as teak decks and brass fixtures.

Cabins and Rates

	Beds	Phone	TV	Sitting Area	Fridge	Tub	Per Diem
Suite	Q or T	●	○	●	○	●	$250–$265
Deluxe Outside	D or T	●	○	○	○	◐	$228–$242
Superior Outside	D or T	●	○	○	○	◐	$221–$235
Large Outside	D or T	●	○	○	○	◐	$214–$228
Outside	D, T, or U/L	●	○	○	○	○	$204–$218
Inside	D, T, or U/L	●	○	○	○	○	$158–$206

Cabins are small and simply furnished but pleasant. Outside cabins on the Daphne Deck look onto a public promenade, and the view from most outside cabins on La Bohème Deck is obstructed by lifeboats.

Outlet voltage: 110/220 AC.

Single supplement: 150% of double-occupancy rate.

Discounts: A third or fourth passenger in a cabin pays $99 per diem. You get a discount of up to $700 per passenger for early booking, up to $250 for arranging your own airfare, and additional discounts for booking consecutive eastern and western Caribbean cruises.

Sports and Fitness   **Health club:** Exercise equipment, two whirlpools, massage.

Walking/jogging: Unobstructed jogging circuit.

Other sports: Aerobics, basketball, golf driving, table tennis, scuba and snorkeling lessons, shuffleboard, skeet shooting, pool.

Facilities   **Public rooms:** Five bars, four entertainment lounges, casino, cinema, dining room, disco, Lido, piano bar, video-game room.

Shops: Gift shop, beauty salon/barber.

Health care: Doctor on call.

Child care: Playroom, baby-sitting, youth programs with counselors during holidays or in summer.

Services: Full-service laundry, dry-cleaning, photographer, film processing.

Other: Safe-deposit boxes, Alcoholics Anonymous.

Access for the Disabled   Public areas are accessible, although bathroom and cabin entrances have door sills. Cabin bathroom doorways are 20″ wide. Passengers who use a wheelchair must travel with an able-bodied adult companion.

Fantasy Cruises

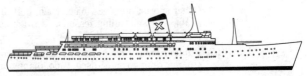

Amerikanis

Ships   SS *Amerikanis*
SS *Britanis*

Evaluation   Fantasy makes no claim to be a luxury line; it is, rather, the budget version of its upscale sister, Celebrity Cruises—both owned by the family-run Chandris Inc. Lively, organized activities and plentiful shore excursions characterize Fantasy cruises, which are among the least expensive available. Not surprisingly, the low prices and many discounts—available to senior citizens, honeymooners, and even groups of friends—attract people on a budget. A large share of passengers are young couples (average age: mid-forties) with children—Fantasy is one of the few lines that lets children under 12 sail free on some cruises.

Unfortunately, it's difficult to forget about money once you're aboard; Fantasy charges for services that are often complimentary on other lines. For instance, passengers must pay for fruit baskets in their cabins, put $5 deposits on library books, and shell out $3 to have the photographer take a particular shot. The pressure from the crew to tip can be annoying, too. Fantasy is also a cash-and-carry cruise line: Only bar drinks can be signed for—everything else must be paid for in cash. Even with the additional charges, however, Fantasy cruises remain among the most competitively priced on the market.

The cruise ships themselves are the oldest in the Americas, but they have a character that is often missing on the large, impersonal cruise ships being built today. If you prefer your cruise ship to have more polish than personality, Fantasy Cruises may not be for you.

Activities   Shipboard life centers on organized group games, including such mainstays as trivia and dance contests, the shipboard version of the Honeymoon Game, and poolside boy/girl teams for beer drinking or greased-pole fights. The atmosphere is convivial and decidedly informal, with passengers often finding themselves caught up in a bridge game with the sociable Greek officers. Impromptu Greek dance classes are not uncommon.

Chart Symbols. *The following symbols are used in the cabin charts that accompany each ship's evaluation.* **D:** *Double bed;* **K:** *King-size bed;* **Q:** *Queen-size bed;* **T:** *Twin bed;* **U/L:** *Upper and lower berths;* ●: *All cabins have this facility;* ○: *No cabins have this facility;* ◐: *Some cabins have this facility*

Dining Dining-room seating arrangements consist of two seatings per meal, with passengers assigned to tables. Cuisine, tailored to the American palate, features such standbys as lobster and steak, cream soups, cakes, and ice cream. Although the food is among the best-prepared and best-presented on any budget line, service is sometimes slow. Special dietary requests should be made in writing at least two weeks before sailing. Two formal evenings are held each week. Early morning tea or coffee and breakfast and lunch buffets are served on the Lido. Other food service includes mid-morning bouillon, afternoon tea, and a midnight buffet. Room service from a limited menu is available 24 hours.

Entertainment Fantasy's entertainment follows the typical mainstream formula in presenting run-of-the-mill acts and entertainers. There are no celebrities or big-name acts. Nevertheless, the variety shows, passenger talent contests, and masquerade contests are all infused with the same bonhomie that enlivens the daytime activities. The ship's entertainment staff make themselves available as dance partners.

Service and Tipping Fantasy Cruises employs a large number of crew members on each of its ships, partially because older vessels require more hands and partially to ensure that passengers receive plenty of attention and service. In fact, the crew may overdo the friendliness: Coupled with the fact that the crew members are constantly soliciting tips, the service may leave some passengers unsatisfied. Tip the room steward and the waiter $2.50 each per passenger per diem, the busboy $1.20, and the maître d' and chief steward $1 each. Tip the wine steward 15%. A 15% service charge is added to any purchase for which you sign at the bar.

For More Information Fantasy Cruises (5200 Blue Lagoon Dr., Miami, FL 33126, tel. 800/437–3111).

SS Amerikanis

Specifications *Type of ship:* Mainstream
Type of cruise: Party
Size: Medium (20,000)
Number of cabins: 310
Outside cabins: 67%

Passengers: 617
Crew: 400 (international)
Officers: Greek
Passenger/crew ratio: 1.5 to 1
Year built: 1952

Itinerary **Fall:** Europe. **Winter:** Seven-day loops out of San Juan call at St. Thomas/St. John, Guadeloupe, Barbados, St. Lucia, Antiqua, and St. Maarten/St. Martin; or at St. Thomas/St. John, Grenada, Caracas/LaGuaira (Venezuela), and Curaçao. **Spring–Summer:** Europe.

Port tax: $90 per passenger.

Overview Built as the *Kenya Castle* in 1952, the *Amerikanis* has been refurbished several times since it was purchased by Chandris in 1968. Despite structural changes, it still has the look of a prewar ocean liner, with a sloping hull, a low superstructure, and a large sloping funnel. An aging ship that has seen better days, the *Amerikanis* was refurbished in 1993—the Mayfair Ballroom has a new stage and dance floor and public areas were repainted and recarpeted. It doesn't have a shopping arcade, it has relatively few bars and public rooms, and its two small restaurants are below decks. Public rooms are comfortable but small. A highlight is the well-stocked library.

Cabins and Rates

	Beds	Phone	TV	Sitting Area	Fridge	Tub	Per Diem
Mini Suite	D or T	●	●	●	○	●	$192–$221
Outside Double	D or T	●	●	○	○	○	$147–$192
Inside Double	D, T, or U/L	●	●	○	○	○	$85–$147
Inside Single	T	●	●	○	○	○	$171–$186

Cabins have recently been given better lighting and new wall coverings, bedspreads, and upholstery—all done in mauve. All cabins on the Sun and Boat decks have picture windows, but they look onto public areas.

Outlet voltage: 220 AC.

Single supplement: 150%–200% of double-occupancy rate.

Discounts: Passengers 65 or older receive a 50% discount when traveling with another full-paying passenger. Children under 2 sail free; children 2–12 traveling with a full-paying adult receive a discount. A third or fourth passenger in a cabin pays about $70 per diem. Airfare is not included in rates.

Sports and Fitness **Health club:** Limited weight-training and exercise equipment, sauna, massage.

Walking/jogging: Circuit on Sun Deck (10 laps=1 mile).

Other sports: Aerobics and other exercise classes, golf putting, table tennis, shuffleboard, skeet shooting, two pools.

Facilities **Public rooms:** Five bars, four entertainment lounges, card room, casino, cinema, disco, library/writing room, TV room, video arcade.

Shops: Gift shop, beauty salon/barber.

Health care: Doctor on call.

Child care: Playroom, preteen youth programs supervised by counselors, baby-sitting arranged privately with crew member.

Services: Full-service laundry, photographer, film processing.

Other: Safe-deposit boxes.

Access for the Disabled None.

SS Britanis

Specifications *Type of ship:* Mainstream
Type of cruise: Party
Size: Medium (26,000 tons)
Number of cabins: 463
Outside cabins: 38.6%

Passengers: 926
Crew: 532 (international)
Officers: Greek
Passenger/crew ratio: 1.7 to 1
Year built: 1932

Itinerary **Fall:** A 52-day circumnavigation of South America calls at each of that continents major ports. **Winter–Summer:** Five-day loops out of Miami call at Key West and Cozumel/Playa del Carmen. Two-day loops out of Miami call at Nassau.

Port tax: $36–$228 per passenger.

Overview Built in 1932 as a trans-Pacific liner and used as a troop carrier during World War II, the *Britanis* is the oldest cruise ship still sailing in the Western Hemisphere. It is also one of only a handful of American-built ships still in service. After many changes in name (the *Monterey,* the *Matsonia,* and the *Lurline*), the *Britanis* was bought and refurbished by Chandris in 1971, but the ship retains the look and feel of an old ocean liner. It is, for example, one of the few passenger ships still sailing that has twin smokestacks, one slightly forward and the other slightly astern. Many original fixtures, such as teak decks and brass fittings, remain, although not all in pristine condition. Much of the interior is art deco.

Cabins and Rates

	Beds	Phone	TV	Sitting Area	Fridge	Tub	Per Diem*
Deluxe Suite	D or T	●	○	○	○	○	$210–$220
Junior Suite	D or T	●	○	○	○	○	$170–$180
Outside Deluxe	T	●	○	○	○	○	$150–$160
Outside Double	D, T, or U/L	●	○	○	○	○	$100–$146
Inside Double	D, T, or U/L	●	○	○	○	○	$80–$140

The *Britanis* has one of the highest percentages of inside, windowless cabins in the industry. As is typical of cabins on converted ocean liners, there is more closet space but fewer amenities—such as radios, TVs, and minibars—than on newer ships.

Outlet voltage: 110 AC.

Single supplement: 150%–200% of double-occupancy rate.

Discounts: Passengers 65 or older receive a 50% discount when traveling with another full-paying passenger. Children under 2 sail free; children 2–12 traveling with a full-paying adult receive a discount. A third or fourth passenger in a cabin pays about $70 per diem. Airfare is not included in rates.

Sports and Fitness **Health club:** Small gym with stationary bikes and fitness machines, sauna.

Walking/jogging: Minimally obstructed circuit on enclosed Promenade Deck (9 laps=1 mile; 6 laps around the Boat Deck=1 mile).

Other sports: Aerobics and other exercise classes, golf putting, table tennis, shuffleboard, skeet shooting, pool.

Facilities **Public rooms:** Five bars, three entertainment lounges, casino, cinema, disco, game room, Lido, library/card room, smoking room, nonsmokers lounge, TV lounge.

Shops: Gift shops, beauty salon/barber.

Health care: Doctor on call.

Child care: Youth programs with counselors during holidays and in summer, baby-sitting arranged privately with crew member.

Services: Full-service laundry, photographer, film processing.

Other: Safe-deposit boxes.

Access for the Disabled None.

Holland America Line

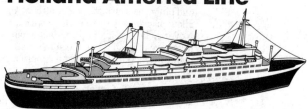

Rotterdam

Ships MS *Maasdam*
MS *Nieuw Amsterdam*
MS *Noordam*
SS *Rotterdam*
MS *Statendam*
MS *Westerdam*

Evaluation Founded in 1873, Holland America is one of the oldest cruise lines extant and has had generations to hone its operations to a consistent level of excellence. Its cruises are conservative affairs renowned for their grace and gentility. No money changes hands (you sign for everything), and loudspeaker announcements are kept to a minimum. A noteworthy feature is the Passport to Fitness program, combining fitness activities and a "heart-healthy" menu. Participation in shore excursions and special activities is emphasized, but passengers are otherwise left to their own devices.

Holland America passengers tend to be better educated, older, and less active than those traveling on party ships, but younger and less affluent than those on a cruise line like Royal Viking. The line won the 1992 *Ocean Cruise News* for offering the best value of any cruise line. Passenger satisfaction is high, as is the percentage of repeat passengers. Holland launched the *Statendam* in March, 1993, the virtually identical *Maasdam* will sail in December 1993, and another sister, the *Ryndam* will debut in late 1994.

Holland is known throughout the industry for its almost fanatical devotion to safety and sanitation. All ships exceed every international safety standard, and kitchens and dining rooms are exceptionally clean. Like only a few other lines, it maintains its own school (in Indonesia) to train staff members, rather than hiring them out of a union hall. If you're looking for a solid, reliable, and refined mainstream cruise, you'll never go wrong taking one of Holland America's ships or shore excursions. If, however, you like dawn-to-midnight entertainment, nonstop partying, or lots of young families on board, you should probably choose another cruise line.

Chart Symbols. *The following symbols are used in the cabin charts that accompany each ship's evaluation.* **D:** *Double bed;* **K:** *King-size bed;* **Q:** *Queen-size bed;* **T:** *Twin bed;* **U/L:** *Upper and lower berths;* ●: *All cabins have this facility;* ○: *No cabins have this facility;* ◑: *Some cabins have this facility*

Activities   Holland offers the full complement of mainstream group activities, such as poolside games, dance classes, trivia contests, and bingo, as well as the more offbeat *karaoke* machines, which allow passengers to sing along with orchestrated recordings. Nevertheless, relaxing in a deck chair and letting the world take care of itself while the ship's staff takes care of you is the prime attraction of a Holland America cruise.

Dining   The focus is on American cuisine, with an occasional Dutch or Indonesian dish for variety. Food is good by cruise-ship standards, served on Rosenthal china. There are two assigned seatings per meal; some breakfasts and lunches are open-seating. Dinner is at 6:15 and 8:15. "Heart-healthy" selections are available in the dining room, and special diets are catered to if requested one month in advance. There are two formal evenings each week, three during a 10-day cruise.

The Lido offers breakfast and lunch buffets and a self-serve ice cream/frozen yogurt parlor at lunch. Other food service includes mid-morning bouillon or iced tea, and a deck lunch of barbecued hot dogs and hamburgers, pasta, or make-your-own tacos. Traditional afternoon tea is served in an inside lounge, as is a midnight buffet. Hot hors d'oeuvres are served during the cocktail hour. Passengers can help themselves to tea and coffee at any time; 24-hour room service is available from a limited menu (full menu at mealtimes).

Entertainment   Apart from a disco, the entertainment is slanted toward an older audience. Main lounge shows, offered twice nightly, feature big-band sounds, magic and dance acts, and revues. You'll also find dance orchestras, a piano bar, string trios, and dance quartets. Cabin TVs, standard on all ships except the *Rotterdam*, have superb closed-circuit service. Rare appearances are made by big-name performers and guest lecturers. The *Statendam*'s 1994 Grand World Cruise will feature a host of prominent speakers; past speakers have included William F. Buckley and *Fortune* magazine's Marshall Loeb. Actor Troy Donahue has given acting lessons on recent *Rotterdam* sailings. On Alaska cruises, an onboard naturalist gives informal talks and lectures.

Service and Tipping   In the 1970s Holland adopted a "no tips required" policy, which has resulted in a level of service that is superior to almost all other cruise lines. Staff members perform their duties with great pride and professionalism. In turn, passengers don't feel the pressure or the discomfort of having crew members solicit tips. As it happens, about 80% of Holland passengers give tips comparable to those recommended on other lines—but entirely at their own discretion. Early sailings on the *Staterdam* revealed holes in Holland's otherwise stellar service, but this is not uncommon on a new ship.

For More Information   Holland America Line (300 Elliott Ave. W, Seattle, WA 98119, tel. 800/426–0327).

MS Maasdam and MS Statendam

Specifications

Type of ship: Upscale Mainstream	*Passengers:* 1,266
Type of cruise: Traditional	*Crew:* 571 (Indonesian/Filipino)
Size: Large (52,000 tons)	*Officers:* Dutch
Number of Cabins: 633	*Passenger/crew ratio:* 2.2 to 1
Outside cabins: 79%	*Year built:* 1993

Itinerary
Maasdam Fall: Ship not yet launched. **Winter–Spring:** A 10-day loop out of Fort Lauderdale will call at Aruba, Cartagena (Colombia), the San Blas Islands, Limón and San José (Costa Rica), and Grand Cayman. A seven-day loop out of Fort Lauderdale will call at Nassau, San Juan, and St. Thomas/St. John. A seven-day Christmas cruise out of Fort Lauderdale will call at Key West, Cozumel/Playa del Carmen (Mexico), and Grand Cayman. Alternating 10-day loops out of Fort Lauderdale will call at St. Maarten/St. Martin, Castries and Soufriere (St. Lucia), Barbados, Cabrits and Roseau (Dominica), St. Thomas/St. John, and Nassau; or Curaçao, Caracas/La Guaira (Venezuela, Grenada, Martinique, St. Thomas/St. John, and Nassau. **Summer:** Alaska, specific ports not announced at press time (Spring 1993).

Port tax: $89–$178 per passenger

Statendam Fall: Alternating 10-day loops out of Fort Lauderdale will call at St. Maarten/St. Martin, Castries and Soufriere (St. Lucia), Barbados, Cabrits and Roseau (Dominica), St. Thomas/St. John, and Nassau; or Curaçao, Caracas/La Guaira (Venezuela), Grenada, Martinique, St. Thomas/St. John, and Nassau. **Winter:** Twelve- and 14-day holiday loops out of Fort Lauderdale will call at St. John/St. Thomas, Barbados, Grenada, La Guaira/Caracas (Venezuela), Aruba, and Grand Cayman. A 98-day world cruise from Los Angeles to New York City will call at 30 ports including the Hawaiian Islands, the South Pacific, Australia, the Philippines, Hong Kong, Thailand, Indonesia, Singapore, Malaysia, India, Sri Lanka, Seychelles, Tanzania, Kenya, Egypt, Israel, Turkey, Greece, Italy, Spain, Morocco, the Madeira Islands, Fort Lauderdale. **Spring–Summer:** Europe.

Port tax: $89–$178 per passenger.

Overview Holland's two newest ships, which will be joined in 1994 by a sister, the *Ryndam*, are elegant and stately—meant to celebrate Holland's esteemed tradition of luxury cruising. With the *Maasdam* due to hit the seas in December 1993, this review focuses on the *Statendam*, which debuted early in 1993. All three ships will be virtually identical.

Decor is traditional, if sedate: Colors in public areas are mellow and well coordinated. Lounges are spacious, walls are curved, dimensions asymmetric. The design encourages mingling and conversation, giving public areas a clubby and uncrowded feel. An immense two-tier dining room is arguably the most elegant space of its kind. A gracious winding staircase connects the two decks, a string quartet serenades diners from the balcony, and wonderful views are had through three sides of floor-to-ceiling windows. Equally dramatic is the three-story atrium lobby, which is anchored by a towering 28-foot-high 17th-century bronze fountain from Italy. Other high highlights are the well-appointed health club and aerobics studio and the popular aft Sun Deck and pool, which are a little less confining than the semi-enclosed Lido. The ship's *Starry Night*–inspired Van Gogh Lounge is a bit much—its walls are a jarring mosaic homage to the great Dutch masterpiece. Two-tiered like the dining room, this enormous show lounge is where all entertainment is staged. From every seat the view is pleasing, except when the lights are on and you can't avoid the dizzying decor. The ships' greatest aesthetic strengths are their incomparable art collections: from ancient maps and prints to contemporary sculptures, you're always walking in the shadows of magnificent artwork.

Service on an early sailing was friendly but uneven—even a little disorganized. Food in the dining room was fine but not up to Holland's high standards; the Lido lunch buffets were adequate, the midnight spreads left quite a lot to be desired in terms of both variety and quality. Ordering room service was a frustrating crapshoot that most passengers lost—food, which rarely resembled the items ordered, came late or not at all. With Holland's outstanding reputation, there's little doubt the early glitches will disappear down the road. One hopes so, because the ships are stunning.

Cabins and Rates

	Beds	Phones	TV	Sitting Area	Fridge	Tub	Per diem
Penthouse Suite	T/Q	●	●	●	○	●	$690–$795
Suite	T/Q	●	●	●	○	●	$468–$530
Deluxe	T/Q	●	●	●	○	●	$355–$424
Outside Double	T/Q	●	●	○	○	●	$288–$375
Inside Double	T/Q	●	●	○	○	●	$243–$323

Penthouse Suites are huge, all Deluxe staterooms and Suites have verandas, whirlpool tubs, VCRs, and minibars. Most cabins have sofa beds. Even the Inside cabins are extremely large at nearly 200 square feet. Closet space is excellent. Color schemes are in muted blues, peaches, and grays, with plenty of wood-paneling.

Outlet voltage: 110 AC.

Single Supplement: 200% of double-occupancy rates in Suites and Deluxe staterooms, 150% elsewhere.

Other discounts: A third or fourth passengers pays about $130–$150 per diem. You get a discount of up to $250 for arranging your own airfare and various discounts for booking early.

Sports and Fitness **Health club:** Nautilus machines, Lifecycles, Lifesteps, treadmills, massage, aerobics studio, saunas, steam rooms.

Walking/jogging: There's an unobstructed circuit.

Other sports: Fitness programs and classes, shuffleboard, skeet shooting, two whirlpools, two pools.

Facilities **Public rooms:** Five lounges, 10 bars, two meeting rooms, restaurant, movie theater, two meeting rooms, library, shopping arcade, photo gallery/shop, disco, casino, show lounge, video-game room.

Shops: Several boutiques and gift shops, beauty salon/barber.

Health care: Doctors and nurses onboard.

Child Care: Youth programs with counselors offered when demand warrants it, baby-sitting arranged privately with crew member.

Services: Full-service laundry, dry-cleaning, laundromat, ironing room, photographer, film-processing.

Other: Safe-deposit boxes.

Access for the Disabled Six cabins are specially equipped for passengers who use wheelchairs. Corridors are wide, elevators and public lavatories are accessible. The crew makes every effort to assist passengers with disabilities.

MS Nieuw Amsterdam and MS Noordam

Specifications *Type of ship:* Upscale mainstream
Type of cruise: Traditional
Size: Medium (33,930 tons)
Number of cabins: 607
Outside cabins: 68%

Passengers: 1,214
Crew: 542 (Indonesian and Filipino)
Officers: Dutch
Passenger/crew ratio: 2.2 to 1
Year built: 1983/1984

Itinerary **Fall:** An 18-day Panama Canal Transit between Vancouver and
Nieuw Amsterdam Tampa calls at Los Angeles, Puerto Vallarta, Ixtapa/Zihuatanejo, Acapulso, along the Canal, the San Blas Islands, Cartagena (Colombia), and Grand Cayman. **Winter:** Seven-day loops leave Tampa Saturdays, calling at Cozumel/Playa del Carmen (Mexico), Ocho Rios or Montego Bay (Jamaica), Grand Cayman, and Key West. **Spring:** Same as Fall. **Summer:** Seven-day cruises between Vancouver and Sitka call at Ketchikan, Juneau, and Glacier Bay National Park. Various land/cruise packages allow you to travel on through Alaska by motorcoach, train, or plane.

Port tax: $95 per passenger.

Noordam **Fall:** Same as *Nieuw Amsterdam*. **Winter–early Spring:** Alternating seven-day loops leave Fort Lauderdale, calling at Nassau, San Juan, and St. Thomas/St. John; or at Cozumel/Playa del Carmen (Mexico), Ocho Rios (Jamaica), and Grand Cayman. **Late Spring:** 10-day cruise between Fort Lauderdale and New Orleans will call at Nassau, Aruba, Ocho Rios (Jamaica), Grand Cayman, and Cozumel/Playa del Carmen (Mexico). **Summer:** Same as *Nieuw Amsterdam*.

Port tax: $95 per passenger.

Overview Originally built for Holland, these ships are virtually identical. Passengers will be struck by how conveniently laid out and comfortable they are. Although the ships are not particularly large, their designers managed to capture a sense of space with extra-wide teak promenades, oversize public rooms, and wide corridors. Dutch nautical antiques, scattered liberally throughout, give the vessels a sense of identity and history. It's hard to pick a favorite room from among the many bars and lounges; however, with their polished hardwood floors and twin balconies, the Admiral's Lounge on the *Noordam* and the Stuyvesant Lounge on the *Nieuw Amsterdam* are always popular.

Cabins and Rates

	Beds	Phone	TV	Sitting Area	Fridge	Tub	Per Diem*
Stateroom Deluxe	K	●	●	●	●	●	$265–$471
Deluxe Outside Double	Q or T	●	●	○	○	●	$234–$393
Large Outside Double	Q or T	●	●	○	○	○	$219–$329
Outside Double	Q or T	●	●	○	○	○	$213–$286
Large Inside Double	Q or T	●	●	○	○	○	$201–$271
Inside Double	T	●	●	○	○	○	$163–$229

Prices in the higher range refer to Alaskan cruises.

Cabins are spotless, comfortable, and relatively large. Views from most cabins on the Boat and Navigation decks (including the Staterooms Deluxe) are partially obstructed.

Outlet voltage: 110 AC.

Single supplement: 200% of double-occupancy rate in Staterooms Deluxe, 150% elsewhere. Holland can arrange for two same-sex adults to share a cabin at the double-occupancy rate.

Discounts: A third or fourth passenger in a cabin pays $60–$108 (Caribbean) or $79–$100 (Alaska) per diem. You get a discount of up to $1,800 per couple on Alaska cruises and up to 43% on Caribbean cruises for booking early. You get up to $250 off for booking your own airfare.

Sports and Fitness **Health club:** Jogging and rowing machines, stationary bicycles, barbells, isometric pulleys, massage, dual saunas, loofah scrubs, Kerstin facials, health-care program.

Walking/jogging: Unobstructed circuit on Promenade Deck (5 laps=1 mile).

Other sports: Exercise classes, golf putting, paddle and deck tennis, shuffleboard, skeet shooting, two pools, whirlpool.

Facilities **Public rooms:** Eight bars, three entertainment lounges, card room, casino, cinema, computer room, disco, Lido, library, video arcade.

Shops: Boutiques, gift shop, beauty salon/barber.

Health care: Doctor on call.

Child care: Youth programs with counselors offered when demand warrants it, baby-sitting arranged privately with crew member.

Services: Full-service laundry, dry-cleaning, laundromat, ironing room, photographer, film processing.

Other: Safe-deposit boxes, Alcoholics Anonymous.

Access for the Four staterooms on each ship have been refitted to better ac-
Disabled commodate wheelchairs. They are Category-B cabins, which
are Deluxe Outside Double rooms on the Navigation Deck. Elevators are wheelchair-accessible.

SS Rotterdam

Specifications *Type of ship:* Upscale   *Passengers:* 1,114
mainstream   *Crew:* 600 (Indonesian
Type of cruise: Traditional   and Filipino)
Size: Large (38,000 tons)   *Officers:* Dutch
Number of cabins: 575   *Passenger/crew ratio:* 1.9 to 1
Outside cabins: 53%   *Year built:* 1959

Itinerary **Fall:** A 58-day world cruise from Vancouver to Los Angeles
calls at about 20 ports, including Seattle, Ketchikan, Glacier
Bay, the Aleutian Islands, Vladivostok, Japan, China, Hong
Kong, Singapore, Bali, the South Pacific, and Honolulu. An 18-
day cruise between Los Angeles and Newport News (VA) calls
at Cabo San Lucas, Acapulco, along the Panama Canal,
Cristóbal (Panama Canal Zone), the San Blas Islands, Cartegena, Ocho Rios (Jamaica), and Fort Lauderdale. **Winter:** A
98-day world cruise is similar to that of the *Statendam.* **Spring:**
A 19-day loop out of Vancouver call at Nawiliwili (Kauai), Kona
(Hawaii), Lahaina (Maui), Honolulu (Oahu), Kahului (Maui),
and Hilo (Hawaii). **Summer:** Seven-day cruises between Vancouver and Seward call at Valdez, Hubbar Glacier, Sitka, Juneau, Ketchikan and along the Inside Passage.

Port tax: $135 (Alaska) per passenger; higher for longer
cruises.

Overview The *Rotterdam,* the flagship of the line, carries the name of four
previous Holland America ships, including the line's very first
vessel. The current *Rotterdam* was launched in 1959 as an
ocean liner, rebuilt in 1969 for cruising, and last refurbished in
1989. At that time the ship was given a brighter look, including
new carpets and upholstery throughout and new tile for the
pool. However, the beautiful wood floors, decks, and paneling
have been retained, as were the shopping arcade and one of the
largest double-decker movie theaters afloat. Although significantly larger than the *Noordam,* the *Rotterdam* carries fewer
passengers. On the upper promenade deck is the impressive
Ritz Carlton ballroom, with two levels connected by a curved
grand staircase. The ceiling lighting in the ballroom is dazzling.

Cabins and Rates

	Beds	Phone	TV	Sitting Area	Fridge	Tub	Per Diem*
Stateroom Deluxe	Q	●	○	●	●	●	$267–$493
Deluxe Outside	D or T	●	○	●	○	●	$218–$414
Large Outside	D or T	●	○	○	○	◑	$204–$371
Outside Double	T	●	○	○	○	○	$189–$336
Economy Outside	U/L	●	○	○	○	○	$165–$279

Large Inside	T	●	○	○	○	●	$189–$293
Inside Double	D or T	●	○	○	○	○	$155–$279
Economy Inside	U/L	●	○	○	○	○	$130–$214

*Prices refer to Alaskan cruises; world cruise per diems are higher.

Views from most cabins on the Sun and Boat decks are partially obstructed. Passengers on B Deck use the upper decks to go from one end of the ship to the other because the dining room blocks passage.

Outlet voltage: 110 AC.

Single supplement: 200% of double-occupancy rate for State-rooms Deluxe, 150% elsewhere. There are several single cabins at $246–$332 per diem (inside) and $332–$418 per diem (outside). Holland can arrange for two same-sex adults to share a cabin at the double-occupancy rate.

Discounts: A third or fourth passenger in a cabin pays $60–$100 per diem. You get a discount of up to $1,800 per couple on Alaska cruises and up to 43% on Caribbean cruises for booking early. You get up to $250 off for arranging your own airfare.

Sports and Fitness   **Health club:** Stationary bicycles, weight machine, exercise board, indoor pool, sauna, massage.

Walking/jogging: Wide, partially enclosed circuit on Upper Promenade.

Other sports: Exercise classes, golf driving, paddle and deck tennis, shuffleboard, skeet shooting, indoor pool, outdoor pool.

Facilities   **Public rooms:** Seven bars, five entertainment lounges, card room, casino, cinema, computer center, disco, Lido, library/writing room, smoking lounge, video arcade.

Shops: Boutique, drugstore, newsstand, gift shop, beauty salon/barber.

Health care: Doctor on call.

Child care: Playroom, teen room, youth programs with counselors during holidays and in summer, baby-sitting arranged privately with crew member.

Services: Full-service laundry, dry-cleaning, laundromat, ironing room, photographer, film processing.

Other: Safe-deposit boxes, Alcoholics Anonymous.

Access for the Disabled   Although some elevators do have doorsills, ramps have been placed over the key ones to improve wheelchair access. Ramps, rails, and special toilets have been fitted in 230 cabins to accommodate the needs of disabled passengers. Passengers should specify their needs when booking.

MS Westerdam

Specifications   *Type of ship:* Upscale mainstream
Type of cruise: Traditional
Size: Large (53,872 tons)

Passengers: 1,494
Crew: 620 (Indonesian and Filipino)
Officers: Dutch

| Number of cabins: 753 | Passenger/crew ratio: 2.4 to 1 |
| Outside cabins: 66% | Year built: 1986 |

Itinerary **Fall:** A 21-day Panama Canal transit between Vancouver and Fort Lauderdale calls at Seattle, Los Angeles, Puerto Vallarta, Zihautenjo/Ixtapa, Acapulco, along the Canal, Cristóbal (Panama Canal Zone), Cartegena (Colombia), Curaçao, St. Croix, and Nassau. **Winter–Spring:** Seven-day loops will leave Fort Lauderdale Saturdays, calling at St. Maarten/St. Martin, St. Thomas/St. John, and Nassau. **Summer:** Seven-day loops out of Vancouver call along the Inside Passage, Ketchikan, Juneau, Glacier Bay National Park, and Sitka.

Port tax: $79 (Caribbean) or $95 (Alaska) per passenger.

Overview Holland America purchased Home Line's two ships in 1988 just to obtain this one, then called the *Homeric.* An additional $80 million investment made the rechristened *Westerdam* the largest, most luxurious ship in Holland's fleet. On the outside, the ship is not a thing of beauty: It has a cluttered, elevated superstructure and an angular, oblique stern. Inside, however, it is unusually comfortable and spacious, largely because it was lengthened by 130 feet during its refurbishment. Into this new space were put a host of bars, cafés, shops, and lounges, as well as a photo-processing studio.

Cabins and Rates

	Beds	Phone	TV	Sitting Area	Fridge	Tub	Per Diem*
Suite	T	●	●	●	○	●	$290–$536
Stateroom Deluxe	T	●	●	●	○	●	$255–$486
Deluxe Outside	Q or T	●	●	●	○	●	$234–$414
Large Outside	D or T	●	●	●	○	◐	$216–$343
Outside Double	D or T	●	●	○	○	○	$204–$300
Economy Outside	T	●	●	○	○	○	$180–$264
Inside Double	T	●	●	○	○	○	$142–$271

*Prices in the higher range refer to Alaskan cruises.

Cabins are large with plenty of storage space; all but the least expensive feature a sitting area with a convertible couch. The use of blond wood and ivory tones adds to the overall sense of airiness.

Outlet voltage: 110 AC.

Single supplement: 200% of double-occupancy rate for Suites or Staterooms Deluxe, 150% elsewhere. Holland will arrange for two same-sex adults to share a cabin at the double-occupancy rate.

Discounts: A third or fourth passenger in a cabin pays $70–$90 (Caribbean) or $79–$100 (Alaska) each per diem. You get a discount of up to $1,800 per couple on Alaska cruises and up to

43% on Caribbean cruises for booking early. You get up to $250 off for arranging your own airfare.

Sports and Fitness **Health club:** Hydrofitness exercise equipment, dual saunas, massage, loofah scrubs, facials, health-care program.

Walking/jogging: Unobstructed circuit on Upper Promenade (4 laps=1 mile).

Other sports: Exercise classes, golf putting, paddle and deck tennis, shuffleboard, skeet shooting (Caribbean), basketball, two pools (one with retractable glass roof), three whirlpools.

Facilities **Public rooms:** Seven bars (including a piano bar), two entertainment lounges, card room, casino, cinema, disco, small meeting room, library, video arcade.

Shops: Boutiques, drugstore, beauty salon/barber.

Health care: Doctor on call.

Child care: Youth programs with counselors on regular basis when the demand warrants it.

Services: Full-service laundry, dry-cleaning, laundromat, photographer, film processing.

Other: Safe-deposit boxes, Alcoholics Anonymous.

Access for the Disabled Elevators are wheelchair-accessible. Four cabins are designed for easier wheelchair maneuvering.

Marquest

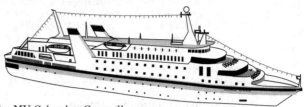

Ship MV *Columbus Caravelle*

Evaluation California-based MarQuest is the North American marketing representative of German-Ukrainian TransOcean Cruise Lines, which owns the *Caravelle*. MarQuest has been catering to adventurous, upscale travelers for more than 25 years, though it remains far from a household name. Typical clients are sophisticated, college-educated, well-traveled individualists interested in "destination-motivated" travel, the type who expect an in-depth experience but with a moderate degree of comfort and service. Many have a strong interest in the sciences and the environment, and roughly 80% have sailed before on other adventure ships, such as the *Frontier Spirit* and the *Explorer*. Passengers are typically between 40 and 70 years old. About half are American, half European; onboard announcements and lectures are given in both German and English.

Activities For this highbrow crowd, no organized activities are offered besides university-level lectures given throughout the day.

Dining The dining room is flanked on three sides by large picture windows that allow you to gaze out upon the open sea. Dinner is single-seating and assigned. The cuisine draws mostly on recipes from Germany and the Ukraine, though American dishes and a light entrée and appetizer are offered at every meal. The kitchen can accommodate special dietary requests when placed a day in advance. At several theme nights, a variety of ethnic dishes are served. Breakfast is a combination of a Continental buffet and American-style bacon and eggs cooked to order. Room service from a limited menu is available 24 hours, and each cabin has a minibar and fresh fruit replenished daily. There's no Lido, although barbecues are sometimes held on deck.

Entertainment The nightly offerings are a cut above those of many other adventure ships: Show-style entertainment and dancing each evening in the main lounge features a four-piece band, a vocalist, and the odd additional performer. The Caravelle Club has a piano bar. Occasionally, local entertainers are invited onboard.

Chart Symbols. *The following symbols are used in the cabin charts that accompany each ship's evaluation.* **D:***Double bed;* **K:***King-size bed;* **Q:** *Queen-size bed;* **T:** *Twin bed;* **U/L:** *Upper and lower berths;* ●: *All cabins have this facility;* ○: *No cabins have this facility;* ◑: *Some cabins have this facility*

Service and Tipping	Though most officers and many crew members are Ukrainian, the food and hotel services are under Western European management. Service is snappy, but some staff possess a limited grasp of English. Generally, servers in the dining room at least understand English, even if they don't speak it fluently. Tip the dining staff and the cabin steward a total of $6 per passenger per diem.
For More Information	MarQuest (101 Columbia St., Suite 150, Laguna Beach, CA 92656, tel. 800/854–4080).

MV Columbus Caravelle

Specifications	*Type of ship:* Specialty		*Passengers:* 250
	Type of cruise: Adventure		*Crew:* 120 (European)
	Size: Small (7,560 tons)		*Officers:* Ukrainian
	Number of cabins: 178		*Passenger/crew ratio:* 2 to 1
	Outside cabins: 100%		*Year built:* 1990

Itinerary **Fall:** A 12-day cruise from Greenland to Acadia National Park (ME) calls at several small ports including St. John (New Brunswick), St. Pierre (Québec), Louisbourg (Cape Breton Island), and Halifax. An 11-day cruise from Newport (RI) to Freeport/Lucaya calls at New York, Philadelphia, Baltimore, Charleston, Jacksonville, and Miami. Various cruises sail through the Panama Canal, Western Caribbean, and down the West coast of South America. **Winter:** 11- to 16-day Antarctic cruises call at various ports and research stations. **Spring:** Seven- to 15-day Brazil and Amazon cruises call at Santos, Recife, Salvador, Fortaleza, Manaus, and many smaller ports. **Summer:** Europe.

Port tax: Varies widely depending upon the itinerary.

Overview The *Caravelle* is one of the largest, most advanced, and most comfortable of the adventure ships. Its ice-hardened hull is designed for Arctic and Antarctic waters, and its state-of-the-art sewage and disposal system is environmentally sound. Among its adventure-oriented facilities and equipment are eight Zodiacs for landing on remote shores or closely following large marine life. Each cruise is accompanied by a staff of naturalists, historians, and other experts. A noteworthy feature, especially for independent travelers who prefer to cruise alone, is that the *Caravelle* has the highest number of single cabins of any ship (70)—and at virtually the same prices as those with double occupancy. Public areas are relatively large.

Cabins and Rates

	Beds	Phone	TV	Sitting Area	Fridge	Tub	Per Diem
Suite	Q	●	●	●	●	●	$243–$301
Outside	T or U/L	●	●	○	●	○	$156–$263
Inside	T	●	●	○	●	○	$127–$179
Inside Single	T	●	●	○	●	○	$124–$209

Though the cabins and suites are smaller than those on conventional ships, they are among the largest on adventure ships.

Suites have a balcony and a bath with whirlpool jets. Lower-deck outside cabins have portholes; those on other decks have picture windows. TVs receive shipboard videotaped programs and some recent films.

Outlet voltage: 220 AC.

Single supplement: Approximately the cost of the least expensive double-occupancy cabin.

Discounts: A third or fourth passenger in a cabin pays about 60% of the double-occupancy rate. Children 12–17 pay $350–$500 per cruise; children under 12 sail free "if sharing a cabin with two adults." Airfare not included in rates.

Sports and Fitness **Health club:** Two exercise bicycles, saunas, whirlpool.

Other sports: Exercise lessons, shuffleboard, pool.

Facilities **Public rooms:** Dining room, main lounge, conference center, two bars, library, photo shop.

Shops: Gift shop, hairdresser.

Health care: Doctor on call.

Child care: Baby-sitting privately arranged with crew member, children-only table in dining room.

Services: Film processing.

Access for the Disabled Two cabins are equipped for passengers who use wheelchairs. The crew is trained to assist disabled passengers in and out of Zodiacs; however, adventure cruises are recommended only to disabled travelers who are reasonably fit and traveling with a an able-bodied companion.

Norwegian Cruise Line

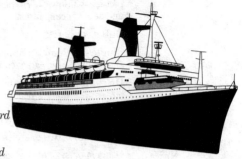

Ships MS *Dreamward*
SS *Norway*
MS *Seaward*
MS *Southward*
MS *Starward*
MS *Westward*
MS *Windward*

Evaluation NCL was the originator of the mainstream formula for cruising: Its ships offer a full schedule of activities and entertainment, generous portions of American-style food, snappy service by an army of stewards and waiters, and a wide range of popular ports. For those who prefer smaller ships, NCL has its White Fleet, consisting of the party ships *Starward* and *Southward*, similar in design, facilities, and personality. For passengers who think bigger is better, the enormous blue-hulled *Norway* is truly one of the grand ladies of the sea. The third NCL subcategory, which aims for the high end of the NCL passenger spectrum, is typified by the medium-size *Seaward* and *Westward*; and the larger *Dreamward* and *Windward*, the latter two having joined NCL in 1993. NCL tries to be everything to everyone, so its passengers tend to span generations, economic brackets, and lifestyles. The newer ships, however, attracts a younger, partying crowd, while the *Norway*, *Seaward*, and *Westward* appeal to an older, more affluent group.

Activities NCL doesn't skimp on activities. It's not unusual to see 30–40 different classes, contests, games, demonstrations, lectures, and performances scheduled for a single day. Having set the industry standard for mainstream cruises, it continues to redefine it to meet America's changing lifestyles: Fitness programs have been beefed up considerably, health food and nouvelle cuisine dishes have been added to the menus, and children's programs have been instituted. Regular theme cruises enliven the usual offerings of bingo, trivia contests, dance classes, wine tastings, and vegetable-carving demonstrations. NCL's most popular theme is the so-called Super Sport series of cruises, during which famous football, basketball, hockey, and baseball players meet and play with passengers. Other theme cruises—Fitness and Beauty, Country and Western,

Chart Symbols. *The following symbols are used in the cabin charts that accompany each ship's evaluation.* **D:** *Double bed;* **K:** *King-size bed;* **Q:** *Queen-size bed;* **T:** *Twin bed;* **U/L:** *Upper and lower berths;* ●: *All cabins have this facility;* ○: *No cabins have this facility;* ◐: *Some cabins have this facility.*

theme cruises—Fitness and Beauty, Country and Western, Floating Jazz Festival, Fifties and Sixties—are scheduled throughout the year. Most upper Caribbean itineraries include an all-day beach party on NCL's own Bahamian island, Great Stirrup Cay, with snorkeling, beach games, and a barbecue.

Dining The cuisine is a combination of American and Continental, usually with at least one Norwegian fish appetizer or entrée at lunch or dinner. The food is plentiful but average; standards are highest on the *Norway*. There are two assigned seatings per meal, although lunch and breakfast may have open seating when in port. "Light entrée" options are available, but special dietary requests should be made one month prior to sailing. Caviar is served at an extra charge. Two formal evenings are held each week. The *Norway* and the *Seaward* each have two dining rooms to which passengers are assigned according to the location of their cabin; each ship also offers an intimate, extra-charge restaurant as an alternative to dinner in the main dining room, as well as an extra-cost ice-cream parlor. The Lido serves a buffet breakfast and lunch; the *Seaward's* Lido also serves dinner. Midnight buffets are served every evening. NCL has broken its long-standing tradition of free room service and now charges $2 per order; 24-hour service is available from a limited menu.

Entertainment Everything one would expect from a mainstream cruise is available in full measure on NCL ships, including Las Vegas–style variety shows, dance orchestras, piano bars, and discos. The *Norway* and the *Seaward* go so far as to feature scaled-down Broadway shows and revues, and the *Norway* has headlined such celebrities as Ricky Skaggs, the Bellamy Brothers, Tanya Tucker, the Tommy Dorsey Orchestra, Mary Wilson, and Paul Revere and the Raiders.

Service and Tipping The general level of service on NCL ships is very good, but *Norway* passengers usually get treated a little better. Tip the room steward and the waiter each $3 per passenger per diem, the busboy $1.50. A 15% service charge is added to the bar tab, and a tip of 50¢ or $1 is expected each time room service is ordered.

For More Information Norwegian Cruise Line (95 Merrick Way, Coral Gables, FL 33134, tel. 800/327-7030).

MS Dreamward and MS Windward

Specifications

Type of ship: Mainstream	*Passengers:* 1,246
Type of cruise: Traditional	*Crew:* 482 (international)
Size: Large (41,000 tons)	*Officers:* Norwegian
Number of cabins: 623	*Passenger/crew ratio:* 2.5 to 1
Outside cabins: 85%	*Year built:* 1992/1993

Itinerary *Dreamward* **Fall–Spring:** Alternating seven-day loops out of Ft. Lauderdale call at Grand Cayman, Cozumel/Playa del Carmen (Mexico), and a private island; or at Nassau, San Juan, and St. Thomas/St. John. **Summer:** Seven-day loops out of New York call at St. George's and Hamilton (Bermuda).

Port tax: $72 (Caribbean) or $82 (Bermuda) per passenger.

Windward **Year-round:** Alternating seven-day loops out of San Juan call at Barbados, Martinique, St. Maarten/St. Martin, and St. Thomas/St. John; or Aruba, Curaçao, Virgin Gorda, Tortola, and St. Thomas/St. John.

Port tax: $72 per passenger.

Overview In December 1992 and June 1993, NCL introduced two identical ships, the *Dreamward* and the *Windward.* This review focuses chiefly on the *Dreamward,* because the *Windward* debuted after our press deadline.

The *Dreamward* utilizes terracing extensively (both forward and aft) to provide unobstructed panoramic views from two dining rooms, the Sun Deck pool, and the show lounge. On these ships, NCL has tossed out the mega-dining room–concept in favor of four smaller formal dining rooms each with a more intimate ambience. The largest, the Terrace, seats only 282 on several levels and has windows on three sides. A variety of special menus and theme meals are available in the various dining rooms; all have children's menus. Dinner has two seatings, but breakfast and lunch are open, so you can try the other restaurants. Hamburgers and hot dogs are served at the casual Sports Bar & Grill. The *Dreamward* offers the usual festive shows, but with a twist: A proscenium stage in the Stardust Lounge allows the production of elaborate full-length Broadway-style shows. After the show, the Stardust Lounge metamorphoses into a late-night lounge and disco. Two-deck-high Casino Royale offers roulette, craps, blackjack and slot machines. In keeping with NCL's "Athlete's Fleet" approach, the *Dreamward* has a series of sports cruises with players on board from championship teams—including football, golf, tennis, hockey, basketball, baseball and volleyball. The Sports Bar & Grill transmits live ESPN and NFL broadcasts on multiple screens. There's plenty of space for relaxing on the five-tier Sun Deck, and the especially broad Promenade Deck is good for walking and jogging.

Cabins and Rates

	Beds	Phone	TV	Sitting Area	Fridge	Tub	Per diem
Grand Deluxe Suite	T/Q	●	●	●	●	●	$406–$427
Suite	T/Q	●	●	●	●	○	$313–$335
Outside	T/Q	●	●	●	○	○	$246–$313
Inside	T/Q	●	●	○	○	○	$182–$232

The *Dreamward* has an unusually high percentage of outside cabins, most with picture windows. Some cabins on the Norway deck have obstructed views. The suites have floor-to-ceiling windows and some have private balconies. Special suite amenities include daily fruit baskets, champagne and trays of hors d'oeuvres, and concierge service. Adjoining suites are available on the Norway, International, and Star decks. Outside cabins have couches that convert into beds. Deluxe suites can accommodate up to four people and adjoining U-shape suites work well for families of up to six.

Outlet voltage: 110 AC.

Single supplement: 150%–200% of double-occupancy rate.

Other discounts: A third or fourth passenger in a cabin (including children) pays $99 per diem. You get up to $300 off for arranging your own airfare.

Sports and Fitness **Health club:** Lifecycles, Lifesteps, exercise equipment, Jacuzzis, a variety of massage treatments.

Walking/jogging: Jogging track on Promenade Deck.

Other sports: Basketball court, exercise course, two pools, golf range.

Facilities **Public rooms:** Four restaurants, six bars, entertainment lounge/theater, nightclub, casino, ice cream parlor (at extra cost), library, video-game room, conference center.

Shops: Gift shops and boutiques, beauty salon/barber.

Health Care: Doctor on call.

Child care: Supervised children's playroom with organized kids' program.

Other: Safe-deposit boxes.

Access for the disabled All decks and activities are wheelchair-accessible, except the Sky Deck and public lavatories. Travel with an able-bodied companion is required. Six specially-equipped cabins are accessible to wheelchairs, others for hearing-impaired passengers.

SS Norway

Specifications *Type of ship:* Mainstream liner
Type of cruise: Traditional/theme
Size: Megaship (76,049 tons)
Number of cabins: 1,024
Outside cabins: 56.9%

Passengers: 2,022
Crew: 900 (international)
Officers: Norwegian
Passenger/crew ratio: 2.3 to 1
Year built: 1962

Itinerary **Year-round:** Alternating seven-day loops leave Miami Saturdays, calling at St. Maarten/St. Martin, St. Thomas/St. John, and Great Stirrup Cay (Bahamas); or at St. Thomas/St. John, San Juan, and Great Stirrup Cay.

Port tax: $72 per passenger.

Overview Deep within the huge hull of the *Norway* beats a Gallic heart. The ship began life in 1962 as the *France*, built with French government subsidies to be the biggest, most beautiful transatlantic liner afloat—a symbol for a country impressed with its own style and stature. Unfortunately, travelers weren't impressed that it took the *France* six days to cross the Atlantic when a jet could fly the distance in seven hours. The ship was sold to Norwegian Cruise Line in 1979 and extensively refitted for vacation cruises.

One of the best-looking ocean liners ever built, the *Norway* has an incredible amount of deck space, as well as a cavernous interior. The enclosed International Deck is so large and wide that its tree-edged walkways, lined with sidewalk cafés, bars, shops, and boutiques, resemble an upscale shopping mall. The port walkway is named Fifth Avenue, and the starboard side, Champs Elysées.

The *Norway* has recently undergone a major refurbishment
that added almost 3,000 tons to its gross tonnage, making it the
largest ship afloat. Among the additions are two new decks, a
6,000-square-foot spa (spa packages include calorie-controlled
lunches), a new extra-charge restaurant, and 124 luxury staterooms (54 with private balconies). Much of the original *France*
is still visible in the wood decks, slate floors, magnificent artwork, sweeping staircases, and sparkling chandeliers. The
Windward and Leeward dining rooms are as large as hotel ban-
quet halls. It's easy to get lost among the plethora of bars and
lounges; many passengers never see all the public rooms by
cruise end.

Cabins and Rates

	Beds	Phone	TV	Sitting Area	Fridge	Tub	Per Diem
Owner's Suite	K	●	●	●	●	●	$747–$806
Grand Deluxe Suite	K	●	●	●	●	●	$686–$735
Pent-house Suite	K or T	●	●	●	●	●	$386–$457
Junior Suite	K, Q, or T	●	●	●	●	●	$323–$348
Deluxe Outside	D or T	●	●	○	●	◐	$306–$330
Superior Outside	T	●	●	○	●	◐	$291–$313
Outside	D, T, or U/L	●	●	○	○	◐	$208–$299
Superior Inside	T	●	●	○	○	◐	$266–$287
Inside	D, T, or U/L	●	●	○	○	◐	$178–$200

Most suites and cabins are larger than those of comparably
priced ships. Suites offer concierge service. Each Owner's
Suite has a private wraparound balcony, a living room, a master
bedroom and second bedroom, a dressing room, a bathroom,
and a whirlpool. Some Grand Deluxe Suites have a separate
living room and a second bedroom, a whirlpool, and a powder
room. Most Penthouse Suites have private balconies. Olympic
Deck cabins look onto the jogging track. Most cabins on the
Fjord and Olympic decks have obstructed or partially obstructed views.

Outlet voltage: 110 AC.

Single supplement: 150%–200% of double-occupancy rate. A
few inside single cabins are available at $207–$271 per diem.

Discounts: A third or fourth passenger in a cabin pays $99 per
diem. You get up to $300 off for arranging your own airfare.

Sports and Fitness　Health club: Fitness center with 14 treatment rooms (for massage, reflexology, herbal treatment, hydrotherapy, thermal
body wraps, and more), two saunas, two steam rooms, body-jet

showers, Cybex Eagle strength-training equipment, Lifecycles and Lifesteps, whirlpool, indoor pool for water exercise. The spa's beauty salon (separate from the ship's main salon) offer facials and other beauty treatments.

Walking/jogging: Unobstructed circuit on Olympic Deck jogging track.

Other sports: Aerobics and other exercise classes, basketball, deck Olympics, golf driving and putting, paddleball, table tennis, shuffleboard, skeet shooting, snorkeling classes and excursions, volleyball, two outdoor pools.

Facilities **Public rooms:** Seven bars, six entertainment lounges, cabaret, casino, disco, ice-cream parlor (extra charge), library, piano bar, theater, video-game room.

Shops: Arcade of gift shops and boutiques, beauty salon/barber.

Health care: Doctor on call.

Child care: Playroom, children's and teens' programs with counselors year-round, special shore excursions for children over age six, baby-sitting arranged privately with crew member. Programs include Circus at Sea, in which kids learn circus routines and then put on a performance (with costumes and makeup) for the adults.

Services: Concierge service in suites, full-service laundry, drycleaning, photographer, film processing.

Other: Safe-deposit boxes (sealed envelopes can be stored in purser's safe), Alcoholics Anonymous.

Access for The *Norway* has a few cabins designed for disabled passen-
the Disabled gers. All public areas except the Sun Deck pool are accessible. The ship's size forces it to anchor offshore at most ports; boarding the tenders can pose a difficulty for disabled passengers. Individuals must provide their own small, collapsible wheelchairs.

MS Seaward

Specifications | | |
|---|---|
| *Type of ship:* Mainstream | *Passengers:* 1,534 |
| *Type of cruise:* Traditional | *Crew:* 624 (international) |
| *Size:* Large (42,000 tons) | *Officers:* Norwegian |
| *Number of cabins:* 767 | *Passenger/crew ratio:* 2.9 to 1 |
| *Outside cabins:* 67.7% | *Year built:* 1988 |

Itinerary **Year-round:** Seven-day loops leave Miami Sundays, calling at Great Stirrup Cay (Bahamas), Ocho Rios (Jamaica), Grand Cayman, and Cozumel/Playa del Carmen.

Port tax: $72 per passenger.

Overview The *Seaward*'s ungainly, top-heavy appearance is much more utilitarian than aesthetic: The ship is blessed with an enormous amount of deck space, which has been used most judiciously, as in the two back-to-back swimming pools (currently the cruising world's largest), surrounded by hundreds of lounge chairs, a bar, and an ice-cream parlor. At the heart of the ship is the spectacular Crystal Court, a two-story entrance hall with cascading water fountains and a marble pool. The main entertainment room, the Cabaret Lounge, seats 740 passengers, though its single-level construction makes viewing difficult for those at the back of the room.

Where the *Seaward* excels is in its dining facilities: The two main dining rooms, the Four Seasons and the Seven Seas, are assigned to passengers according to their cabin. For a more informal atmosphere, there are two indoor/outdoor cafés, The Big Apple and East Side/West Side. For those with the palate and the pocketbook, the *Seaward's* intimate top-deck bistro, the Palm Tree, serves à la carte dinners for an additional charge. Throughout the ship, plentiful use is made of NCL's new color scheme of muted corals and blues, as well as mirrored walls and nautical brass trim.

Cabins and Rates

	Beds	Phone	TV	Sitting Area	Fridge	Tub	Per Diem
Deluxe Outside Suite	T/D	●	●	●	●	●	$358–$383
Large Outside	T/D	●	●	○	○	○	$330–$347
Outside	T/D	●	●	○	○	○	$306–$329
Inside	T/D or U/L	●	●	○	○	○	$178–$260

Some cabins on the Norway and Star decks have obstructed or partially obstructed views.

Outlet voltage: 110 AC.

Single supplement: 150%–200% of double-occupancy rate. A few inside single cabins are available at $207–$271 per diem.

Discounts: A third or fourth passenger in a cabin pays $99 per diem. You get up to $300 off for arranging your own airfare.

Sports and Fitness **Health club:** Exercise equipment, massage, sauna.

Walking/jogging: Unobstructed circuit on Promenade Deck (4 laps=1 mile).

Other sports: Aerobics and other exercise classes, basketball, golf driving, table tennis, shuffleboard, skeet shooting, snorkeling lessons and excursions, volleyball, two pools, two whirlpools.

Facilities **Public rooms:** Six bars, five entertainment lounges, disco, piano bar, cabaret, card room, casino, extra-charge restaurant and ice-cream parlor.

Shops: Several stores, beauty salon/barber.

Health care: Doctor on call.

Child care: Youth programs with counselors year-round, special shore excursions for children over age six baby-sitting arranged privately with crew member. Programs include Circus at Sea, in which kids learn circus routines and then put on a performance for the adults.

Services: Full-service laundry, dry-cleaning, photographer, film processing.

Other: Safe-deposit boxes (envelopes may be stored in purser's safe), Alcoholics Anonymous.

Access for the Disabled The *Seaward* has excellent facilities for the disabled. Certain cabins are specially equipped, and no area of the ship is inaccessible to passengers in wheelchairs. Passengers must provide their own small, collapsible wheelchairs.

MS Southward

Specifications

Type of ship: Mainstream *Passengers:* 752
Type of cruise: Party *Crew:* 320 (international)
Size: Small (16,607 tons) *Officers:* Norwegian
Number of cabins: 377 *Passenger/crew ratio:* 2.4 to 1
Outside cabins: 69.5% *Year built:* 1971

Itinerary **Year-round:** Three- and four-day loops leave Los Angeles Fridays and Mondays, calling at Catalina Island, Ensenada, and sometimes San Diego.

Port tax: $43–$48 per passenger.

Overview Built for NCL and last refurbished in 1987, the *Southward* is similar in proportions and style to the *Starward*. Though it is more than 20 years old, it is still a comfortable, attractive ship with long, low lines and a sleek bow.

Cabins and Rates

	Beds	Phone	TV	Sitting Area	Fridge	Tub	Per Diem
Outside Deluxe Suite	D or T	●	○	●	●	●	$243–$299
Outside	D & U or T/D	●	○	○	○	○	$136–$240
Inside	D & U	●	○	○	○	○	$174–$232

Most cabins are small, though a few have extra room. Outside cabins have portholes. Some of the cheapest accommodations are actually outside cabins (categories 8, 9, and 10), but they have only one oversize.

Outlet voltage: 110 AC.

Single supplement: 150%–200% of double-occupancy rate.

Discounts: A third or fourth passenger in a cabin pays $65 (four days) or $83 (three days) per diem. You get up to $300 off for arranging your own airfare.

Sports and Fitness **Health club:** Exercise equipment, sauna, massage.

Walking/jogging: Unobstructed circuit on Boat Deck.

Other sports: Aerobics and other exercise classes, basketball, table tennis, shuffleboard, snorkeling lessons and excursions, pool.

Facilities **Public rooms:** Four bars, three entertainment lounges, card room, casino, cinema, disco, Lido.

Shops: Three gift shops, beauty salon/barber.

Health care: Doctor on call.

Child care: Playroom, youth programs with counselors during holidays and in summer, special shore excursions for children over age six, baby-sitting arranged with crew member. Programs include Circus at Sea, in which children learn circus routines and then put on a performance for the adults.

Services: Full-service laundry, photographer, film processing.

Other: Safe-deposit boxes (sealed envelopes can be stored in the purser's safe), Alcoholics Anonymous.

Access for the Disabled The major areas of the ship are wheelchair-accessible, but there are no specially equipped cabins. Disabled passengers must provide their own small, collapsible wheelchairs.

MS Starward

Specifications *Type of ship:* Mainstream
Type of cruise: Party
Size: Small (16,107 tons)
Number of cabins: 379
Outside cabins: 58.3%

Passengers: 758
Crew: 315 (international)
Officers: Norwegian
Passenger/crew ratio: 2.4 to 1
Year built: 1968

Itinerary **Year-round:** Seven-day loops leave Los Angeles Sundays, calling at Cabo San Lucas, Mazatlán, and Puerto Vallarta.

Port tax: $83 per passenger.

Overview The *Starward*, the oldest of the White Fleet built for NCL, was last refurbished in 1987. Its main difference from its sister ship is that it has two swimming pools rather than one. On the top deck, a large glass pyramid, closed on three sides, covers an attractive bar/lounge and one of the pools. Not everyone manages to find this shady spot on the top deck, but those who do will enjoy curling up with a book and gazing out at the sea.

Cabins and Rates

	Beds	Phone	TV	Sitting Area	Fridge	Tub	Per Diem
Deluxe Outside Suite	D	●	○	●	●	●	$292–$321
Outside Suite	D	●	○	●	○	○	$262–$280
Outside	D & U, T/D, or U/L	●	○	○	○	○	$128–$246
Inside	D & U or T	●	○	○	○	○	$161–$199

The lowest-priced cabins are actually small outside rooms with upper and lower berths. The cabins on the Boat Deck look onto a public promenade.

Outlet voltage: 110 AC.

Single supplement: 150%–200% of double-occupancy rate.

Discounts: A third or fourth passenger in a cabin pays $106 per diem. You get up to $300 off for arranging your own airfare.

Sports and Fitness **Health club:** Exercise equipment, sauna, massage.

Walking/jogging: Boat Deck.

Other sports: Aerobics and other exercise classes, basketball, table tennis, skeet shooting, scuba and snorkeling lessons and excursions, two pools.

Facilities **Public rooms:** Four bars, four entertainment lounges, card room/library, casino, cinema, disco, Lido.

Shops: Boutique/gift shop, beauty salon/barber.

Health care: Doctor on call.

Child care: Playroom, youth programs with counselors during holidays and in summer, special shore excursions for children over age six, baby-sitting arranged privately with crew member. Programs include Circus at Sea, in which children learn circus routines and then put on a performance for the adults.

Services: Full-service laundry, photographer, film processing.

Other: Safe-deposit boxes (sealed envelopes can be stored in purser's safe), Alcoholics Anonymous.

Access for the Disabled The major areas of the ship are wheelchair-accessible, but no cabins are specially equipped. Passengers must provide their own small, collapsible wheelchairs.

MS Westward

Specifications *Type of ship:* Mainstream *Passengers:* 829
Type of cruise: Traditional *Crew:* 325 (international)
Size: Medium (28,000 tons) *Officers:* Norwegian
Number of cabins: 390 *Passenger/crew ratio:* 2.5 to 1
Outside cabins: 85% *Year built:* 1972

Itinerary **Year-round:** Three- and four-day loops leave Fort Lauderdale Fridays and Mondays, calling at Nassau, Great Stirrup Cay (Bahamas), and sometimes Freeport/Lucaya.

Port tax: $43 per passenger.

Overview The *Westward* is actually a reincarnation of the *Royal Viking Star,* renamed when the ship moved over from its sister division. The ship was originally built in 1972, expanded in 1981, then refurbished when it became the *Westward* in April 1991. Passengers tend to be middle-aged couples, the kind of folks you'd see strolling off the tennis courts or golf course. As on NCL's other ships, there's an extensive list of activities—favorites include a mini-Olympics and, on every cruise, the chance to meet a pro football player—as well as a full complement of interesting shore excursions.

Cabins and Rates

	Beds	Phone	TV	Sitting Area	Fridge	Tub	Per Diem
Penthouse Suite	T or D	●	●	●	●	●	$392–$442
Suite	T	●	●	●	●	●	$320–$385
Deluxe Outside	T	●	●	●	●	●	$300–$320
Outside	T	●	●	○	○	●	$225–$302

Inside	T	●	●	○	○	●	$179– $218

These are among the most spacious cabins of the ships afloat. Most are decorated in warm sunset colors and have bathtubs. Each Penthouse Suite has a large, open sitting area, a separate bedrooms, floor-to-ceiling windows, and a private balcony. Smaller suites also feature separate bedrooms, and concierge service is available to some.

Outlet voltage: 110 AC.

Single supplement: 200% of double-occupancy rate.

Discounts: A third or fourth passenger in a cabin pays $65 (four days) or $83 (three days) per diem. You get up to $300 off for arranging your own airfare.

Sports and Fitness   **Health club:** Circuit-training equipment, two saunas, two steam baths, six massage rooms.

Other sports: Aerobics, paddle-tennis, golf driving range, two heated pools.

Facilities   **Public rooms:** Four lounges, theater, casino, library, card room, video arcade, disco.

Shops: Shopping arcade with several gift shops, beauty salon, barber shop.

Health care: A doctor is on call.

Child care: Playroom, children's program (ages 6–17) with supervised activities during holidays and in summer.

Access for the Disabled   The *Westward* has no wheelchair-accessible cabins; cabins have a step up into the bathroom, and doors aren't wide enough for a wheelchair. In spite of that drawback, an average of five people who use wheelchairs sail on the ship each week. The *Westward* does have ramps into the public areas and elevators that are wheelchair-accessible, and the staff go out of their way to accommodate special requests.

Premier Cruise Lines

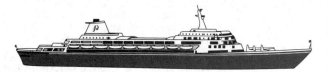

Ships *Star/Ship Atlantic*   Starship Oceanic
Star/Ship Majestic
Star/Ship Oceanic

Evaluation As the official cruise line of Walt Disney World, Premier is ideal for families. It has the best child care and youth programs in the industry—Mickey Mouse, Goofy, and other Disney folk even sail along. A recreation center on each ship for children age two and over has its own wading pool and sun deck and provides supervised programs on and off the ship, and teenagers have their own programs and playroom as well. To accommodate all these families, the ships have a high percentage of cabins with berths for three, four, and even five passengers. There's even a special price structure for single parents.

If you don't like children, don't sail with Premier, but you don't have to have them to enjoy these lively, unpretentious cruises. Increasingly, they are popular with honeymooners who want to combine a cruise with a visit to Walt Disney World. The three- or four-day stay at Walt Disney World includes hotel accommodations at a Disney resort, a Three Park Passport for unlimited admission to all Disney World theme parks, a breakfast with Disney characters, airfare, a seven-day car rental with unlimited mileage, and a tour of the Kennedy Space Center's Spaceport USA. Fare for the seven-day Disney and cruise package ranges from $789 to $1,739 per person. All three ships visit Nassau and Freeport/Port Lucaya. On its four-day cruise, the *Majestic* also visits Key West.

Activities For adults Premier offers traditional cruise activities—"horse racing," bingo, pool games, trivia contests, bridge tournaments—as well as extensive fitness programs and facilities. Young children and teenagers have their own activities centers, video-game room, and counselor-supervised programs.

Dining Food is good basic fare. The waiters are exceptionally good with children, but don't look for elegance or snappy service, especially with the high number of children served. If you are traveling with small children, it's smart to sign up for the first seating. If you wish a more sedate environment, you would be wise to select the late seating.

Chart Symbols. *The following symbols are used in the cabin charts that accompany each ship's evaluation.* **D:** *Double bed;* **K:** *King-size bed;* **Q:** *Queen-size bed;* **T:** *Twin bed;* **U/L:** *Upper and lower berths;* ●: *All cabins have this facility;* ○: *No cabins have this facility;* ◐: *Some cabins have this facility*

Dining-room arrangements consist of two assigned seatings per meal (6 and 8:15). The menu, decor, and waiters' costumes change nightly to reflect a theme—French, Italian, Caribbean, American. Special dietary requests should be made in writing at least four weeks prior to sailing. A children's menu is available, with such favorites as hamburgers, hot dogs, and macaroni-and-cheese. There is one semiformal evening on each cruise.

Early morning coffee is served on the Pool Deck, as are extensive breakfast and lunch buffets. Other food service includes a make-your-own sundae bar, afternoon tea, midnight buffet, and a late-night omelet bar. There is no room service.

Entertainment Disney characters appear several times a day to play with children (and adults, who seem to get into the act when no one is looking). Otherwise, Premier entertainment is traditional, featuring variety shows, magicians, films, and a masquerade party. After the sun goes down, Premier presents Vegas-style revues, cabaret acts, piano playing, and other adult forms of entertainment. (The comedy, however, is strictly PG–13, instead of the R-rated material most party ships offer late-night passengers.) Premier also features large casinos with row upon row of slot machines.

Service and Tipping Generally, the crew is superb at handling children and all their wants. They're patient, always smiling, and ready to give a helping hand. Tip the room steward and the waiter each $3 per passenger per diem, the busboy $1.50, both slightly more for the four-night cruise. Tip the headwaiter $2 per passenger per cruise for a three-night cruise, $3 for a four-night cruise. When you sign for bar and wine bills, a 15% service charge is automatically added.

For More Information Premier Cruise Lines (Box 517, Cape Canaveral, FL 32920, tel. 800/473–3262).

Star/Ship Atlantic

Specifications

Type of ship: Mainstream	*Passengers:* 1,500
Type of cruise: Traditional/family	*Crew:* 550 (international)
	Officers: Greek
Size: Large (36,500 tons)	*Passenger/crew ratio:* 3.2 to 1
Number of cabins: 549	*Year built:* 1982
Outside cabins: 73%	

Itinerary Three- and four-day loops leave Port Canaveral Fridays and Mondays, calling at Nassau and Freeport/Lucaya.

Port tax: $58 per passenger.

Overview The *Atlantic* is a generic-looking cruise ship that previously sailed as the *Atlantic* for Home Lines. During a major refurbishment in 1989, the public rooms and casino were enlarged, extra cabins were added, and more facilities for children were installed. Like its sister ship *Oceanic*, it features a retractable transparent roof over the Riviera Pool. Most daytime activities are centered on the Promenade Deck, which has an ice-cream parlor, a well-equipped sports-and-fitness center, and two pools with adjacent sun areas.

Children age two or older can enjoy Pluto's Playhouse in the Children's Recreation Center (the largest of any ship sailing the Bahamas), as well as a shallow children's pool. For older children, the Space Station Teen Center has a jukebox and a dance floor, and the Star Fighter Arcade is packed with state-of-the-art video games.

Cabins and Rates

	Beds	Phone	TV	Sitting Area	Fridge	Tub	Per Diem
Apartment Suite	Q or T	●	●	●	○	●	$358–$385
Suite	Q or T	●	●	●	○	●	$325–$351
Deluxe Outside	Q or T	●	●	●	○	◕	$265–$285
Outside	Q, T, or U/L	●	●	●	○	●	$245–$265
Inside	D, T, or U/L	●	○	○	○	◐	$148–$251

Cabins are simply furnished, but many can accommodate three or four passengers.

Outlet voltage: 110 AC.

Single supplement: 100%–175% of double-occupancy rate.

Discounts: A third or fourth passenger in a cabin pays from $40 to $600 per cruise depending upon the cabin class. You can save up to $400 for booking early and $150 for arranging your own airfare. Senior citizens receive a 10% discount.

Sports and Fitness **Health club:** Life Cycles, Universal weights, minitrampolines, sit-up boards, massage.

Walking/jogging: Jogging track overlooking Pool Deck.

Other sports: Aerobics and other exercise classes, basketball, table tennis, snorkeling lessons, shuffleboard, skeet shooting, volleyball, whirlpools, three pools, wading pool.

Facilities **Public rooms:** Four bars, three entertainment lounges, casino, cinema, disco, ice-cream parlor, video arcade.

Shops: Large gift shop, beauty salon/barber.

Health care: Doctor on call.

Child care: Children's recreation center (age two and up), with wading pool, sun deck, supervised programs on and off ship; teen programs and playroom; baby-sitting for children over age two.

Services: Full-service laundry, photographer.

Other: Safe-deposit boxes.

Access for the Disabled Wheelchair access is limited. Passengers in wheelchairs may have difficulty boarding the tenders that ferry passengers to the beach party.

Star/Ship Majestic

Specifications *Type of ship:* Mainstream
Type of cruise: Traditional/family
Size: Small (17,750 tons)

Passengers: 1,006
Crew: 380 (international)
Officers: Greek
Passenger/crew ratio: 2.7 to 1

Number of cabins: 380   *Year built:* 1972
Outside cabins: 67%

Itinerary **Year-round:** Three-day loops leave Port Everglades Thursdays, calling at Nassau and Freeport/Lucaya; four-day loops leave Port Everglades Sundays, calling at Freeport/Lucaya and Key West.

Port tax: $58 per passenger.

Overview Acquired by Premier in 1988, the *Majestic* previously sailed for Princess Cruises as the *Sun Princess* and, before that, as the *Spirit of London.* Because it is less than half the size of Premier's other two ships, it can include in its unique itinerary islands generally not visited by cruise ships. It accommodates up to 1,006 passengers. Most of the public rooms are significantly smaller than their counterparts on the *Atlantic.* Extensive use of mirror paneling helps lighten the sense of confinement. Because a large percentage of passengers are children, some adults may find the ship noisy and crowded, particularly during school holidays.

Cabins and Rates

	Beds	Phone	TV	Sitting Area	Fridge	Tub	Per Diem
Suite	D, Q, or T	●	○	●	●	●	$325–$351
Deluxe Outside	T/D	●	○	○	○	○	$265–$285
Outside	Q or T/D	●	○	○	○	○	$245–$265
Inside	D, T, or U/L	●	○	○	○	○	$148–$251

Cabins are simply furnished, but many can accommodate three or four passengers.

Outlet voltage: 110 AC.

Single supplement: 100%–175% of double-occupancy rate.

Discounts: A third or fourth passenger in a cabin saves from $40 to $600 per cruise depending upon the cabin class. You can save up to $400 for booking early and $150 for arranging your own airfare. Senior citizens receive a 10% discount.

Sports and Fitness **Health club:** Life Cycles, Universal weights, mini-trampolines, sit-up boards, massage.

Other sports: Aerobics and other exercise classes, basketball, table tennis, snorkeling lessons, shuffleboard, skeet shooting, volleyball, pool, wading pool.

Facilities **Public rooms:** Four bars, three entertainment lounges, casino, cinema, ice-cream parlor, piano bar, video arcade.

Shops: Gift shop, beauty salon/barber.

Health care: Doctor on call.

Child care: Children's recreation center (age two and up), with wading pool, sun deck, supervised programs on and off ship; teen programs and playroom; baby-sitting for children over age two.

Services: Full-service laundry, photographer.

Other: Safe-deposit boxes.

Access for the Disabled Wheelchair access is limited. Passengers who use wheelchairs may have particular difficulty aboard the *Majestic* because tenders are frequently used to transport passengers ashore.

Star/Ship Oceanic

Specifications *Type of ship:* Mainstream   *Passengers:* 1,600
Type of cruise: Traditional/   *Crew:* 565 (international)
family   *Officers:* Greek
Size: Large (40,000 tons)   *Passenger/crew ratio:* 3 to 1
Number of cabins: 590   *Year built:* 1965
Outside cabins: 44%

Itinerary Same as *Star/Ship Atlantic,* above.

Port tax: $58 per passenger.

Overview In the tradition of having prominent ladies christen ships, Minnie Mouse was the celebrity wielding the champagne bottle when the *Star/Ship Oceanic* was inaugurated as a Premier ship in 1986; it previously sailed for Home Lines and was completely refurbished in January 1993. The exterior is stunning, with the classic lines of a transatlantic liner. Much of the daytime activity centers on the Pool Deck; its two pools can be covered by a retractable, transparent dome in the event of rain. The Seven Continents Restaurant is huge and well lighted, with wide aisles and ample space between the tables, but it tends to become noisy. The casino is one of the largest on any cruise ship; children under 18 are forbidden to play the slot machines, but a video arcade is nearby.

Cabins and Rates

	Beds	Phone	TV	Sitting Area	Fridge	Tub	Per Diem
Apartment Suite	Q or T	●	●	●	○	●	$358–$385
Suite	D or T	●	●	●	○	●	$325–$351
Deluxe Outside	T	●	○	●	○	●	$265–$285
Outside	D, T, or U/L	●	○	◑	○	●	$245–$265
Inside	D, T, or U/L	●	○	○	○	◑	$148–$251

Cabins are simply furnished; many accommodate three or four passengers.

Outlet voltage: 110 AC.

Single supplement: 100%–175% of double-occupancy rate.

Discounts: A third or fourth passenger in a cabin saves from $40 to $600 per cruise depending upon the cabin class. You can save up to $400 for booking early and $150 for arranging your own airfare. Senior citizens receive a 10% discount.

Sports and Fitness **Health club:** Life Cycles, Universal weight equipment, minitrampolines, sit-up boards, massage.

Walking/jogging: Jogging track overlooking Pool Deck.

Other sports: Aerobics and other exercise classes, basketball, table tennis, pool volleyball, snorkeling lessons, shuffleboard, skeet shooting, tennis practice, volleyball, two adjacent swimming pools, wading pool, three whirlpools.

Facilities **Public rooms:** Five bars, four entertainment lounges, casino, cinema, disco, ice-cream parlor, large indoor cafeteria, reading room, video arcade.

Shops: Gift shop, beauty salon/barber.

Health care: Doctor on call.

Child care: Children's recreation center (age two and up), with wading pool, sun deck, supervised programs on and off ship; teen programs and playroom; baby-sitting for children over age two.

Services: Full-service laundry, photographer.

Other: Safe-deposit boxes.

Access for the Disabled Wheelchair access is limited. The beach party is reached by tender, which could pose problems for anyone in a wheelchair.

Princess Cruises

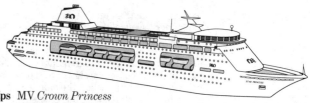

Star Princess

Ships MV *Crown Princess*
TSS *Fair Princess*
MV *Golden Princess*
MV *Island Princess*
MV *Pacific Princess*
MV *Regal Princess*
MV *Royal Princess*
TSS *Sky Princess*
MV *Star Princess*

Evaluation Most of us remember Princess ships from the cheerful TV series in which several took turns portraying the "Love Boat." In the real world, however, Princess Cruises is an upscale British company whose strengths are high-quality service and a graceful, elegant style. Passengers tend to be older, experienced travelers who expect superior service and won't accept less. In 1988 Princess acquired Sitmar, an upscale Italian line, which seems to have infused its parent company with a refreshing hint of Italian exuberance.

Passengers are treated like members of an elite club. Shipboard purchases can be signed for and accounts settled at the end of the cruise. Even on the last day, when most lines hustle people off to make room for the next group, Princess serves a lunch buffet for those whose flights leave later in the day.

In fall 1995, Princess will usher in the mammoth 77,000-ton *Sun Princess*, a 14-story megaship that will carry 1,950 passengers. At a cost of $300 million, the *Sun* will feature a variety of dining rooms and entertainment lounges, a state-of-the-art conference center, and equally stupendous health center and spa.

Activities Many Princess passengers are content to take it easy, although there's plenty to keep them busy if they prefer. All the expected mainstream activities are offered—dance lessons, bingo, "horse racing," bridge and backgammon tournaments. Fitness facilities include an exercise manager who can create a customized fitness program just for you. An extensive watersports program includes scuba-diving classes held in the pools.

Chart Symbols. *The following symbols are used in the cabin charts that accompany each ship's evaluation.* **D:** *Double bed;* **K:** *King-size bed;* **Q:** *Queen-size bed;* **T:** *Twin bed;* **U/L:** *Upper and lower berths;* ●: *All cabins have this facility;* ○: *No cabins have this facility;* ◐: *Some cabins have this facility*

On the former Sitmar ships, youth centers, with a children's pool and sun deck, provide daily supervised activities year-round; this is available on the other ships when the numbers warrant it.

Dining Food is better than on comparably priced ships. The Italian staff supervise meals with élan and pride. Each night at dinner the headwaiter prepares a fresh pasta dish tableside. Caviar, or just about anything else, may be ordered even when it is not on the menu. Dining arrangements consist of two seatings per meal, with passengers assigned to tables; breakfast and lunch may be open seating when the ship is in port. Special dietary requests are well handled, but they should be made in writing three weeks before sailing. Alternative low-fat, low-choles-terol, and low-sodium selections are offered at every meal.

Two formal evenings are held on seven-day cruises, three on nine- to 16-day cruises. On Princess, formal *does* mean a tux-edo, dinner jacket, or dark suit for men. The Lido serves a breakfast and lunch buffets. Other food service includes mid-morning bouillon, afternoon tea, and a midnight buffet; 24-hour room service is limited to sandwiches and beverages except during meal hours. The *Crown, Fair, Regal, Sky,* and *Star* have free pizza parlors open throughout the afternoon and evening. On the *Crown, Royal,* and *Star,* a patisserie serves desserts and specialty coffees for an extra charge.

Entertainment Princess emphasizes entertainment suitable for the entire family. Although well-known entertainers appear regularly, don't expect Las Vegas–style extravaganzas. Offerings include variety shows, cabarets, a piano bar, a dance orchestra and combo, and a disco. Local musicians sometimes come aboard and perform.

Service and Tipping Princess places heavy emphasis on keeping passengers happy and satisfied. Generally, the service is excellent and unobtru-sive, though passengers occasionally complain of stuffiness among crew members. The room service is exceptional. Tip the room steward and waiter $3 each per passenger per diem, the waiter's assistant $1.75. The maître d' and the headwaiter may be tipped at the passenger's discretion for a job well done. A 15% gratuity is automatically added to bar and wine charges.

For More Information Princess Cruises (10100 Santa Monica Blvd., Los Angeles, CA 90067, tel. 310/553–1770).

MV Crown Princess and MV Regal Princess

Specifications *Type of ship:* Upscale mainstream
Type of cruise: Traditional
Size: Megaship (70,000 tons)
Number of cabins: 795
Outside cabins: 80%

Passengers: 1,590
Crew: 696 (international)
Officers: Italian
Passenger/crew ratio: 2.2 to 1
Year built: 1990/1991

Itinerary
Crown Princess **Fall:** Seven-day alternating loops leave Port Everglades, call-ing at San Juan, St. Maarten/St. Martin, St. Thomas/St. John, and Princess Cays (Bahamas); or Montego Bay (Jamaica), Grand Cayman, and Cozumel/Playa del Carmen (Mexico). **Winter:** Ten- and 11-day loops leave Port Everglades, calling at Princess Cays, St. Thomas/St. John, Ocho Rios (Jamaica), Grand Cayman, and Cozumel/Playa del Carmen; or St.

Maarten/St. Martin, St. Barts, Martinique, Barbados, Dominica, St. Thomas/St. John, and Princess Cays. **Spring–Summer:** Alaska, ports not yet announced.

Port tax: $84–$155 per passenger.

Regal Princess **Fall:** Same as *Crown Princess*. **Winter:** Ten- and 11-day loops out of Port Everglades call at St. Maarten/St. Martin, St. Thomas/St. John, Martinique, Barbados, and Princess Cays (Bahamas); or Princess Cays, St. Thomas/St. John, Tortola, St. Croix, Ocho Rios (Jamaica), Grand Cayman, and Cozumel/Playa del Carmen (Mexico). **Spring–Summer:** Same as *Crown Princess*.

Port tax: $84–$155 per passenger.

Overview Supposedly modeled on the curves of a dolphin, Princess Cruises' two flagships look more like oversize seafaring versions of the Japanese bullet train. The unusual exteriors, designed by Italian architect Renzo Piano (known for Paris's controversial Pompidou Center), are a blend of the traditional and the avant-garde. The company's biggest and best-equipped ships, the *Crown* and the *Regal* each feature a dramatic domed entertainment area, a million-dollar art collection, and a three-story atrium foyer. The ships are almost as large as Royal Caribbean Cruise Line's 74,000-ton megaship, *Majesty of the Seas,* but they hold about 1,200 fewer passengers and only 140 fewer crew members. The ships also have a high percentage of outside cabins, many of which have private verandas. These comfortable ships manage to avoid overwhelming passengers with their sheer size by creating a soft warm interior with stuffed art-deco furnishings; light-wood panels; polished metals; and muted coral, blue, and aqua tones.

Cabins and Rates

	Beds	Phone	TV	Sitting Area	Fridge	Tub	Per Diem
Suite	Q	●	●	●	●	●	$381–$463
Mini-suite	T/Q	●	●	●	●	●	$320–$407
Outside	T/Q	●	●	●	●	○	$213–$345
Outside	U/L	●	●	●	●	○	$210–$250
Inside	T/Q	●	●	●	●	○	$199–$270

Each cabin has a walk-in closet, a refrigerator, a separate dressing area, and a safe. Outside cabins have large picture windows. Most outside cabins on the Aloha and Baja decks (including all suites and minisuites) have private verandas. The view from the F-category outside cabins on Dolphin Deck is obstructed.

Outlet voltage: 110 AC.

Single supplement: 200% of double-occupancy rate for suite, and minisuites, 140%–160% for other cabins.

Discounts: A third or fourth passenger in a cabin pays $86–$116 per diem. You get a discount for early booking on summer

Alaska cruises and Panama Canal repositioning transits, and for arranging your own airfare.

Sports and Fitness **Health club:** Sizable below-decks facility with aerobics room, steam room, sauna, weight machines, stationary bikes, other exercise equipment, massage, beauty parlor.

Walking/jogging: Unobstructed, tractioned running track on Sun Deck (6 laps=1 mile).

Other sports: Exercise classes, golf driving, ping-pong, scuba and snorkeling lessons (scuba certification available), shuffleboard, skeet shooting, two pools (one with a waterfall, the other with a swim-up bar), two whirlpools.

Facilities **Public rooms:** Nine bars, five entertainment lounges, card room, casino, champagne/caviar bar, cinema/conference center, dining room, disco, domed observation lounge, Lido, library, patisserie/specialty-coffee bar (*Crown*), piano bar, pizzeria.

Shops: Two-level arcade of boutiques, gift shops, drugstore, hairdresser.

Health care: Two doctors and two nurses on call.

Child care: Children's program with youth counselor when 15 or more children on board.

Services: Laundry, dry-cleaning, photographer, film processing.

Other: Alcoholics Anonymous.

Access for the Disabled Ten cabins have been designed for wheelchair access.

TSS Fair Princess

Specifications | | |
|---|---|
| *Type of ship:* Upscale mainstream | *Passengers:* 890 |
| | *Crew:* 445 (European) |
| *Type of cruise:* Traditional/senior | *Officers:* Italian |
| | *Passenger/crew ratio:* 2 to 1 |
| *Size:* Medium (25,000 tons) | *Year built:* 1957 |
| *Cabins:* 445 | |
| *Outside cabins:* 51.2% | |

Itinerary **Fall:** Part of season in Far East. A nine-day Pacific crossing between Honolulu and Los Angeles calls at Kauai, Lahaina (Maui), Kona (Big Island), and Ensenada (Mexico). **Winter:** Ten-day loops out of Los Angeles call at Puerto Vallarta, Zihuatanejo/Ixtapa, Acapulco, Mazatlán, and Cabo San Lucas. **Spring–Summer:** Seven-day cruises between Vancouver and Anchorage call at Ketchikan, Juneau, Skagway, Glacier Bay, College Fjord, and Columbia Glacier.

Port tax: $74–$155 per passenger.

Overview A former Sitmar ship, the *Fair* was built in 1957 as an ocean liner and refurbished in 1993. It has retained much of its original look, with teakwood decks, glass-paneled library bookshelves, muted pastel interiors, and wood paneling. As is often the case on converted ocean liners, however, public space is relatively limited.

Cabins and Rates

	Beds	Phone	TV	Sitting Area	Fridge	Tub	Per Diem*
Suite	D	●	●	●	●	●	$327–$501
Mini-suite	T	●	●	●	○	○	$256–$428
Outside	T or U/L	●	○	○	○	○	$171–$350
Inside	T or U/L	●	○	○	○	○	$128–$270

Mexico cruises cost the least, Alaskan cruises the most.

Because the ship was built as a liner, cabins are larger than average and include such features as oversize closets, full-length mirrors, and wood trim. Outside views from cabins on the Aloha Deck are obstructed by lifeboats; cabins on the Baja Deck look onto a public promenade. All cabins—except suites, minisuites, and cabins in categories K, N, and P—have two extra upper berths.

Outlet voltage: 110 AC.

Single supplement: 200% of double-occupancy rate for Suites and Mini-suites, 140%–160% for other cabins.

Discounts: A third or fourth passenger in a cabin pays $71–$143 per diem. You get a discount for early booking on Alaska cruises and other select sailings, and for arranging your own airfare.

Sports and Fitness   **Health club:** Rowing machines, Life Cycles, sit-up boards, Paramount Fitness Trainer, sauna, massage, Nautilus bicep machine, punching bag.

Walking/jogging: Partly obstructed circuit on Baja Deck.

Other sports: Aerobics and other exercise classes, table tennis, shuffleboard, volleyball, three pools.

Facilities   **Public rooms:** Six bars, four entertainment lounges (main showroom, cabaret, disco, nightclub), card room, casino, cinema/theater, library, Lido, piano bar, pizzeria.

Shops: Five boutiques/gift shops, beauty salon/barber.

Health care: Doctor and two nurses on call.

Child care: Youth center (open 9 AM–midnight to children over six months) with video and other games, wide-screen TV, children's pool, sun deck; counselors and children's programs year-round.

Services: Full-service laundry, laundromat, ironing room, photographer, film processing.

Other: Safe-deposit boxes, Alcoholics Anonymous.

Access for the Disabled   Ramps have been installed throughout the two ships; however, some areas remain inaccessible. Most of the elevators are wheelchair- accessible.

MV Golden Princess

Specifications *Type of ship:* Upscale mainstream *Passengers:* 830
Type of cruise: Traditional/senior *Crew:* 410 (European)
Size: Medium (28,000 tons) *Officers:* European
Number of Cabins: 415 *Passenger/crew ratio:* 2 to 1
Outside cabins: 85% *Year built:* 1973

Itinerary **Fall–Spring:** Seven- and 10-day loops out of Los Angeles call at Cabo San Lucas, Mazatlán, Puerto Vallarta, Acapulco, and Zihuatanejo/Ixtapa. In spring and fall, several nine-, 10-, and 11-day cruises sail from Vancouver, Tahiti, and Mexico, calling at the Hawaiian islands of Kuaui, Honolulu (Oahu), Lahaina (Maui), and Kona and Hilo (Hawaii). **Summer:** Same as *Fair Princess*.

Port tax: $74–$155 per passenger

Overview At press time (spring 1993), the *Golden Princess* was still several weeks away from replacing the *Dawn Princess,* and a full firsthand review was not possible. The *Golden* will take over the *Dawn*'s itinerary, and Princess is investing a great deal in its refurbishment. The *Golden* sailed formerly with Royal Viking Line as the *Royal Viking Sky;* it was later operated by NCL as the *Sunward* and recently in Europe by Birka Lines as the *Birka Queen.* In its previous lives, the *Golden* was one of the most luxurious ships of its kind, and its 1993 inaugural voyage is expected to show off one of the better ship reincarnations in years.

Cabins and Rates

	Beds	Phones	TV	Sitting Area	Fridge	Tub	Per Diem
Suite	D/T	●	●	●	●	●	$401–$708
Outside Deluxe	D/T	●	●	●	●	●	$266–$463
Outside	D/T	●	●	○	○	●	$198–$331
Inside	D/T	●	●	○	○	●	$174–$285

Suites have verandas. Outside Deluxe staterooms have large picture windows.

Outlet voltage: 110 AC.

Single Supplement: 200% of double-occupancy rate for suites, 150%–160% for other cabins.

Other discounts: A third or fourth passengers pays about $87–$141 per passenger per diem. You get a discount of up to $250 for arranging your own airfare. You get an additional discount for booking early.

Sports and Fitness **Health club:** Lifecycles, Lifesteps, rowing machines, free weights, saunas.

Walking/jogging: There's an unobstructed circuit.

Other sports: Shuffleboard, golf driving, ping-pong, basketball, paddle tennis, two whirlpools, two pools.

Facilities **Public rooms:** Several lounges and bars, restaurant, Lido buffet, small conference room, library, shopping arcade, photo gallery/shop, disco, casino, show lounge.

Shops: Several boutiques and gift shops, beauty salon/barber.

Health care: Doctor on call.

Child Care: Youth programs with counselors offered when demand warrants it.

Services: Full-service laundry, dry-cleaning, photographer.

Other: Safe-deposit boxes.

Access for the Disabled Information on the *Golden*'s access for travelers with disabilities was not available at press time (spring 1993).

MV Island Princess and MV Pacific Princess

Specifications *Type of ship:* Upscale mainstream
Type of cruise: Traditional
Size: Medium (20,000 tons)
Cabins: 305
Outside cabins: 77.5%

Passengers: 610
Crew: 350 (international)
Officers: British
Passenger/crew ratio: 1.7 to 1
Year built: 1972/1971

Itinerary **Island Princess** **Fall:** Mediterranean. **Winter:** Australia and South Pacific. **Spring:** A 14-day Panama Canal Transit between Los Angeles and San Juan calls at Puerto Caldera (Costa Rica), along the Canal, St. Maarten/St. Martin, and St. Thomas/St. John. An 11-day Amazon sailing between San Juan and Manaus (Brazil) call at St. Thomas/St. John, Martinique, Barbados, Devil's Island (off French Guiana); Santana, Santarém, Alter do Chão, and Boca do Valer (Amazon River, Brazil). A 14-day sailing between Manaus and Buenos Aires calls at the Brazilian ports of Santana, Recife, Rio de Janeiro, and Santos and at Montevideo. **Summer:** Outside Western Hemisphere.

Port tax: $51–$123 per passenger.

Pacific Princess **Fall:** Part of season outside Western Hemisphere. A 14-day Panama Canal Transit between San Juan and Los Angeles calls at St. Thomas/St. John, St. Maarten/St. Martin, along the Canal, Puerto Caldera (Costa Rica), Acapulco. **Winter–Summer:** Outside Western Hemisphere.

Port tax: $51–$123 per passenger.

Overview Though the *Island Princess* and *Pacific Princess* are the smallest vessels in the fleet, they are spacious and attractive. Both also carry large crews, which results in superior service—from the fresh flowers everywhere to the white-gloved stewards who are always close by.

Most outdoor activities are centered on the cloverleaf-shaped swimming pool, protected by a retractable canopy called the Sun Dome. The interiors are modern and impressive—particularly the two-story lobby, with its spectacular staircase, floor-to-ceiling mirrors, and glass paneling. The dining rooms are well-lit and roomy, with plenty of tables for two.

In an effort to remain popular in the competitive cruise market, both ships completed $20-million refurbishments recently—the *Pacific Princess* in September 1992, the *Island Princess* in April 1993. The ships now have completely new interiors, including electrically controlled sliding glass doors leading to the pool deck, a new Veranda buffet, new colors and patterns, and a new collection of contemporary art. The jogging track has been resurfaced for better traction.

Cabins and Rates	Beds	Phone	TV	Sitting Area	Fridge	Tub	Per Diem*
Suite	T	●	○	●	●	●	$502–$726
Mini-suite	D or T	●	○	●	●	●	$435–$644
Outside Deluxe Single	T	●	○	○	●	○	$449–$658
Outside Deluxe	T	○	○	●	●	○	$346–$540
Inside Deluxe	T	○	○	●	●	○	$320–$503
Outside	T	○	○	○	○	○	$264–$463
Inside	T	○	○	○	○	○	$206–$390

Panama Canal Transits cost the least, South American cruises the most.

Some cabins on the Promenade Deck look onto a public area.

Outlet voltage: 110 AC.

Single supplement: 200% of double-occupancy rate for suites and mini-suites, 140%–160% for other cabins.

Discounts: A third or fourth passenger in a cabin pays $132–$169 (*Pacific Princess*) or $285–$350 (*Island Princess*). You get a discount for early booking on most itineraries, and for arranging your own airfare.

Sports and Fitness **Health club:** Life Cycles, rowing machines, weights, weight machines, saunas, massage.

Walking/jogging: Observation Deck (18 laps=1 mile).

Other sports: Aerobics and other exercise classes, golf driving, table tennis, shuffleboard, skeet shooting, two pools.

Facilities: **Public rooms:** Six bars, four entertainment lounges, card room, three casinos, cinema/theater, disco, library/writing room, Lido.

Shops: Gift shop, beauty salon/barber.

Health care: Doctor and two nurses on call.

Child care: Daytime youth programs with counselors when more than 15 children on board.

Services: Full-service laundry, dry-cleaning, photographer.

Other: Safe-deposit boxes, Alcoholics Anonymous.

Access for the Disabled Public lavatories and some cabins are equipped with wide toilet stalls and hand bars to accommodate disabled passengers. All four elevators are wheelchair-accessible.

MV Royal Princess

Specifications *Type of ship:* Luxury mainstream
Type of cruise: Traditional
Size: Large (45,000 tons)
Cabins: 600
Outside cabins: 100%

Passengers: 1,200
Crew: 520 (international)
Officers: British
Passenger/crew ratio: 2.4 to 1
Year built: 1984

Itinerary **Fall–Spring:** Ten- and 11-day Panama Canal Transits between Acapulco and San Juan call at Puerto Caldera (Costa Rica), along the Canal, Cartagena (Colombia), St. Maarten/St. Martin, and St. Thomas/St. John; or St. Thomas/St. John, Martinique, Grenada, Caracas/La Guaira, Curaçao, and along the Canal. **Summer:** Europe.

Port tax: $125–$195 per passenger.

Overview The *Royal Princess* was one of the first ships to offer outside cabins and staterooms. Furthermore, many cabins have private verandas, although views from some are obstructed by lifeboats. Add to this 2 acres of open deck space, and you see why this is one of the most opulent, extravagant mainstream ships afloat—and the hallmark of Princess Cruises.

The Horizon Lounge and Bar offers a breathtaking, 360-degree view of the sea from its position atop the ship. Lovely as it is, the lounge is rarely crowded. Most other public rooms are clustered on the Riviera Deck. The two main showrooms—the circular International Lounge and the cabaret-style Riviera Club—boast excellent acoustics.

Cabins and Rates

	Beds	Phone	TV	Sitting Area	Fridge	Tub	Per Diem
Penthouse	Q	●	●	●	●	●	$715–$865
Suite	Q	●	●	●	●	●	$565–$692
Mini-suite	Q	●	●	●	●	●	$465–$607
Outside	T/Q	●	●	○	●	●	$265–$530

Penthouses, suites, minisuites, and Aloha Deck outside cabins have private verandas. Categories H, HH, I, J, JJ, and K are outside cabins with partially or entirely obstructed views. Even the smallest cabins are well equipped, with details and amenities not found in the suites of many other ships, such as double sinks, shower/bathtubs, refrigerators, and large windows. Higher-priced cabins have wall safes, and penthouses have whirlpools. Every cabin receives a fresh-fruit basket that is refilled throughout the cruise.

Outlet voltage: 110 AC.

Single supplement: 200% of double-occupancy rate for suites or outside cabins with verandas, 140%–160% for other cabins.

Discounts: A third or fourth passenger in a cabin pays $132–$150 per diem. You get a discount for early booking on Panama Canal Transits, and for arranging your own airfare.

Sports and Fitness **Health club:** Four high-tech stationary bikes, rowing machines, whirlpool; adjacent beauty center with two saunas, two massage rooms, spa treatments.

Walking/jogging: Unobstructed circuit (3.5 laps=1 mile).

Other sports: Aerobics and other exercise classes, golf driving, table tennis, pool sports, shuffleboard, skeet shooting, four pools (one for laps, a much smaller one surrounded by dipping pools and a whirlpool).

Facilities **Public rooms:** Seven bars, four entertainment lounges, card room, casino, cinema/theater, disco, library, enclosed Lido, video arcade.

Shops: Gift shop, beauty salon/barber.

Health care: Two doctors and two nurses on call.

Child care: Daytime youth programs with counselors when more than 15 children on board.

Services: Full-service laundry, dry-cleaning, laundromat, photographer, film processing.

Other: Safe-deposit boxes, Alcoholics Anonymous.

Access for the Disabled Ten cabins per cruise are available to disabled passengers. All public areas, except the laundromat, are wheelchair-accessible. Several public lavatories are specially equipped.

TSS Sky Princess

Specifications *Type of ship:* Upscale mainstream
Type of cruise: Traditional
Size: Large (46,000 tons)
Cabins: 600
Outside cabins: 64%

Passengers: 1,200
Crew: 535 (international)
Officers: British
Passenger/crew ratio: 2.2 to 1
Year built: 1984

Itinerary **Fall:** Eleven-day Panama Canal Transits between Port Everglades and Acapulco call at Puerto Caldera (Costa Rica), along the Canal, Cartagena (Colombia), Ocho Rios (Jamaica), and Princess Cays (Bahamas). Fifteen-day Panama Canal Transits between Port Everglades and Los Angeles call at the above ports, as well as Cabo San Lucas. **Winter:** Seven-day loops out of Port Everglades call at Princess Cays, Montego Bay (Jamaica), Grand Cayman, and Cozumel/Playa del Carmen (Mexico). **Spring:** Same as Fall. **Summer:** Ten-day loops leave San Francisco, calling at Vancouver, Juneau, Glacier Bay, Sitka, and Victoria.

Port tax: $74–$155 per passenger.

Overview Formerly Sitmar's *Fairsky*, the *Sky Princess* underwent a major refurbishment in 1992. A huge showroom—with a tiered floor, a large stage, and new light and sound systems—was installed. In addition to redecorating the entire ship, Princess expanded the shopping area. Three swimming pools are on deck, with plenty of space for sunning.

Cabins and Rates

	Beds	Phone	TV	Sitting Area	Fridge	Tub	Per Diem*
Suite	D	●	●	●	●	●	$500–$631
Mini-suite	T	●	●	●	●	○	$399–$425
Outside	T	●	●	○	○	○	$250–$331
Inside	T	●	●	○	○	○	$171–$263

* *Alaska cruises cost the most, Panama Canal Transits the least.*

Suites have verandas. Many cabins have two upper berths to accommodate third and fourth passengers.

Outlet voltage: 110 AC.

Single supplement: 200% of double-occupancy rate for suites and minisuites, 140%–160% for other cabins.

Discounts: A third or fourth passenger in a cabin pays $122–$131. You get a discount for early booking on all Alaska cruises and most Panama Canal Transits, and for arranging your own airfare.

Sports and Fitness **Health club:** Nautilus machines; sit-up board, three Life Cycles, two stationary bikes, ballet barre, sauna, massage room, large whirlpool.

Walking/jogging: ⅟₁₅-mile jogging track above the Sun Deck.

Other sports: Aerobics and other exercise classes, paddle and table tennis, pool games, shuffleboard, skeet shooting, volleyball, three pools (one for children), scuba certification.

Facilities **Public rooms:** Seven bars, five entertainment lounges, card room, casino, cinema, disco, library, Lido, piano bar, pizzeria, video arcade.

Shops: Four boutiques/gift shops, beauty salon/barber.

Health care: Doctor and two nurses on call.

Child care: Youth center (open 9 AM–midnight) with separate rooms for teens and younger children (older than six months), games, video games, wide-screen TV, children's pool, sun deck, programs supervised by counselors year-round.

Services: Full-service laundry, dry-cleaning, laundromat, photographer, film processing.

Other: Safe-deposit boxes, Alcoholics Anonymous.

Access for the Disabled Six cabins are designed for passengers in wheelchairs. All six elevators are wheelchair-accessible.

MV Star Princess

Specifications *Type of ship:* Upscale mainstream
Type of cruise: Traditional
Size: Megaship (63,500 tons)

Passengers: 1,494
Crew: 600 (international)
Officers: Italian
Passenger/crew ratio: 2.5 to 1
Year built: 1989

Cabins: 736
Outside cabins: 77.6%

Itinerary **Year-round:** Seven-day loops out of San Juan call at Barbados, Martinique, Mayreau (Grenadines), St. Maarten/St. Martin, and St. Thomas/St. John.

Port tax: $89 per passenger.

Overview The *Star Princess*, the first new ship to be built after Sitmar and Princess merged, is striking for its size alone: It has 12 public decks. Princess resisted the temptation to cram in as many cabins and staterooms as possible, and as a result, the ship is extremely spacious. Its centerpiece is The Plaza, a dramatic three-deck-high atrium topped by a dome. Perhaps the most engaging public room is the Windows on the World Lounge, with its 360-degree view of the sea. A million-dollar collection of contemporary art is placed throughout the ship, both in the public rooms and in individual cabins. Daytime activities revolve around the Pool Deck, where two swimming pools and four whirlpools are connected by a walkway and waterfalls, and passengers can swim to the splash bar.

Cabins and Rates

	Beds	Phone	TV	Sitting Area	Fridge	Tub	Per Diem
Suite	Q	●	●	●	●	●	$462–$669
Mini-suite	T/Q	●	●	●	●	●	$398–$539
Outside	T/Q	●	●	○	●	○	$250–$319
Inside	T/Q	●	●	○	●	○	$171–$254

Standard cabins are spacious, with twin beds that convert to queen-size, a built-in safe, minifridges, and remote-control color TVs. The suites have separate sitting areas, marble baths, and king-size beds. Outside cabins have large picture windows; the suites and minisuites have verandas with sliding glass doors. Some outside cabins have obstructed views. Most cabins have upper berths to accommodate a third or fourth passenger.

Outlet voltage: 110 AC.

Single supplement: 200% of double-occupancy rate for suites and minisuites, 140%–160% for other cabins.

Discounts: A third or fourth passenger in a cabin pays $109–$134 per diem. You get a discount for early booking on Alaska cruises and some Panama Canal Transits, and for arranging your own airfare.

Sports and Fitness **Health club:** Nautilus equipment, aerobics area, sauna, steam room, massage, beauty treatments.

Walking/jogging: Sun Deck (5 laps=1 mile).

Other sports: Exercise classes, shuffleboard, skeet shooting, volleyball, three pools, four whirlpools, scuba certification.

Facilities   **Public rooms:** Seven bars, seven lounges, card room, casino, cinema/theater, disco, library, Lido, patisserie/specialty-coffee café, piano bar, pizzeria, wine bar.

Shops: Four boutiques/gift shops, beauty salon/barber.

Health care: Two doctors and two nurses on call.

Child care: Youth center (open 9 AM–midnight) for children over six months, with games, video games, wide-screen TV, children's pool and sun deck, programs supervised by counselors year-round.

Services: Full-service laundry, dry-cleaning, laundromat, ironing room, photographer, film processing.

Other: Safe-deposit boxes, Alcoholics Anonymous.

Access for the Disabled   Ten cabins are equipped for disabled passengers. All nine elevators are wheelchair-accessible.

Regency Cruises

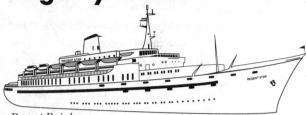

Ships *Regent Rainbow*
Regent Sea
Regent Star
Regent Sun

Evaluation Relatively new on the mainstream cruising scene, Regency has carved a niche for itself by offering affordable cruises to unusual destinations. Passengers tend to be sophisticated, experienced cruisers who want to see more than the typical Caribbean loop but can't afford most exotic cruises. Others are first-timers after an inexpensive vacation. While the Alaska cruises draw mostly families and younger folks. Regency rewards all with good value.

Founded in 1984, the company showed a profit almost immediately, refitting older vessels instead of building new ones. For cruise buffs, sailing on ships that were once famous liners can be a great thrill. All these charming, mature ships are comfortable and friendly rather than modern and glitzy. Like many older ships, they also have spacious cabins, classic lines, a full-screen theater, and a full-size gym and casino.

In addition to Regency's low published rates, substantial discounts are given for advance or last-minute bookings, back-to-back or repeat cruises, or trips during the shoulder season. Special deals like second-honeymoon packages, which include a number of romantic perks, are a nice touch. Fortunately, Regency doesn't *feel* like a budget operation. As on the more expensive lines, passengers sign for all on-board purchases, settling their accounts when they debark. European-style service and outstanding Continental cuisine are among the other features usually associated with higher-priced cruise lines.

Activities Regency offers bingo, crafts classes, dance lessons, duplicate bridge, wine tasting, pool games, scavenger hunts, trivia quizzes, and other typical activities. In the Caribbean, optional snorkeling and scuba programs, with onboard instruction, and supervised underwater tours are available. Lectures on scenery and wildlife are given by trained naturalists during the Alaska cruises—which are also noted for offering as many as

Chart Symbols. *The following symbols are used in the cabin charts that accompany each ship's evaluation.* **D:** *Double bed;* **K:** *King-size bed;* **Q:** *Queen-size bed;* **T:** *Twin bed;* **U/L:** *Upper and lower berths;* ●: *All cabins have this facility;* ○: *No cabins have this facility;* ◑: *Some cabins have this facility*

eight or nine shore excursions per port. Gentlemen hosts are on board many sailings as dancing and bridge partners.

Dining Cuisine tends to be above average. Portions are hearty. "Lean and light" alternatives are usually available. Breakfast and lunch are usually open seating. The Lido café serves good breakfast and lunch buffets, and an outdoor grill offers hot dogs, hamburgers, and chicken for lunch. Other food offerings are mid-morning bouillon, afternoon tea, hot and cold hors d'oeuvres before dinner, and a gracious midnight buffet; snack hours are long and fill the gaps between meals. Room service is prompt, accurate, and available 24 hours from a limited menu. Write one month ahead for special diet requests or kosher selections. The sugar-free desserts are excellent. There are two assigned seatings at dinner (6 and 8:15).

Entertainment You'll see nightly variety shows, disco, dance orchestras, and movies. At some ports, local folkloric dancers come aboard to perform. Other lively and not-so-lively participatory games and activities include "horse racing," passenger talent shows, Liar's Club, and the well-attended "Mr. and Mrs." newlyweds game. A singles party is held early in the cruise. Overall, the entertainment is wholesome (no off-color jokes or Las Vegas–style dancers) and appropriate for children. About five recent films are shown weekly in the ships' theaters.

Service and Tipping With relatively low crew-to-passenger ratios, service is superior to other mainstream lines. Because Regency respects its employees, treats them well, and even provides entertainment for them, there is a low personnel turnover. This fosters dignified, competent service that is even over-conscientious at times. Most of the staff is recruited from Europe, and although language lessons are given on board, new employees sometimes have an initial problem with English. Tip the cabin stewardess and the dining room waiter $2.50 each per passenger per diem, the busboy $1.50.

For More Information Regency Cruises (260 Madison Ave., New York, NY 10016, tel. 212/972–4499 or 800/341–5566).

Regent Rainbow

Specifications | | |
|---|---|
| *Type of ship:* Economy mainstream | *Passengers:* 960 |
| *Type of cruise:* Traditional | *Crew:* 420 (mostly European) |
| *Size:* Medium (25,000 tons) | *Officers:* Greek |
| *Number of cabins:* 484 | *Passenger/crew ratio:* 2.3 to 1 |
| *Outside cabins:* 68% | *Year built:* 1957 |

Itinerary **Year-round:** Two-day "cruises to nowhere" leave Tampa Fridays, returning on Sunday. Five-day loops leave Tampa Sundays, calling at Cozumel/Playa del Carmen (Mexico) and Key West.

Port tax: $52 per passenger.

Overview The *Rainbow* was introduced in January 1993, luring first-time cruisers interested in shorter vacations with two-day cruises to nowhere. The theory is that if passengers enjoy the two-day cruises, they'll come back for a five-day stint. It will be interesting to see whether this strategy works over the long haul.

Regency put $75 million into restoring the former *Santa Rosa*, and they've done a commendable job. In the Chanterelle dining room, with an orchestra balcony and a stained-glass ceiling, you'll feast (at two seatings) on excellent cuisine prepared by expertly trained French chefs. Breeze up to the Bridge Deck for dancing to an orchestra in the Starlight Lounge or bopping the night away in the Sky Room disco. A casino provides all the usual tables, from blackjack to Caribbean stud poker. A well-appointed fitness center has saunas and a massage room.

Cabins and Rates

	Beds	Phone	TV	Sitting Area	Fridge Diem	Tub	Per
Suites	D	●	●	●	○	○	$185–$218
Deluxe Outside	D,T	●	●	○	○	●	$175–$188
Superior Outside	D,T	●	●	○	●	○	$161–$173
Outside	D,T	●	●	○	●	○	$148–$150
Inside	D,T	●	●	○	●	○	$98 $125

Many cabins have large picture windows. All have color TV, telephone, radio, and climate control.

Outlet voltage: 110 AC.

Single supplement: 140%–200% of double-occupancy rate. Regency will match same-sex single passengers; if no roommate is found, the single passenger still pays just half the double-occupancy rate.

Discounts: A third or fourth passenger in a cabin pays about $100–$120 per diem.

Sports and Fitness **Health club:** Sauna, massage.

Walking/jogging: Promenade Deck jogging track.

Other sports: Two pools.

Facilities **Public rooms:** Six lounges, disco, casino, card room, library, conference room, dining room.

Shops: Boutiques, beauty salon/barber.

Health care: Infirmary, doctor on call.

Child care: Supervised children's playroom.

Services: Full-service laundry, photographer.

Access for the Disabled There are four fully equipped disabled-accessible staterooms.

Regent Sea

Specifications *Type of ship:* Mainstream
Type of cruise: Traditional/
Size: Medium (22,000 tons)
Number of cabins: 361
Outside cabins: 92%

Passengers: 729
Crew: 365 (European/
international)
Officers: Greek
Passenger/crew ratio: 2 to 1
Year built: 1957

Itinerary **Fall:** Two 10-day Hawaii cruises are offered. One sails between Vancouver and Honolulu. The second sails between San Diego and Honolulu. Both call at Hilo and Kona (Hawaii), Honolulu (Oahu), and Lahaina and Nawilliwili (Kauai). A 50-day circumnavigation of South America (with smaller segments available) starts and ends in Tampa. **Winter–Spring:** Seven-day loops leave Tampa Sundays, calling at Cozumel/Playa del Carmen, Montego Bay (Jamaica), and Grand Cayman. **Summer:** Seven-day, one-way cruises between Vancouver and Anchorage/Whittier call at Ketchikan, Juneau, Skagway, Sitka, along the Inside Passage, and Columbia Glacier/College Fjord. Sometimes Glacier Bay National Park is a substitute port.

Port tax: $69 (Caribbean), $119 (Alaska), or $77–$227 (South America) per passenger.

Overview The *Gripsholm,* a legendary Swedish-American luxury liner, fell on hard times and underwent several incarnations before Regency purchased it and transformed it into the *Regent Sea.* The vessel retains its classic lines and much of its original handsome woods and fixtures. It's also one of the few remaining cruise ships with twin smokestacks and a wraparound, glass-enclosed promenade. The latter allows you to enjoy Alaska's spectacular scenery without having to brave its frigid climate.

The public rooms (except the dining room, theater, and gymnasium) are on one deck, which makes it easy to get your bearings. But, as on many older ships, the dining room cuts the Main Deck in half, forcing passengers to go up a deck, across, and then down again to get past the dining room when it's closed. Although the *Sea* is well maintained and appointed, don't look for luxury. The decor is a blend of traditional and modern, with a fairly successful marriage of old wood and highly polished mirrors and brass. Most cabins are outside.

Cabins and Rates

	Beds	Phone	TV	Sitting Area	Fridge	Tub	Per Diem*
Suites	T or D	●	○	●	◑	●	$300–$419
Deluxe Outside	T or D	●	○	●	○	●	$270–$382
Superior Outside	T or D	●	○	●	○	●	$244–$339
Outside	T or U/L	●	○	○	○	◑	$169–$315
Inside	T or D	●	○	○	○	○	$188–$246

Alaska cruises cost the most, Caribbean cruises the least.

Cabins are quite large compared with those on similarly priced ships, and storage space is unusually abundant. Most cabins are outside, but lifeboats obstruct the view of some on the Sun Deck, where all suites and cabins look onto a public promenade (privacy is afforded in these cases with one-way-mirror windows). It takes a few detours to reach the forward cabins on the Bolero and Allegro decks (the bottom two decks), accessible only by the forward stairways.

Outlet voltage: 110 AC.

Single supplement: 130%–200% of double-occupancy rate. Regency will match same-sex single passengers; if no roommate is found, the passenger still pays just half the double-occupancy rate.

Discounts: A third or fourth passenger in a cabin pays $104–$119 per diem. A child under 18 in a cabin with two adults pays $85–$104 per diem.

Sports and Fitness   **Health club:** Exercise equipment, whirlpools, men's and women's saunas, massage.

Walking/jogging: Unobstructed circuit on Sun Deck.

Other sports: Aerobics and other exercise classes, golf driving range, scuba and snorkeling lessons, shuffleboard, ping-pong, trapshooting, pool.

Facilities   **Public rooms:** Three bars, three entertainment lounges, card room, casino, cinema, dining room, disco, library, Lido.

Shops: Boutiques, beauty parlor/barber.

Health care: Doctor on call.

Child care: Youth programs with counselors during holidays, baby-sitting arranged privately with staff member.

Services: Full-service laundry, photographer.

Other: Safe-deposit boxes, Alcoholics Anonymous.

Access for the Disabled   Two cabins have been refitted with wider doors and bathrooms for wheelchair access. All elevators and public rooms are reached from a level deck.

Regent Star

Specifications   *Type of ship:* Mainstream
Type of cruise: Traditional/
Size: Medium (24,500 tons)
Number of cabins: 485
Outside cabins: 56.9%

Passengers: 950
Crew: 450 (European/
 international)
Officers: Greek
Passenger/crew ratio:
 2 to 1
Year built: 1957

Itinerary   **Fall–Winter:** Seven-day loop cruises leave Tampa Sundays, calling at Cozumel/Playa del Carmen (Mexico), Montego Bay (Jamaica), and Grand Cayman. A seven-day loop leaves Montego Bay, calling at Cartagena (Colombia), Aruba, Curaçao, Gatun Lake (along Panama Canal), and Puerto Moin (Costa Rica). **Spring–Summer:** Seven-day one-way cruises between Vancouver and Anchorage/Whittier call at Ketchikan, Juneau, Skagway, Sitka, along the Inside Passage, and Columbia Glacier/College Fjord. Sometimes Glacier Bay National Park is a substitute port.

Port tax: $104 (Caribbean) or $119 (Alaska) per passenger.

Overview   The *Star*—formerly the *Statendam*—is a handsome vessel that has delighted cruisers for decades. Although only 500 tons larger than the *Sea*, the *Regent Star* carries 231 more passengers. However, the public rooms, including the main dining room, are large and roomy, and the almost two-to-one ratio of passengers to crew assures personal attention. The *Star*'s interior is streamlined and contemporary, and most of the public rooms, including the Cordon Bleu dining room, feature large windows.

Cabins and Rates		Beds	Phone	TV	Sitting Area	Fridge	Tub	Per Diem*
	Deluxe Outside	D or T	●	○	●	◐	◐	$271–$404
	Superior Outside	D or T	●	○	●	○	◐	$244–$356
	Outside	D, T, or U/L	●	○	○	○	◐	$222–$321
	Inside	D, T, or U/L	●	○	○	○	◐	$176–$335

*Alaska cruises cost the most, Caribbean cruises the least.

Views from cabins on the Bridge Deck are obstructed by lifeboats. On the Upper Promenade Deck cabins look onto a public promenade; one-way-mirror windows afford privacy.

Outlet voltage: 110 AC.

Single supplement: 130%–200% of double-occupancy rate. Regency will match same-sex single passengers; if no roommate is found, the single passenger still pays just half the double-occupancy rate.

Discounts: A third or fourth passenger in a cabin pays $104–$118 per diem. A child under 18 in a cabin with two adults pays $85–$104 per diem. Cabin S18 is a sitting room that can booked for an extra $985 (with no additional passengers) or $1,065 (for each additional passenger) with cabin S16 or S17 to form a large suite.

Sports and Fitness   **Health club:** Lower-deck gym with exercise equipment, indoor pool, sauna, massage.

Walking/jogging: The promenade is wide and glass-enclosed and okay for walking. There is nowhere to jog.

Other sports: Exercise classes, ping-pong, scuba and snorkeling lessons, shuffleboard, trapshooting, outdoor pool, two whirlpools, golf driving range, basketball hoop.

Facilities   **Public rooms:** Three bars, three entertainment lounges, card room, casino, cinema, library, dining room, disco, Lido.

Shops: Boutiques, hairdresser/barber.

Health care: Doctor on call.

Child care: Youth programs with counselors during holidays, baby- sitting arranged privately with staff member.

Services: Laundry, photographer.

Other: Safe-deposit boxes, Alcoholics Anonymous.

Access for the Disabled   Two cabins have been refitted with wider doors and bathrooms for wheelchair access. All elevators and public rooms are reached from a level deck. The Sports Deck is inaccessible.

Regent Sun

Specifications   *Type of ship:* Mainstream   *Passengers:* 836

Type of cruise: Traditional	*Crew:* 390 (European/
Size: Medium (25,500 tons)	international)
Number of cabins: 419	*Officers:* Greek
Outside cabins: 81.9%	*Passenger/crew ratio:*
	2.14 to 1
	Year built: 1964

Itinerary **Late Fall–Spring:** Ten- and 11-day alternating loops leave San Juan, calling at Grenada, Trinidad, Barbados, Martinique, St. Kitts, St. Maarten/St. Martin, and St. Thomas/St. John; or St. Lucia, Barbados, Caracas/La Guaira (Venezuela), Bonaire, Aruba, St. Barts, and St. Thomas/St. John. **Summer–early Fall:** Seven-day cruises between New York and Montréal call at Newport (RI), Portland (ME), Halifax, Québec City, and along the Saguenay Fjord on the northbound trip; or at Québec City, Sydney (Cape Breton Island, Nova Scotia), Bar Harbor, and Provincetown (MA) on the southbound trip.

Port tax: $91–$94 (Caribbean) or $98 (Northeast) per passenger.

Overview The *Regent Sun*—formerly Royal Cruise Line's *Royal Odyssey* and still retaining original Israeli art from its days as the *Shalom*—became Regency Cruises' flagship in 1988. Though it is a relatively seasoned ship, Regency keeps its appearance pristine. The Casino Royale is minuscule compared with other ships' casinos; its glass enclosure effectively prevents underage children from playing the slot machines. Bars are not uniformly active: The Monte Carlo Court is busy when a band is playing or when the pre-dinner hors d'oeuvres are served, but the Panorama Lounge is rarely crowded. The Yacht Club is a small lounge suitable for a quiet drink. The Regency Lounge, which is the main showroom, offers good visibility, padded seats, and easy access. The Cordon Rouge Dining Room is small, pretty, and well laid-out, offering a range of seating options.

Cabins and Rates

	Beds	Phone	TV	Sitting Area	Fridge	Tub	Per Diem*
Suite	K or T	●	○	●	○	◑	$270–$354
Deluxe Outside	D or T	●	○	●	○	◑	$250–$305
Superior Outside	D or T	●	○	●	○	○	$231–$286
Outside	T	●	○	○	○	○	$213–$268
Inside	T	●	○	○	○	○	$170–$231

*Northeast cruises cost the most, Caribbean cruises the least.

Cabins are average size, modestly but tastefully furnished, each with a mirrored vanity. Lifeboats obstruct the view from many cabins on Riviera Deck. Some cabins on Promenade Deck look onto a public walkway; one-way-mirror windows provide privacy.

Outlet voltage: 110 AC.

Single supplement: 130%–200% of double-occupancy rate. Regency will match same-sex single passengers; if no roommate is found, the single passenger still pays just half the double-occupancy rate.

Discounts: A third or fourth passenger in a cabin pays $98–$106 per diem. A child under 18 in a cabin with two adults pays $42–$89 per diem.

Sports and Fitness

Health club: Stationary bikes, rowing and Universal machines, treadmill, free weights, indoor swimming pool, men's and women's saunas, massage.

Walking/jogging: No deck has an unobstructed circuit.

Other sports: Aerobics and other exercise classes, deck tennis, miniature golf and driving cage, ping-pong, shuffleboard, snorkel and scuba lessons, trapshooting, outdoor pool.

Facilities

Public rooms: Five bars, four entertainment lounges, card room, casino, cinema, computer room, dining room, disco/Lido, library.

Shops: Boutique, beauty parlor/barber.

Health care: Doctor on call.

Child care: Youth programs with counselors during holidays and in summer, baby-sitting arranged privately with staff member.

Services: Laundry, photographer.

Other: Safe-deposit boxes, Alcoholics Anonymous.

Access for the Disabled

Two cabins have wider doors and bathrooms for wheelchair access. Elevators and public rooms are reached from a level deck. The Bridge Deck, where the deck-tennis court and golf driving cage are located, is inaccessible. There is a small single step to get into the gym.

Renaissance Cruises

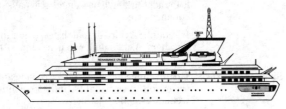

Ships *Renaissance III*
Renaissance VI

Evaluation Renaissance Cruises offers two very different cruise experiences in one. Its ships are yachtlike vessels modeled after Cunard's *Sea Goddess*es. But its ports are chosen for the sake of adventure and education. The only organized onboard activities are lectures about the culture, history, and nature of the areas visited. Passengers are typically intellectual, culturally minded individuals who want to learn about the world as they travel in supreme comfort. Like other cultural cruises, Renaissance provides passengers with pre-trip reading lists. Most passengers are experienced cruisers in their late fifties to early sixties. A number of special-interest tour operators, such as the Smithsonian Institution, use Renaissance vessels for educational cultural tours.

Renaissance describes its fleet of eight ships, six of which sail outside the Western Hemisphere, as "modular." Shortly after the company formed in 1989, it began an unusual and ambitious program to build eight nearly identical ships at the same Italian shipyard, to be launched over a period of three years. Besides saving Renaissance considerable expense, this plan provided passengers with a familiarly laid-out vessel whenever and wherever they cruise with the line.

Activities Don't look for pool games, trivia contests, or other traditional cruise pastimes. Renaissance passengers prefer more introspective activities, such as sitting on a deck chair reading selections from the ship's library, or attending one of the numerous lectures usually related to the culture and history of ports of call. However, Renaissance does have a small casino and extensive water-sports facilities—including a platform that lowers for sailing, snorkeling, and other activities.

Dining The cuisine is international, with a focus on nouvelle light dishes with fresh ingredients. Meals in the restaurant are at two open seatings. The extensive wine cellar is moderately priced. Early morning coffee, breakfast, and lunch are available on deck, weather permitting. A late-night snack is served; 24-hour room service from a limited menu is available. A ques-

---

Chart Symbols. *The following symbols are used in the cabin charts that accompany each ship's evaluation.* **D:** *Double bed;* **K:** *King-size bed;* **Q:** *Queen-size bed;* **T:** *Twin bed;* **U/L:** *Upper and lower berths;* ●: *All cabins have this facility;* ○: *No cabins have this facility;* ◑: *Some cabins have this facility*

tionnaire is mailed to passengers before their trip so that the
cabin refrigerator may be stocked with their favorite beverages and snacks. (There is a charge for whatever is consumed
from the refrigerator.) Men are expected to wear a jacket and
tie to dinner.

Entertainment Renaissance Cruises believes in leaving passengers alone to
enjoy themselves. The library is well stocked with best-sellers,
old favorites, reference works, and recently released videos.
The only other forms of entertainment provided are a small
dance band and a piano bar. Local entertainers are sometimes
brought on board to perform.

Service and Tipping Service is elegant, unobtrusive, and omnipresent, though not
on the level of Seabourn cruises. Tip the stewardess $3 per
passenger per diem, the dining room staff $5 (dining room tips
are pooled). A 15% gratuity is automatically added to the bar
bill. All tips may be charged to your shipboard account, if you'd
rather not use cash.

For More Renaissance Cruises (1800 Eller Dr., Suite 300, Box 350307,
Information Fort Lauderdale, FL 33335–0307, tel. 800/525–2450).

Renaissance III and VI

Specifications *Type of ship:* Luxury   *Passengers:* 104 (*III*)/
yachtlike   114 (*VI*)
Type of cruise: Cultural   *Crew:* (European) 67 (*III*)/
Size: Small (4,500 tons)   72 (*VI*)
Officers: Italian   *Passenger/crew ratio:* 1.6 to 1
Number of cabins: 50   *Year built:* 1990–1991(*III*)/57
Outside cabins: 100%   (*VI*)

Itinerary **Year-round:** Throughout the year, different Renaissance ships
sail in locales outside the Western Hemisphere. Two eight-day
loops leave Antigua, calling at St. Kitts, St. Croix, Virgin
Gorda, St. Maarten/St. Martin, and St. Barts; or Dominica, St.
Lucia, St. Vincent, Bequia (Grenadines), Martinique, and
Montserrat.

Port tax: $195 per passenger.

Overview Renaissance ships aren't graced with long, lean lines; instead,
they look something like a cross between an oversize yacht and
a giant houseboat with wings. The interiors are beautiful, the
furnishings lavish. Subtle earth tones dominate, and many of
the walls are paneled in rich, dark woods accented by polished
brass. Throughout the ship extensive and effective use is made
of mirrors, polished teak, marble, and tasteful modern art. The
atmosphere is refined and warm, and (because the ship is
small) friendly. However, the cruise line has only a satisfactory
reputation for tending to its exterior as meticulously as other
lines do; note the absence of crew members busily painting
away scrape marks whenever the vessels are in port, as is the
tradition in upscale cruising. Though similar to the *Sea Goddess*es and Seabourn ships in design, the Renaissance fleet is
not as beautiful, the lifestyle not as elegant, and the service a
bit short of flawless. But the price is lower, too, the itineraries
are some of the most unusual you'll find, and the lecturers are
stellar.

Cabins and Rates

	Beds	Phone	TV	Sitting Area	Fridge	Tub	Per Diem
Renaissance Suite	T/Q	●	●	●	●	○	$499
Veranda Suite	T/Q	●	●	●	●	○	$437
Deluxe Suite	T/Q	●	●	●	●	○	$374
Superior Suite	T/Q	●	●	●	●	○	$312
Standard Suite	T/Q	●	●	●	●	○	$249

Suites are large compared with those on other small upscale cruise ships, and mirror tiling makes them seem even larger. Bathrooms have teak floors and marble paneling and are equipped with hair dryers; none have bathtubs, however—an unusual omission for this type of ship. Beds can be configured as either twins or queen-size. Rooms have VCRs and a lockable drawer. Most cabins on the Erikson, Marco Polo, and Columbus decks look onto public promenades. Renaissance Suites have oversize walk-in closets and private verandas that look out to sea with no obstructions.

Outlet voltage: 110 AC.

Single supplement: $995 over the double-occupancy rate.

Discounts: A third or fourth passenger in a cabin pays $995 per cruise. Airfare is not included in rates.

Sports and Fitness **Health club:** Exercise equipment, massage, sauna.

Walking/jogging: Unobstructed circuits on Erikson, Marco Polo, and Columbus decks.

Other sports: Zodiacs, sailfish, snorkeling, scuba diving, pool, whirlpool; a water-sports platform that lowers from the stern allows access to the water when the ship is at anchor.

Facilities **Public rooms:** Three bars, one main lounge, blackjack table, slot machines, library, piano bar.

Shops: Gift shop, hairdresser.

Health care: Doctor on call.

Child care: None.

Services: Full-service laundry.

Access for the Disabled There are ledges at the entrance to cabin bathrooms and at the doors that lead from the outer decks to the inside of the ship. There is no official policy regarding disabled passengers, but Renaissance advises that these cruises may be too strenuous for nonambulatory passengers.

Royal Caribbean Cruise Line

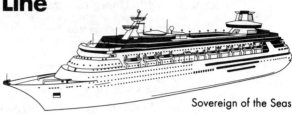

Sovereign of the Seas

Ships MS *Majesty of the Seas*
MS *Monarch of the Seas*
MS *Nordic Empress*
MS *Nordic Prince*
MS *Song of America*
MS *Song of Norway*
MS *Sovereign of the Seas*
MS *Sun Viking*
MS *Viking Serenade*

Evaluation RCCL is a well-run and experienced cruise line that the competition attempts, with varying degrees of success, to emulate. Most of its vessels have won the "Ship of the Year" award given by the World Ocean & Cruise Liner Society. The ships were designed specifically for cruising. While the fleet comprises ships of almost every size, the company's philosophy remains consistent: Offer every imaginable activity in a resort atmosphere interspersed with calls at a variety of ports. RCCL draws customers from every age group and economic bracket, all lured by the prospect of a cruising experience that is above average but certainly not upscale.

Cantilevered from the top of the funnel is the hallmark of an RCCL ship: the glass-enclosed Viking Crown Lounge, with its bird's-eye view. Inside, the cabins are comfortable but neither luxurious nor spacious. Public rooms sport a musical-comedy theme, such as the Annie Get Your Gun Lounge and the HMS Pinafore Dining Room on the *Sun Viking.*

Activities Life on board is similar to that of the party ships run by Carnival but slightly more sophisticated and conservative. Among the many activities offered are cash bingo (plus free poolside bingo for prizes), board and card games, arts and crafts, pool games, dance classes, golf driving and putting, and "horse racing." In response to current fitness trends, the ships also feature numerous exercise activities and well-equipped gyms. Most ships have daylong beach parties in a private cove at CocoCay, a private Bahamian island.

Chart Symbols. *The following symbols are used in the cabin charts that accompany each ship's evaluation.* **D:** *Double bed;* **K:** *King-size bed;* **Q:** *Queen-size bed;* **T:** *Twin bed;* **U/L:** *Upper and lower berths;* ●: *All cabins have this facility;* ○: *No cabins have this facility;* ◐: *Some cabins have this facility*

Dining Food is American and above average, served at two assigned seatings per meal. Dining rooms can be noisy and crowded, and sometimes service is slow. The waiters are friendly to passengers regularly assigned to their tables but less so at midnight buffets or open-seating meals. Alternative menu selections conform to American Heart Association guidelines, but RCCL is not equipped to handle special dietary requests, other than providing vegetarian and children's dishes at all meals. On that note, RCCL began offering vegetarian menus on all of its ships in 1993. Two formal evenings are held on each seven-day cruise, one on three- and four-day cruises.

The Lido-style indoor/outdoor café serves early morning coffee, a buffet breakfast, and lunch. Other food service includes afternoon tea (with a make-your-own sundae bar), a midnight buffet, and late-night sandwich service in the lounges. Room service is available 24 hours from a limited menu (full menu on the *Nordic Empress*'s Concierge Deck). The *Sovereign of the Seas* sells specialty coffees at the shopping arcade "sidewalk" café.

Entertainment This is one of RCCL's strong suits. The company conforms to the established formula for cruise-ship entertainment, but with a dash of pizzazz and professionalism that other lines often lack. Passengers can expect plenty of glitz and glamour: On the *Majesty of the Seas, Monarch of the Seas,* and *Sovereign of the Seas,* two celebrity acts are featured on every cruise. Nightly variety shows, late-night comedy and solo cabaret acts, steel-drum combos, passenger talent shows, and theme parties are staged on each cruise.

Service and Tipping The crew is generally enthusiastic and personable, although service can be slow. Unfortunately, crew members display little subtlety in soliciting tips. Tip the room steward and the waiter each $3 per passenger per diem, the busboy $1.50; the head-waiter gets $2.50 per passenger per cruise (for excellent service only). Tips for bar staff should be given at the time of service.

For More Information Royal Caribbean Cruise Line (1050 Caribbean Way, Miami, FL 33132, tel. 800/327–6700).

MS Majesty of the Seas, MS Monarch of the Seas, and MS Sovereign of the Seas

Specifications *Type of ship:* Mainstream
Type of cruise: Party
Size: Megaship;
73,941/73,941/73,192 tons
Number of cabins:
1,177/1,177/1,138
Outside cabins: 63%

Passengers: 2,766/2,354/2,278
Crew: 822/822/808
(international)
Officers: Norwegian
Passenger/crew ratio: 2.8 to 1
Year built: 1992/1991/1988

Itinerary **Year-round:** Seven-day loops leave Miami Sundays, calling at
Majesty of the Seas Grand Cayman, Cozumel/Playa del Carmen (Mexico), Ocho Rios (Jamaica), and CocoCay (Bahamas).

Port tax: $71 per passenger.

Monarch of the Seas **Year-round:** Seven-day loops leave San Juan Sundays, calling at Martinique, Barbados, Antigua, St. Maarten/St. Martin, and St. Thomas/St. John.

Port tax: $71 per passenger.

Sovereign of the **Year-round:** Seven-day loops leave Miami Saturdays, calling at
Seas CocoCay (Bahamas), San Juan, and St. Thomas/St. John.

Port tax: $71 per passenger.

Overview *Majesty of the Seas* and *Monarch of the Seas*, identical sister
ships, are two of the largest vessels built specifically for cruising. The slightly smaller *Sovereign of the Seas* was the proto-
type for the fleet and has only a few design differences: The
layout of some public rooms is different, and the larger ships
have just one theater, 39 more cabins, and teen nightclubs. The
ships incorporate an incredible range of facilities and amenities
requested by passengers in a special survey. All three are like
floating Atlantic City resorts.

Each ship is as tall as the Statue of Liberty and three football
fields long. The Viking Crown Lounge is 14 stories above sea
level, higher than any lounge on any other line's ship. Given
such enormous dimensions, RCCL ships are often described in
superlatives. Their immense size, however, also means that you
can spend seven days on board and never feel that you're really
at sea. Lines, too, can be long, and the service impersonal. Nevertheless, these are excellent ships for first-time passengers
because they have everything a cruise was ever meant to have.

The heart of each ship is a dramatic four-story atrium accented
with brass railings and curving stairways as well as the signature glass elevators. An arcade with more than a dozen shops
sells everything from fur coats to jewelry. During mealtimes
and in the afternoon, passengers are serenaded with music.
The dining room serves a different international menu each
evening; waiters dress accordingly, and musicians strolls
among the tables playing music to match the cuisine.

Cabins and Rates

	Beds	Phone	TV	Sitting Area	Fridge	Tub	Per Diem
Royal Suite	T/Q	●	●	●	●	●	$485–$513
Suite	T/Q	●	●	●	○	●	$356–$395
Deluxe Outside	T/Q	●	●	●	○	●	$324–$366
Standard Outside	T/Q	●	●	○	○	◗	$249–$295
Inside	T/Q	●	●	○	○	○	$177–$280

Cabins on the Promenade Deck look onto a public area. Concierge service is provided for passengers in suites. Many cabins
have one or two upper berths in addition to the normal configuration.

Outlet voltage: 110/220 AC.

Single supplement: 150% of double-occupancy rate; however,
less expensive singles can be had if you're willing to wait for
your cabin assignment until embarkation time.

Discounts: A third or fourth passenger in a cabin pays about
$100 per diem. Senior citizen discounts are offered on specific
sailings. You get a discount for arranging your own airfare, and

for early booking—the earlier you book, the lower your cabin rate (excluding inside cabins and suites).

Sports and Fitness **Health club:** Rowing machines, treadmills, stationary bikes, massage, men's and women's saunas, outdoor whirlpool.

Walking/jogging: The Promenade has a springy surface for fitness walks (3.5 laps=1 mile).

Other sports: Aerobics and fitness program, basketball, golf driving and putting, table tennis, shuffleboard, skeet shooting, snorkeling lessons, two pools.

Facilities **Public rooms:** Seven entertainment lounges, 10 bars, card room, casino, champagne bar, two cinemas on *Sovereign* and one on *Majesty* and *Monarch*, disco, library, indoor/outdoor double-tier Lido, piano bar, specialty coffee café (*Sovereign*) (extra charge), video-game room, teen centers (*Majesty, Monarch*).

Shops: At least 10 boutiques and gift shops, beauty salon/barber.

Health care: Two doctors and four nurses on call.

Child care: Playroom, youth programs run by counselors, baby-sitting privately arranged with crew member.

Services: Full-service laundry, dry-cleaning, photographer, film processing.

Other: Safe-deposit boxes.

Access for the Disabled These ships are well suited for wheelchairs, with 18 accessible elevators, wide corridors, and specially equipped public lavatories. Two inside and two outside cabins are designed for the disabled. The tenders ferrying passengers to the CocoCay beach party are easy to board; if seas are rough, crew members will carry disabled passengers and their wheelchairs on board. CocoCay is all sand, however, which makes moving about in a wheelchair difficult.

MS Nordic Empress

Specifications | | |
|---|---|
| *Type of ship:* Mainstream | *Passengers:* 1,600 |
| *Type of cruise:* Party | *Crew:* 671 (international) |
| *Size:* Large (48,563 tons) | *Officers:* International |
| *Number of cabins:* 800 | *Passenger/crew ratio:* 2.3 to 1 |
| *Outside cabins:* 60% | *Year built:* 1990 |

Itinerary **Year-round:** Four-day loops leave Miami Mondays, calling at Nassau, CocoCay (Bahamas), and Freeport/Lucaya. Three-day loops leave Miami Fridays, calling at Nassau and CocoCay. **Port tax:** $43–$47 per passenger.

Overview The *Nordic Empress*—a distinctive but ungainly ship that looks like an oversize houseboat with huge rear bay windows—was designed to target the three- and four-day cruise market. Although it falls into the party-ship category, the *Empress* is more sophisticated than Carnival ships and does not reach the high-energy levels of its less-expensive competitor.

The interior, filled with large and festive public rooms, is a glittering combination of art deco and futuristic designs that can seem brash. At the center of the ship is an incredible five-story atrium that dazzles with light, glass, chrome, and even cascading waterfalls. Vying for attention is the industry's only triple-level casino and a spacious double-decker dining room with a sensational view of the sea. The commodious Showroom and the disco also rise two decks. Because of the stern windows, the *Empress*'s Windjammer Café is forward rather than aft, where most traditional Lidos are situated. The unusually configured and decorated Sun Deck is more like a private club, with its saillike canopies, gazebos, and fountains.

Cabins and Rates

	Beds	Phone	TV	Sitting Area	Fridge	Tub	Per Diem
Royal Suite	Q	●	●	●	●	●	$404–$424
Suite	Q	●	●	●	●	●	$291–$319
Deluxe Outside	T/Q	●	●	○	○	●	$276–$299
Standard Outside	T/Q	●	●	○	○	○	$249–$269
Inside	T/Q	●	●	○	○	○	$221–$242
Economy Inside	T/Q	●	●	○	○	○	$159–$181

Cabins are average in size but have spacious closets. Interiors are in Scandinavian blond woods and white trim with light pastels and contemporary furnishings. Bathrooms are bright, compact, and intelligently laid out. Some cabins are not insulated well against noise. Views from some cabins on Mariner Deck are obstructed by lifeboats. Suites have private verandas.

Outlet voltage: 110/220 AC.

Single supplement: 150% of double-occupancy rate; however, less expensive singles can be had if you're willing to wait for your cabin assignment until embarkation time.

Discounts: A third or fourth passenger in a cabin pays about $65 per diem. Senior citizen discounts are offered on specific sailings. You get a discount for arranging your own airfare, and for early booking—the earlier you book, the lower your cabin rate (excluding inside cabins and suites).

Sports and Fitness **Health club:** Gym with aerobics area, rowing machine, stationary bicycles, free weights, sauna, steam room, and massage.

Walking/jogging: Sun Deck (5 laps=1 mile).

Other sports: Aerobics and other exercise classes, computerized golf driving, skeet shooting, table tennis, shuffleboard, pool, children's pool, four whirlpools.

Facilities **Public rooms:** Six bars, three entertainment lounges, casino, disco, conference center, ice cream bar, video arcade.

Shops: Gift shop, beauty salon/barber.

Health care: Doctor and two nurses on call.

Child care: Kid/Teen Center playroom on Sun Deck has supervised programs for preteens during holidays and summer vacations; baby-sitting arranged privately with crew member.

Services: Full-service laundry, photographer.

Other: Safe-deposit boxes.

**Access for
the Disabled** The *Nordic Empress* is well suited for wheelchairs, although official company policy requires that an able-bodied companion accompany passengers who use wheelchairs. Four cabins are equipped for wheelchairs, with wide doors, level floors, and oversize bathrooms with rails. Most elevators accommodate regular-size wheelchairs.

MS Nordic Prince and MS Song of Norway

Specifications *Type of ship:* Mainstream
Type of cruise: Traditional/ party
Size: Medium (23,000 tons)
Number of cabins: 506/502
Outside cabins: 65.2%

Passengers: 1,012/1,004
Crew: 434/423 (international)
Officers: Norwegian
Passenger/crew ratio: 2.4 to 1
Year built: 1971/1970, rebuilt 1980/1978

**Itinerary
*Nordic Prince*** **Fall–Spring:** Seven-day loops leave Los Angeles Sundays, calling at Cabo San Lucas, Mazatlán, and Puerto Vallarta. **Summer:** Seven-day cruises between Vancouver and Skagway leave Sundays, calling along the Inside Passage and the Tracy Arm Fjord, at Haines, Juneau, and Ketchikan, and along the Misty Fjords.

Port tax: $55–$91 per passenger.

Song of Norway **Fall:** Europe. **Winter–Spring:** Ten- and 11-day cruises between San Juan and Acapulco call at Puerto Caldera (Costa Rica), along the Panama Canal, Curaçao, and St. Thomas/St. John.

Port tax: $91 per passenger.

Overview Built in the early 1970s, both ships were split and stretched 10 years later to accommodate more passengers and increase the size and number of public rooms. Essentially identical in layout, they have a superb Sun Deck with an unusually large pool for swimming laps.

Cabins and Rates

	Beds	Phone	TV	Sitting Area	Fridge	Tub	Per Diem
Owner's Suite	D or T	●	●	●	●	●	$377–$389
Deluxe Outside	D or T/D	●	○	○	○	○	$313–$325
Standard Outside	D/U or T	●	○	○	○	○	$249–$260
Standard Inside	D/L or T	●	○	○	○	○	$199–$210
Economy Inside	D, D/U, or T	●	○	○	○	○	$163–$175

*Mexican Riviera cruises cost the least, Alaska cruises the most.

Cabins are above the waterline, but thoses on the Promenade Deck look onto a public area. On the *Empress,* cabins 604 and 704 are larger outside staterooms with one double bed plus upper and lower berths.

Outlet voltage: 110 AC.

Single supplement: 150% of double-occupancy rate; however, less expensive singles are available if you are willing to wait for your cabin assignment until embarkation time.

Discounts: A third or fourth passenger in a cabin pays $87–$150 per diem.Senior citizen discounts are offered on specific sailings. You get a discount for arranging your own airfare, and for early booking—the earlier you book, the lower your cabin rate (excluding inside cabins and suites).

Sports and Fitness **Health club:** Stationary bikes, rowing machines, treadmills, separate men's and women's saunas and massage rooms.

Walking/jogging: Unobstructed circuit on Compass Deck, above Sun Deck.

Other sports: Aerobics, basketball, dancercise, golf driving and putting, table tennis, shuffleboard, skeet shooting, yoga, snorkeling lessons, pool.

Facilities **Public rooms:** Five bars, three entertainment lounges, casino, disco, Lido.

Shops: Gift shop, beauty salon/barber.

Child care: Youth programs with counselors during holidays or in summer, baby-sitting arranged privately with crew member.

Health care: Doctor on call.

Services: Full-service laundry, dry-cleaning, photographer, film processing.

Other: Safe-deposit boxes.

Access for the Disabled Wheelchair access is limited. The Viking Crown Lounge is inaccessible via wheelchair. Doorways throughout the ship have lips, and public bathrooms are not specially equipped. Disabled passengers must bring their own traveling wheelchair, and they must be escorted by an able-bodied companion.

MS Song of America

Specifications *Type of ship:* Mainstream
Type of cruise: Traditional/party
Size: Large (37,584 tons)
Number of cabins: 701
Outside cabins: 57%

Passengers: 1,402
Crew: 535 (international)
Officers: Norwegian
Passenger/crew ratio: 2.6 to 1
Year built: 1982

Itinerary **Fall:** Ten-day loops out of New York call at St. George's and Hamilton (Bermuda). **Winter–Spring:** Ten- and 11-day cruises between San Juan and Miami call at St. Thomas/St. John, St. Maarten/St. Martin, St. Lucia, Tobago, Guadaloupe, Dominica, St. Croix, and CocoCay (Bahamas). **Summer:** Same as Fall.

Port tax: $92 per passenger.

Overview The *Song of America* is unusually handsome. Despite its size, it looks more like a yacht than a cruise ship, though its width gives it space and stability that a yacht could never manage. Plentiful chrome, mirrors, and overhead lights give the ship a flashier look than other RCCL vessels, but the overall effect is clean, crisp, and airy. As on its sister ships, public rooms on the *Song of America* are patterned after famous musical comedies, including the Guys and Dolls Night Club.

Cabins and Rates

	Beds	Phone	TV	Sitting Area	Fridge	Tub	Per Diem
Owner's Suite	D or T	●	●	●	●	●	$413–$435
Suite	T	●	●	●	●	●	$370–$392
Deluxe Outside	T	●	●	○	○	○	$285–$306
Standard Outside	T or T/D	●	●	○	○	○	$249–$270
Inside	T or T/D	●	●	○	○	○	$177–$256

Cabins are above the waterline, but suites on the Promenade Deck look onto a public area.

Outlet voltage: 110/220 AC.

Single supplement: 150% of double-occupancy rate; however, less expensive singles are available if you are willing to wait for your cabin assignment until embarkation time.

Discounts: A third or fourth passenger in a cabin pays $99 per diem. Senior citizen discounts are offered on specific sailings. You get a discount for arranging your own airfare, and for early booking—the earlier you book, the lower your cabin rate (excluding inside cabins and suites).

Sports and Fitness

Health club: Rowing machines, treadmills, stationary bikes, massage, men's and women's saunas.

Walking/jogging: Unobstructed circuits on Sun Deck and Promenade Deck.

Other sports: Aerobics, golf putting, table tennis, ring toss, snorkeling lessons, shuffleboard, skeet shooting, two pools.

Facilities

Public rooms: Six bars, four entertainment lounges, card room, casino, cinema, disco, Lido, piano bar.

Shops: Gift shop, drugstore, beauty salon/barber.

Health care: Doctor on call.

Child care: Youth programs with counselors during holidays and in summer, baby-sitting arranged privately with crew member.

Services: Full-service laundry, dry-cleaning, photographer, film processing.

Other: Safe-deposit boxes.

Access for the Disabled

Wheelchair access is limited. Doorways have lips, and public bathrooms are not specially equipped. Disabled passengers must bring a portable wheelchair and be escorted by an able-bodied companion. Tenders are easy to board; if seas are rough, crew members will carry disabled passengers and their wheelchairs on board. Labadie is all sand, however, which makes moving about in a wheelchair difficult.

MS Sun Viking

Specifications *Type of ship:* Mainstream   *Passengers:* 714

Type of cruise: Traditional	*Crew:* 341 (international)
Size: Small (18,556 tons)	*Officers:* Norwegian
Number of cabins: 357	*Passenger/crew ratio:* 2.3 to 1
Outside cabins: 68.9%	*Year built:* 1972

Itinerary **Fall:** Europe. **Winter:** Seven-day loops leave San Juan call at St. Croix, St. Barts, Guadeloupe, St. Maarten/St. Martin, and St. Thomas/St. John. **Spring–Summer:** Europe.

Port tax: $71 per passenger.

Overview The *Sun Viking* is RCCL's smallest ship. Unlike other RCCL ships, the *Viking* has never been lengthened—meaning fewer public rooms, less space to play in, and small cabins. Nevertheless, passengers are lured back to it time and again because they feel more in touch with the sea here than on a larger vessel. Certainly, passengers and crew get to know one another better. As on all RCCL ships, the *Sun Viking* has the trademark Viking Crown Lounge wrapped high around the funnel. Don't expect to find a busy, partying atmosphere on this ship. One important feature is the swimming pool, which has a shallow area around the perimeter for wading.

Cabins and Rates

	Beds	Phone	TV	Sitting Area	Fridge	Tub	Per Diem
Owner's Suite	D or T	●	○	●	●	●	$395–$423
Deluxe Outside	T	●	○	○	●	○	$323–$352
Standard Outside	D/U or T	●	○	○	○	○	$259–$287
Inside	D/L or T	●	○	○	○	○	$180–$275

Cabins are above the waterline, but they are significantly smaller than those on comparable ships. Suites and cabins on the Promenade Deck look onto a public area.

Outlet voltage: 110 AC.

Single supplement: 150% of double-occupancy rate; however, less expensive singles are available if you're willing to wait for your cabin assignment until embarkation.

Discounts: A third or fourth passenger in a cabin pays $106 per diem. Senior citizen discounts are offered on specific sailings. You get a discount for arranging your own airfare, and for early booking—the earlier you book, the lower your cabin rate (excluding inside cabins and suites).

Sports and Fitness **Health club:** Exercise equipment, men's and women's saunas.

Walking/jogging: Unobstructed circuits on Promenade and Compass decks.

Other sports: Aerobics and other exercise classes, basketball, golf driving and putting, table tennis, ring toss, shuffleboard, skeet shooting, pool.

Facilities **Public rooms:** Six bars, three entertainment lounges, small casino (slot machines), disco, Lido.

Shops: Boutique, gift shop, beauty salon/barber.

Health care: Doctor on call.

Child care: Youth programs run by counselors during holidays and in summer, baby-sitting arranged privately with crew member.

Services: Full-service laundry, dry-cleaning, photographer, film processing.

Other: Safe-deposit boxes.

Access for the Disabled Wheelchair access is limited, with lips to bathrooms and in doorways throughout the ship. Public bathrooms are not specially equipped. The Viking Crown Lounge is inaccessible to wheelchairs. A portable wheelchair and an able-bodied traveling companion are required.

MS Viking Serenade

Specifications *Type of ship:* Mainstream
Type of cruise: Traditional/party
Size: Large (40,132 tons)
Number of cabins: 756
Outside cabins: 63%

Passengers: 1,512
Crew: 612 (international)
Officers: International
Passenger/crew ratio: 2.4 to 1
Year built: 1982, rebuilt 1991

Itinerary **Year-round:** Three- and four-day loops leave Los Angeles, calling at Catalina Island, San Diego, and Ensenada.

Port tax: $35–$40 per passenger.

Overview Formerly Admiral Cruises' *Stardancer,* the *Viking Serenade* was completely rebuilt shortly after RCCL acquired Admiral. It was originally designed as the world's only cruise ship/car ferry, which explains why it looks more like a barge than a cruise ship. However, RCCL spent $75 million to convert the car deck into cabins, add a three-story atrium, renovate the existing cabins and public rooms, and add the company's signature observation deck, the glass-enclosed Viking Crown Lounge. Other features are a much-enlarged casino, a shopping arcade, a teen disco, and a state-of-the-art fitness center. Designs and furnishings are bright and contemporary. Brass, glass, mirrors, and stainless steel are used extensively.

Cabins and Rates

	Beds	Phone	TV	Sitting Area	Fridge	Tub	Per Diem
Royal Suite	Q	●	●	●	●	●	$436–$461
Suite	Q	●	●	●	●	●	$323–$348
Deluxe Outside	T	●	●	●	●	●	$286–$311
Standard Outside	T	●	●	○	○	○	$223–$268
Inside	T	●	●	○	○	○	$143–$231

The *Serenade* has almost as many inside cabins as any ship afloat. The larger outside staterooms on Club Deck have partially obstructed views.

Outlet voltage: 110/220 AC.

Single supplement: 150% of double-occupancy rate; however, less expensive singles are available if you are willing to wait for your cabin assignment until embarkation time.

Discounts: A third or fourth passenger in a cabin pays $99 per diem. Senior citizen discounts are offered on specific sailings. You get a discount for arranging your own airfare, and for early booking—the earlier you book, the lower your cabin rate (excluding inside cabins and suites).

Sports and Fitness **Health club:** Top-deck spa with rowing machines, stationary bikes, free weights, sauna.

Walking/jogging: Jogging track with four parcours stations (8 laps=1 mile).

Other sports: Aerobics and other exercise classes, ping-pong, shuffleboard, trapshooting, pool with retractable dome.

Facilities **Public rooms:** Six bars, four entertainment lounges, casino, disco, Lido, card room/library.

Shops: Gift shop, beauty salon/barber.

Health care: Doctor on call.

Child care: Playroom; teen club with soda bar, video games, and dance floor; children's programs with counselors year-round.

Services: Full-service laundry, dry cleaning, photographer.

Other: Safe-deposit boxes.

Access for the Disabled Four cabins have been outfitted for wheelchair access. All public areas are wheelchair-accessible.

Royal Cruise Line

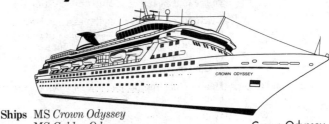

Crown Odyssey

Ships MS *Crown Odyssey*
MS *Golden Odyssey*

Evaluation Although it's a maritime tradition to give ships aristocratic names, few shipping companies live up to the superlatives that such appellations imply. Royal Cruise Line is an exception, however, for its reputation is as good as its name. The royal treatment—luxurious cabins and amenities and, above all, superb service by the predominantly Greek staff—is in store for all passengers who board its ships. Royal was voted number-one cruise line by readers of *Condé Nast Traveler* magazine in 1991. It's no surprise that, on average, 40%–50% of guests—and as many as 85% on certain cruises—are repeat passengers. New itineraries, in particular, draw plenty of repeaters eager to sail again with Royal. Guests tend to be retired (mid-fifties), successful, and well-traveled. Children are rarely taken on Royal cruises, and only during school vacations.

Sensitivity to the needs of its passengers and willingness to go the extra mile mark Royal's programs and activities. For instance, its host program is aimed at the many older, single women who travel on Royal ships: Senior gentlemen travel as unsalaried guests to act as partners for dining, bridge, or dancing—all extremely popular activities on board. These men are carefully screened; they are forbidden to play favorites or become romantically involved.

In addition to excellent service, Royal is known for its wide-ranging itineraries, well-organized shore excursions, fine cuisine, and professional entertainment. In addition to the two ships reviewed here, the *Royal Odyssey*, added to the fleet in 1991, sails outside the Western Hemisphere.

Activities A variety of cruise activities are offered, including dance and language classes, card and board games (with such prizes as a free cruise), trivia contests, and visits to the navigation bridge. Occasionally, there are special theme sailings, such as "Big Band" cruises. The New Beginnings program offers lectures on fitness, nutrition, and self-improvement. Other lectures cover subjects ranging from the ports visited to estate planning

Chart Symbols. *The following symbols are used in the cabin charts that accompany each ship's evaluation.* **D:** *Double bed;* **K:** *King-size bed;* **Q:** *Queen-size bed;* **T:** *Twin bed;* **U/L:** *Upper and lower berths;* ●: *All cabins have this facility;* ○: *No cabins have this facility;* ◖: *Some cabins have this facility*

and investments. Shore excursions are outstanding; at least 70% of passengers partake in one or more tours.

Dining Food is exquisitely prepared and elegantly presented. Although Greek specialties are always available, cuisine is usually traditional and Continental. The dining-room stewards are superb: After the first meal, they know each passenger's preferences and serve meals accordingly. If you take skim milk in your coffee, a pitcher of it will be brought automatically. Every menu carries a low-calorie, low-cholesterol selection approved by the American Heart Association; a booklet in each cabin explains the ship's alternative dining program, offers tips on battling appetite, and provides a photo of each dish along with a nutritional breakdown. Entrées that meet AHA guidelines include skewered scallops with asparagus spears, chicken Salinas (with cold artichoke hearts and lemon), and broiled marinated salmon with apricots. Other dietary requests should be made in writing five weeks before sailing.

Two formal evenings are held each cruise; other evenings are semiformal. Early morning coffee, breakfast, and lunch buffets are served on deck and in one of the lounges. Other service includes mid-morning bouillon, afternoon tea, and a late-night buffet. Room service is available around the clock, though selection is dictated by kitchen hours.

Entertainment Style, not glitz, is the tone of Royal's entertainment, which caters to the tastes of its older clientele. In addition to a nightly variety show and first-run movies, there are cabarets, piano and harp duos, and dancing (ballroom or disco). Big-name entertainers are sometimes on board, as are literary or film celebrities. On Greek Night, passengers may be surprised to see their dining-room steward playing the bouzouki or singing. This is one of the most popular events of the cruise, although passenger talent night and the costume party also pack them in. A singles cocktail party and a repeaters party (for passengers who have sailed with Royal before) are other regular features.

Service and Tipping Royal prides itself on a highly professional staff noted for their warm, personal style. The dining-room staff, in particular, love to spoil the passengers. Most of the crew have been working together on Royal ships since the company was formed in 1971. In fact, Theo's Bar on the *Crown Odyssey* is named for a popular bartender on the *Golden Odyssey*. A majority of the waiters and stewards were trained in first-class European hotels, and the level of service reflects this. Tips are pooled and distributed among the crew. Tip $9–$10 per passenger per diem.

For More Information Royal Cruise Line (1 Maritime Plaza, San Francisco, CA 94111, tel. 415/956–7200).

MS Crown Odyssey

Specifications *Type of ship:* Luxury mainstream
Type of cruise: Traditional/senior
Size: Medium (34,250 tons)
Number of cabins: 526
Outside cabins: 78%

Passengers: 1,052
Crew: 470 (Greek)
Officers: Greek
Passenger/crew ratio: 2.2 to 1
Year built: 1988

Itinerary Fall: Europe. **Winter:** Eight- and 16-day cruises between Ensenada or Los Angeles and Honolulu call at Kahului and Lahaina (Maui), Hilo (Hawaii), and Nawiliwili (Kauai). Eight-day loops leave Los Angeles, calling at Puerto Vallarta, Zihuatanejo/Ixtapa, Acapulco, Mazatlán, and Cabo San Lucas. Various Panama Canal Transits between Los Angeles and San Juan call along the Mexican Riviera, Puerto Caldera (Costa Rica), Aruba, Curaçao, St. Croix, St. Thomas/St. John, and along the Canal. **Spring–Summer:** Europe.

Port taxes: Vary widely according to itinerary.

Overview The *Crown Odyssey* is an ultramodern vessel, more like a floating town than a classic cruise ship—and the crew make you feel like its mayor. The art deco interior is a mosaic of textures and materials, including marble, wood, glass, stainless steel, and brass. Passengers have 10 decks to wander. At the mirrored entrance to Theo's Bar is the centerpiece of the ship: a modern sculpture of a peacock in a glass cage. (Fiber optics in the peacock's fantail change color constantly.) Equally spectacular is the Top of the Crown Lounge, with its 360-degree view of the sea and the ship's interior through floor-to-ceiling windows.

Much emphasis is placed on physical fitness. The Health Center, styled after a Roman bath, has tile walls with inlaid mosaics and Italian white rattan furniture. Its offerings include low-impact programs for older passengers, a health bar, indoor whirlpools, and even an indoor pool. Dining in the Seven Continents restaurant is an experience difficult to top. Royal Doulton china, European linen, and silver set the tone for meals that are superbly prepared and deftly served.

Cabins and Rates

	Beds	Phone	TV	Sitting Area	Fridge	Tub	Per Diem
Superior Deluxe Apartment	T/D	●	●	●	●	●	$447–$879
Superior Deluxe Suite	T/D	●	○	●	○	●	$390–$769
Superior Deluxe Junior Suite	T/D	●	○	●	○	●	$354–$698
Superior Deluxe Outside	T/D	●	○	○	○	●	$331–$643
Deluxe Junior Suite	T/D	●	○	●	○	●	$320–$615
Deluxe Outside	T	●	○	○	○	◑	$183–$573
Deluxe Inside	T/D	●	○	○	○	◑	$156–$363

Suites are spacious and comfortable. Wood paneling and trim are used extensively in cabins and suites, which also the latter of which provide fully mirrored closets, and phones for worldwide communications. The 16 Penthouse Deck suites are decorated in themes suggested by their names (Taj Mahal, Bel Air, Shangri-la) and have private balconies, marble bathrooms, walk-in closets, whirlpool baths, and butler service. Some Superior Deluxe Apartments can be combined with an adjoining cabin to provide 1,000 square feet of space. Superior Deluxe Suites and Junior Suites on the Riviera Deck have bay windows with panoramic views. Views from most cabins on the Lido Deck are partially or fully obstructed by lifeboats.

Outlet voltage: 110/220 AC.

Single supplement: 160%–200% of double-occupancy rate; some cabins available at $75 per diem additional on selected sailings.

Discounts: A third or fourth passenger in a cabin pays 60% of the double-occupancy rate. You get a discount of 10%–50% for early booking. Repeat passengers and those who book their own flights are eligible for additional discounts and amenities.

Sports and Fitness   **Health club:** Eight-station Universal gym with full-time fitness instructor, four Life Cycles, treadmill, rower, free weights, ballet barre, indoor pool, two whirlpools, massage, health bar, men's and women's saunas, full-service beauty center (herbal wraps, facials, and more).

Walking/jogging: Penthouse Deck parcours trail; unobstructed circuits on Penthouse and Horizon decks.

Other sports: Aqua parcours, table tennis, shuffleboard, exercise classes (some geared toward older passengers), outdoor pool, children's pool, two outdoor whirlpools.

Facilities   **Public rooms:** Six bars, five entertainment lounges, card room, casino, cinema, large-screen TV, disco, library, open Promenade Deck.

Shops: Two boutiques, sundries shop, beauty salon/barber.

Health care: Doctor on call.

Services: Full-service laundry, photographer, film processing.

Other: Safe-deposit boxes.

Access for the Disabled   Four cabins designed to accommodate disabled passengers (and allowing full rotation of a standard wheelchair) feature such details as sit-down showers, grip bars around the shower and toilet areas, and tilting mirrors.

MS Golden Odyssey

Specifications

Type of ship: Luxury mainstream
Type of cruise: Traditional/senior
Size: Small (10,500 tons)
Number of cabins: 237
Outside cabins: 80.6%

Passengers: 460
Crew: 200 (Greek)
Officers: Greek
Passenger/crew ratio: 2.3 to 1
Year built: 1974

Itinerary   **Fall–early Winter:** Seven- and 14-day cruises with varying itineraries run between New York and Montréal, calling at Bar Harbor, Halifax, along the Gulf of St. Lawrence and the Saguenay Fjord, Québec City, Sydney (Cape Breton Island, Nova Scotia), Boston, along the Cape Cod Canal, and Newport (RI). A repositioning cruise between New York and Nassau calls along the U.S. East Coast. Various Panama Canal Transits between Aruba or Curaçao and Acapulco call at Caracas/La Guaira, along the Canal, the San Blas Islands (near Panama), and Puerto Caldera (Costa Rica). **Late Winter:** Loops out of New Orleans call in the Western Caribbean. **Spring:** Eleven-day Amazon cruises between Aruba and Manaus call at various southern Carribean and South American ports. Eight-day cruises between San Francisco and Acapulco call at various Carribean and Mexican Riviera ports. Panama Canal Transits (*see* Fall–early Winter, *above*). **Summer:** Seven-day cruises between Vancouver and Anchorage and 10-day cruises between San Francisco and Anchorage call at Anchorage/Seward, Columbia Glacier/College Fjord, along Prince William Sound, Hubbard Glacier, along Yakutat Bay, Skagway, Juneau, along the Tracy Arm Fjord, and Ketchikan.

Port tax: Vary widely according to the itinerary.

Overview   Built for Royal in 1977 and refurbished in 1987, the *Golden Odyssey* became the model for an entire generation of small, upscale cruise ships. Despite its size, the ship has plenty of deck space, with room for a good-size swimming pool. The interior is a mix of new and old: Teak and other fine woods are used throughout, accented with frosted glass, mirrors, mother-of-pearl inlays, green marble, and original artwork. The *Golden Odyssey* is about one-third the size of the newer *Crown Odyssey*, and with only 460 passengers (to the *Crown*'s 1,052), it has a much more intimate and informal feel. Fewer activities are offered, and passengers are generally happier curled up in their favorite lounge chair than skeet shooting or shuffleboarding.

Cabins and Rates

	Beds	Phone	TV	Sitting Area	Fridge	Tub	Per Diem
Superior Deluxe Suite	T	●	○	●	○	●	$429–$814
Superior Deluxe Outside	T	●	○	○	○	●	$360–$730
Deluxe Outside	T	●	○	○	○	○	$300–$650
Deluxe Inside	T	●	○	○	○	○	$197–$480

Cabins are smaller than those on many newer luxury ships. They're decorated in cranberry, aqua, rose, and lavender hues, with pull-out tables and private telephones. Accommodations range from the Superior Deluxe Suites, with four picture windows and sitting areas, to Deluxe Outside Staterooms, with double windows or portholes, to Deluxe Inside Staterooms, which average 127 square feet. Cabins on the Riviera Deck look onto a public promenade.

Outlet voltage: 110/220 AC.

Single supplement: 160%–200% of double-occupancy rate; $75 per diem on selected sailings.

Discounts: A third or fourth passenger in a cabin pays 60% of the double-occupancy rate. You get a discount of 10%–50% for early booking. Repeat passengers and those who book their own flights are eligible for additional discounts and amenities.

Sports and Fitness **Health club:** Exercise bikes, Stairmaster, treadmill, weight machines, rowing machine, ballet barre, sauna.

Walking/jogging: Promenade Deck.

Other sports: Aqua parcours, exercise classes, table tennis, shuffleboard, pool.

Facilities **Public rooms:** Three bars, two entertainment lounges, card room, small casino (slots and blackjack only), cinema, disco, library/writing room, outdoor Lido.

Shops: Gift shop, beauty salon/barber.

Health care: Doctor on call.

Services: Full-service laundry and pressing, photographer, film processing.

Other: Safe-deposit boxes.

Access for the Disabled While there are no special facilities, cabins can accommodate wheelchairs (23″ portable). Most public rooms are wheelchair-accessible, and portable ramps are available.

Royal Viking Line

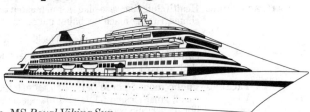

Ship   MS *Royal Viking Sun*

Evaluation   Attentive service, interesting itineraries, and an emphasis on comfort are the hallmarks of a Royal Viking cruise. Passengers tend to be older (fifties to mid-seventies), experienced, and sophisticated, with enough time and money to take long voyages. More adventurous itineraries attract a somewhat younger crowd. Foreign travelers make up about 20% of Royal Viking's clientele and are assisted by an international hostess. Life on board tends toward the formal, and neat attire is required at all times.

In keeping with other upscale cruise lines, Royal Viking does whatever is necessary, and more, to make a cruise memorable. Senior gentlemen, all of whom have been carefully screened, mingle among the passengers, ensuring that single women don't miss out on activities like bridge or dancing for want of a partner. Staterooms have all the amenities that could be expected, including walk-in closets, refrigerators, and TVs and VCRs; many cabins have verandas.

Activities   Mainstream activities include trivia quizzes, duplicate bridge, dance and golf lessons, "horse racing," a needlepoint club, and a fashion show. Guest experts lecture on a variety of subjects ranging from computers to fashion to history, and chefs from famous restaurants sometimes give cooking demonstrations. Introduced in 1992 was the World Affairs Program, an enrichment series offered in cooperation with Georgetown University, in which experts give lectures and host roundtable discussions on topics relevant to ship destinations. If you're feeling lazy, you can watch these talks on your cabin TV, along with the port talks and "Sunrise," a morning show presented by cruise director Paul McFarland. Get-togethers are held for singles and repeat passengers.

Dining   Royal Viking touts its cuisine as some of the best in the industry, and that's not an idle boast. It is the only cruise line awarded membership in both the Les Toques Blanches society and the Master Chefs Institute. Much care and attention is devoted to preparation, and passengers never see the same menu twice. All meals in the dining room are served in a single,

---

Chart Symbols. *The following symbols are used in the cabin charts that accompany each ship's evaluation.* **D:** *Double bed;* **K:** *King-size bed;* **Q:** *Queen-size bed;* **T:** *Twin bed;* **U/L:** *Upper and lower berths;* ●: *All cabins have this facility;* ○: *No cabins have this facility;* ◑: *Some cabins have this facility*

assigned seating. Caviar may be ordered at any dinner, even when it isn't on the menu, and just about any special order can be prepared with 24 hours' notice. However, special dietary requests (such as for diabetics or vegetarians) should be made in writing at least four weeks before sailing. An American Heart Association–approved meal is featured on every menu—including diet chocolate mousse. Two formal evenings are held each week, but passengers are expected to dress smartly even on informal evenings.

The Garden Café serves early morning coffee, morning snacks, and an extensive buffet lunch. Other food service includes mid-morning bouillon, afternoon snacks, elegant afternoon teas, evening sandwiches, and a midnight buffet. On Norwegian Day, passengers feast on a midday Norwegian Grand Buffet and enjoy Norwegian folk entertainment in the evening. Room service is always available, with a limited menu other than at mealtimes.

Entertainment Shipboard entertainment caters to an older audience. In addition to heavily attended mainstream production shows, there are occasional talent shows, masquerade parties, cabarets, or game shows. Classical-music recitals and performances by solo harpists and pianists are popular. Hollywood celebrities and big-name entertainers are occasionally featured. Two movies are shown daily, and the library is stocked with 700 videotapes for cabin VCRs. Passengers looking for Las Vegas–style entertainment or loud parties will be disappointed.

Service and Tipping Royal Viking treats its staff better than do most cruise lines, and this is reflected in the service. Staff are capable and courteous, and they don't solicit tips as obviously as some ship crews do. The concierge service is especially noteworthy. Concierges are happy to handle any request, whether you want to find a bed-and-breakfast for a post-cruise stay, hire a baby-sitter, or charter a plane. Gratuities for cabin stewards and waiters are included in the cruise fare. Maître d's, butlers, and night stewards may be tipped for unusual service. A 15% service charge is automatically added to bar and wine purchases.

For More Information Royal Viking Line (Kloster Cruise Limited, 95 Merrick Way, Coral Gables, FL 33134, tel. 800/422–8000).

MS Royal Viking Sun

Specifications

Type of ship: Luxury mainstream	*Passengers:* 740
	Crew: 460 (European)
Type of cruise: Traditional/ senior	*Officers:* Norwegian
	Passenger/crew ratio: 1.6 to 1
Size: Large (38,000 tons)	*Year built:* 1988
Number of cabins: 370	
Outside cabins: 94.8%	

Itinerary Fall: Europe. **Winter–Spring:** Ten- and 15-day cruises between San Francisco and Fort Lauderdale call at Galveston, New Orleans, Cozumel/Playa del Carmen (Mexico), Belize City, Key West, Aruba, Puerto Caldera (Costa Rica), Acapulco, Zihuatanejo/Ixtapa, Cabo San Lucas, and Los Angeles. A 16-day Christmas cruise between Fort Lauderdale and Cozumel/Playa del Carmen calls at Tortola, St. Lucia, Barbados, Tobago, Grenada, Aruba, and Limón (Costa Rica). A 108-day world cruise circumnavigates South American, then sails around the South Pacific, to New Zealand, Australia, Indonesia, Singapore, Thailand, Hong Kong, Korea, Japan, Hawaii, and San Francisco. **Summer:** Europe.

Port tax: Varies widely depending upon the itinerary.

Overview The *Sun*, Royal Viking's flagship, is a relatively new vessel, and no expense was spared in its outfitting. The interior is luxurious and spacious, designed for maximum comfort even on very long voyages. A feeling of light and space is created by the use of floor-to-ceiling windows, and two glass-walled elevators look onto the ship's interior. The ship also has its share of small, private lounges, including the Oak Room, with a wood-burning fireplace, leather upholstery, and wood paneling. At the bow is the Stella Polaris Room, an observation lounge with 360-degree views. The *Sun's* passenger-to-crew ratio is just about the lowest among cruise ships, which translates into service almost unrivaled.

Cabins and Rates

	Beds	Phone	TV	Sitting Area	Fridge	Tub	Per Diem
Penthouse	T/K	●	●	●	●	●	$1,030–$1,175
Deluxe Bedroom	T/K	●	●	●	●	◐	$521–$936
Outside Double	T/K	●	●	●	●	◐	$390–$551
Inside Double	T	●	●	○	●	◐	$336–$400

Cabins are oversize, beautifully furnished, and equipped with all the amenities, including walk-in closets, bathrobes, lockable drawers, TVs, and VCRs. Penthouses, Deluxe Bedrooms, and some Outside Doubles have verandas. The remarkable Owner's Suite features butler service, a large veranda, and two bathrooms, one with a whirlpool in a glassed-in alcove looking out at the ocean. Cabins on the Promenade Deck look onto a public area.

Outlet voltage: 110/220 AC.

Single supplement: 125%–200% of double-occupancy rate.

Discounts: A third passenger in a cabin pays the minimum fare. A child under 12 sharing a cabin with two adults pays half the minimum. Various discounts are offered for repeaters, first-time cruisers, and early booking. You get a discount of $300 for arranging your own airfare.

Sports and Fitness **Health club:** Life Rowers, Life Cycles, free weights, a variety of other equipment, saunas, massage.

Walking/jogging: Unobstructed circuit on Promenade Deck (4 laps=1 mile).

Other sports: Aerobics and other exercise classes, badminton, croquet, golf driving, putting course, computerized golf simulator, table tennis, shuffleboard, quoits, trapshooting, two pools (one with wet bar), whirlpool.

Facilities **Public rooms:** Six bars, four entertainment lounges, card room, casino, cinema, disco, library, piano bar, wine bar, videotape library.

Shops: Gift shop, beauty salon (with facials and massages), barber.

Health care: Doctor and two nurses on call.

Child care: Children's programs during major holidays and in summer, baby-sitting arranged through concierge.

Services: Concierge, full-service laundry, dry-cleaning and pressing, laundromat, ironing room, photographer, film processing.

Other: Safe-deposit boxes, Alcoholics Anonymous.

Access for the Disabled Four staterooms have L-shaped bed configurations for greater wheelchair maneuverability and are specially equipped. Anyone confined to a wheelchair must travel with an able-bodied companion and provide his or her own 22" wheelchair.

Seabourn Cruise Line

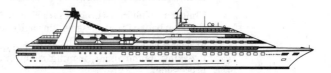

Ships *Seabourn Pride*

Evaluation Of the millions of people who go on cruises, only a few can afford the type of voyage offered by Seabourn. Patterned after the luxury cruises offered by Cunard's *Sea Goddess*es, Seabourn set new standards in ship comfort and design—although it has yet to match its competitor's level of service. Certainly, no expense was spared in the construction and decoration of the *Seabourn Pride*. From the crystal glasses in cabins to the huge expanse of marble in the circular atrium, Seabourn represents the pinnacle of cruising elegance. The *Pride* is among the most spacious ships afloat, too, and notably so in the cabins, which are the highlight of the ship. Each cabin is an outside suite complete with 5-foot-high picture windows, sitting area, stocked bar and refrigerator, TV and VCR, large marble bath with twin sinks and tub/shower, and walk-in closets. Here as in the rest of the ship, glass, blond woods, and mirrors are used to great effect.

Passengers pay an extremely high price for such amenities. As a result, the majority are middle-age or older. While this is reflected in activities and entertainments in general, there is plenty in the way of water sports to keep even the passengers in their thirties busy. The *Pride*'s equally sumptuous sister ship, the *Seabourn Spirit*, will cruise in Southeast Asia and the Mediterranean in 1994. In 1993 Seabourn was named the world's best cruise line by *Condé Nast Traveler* magazine.

Activities The few organized activities include lectures on subjects ranging from Spanish treasure fleets to art appreciation, as well as shuffleboard and skeet shooting. There's a small casino, a library with a good selection of books and videos, and a card room. The most exciting activities take place off the back of the ship. Anchored in the calm waters of a cove or bay, the ship can lower its stern to create a platform with a central swimming area protected by wire netting; from this platform passengers can swim, sail, waterski, or windsurf. For more sedate explorations, the ship also carries paddleboats and a glass-bottom boat.

Chart Symbols. *The following symbols are used in the cabin charts that accompany each ship's evaluation.* **D:** *Double bed;* **K:** *King-size bed;* **Q:** *Queen-size bed;* **T:** *Twin bed;* **U/L:** *Upper and lower berths;* ●: *All cabins have this facility;* ○: *No cabins have this facility;* ◑: *Some cabins have this facility*

Dining The dining room is formal and large, with tables spaced so far apart they would make a New York restaurateur swoon. Tables are unassigned, and passengers may dine at any time during meal hours (dinner is from 7:30 to 10). Typically, passengers line up fellow table mates in the afternoon, perhaps meeting before dinner for drinks at the bar—it can be a bit like arranging a new dinner party every day. The cuisine has a French accent and is strongly nouvelle-influenced in presentation and portions. Meals are prepared to order, and passengers are free to ask for dishes not on the menu. The outstanding food is complemented by a superb wine list.

Although *low cholesterol* is not a term with which the kitchen seems overly familiar, the Seabourn Spa does make menu recommendations. Special dietary requests, however, should be made at least four weeks before sailing. Two formal evenings are held each week, but gentlemen are expected to wear a jacket and tie on other nights, long pants for all other meals. The formality of the dining room, which works so successfully for dinner, seems stuffy at breakfast and lunch.

For more informal meals, the Veranda Café is a delightful spot. With its rattan furniture and tightly packed tables, it is the ship's cheeriest room. Located on the same deck as the pool, the café serves opulent buffet breakfasts and lunches, as well as a few items cooked to order, like eggs, hot dogs, and hamburgers. Pasta dinners are also frequently served.

Room service is superb and available 24 hours. At least once during your cruise, be sure to have dinner in your cabin; it's a romantic, candlelit affair with personal service and beautifully prepared cuisine. Breakfast in the cabin is also presented with grace and panache.

Entertainment Evening performances are geared to a middle-age and older crowd, with an emphasis on song-and-dance numbers. A pianist plays in the club, and most evenings a short revue is accompanied by a musical quartet.

Service and Tipping The passenger-to-crew ratio is among the lowest of any ship. The no-tipping policy has helped produce a highly professional yet personable crew who accommodate passenger requests when possible. Individually, crew members are nonpareil.

For More Information Seabourn Cruise Line (55 Francisco St., San Francisco, CA 94133, tel. 800/351–9595).

Seabourn Pride

Specifications

Type of ship: Luxury, yachtlike	*Passengers:* 204
	Crew: 140 (international)
Type of cruise: Traditional	*Officers:* Norwegian
Size: Small (10,000 tons)	*Passenger/crew ratio:* 1.5 to 1
Number of cabins: 106	*Year built:* 1988
Outside cabins: 100%	

Itinerary **Fall:** Fourteen-day loops leave Boston, calling along the Saguenay Fjord and the Gulf of St. Lawrence and at North East Harbor (ME), St. John (New Brunswick), Lunenburg and Cape Breton Island's Baddeck and Louisbourg (Nova Scotia), St. Pierre (Québec), Québec City, Newfoundland, Halifax, and Camden (ME). There's a repositioning cruise from New York to St. Thomas/St. John. **Winter–early Spring:** Fourteen-day loops leave Fort Lauderdale, calling at the Dominican Republic, Tortola, St. Maarten/St. Martin, St. Barts, St. Thomas/St. John, Mayreau (Grenadines), Antigua, and Virgin Gorda. Sixteen-day Panama Canal Transits call at many of the above ports, plus Aruba, Puerto Caldera (Costa Rica), and Acapulco. A 16-day Amazon cruise calls at many of those ports, plus Manaus, Devil's Island, Munguba (on the Jari River), and, on the Amazon River, Parintins—where passengers are treated to a raucous carnival held just for Seabourn—and Anavilhanas Archipelago. **Late Spring–Summer:** Europe.

Port tax: $105–$165 per passenger.

The above cruises are available in segments; for instance, most 14-day loop cruises may be purchased in seven-day, one-way segments; and many 16-day cruises may be purchased in eight-day segments. Consecutive cruises can be combined.

Overview   Aesthetically, the *Seabourn Pride* may be the finest cruise ship afloat. With its sleek lines and twin funnels that resemble airfoils, the *Pride*'s profile makes other cruise vessels look cluttered and ungainly. Generous use of glass, brass, and marble gives the interior a similarly clean look, a sensation heightened by the ship's spaciousness. Peaches, blues, and soft beiges dominate, with additional splashes of color provided by paintings. From morning until sunset, passengers taking a break from sunbathing gather around the Sky Bar—a simple outdoor bar that is the premier daytime attraction.

The other most popular spot is the Club/Casino, with its piano bar and the sloping picture windows that form the stern wall. Spotlights, potted plants, and glass partitions make this an attractive room for preprandial cocktails and after-dinner dancing. The darker Magellan Lounge on the deck below has none of the Club/Casino's charm, but its gently tiered floor makes it ideal for musical revues and lectures. Two decks up is the magnificent Constellation Lounge; from its position above the bridge it has a commanding view of the sea through a semicircle of large picture windows. Little more than gimmicks are the tiny Star Observatory—a couch-lined structure that resembles a UFO and looks as though it were welded in place above the whirlpools as an afterthought—and the underwater-viewing room, with a window that looks through the bottom of the ship.

Cabins and Rates

	Beds	Phone	TV	Sitting Area	Fridge	Tub	Per Diem
Owner's Suite	Q or T	●	●	●	●	●	$910–$1,465
Regal Suite *Type C*	Q or T	●	●	●	●	●	$830–$1,335
Regal Suite *Type B*	Q or T	●	●	●	●	●	$670–$1,080
Seabourn Suite *Type A*	Q or T	●	●	●	●	●	$510–$825

Cabin refrigerators/bars are stocked with a large selection of liquors, beer, and soft drinks; there's a charge for liquor refills. Unlimited soft drinks are complimentary here, as throughout the ship. All cabins have coffee tables, which convert to dining tables, and safes. The Owner's Suites at the front of the ship have curved bow windows that make you feel as though you're on your own yacht, but midship Owner's Suites are larger.

Outlet voltage: 110/220 AC.

Single supplement: 110% double-occupancy rate; 200% for Owner's and Regal Suites.

Discounts: A third passenger in a suite pays 50% the double-occupancy rate. You get a $300–$650 discount for arranging your own airfare. Seabourn provides free travel insurance, covering trip cancellation or interruption, baggage loss, and travel delay. A "frequent cruiser" program exists for repeat clients.

Sports and Fitness **Health club:** Aerobics rooms, exercise equipment (including Nautilus), weight-training classes, massage, steam room, sauna, health and beauty treatments (herbal wraps, facials, dietary counseling, personalized fitness programs).

Walking/jogging: Unobstructed, though abbreviated, circuit on Leif Erikson Deck.

Other sports: Aerobics and other exercise classes, shuffleboard, skeet shooting, small pool, three whirlpools, sailing, windsurfing, waterskiing, snorkeling.

Facilities **Public rooms:** Three bars, two lounges, card room, casino, business center, star observatory, library with books and videos, indoor/outdoor Lido, piano bar, underwater observatory.

Shops: Clothing boutique, gift shop, beauty salon/barber.

Health care: Doctor on call.

Child care: Baby-sitting arranged with purser's office. Children under 18 must be accompanied by an adult and have written permission from a legal guardian.

Services: Full-service laundry, dry-cleaning, overnight shoeshine service, laundromat, photographer, film processing.

Access for the Disabled Three Seabourn Suites (type A) are organized for easier wheelchair access. All elevators and public areas are wheelchair-accessible, and public lavatories are specially equipped. Disabled passengers are required to travel with an able-bodied adult. In small ports to which passengers must be ferried by tender, those in wheelchairs may have trouble getting ashore.

Seawind Cruise Line

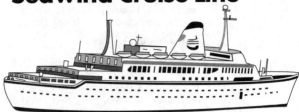

Ship TSS *Seawind Crown*

Evaluation This single-ship cruise line, begun in October 1991, has enjoyed unusually high occupancy rates right from the start. The Portuguese *Seawind Crown* was built in 1961, bought and refitted by a Panamanian compnay in 1989, and subsequently taken over in 1991 by the Swedish conglomerate Nordisk AB, owner of the Seawind Cruise Line. Despite the high cost of flying passengers free from 28 U.S. gateways to its unusual home port of Aruba, the line offers relatively low prices, thanks in part to an advance-booking program that can save you up to $900 per passenger. In addition to solid service and an unusual southern Caribbean itinerary, *Seawind Crown* offers a high passenger-to-space ratio. Though the ship carries just 624, the personal attention and vibrant atmosphere you find here is what you might expect on a megaship.

Activities Though English is the ship's first language, activities are conducted in English, Spanish, and Portuguese to accommodate the large number of South American passengers. Offerings are typical: bingo, singles get-togethers, deck games, shopping programs. Of particular note is a program of wedding-vow renewal, offered to couples married 10 years or longer; the lovely ceremonies take place Saturdays in the St. Nicholas Chapel or on deck.

Dining Food service is provided by Worldwide Catering, the company that originated RCCL's laudable in-house dining concession. And not surprisingly, the overall dining experience receives very high marks from passengers. Chefs are members of the Confrérie de "La Chaine Des Rôtisseurs," the world's oldest and most famous gourmet society. The cuisine has Portuguese and Greek influences, and a few spicy, exotic dishes, such as lamb kebabs or Greek salad, are offered at every meal. Lunch and dinner are presented at two seatings in the elegantly appointed Vasco da Gama Dining Room. Other options include morning buffets, snacks, and elaborate midnight buffets. Other than Continental breakfast, there is very limited room service. Dinner is at two assigned seatings (6 and 8:15).

Chart Symbols. *The following symbols are used in the cabin charts that accompany each ship's evaluation.* **D:** *Double bed;* **K:** *King-size bed;* **Q:** *Queen-size bed;* **T:** *Twin bed;* **U/L:** *Upper and lower berths;* ●: *All cabins have this facility;* ○: *No cabins have this facility;* ◐: *Some cabins have this facility*

Entertainment This small ship offers a similarly small but ambitious troupe of entertainers, including four regular dancers, a handful of guest singers, and typically a visiting magician or comedian. Latin and Caribbean music are performed throughout the day on various decks and in various lounges.

Service and Tipping Seawind's staff is particularly gracious, due in part to the intimate onboard ambience—you'll probably get to know several staff members fairly well on a seven-day cruise. Tip your waiter $3 per diem per passenger, the busboy $1.50, the cabin steward $3; the headwaiter gets $5 per week per passenger. A service charge is automatically added to the bar bill.

For More Information Seawind Cruise Line (1750 Coral Way, Miami, FL 33145, tel. 800/258–8006).

TSS Seawind Crown

Specifications *Type of ship:* Mainstream economy
Type of cruise: Traditional
Size: Medium (24,000 tons)
Number of cabins: 312
Outside cabins: 68%

Passengers: 624
Crew: 300 (international)
Officers: Greek and Portuguese
Passenger/crew ratio: 2.1 to 1
Year built: 1961

Itinerary **Year-round:** Seven-day loops leave Aruba Sundays, calling at Caracas/LaGuaira (Venezuela), Curaçao, Grenada, Barbados, and St. Lucia.

Port tax: $102 per passenger.

Overview Probably the ship's outstanding feature is its proportions: There's more than 43,000 square feet of deck space, and many cabins are 500 square feet—more than double what you find on many ships. Among the ship's offerings are an array of bars and lounges, an extensive shopping gallery, and a well-equipped exercise room. An asset for southern Carribean enthusiasts is that the *Crown* spends several more hours in Curaçao and Grenada than do most ships. Originally designed for Scandinavians and Germans, the ship has a decidedly European ambience and attracts a fair number of European passengers.

Cabins and Rates

	Beds	Phone	TV	Sitting Area	Fridge	Tub	Per Diem
Deluxe Suites	D	●	●	●	●	○	$342–$385
Outside Cabins	D,T, or U/L	●	●	○	●	◐	$199–$299
Inside Cabins	D,T, or U/L	●	●	○	●	○	$128–$213

Cabins are enormous and equipped with a telephone, minifridge, and closed-circuit TV. Cabins are adequately appointed in pastel hues—but it's function over form here.

Outlet voltage: 220 AC.

Single supplement: 150%–200% of double-occupancy rate.

Discounts: A third or fourth passenger in a cabin pays about $115 per diem. You get a discount of up to $200 for arranging your own airfare, and an 18%–25% discount for booking 90 days in advance. Children under age two sail free.

Sports and Fitness   **Health club:** Rowing machines, treadmill, sauna, massage.

Walking/jogging: Two unobstructed circuits.

Other sports: Volleyball, squash, two pools.

Facilities   **Public rooms:** Six bars and lounges, disco, casino, cinema, restaurant, chapel, card room, library.

Shops: Boutiques gallery, beauty salon/barber.

Health care: Fully staffed hospital.

Child care: Playroom, daily chaperoned children's activities.

Services: Photo service, Photo shop.

Access for the Disabled   There are four elevators and two handicapped-accessible cabins. Passengers who use wheelchairs must state this at the time of booking and must travel with an able-bodied adult.

Special Expeditions

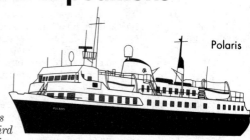

Polaris

Ships MS *Polaris*
MV *Sea Bird*
MV *Sea Lion*
SY *Sea Cloud*

Evaluation Special Expeditions is an adventure cruise line that attracts
passengers who want more than pampering. The focus is on
nature and on traveling to remote destinations and seldom-fre-
quented ports. Its cruises are friendlier and significantly less
expensive than those offered by other adventure companies
and are characterized by a slightly younger, less affluent, more
easygoing crowd. Cruises are joined by scientists, naturalists,
and others with specialties related to the itinerary who lecture
on board ship and accompany passengers on shore visits. Unlike guest experts on some ships who are treated either as employees or celebrities, specialists on Special Expeditions
cruises eat and socialize with passengers. You'll feel less like a
paying spectator and more like part of a grand adventure.

And these cruises *are* an adventure, offering remarkable and
intimate glimpses of nature. Small Zodiacs are used to make
wet landings on even deserted, rocky beaches. Bring or borrow
tall rubber boots, rubberized raincoats and rain hats, and some
old clothing. Because all shore excursions, snorkeling, entrance fees, and lectures are included in the fare, few financial
surprises await you.

In addition to the *Polaris, Sea Bird, Sea Lion,* and *Sea Cloud,*
Special Expeditions charters other vessels for unusual destinations, such as the Galápagos Islands. They also offer land
tours of the American Southwest and African photo safaris.

Activities These are extremely unstructured cruises. Sailing schedules
and shore excursions are all subject to change. Sometimes the
captain makes the decision about where to go next; at other
times, passengers vote. For instance, passengers might decide
whether the ship should follow a pod of whales or head for a
nearby fishing village. In tropical waters more emphasis is
placed upon individual leisure activities, like snorkeling and
sailing. Shipboard activities consist mainly of numerous lec-

---

Chart Symbols. *The following symbols are used in the cabin charts
that accompany each ship's evaluation.* **D:** *Double bed;* **K:** *King-size
bed;* **Q:** *Queen-size bed;* **T:** *Twin bed;* **U/L:** *Upper and lower berths;*
●: *All cabins have this facility;* ○: *No cabins have this facility;* ◖:
Some cabins have this facility

tures given by the staff of naturalists and historians on the wildlife and culture of the ports of call.

Dining The cuisine is northern German and Scandinavian, with lots of fish and schnitzel dishes, sausages, and cheeses. Meals are served in a single open seating. Special dietary requests are not easily handled. Passengers are expected to dress smartly on two designated evenings. Passengers can help themselves to coffee and cookies at any time. Room service is available only if you are ill.

Entertainment Although there is no organized entertainment, the captain will occasionally invite local performers to dinner and have them play or sing in the lounge afterward. Otherwise, passengers play cards or board games at night or read. Most passengers hit the sack early to rest up for the next day's adventures.

Service and Tipping Besides the sheer adventure of a Special Expeditions cruise, it is the warmth, competence, and intelligence of the crew that passengers remember. Crew members are very special; they engender trust, respect, and friendship. Tips are given anonymously by placing cash (or not-so-anonymous personal checks) in an envelope at the information desk, where they're then pooled and divided among the crew. Tip $8 per passenger per diem.

For More Information Special Expeditions (720 5th Ave., New York, NY 10019, tel. 800/762–0003).

MS Polaris

Specifications

Type of ship: Adventure	*Passengers:* 84
Type of cruise: Cultural	*Crew:* 44 (Filipino
Size: Very small (2,214	and Swedish)
tons)	*Officers:* Swedish
Number of cabins: 41	*Passenger/crew ratio:* 1.9 to 1
Outside cabins: 100%	*Year built:* 1960

Itinerary **Fall:** A variety of Amazon cruises depart from various river ports, calling at Belém (Brazilian coast), Devil's Island, along the Orinoco River and River and at Ciudad Guayana/Angel Falls (Venezuela), Rio Negro, Iquitos (Amazon River, Peru), and all along the upper Amazon. **Winter–Spring:** Central American cruises may call at the Darian Jungle, Panama City and Chiriqui Lagoon (Panama), the San Blas Islands (near Panama), and at various ports in Costa Rica, Nicaragua, Honduras, and Belize. A Mayan Coast/Caribbean cruise calls throughout Central America, as well as at Cartagena (Colombia), Bonaire, Isla Blanquilla (Lesser Antilles), Trinidad, the Grenadines, St. Lucia, Dominica, Iles des Saintes (Guadeloupe), and Antigua. **Summer:** Europe.

Port tax: Included in fare.

Overview The ungainly lines of the *Polaris* reveal its former life as a Scandinavian ferry, and the ship lacks a wealth of amenities. Nevertheless, it is well suited for adventure cruises. The main public room is more like an oversize living room than a cruiseship lounge. An even smaller lounge in the stern doubles as the library, which is well-stocked with reference books, bestsellers, and atlases. The dining room, split into smoking and nonsmoking sections, commands a magnificent view of the sea.

In addition to a fleet of Zodiacs and snorkeling equipment, the ship also carries a glass-bottom boat for underwater viewing.

Cabins and Rates

	Beds	Phone	TV	Sitting Area	Fridge	Tub	Per Diem
Category 5	T	○	○	●	○	○	$504–$583
Category 4	T	○	○	●	○	○	$427–$489
Category 3	T	○	○	○	○	○	$403–$461
Category 2	T	○	○	○	○	○	$357–$405
Category 1	T	○	○	○	○	○	$318–$359

Cabins are tiny, narrow, and poorly lighted, but they all have sea views.

Outlet voltage: 220 AC (bathrooms 110 AC).

Single supplement: 150% of double-occupancy rate in categories 1 and 2.

Discounts: A third or fourth passenger in a cabin pays half the double-occupancy rate. Airfare is not included in rates.

Facilities **Public rooms:** Lounge/bar, library, sauna; navigation bridge open to passengers.

Shops: Small gift shop, beauty salon/barber.

Health care: Doctor on call.

Services: Full-service laundry.

Other: Electrical adapters. Valuables may be kept in purser's safe.

Access for the Disabled Adventure cruises are not recommended for the disabled or for those in poor health.

MV Sea Bird and MV Sea Lion

Specifications *Type of ship:* Adventure
Type of cruise: Cultural
Size: Very small (99.7 tons)
Number of cabins: 37
Outside cabins: 100%

Passengers: 70
Crew: 21 (American)
Officers: American
Passenger/crew ratio: 3.3 to 1
Year built: 1982/1981

Itinerary **Fall:** Both ships make a number of Columbia River and Snake River as well as Sacramento Bay and San Francisco cruises, calling at Pasco (WA), along the Palouse River, Astoria (OR), and Olympic National Park. **Winter:** Cruises throughout the Gulf of California search for whales and other wildlife. **Spring:** Same as Fall and Winter. **Summer:** A 10-day Alaska cruise between Sitka and Prince Rupert calls at Admiralty Island, along the Seymour Canal and the Tracy Arm Fjord, Point Adolphus, Elfin Cove, Glacier Bay National Park, along Le Conte Bay, Petersburg, and along the Misty Fjords. Less frequent 14-day cruises between Sitka and Vancouver call along the Johnstone Strait, at various Queen Charlotte Islands, and at several of the above-mentioned ports.

Port tax: Included in fare.

Overview The tiny *Sea Lion* and *Sea Bird* look like hybrids of ferries and riverboats. While technically oceangoing vessels, they mostly sail on rivers and inside passages. With shallow drafts, they can sail in waters that would ground larger ships, even the *Polaris*. On the other hand, they are very friendly, homey vessels. The *Sea Lion* and the *Sea Bird* carry almost the same number of passengers as the *Polaris*, despite their smaller size. The ships' storage capacity, the size of the crews, and the number of public areas have been cut back as a result. Lectures, films, and other entertainment are held in the single lounge/bar. These ships are not for claustrophobics, or for those who easily become seasick. They rock noticeably in rough waters. Packets of Dramamine are kept in a bowl outside the purser's office.

Cabins and Rates

	Beds	Phone	TV	Sitting Area	Fridge	Tub	Per Diem
Category 4	T/D	○	○	●	○	○	$248–$420
Category 3	D	○	○	●	○	○	$225–$375
Category 2	T	○	○	○	○	○	$208–$354
Category 1	D or T	○	○	○	○	○	$173–$297

The cabins are among the smallest afloat.

Outlet voltage: 110 AC.

Single supplement: 150% of double-occupancy rate.

Discounts: A third or fourth passenger in a cabin pays half the double-occupancy rate in category 1 and 2 cabins only; it's 200% elsewhere. Airfare is not included in rates.

Facilities **Public rooms:** Lounge/bar; navigation bridge open to passengers.

Shops: Gift shop.

Health care: Doctor on board only on the Baja cruise; otherwise, the ship, never far from land, will dock in a U.S. or Canadian port if care is required.

Services: Full-service laundry.

Other: Electrical adapters, purser's safe.

Access for the Disabled Adventure cruises are not recommended for the disabled.

SY Sea Cloud

Specifications *Type of ship:* Sailing yacht
Type of cruise: Cultural/adventure
Size: Small (2,323 tons)
Number of cabins: 35
Outside cabins: 100%

Passengers: 70
Crew: 65 (German)
Officers: German
Passenger/crew ratio: 1 to 1
Year built: 1932

Itinerary **Fall:** Outside Western Hemisphere. **Winter:** Twelve-day loops leave Antigua, calling at St. Lucia, Bequia and Carriacou

(Grenadines), Grenada, Dominica, St. Kitts, and Anguilla. Ten-day cruises sail between Antigua and St. Maarten/St. Martin, calling at several of the above ports. **Spring–Summer:** Outside Western Hemisphere.

Port tax: Included in fare.

Overview The four-masted *Sea Cloud*, perhaps the most beautiful barque afloat, is a vision of maritime grace and elegance. When it was built, as the *Hussar V*, for the heiress Marjorie Merriweather Post and financier E. F. Hutton, it was the world's largest privately owned yacht. It's led a colorful life since then: as a naval weather station during World War II, as the yacht of Dominican dictator Molina Trujillo, and as carrier of numerous Hollywood stars and even the Duke and Duchess of Windsor. Eventually, a dispute over ownership left the ship rotting and derelict until a group of German investors refurbished and relaunched it in 1978.

Every attempt has been made to keep the *Sea Cloud* true to its origins, an artifact of a grander, more glamorous era. Every inch of this classic sailing yacht is finely polished and crafted. It's truly a sight to watch crew members scamper up the 20-story masts to unfurl the ship's 29 billowing sails (which cover 32,000 square feet). Auxiliary engines are fired up when necessary, but cruising under sail is much quieter, smoother, and more romantic.

Many of the original wood panels, desks, antiques, and other furnishings have been meticulously retored. Life on board is casual, laid-back, and unhurried, with few organized activities. The *Sea Cloud* allows you to feel the waves under you, to list side to side with the winds, to experience the energy of the sea. Bring plenty of Dramamine.

Cabins and Rates

	Beds	Phone	TV	Sitting Area	Fridge	Tub	Per Diem
Owner's Suite	D	○	○	●	○	●	$855–$871
Deluxe	D/T	○	○	●	○	●	$783–$798
Superior	D	○	○	○	○	○	$599–$614
Superior Single	T	○	○	○	○	○	$799–$816
Type A	D	○	○	○	○	○	$549–$558
Type A Single	T	○	○	○	○	○	$710–$724
Type B	D or T	○	○	○	○	○	$495–$498
Type B Single	D or T	○	○	○	○	○	$620–$724

Cabins and suites are individually decorated and laid out, as expected on a private yacht. Most prized are the Owner's Suites, with original chandeliers and nonworking fireplaces, which belonged to the original owners. Suites and Deluxe Staterooms have safes. Closet space is generous, and newer cabins have windows rather than portholes. Views from some Upper Deck cabins are partially obstructed by lifeboats. Cabins on the Promenade Deck look out onto public areas.

Outlet voltage: 220 AC.

Single supplement: 200% of double-occupancy rate; some singles are available.

Discounts: A third or fourth passenger in a cabin pays half the double-occupancy rate. Airfare is not included in rates.

Sports and Fitness **Walking/jogging:** Unobstructed circuit on Promenade Deck.

Other sports: Snorkeling.

Facilities **Public rooms:** Dining room, library, lounge, lido bar on Sun Deck; navigation bridge open to passengers.

Shops: Gift shop.

Health care: Doctor on call.

Services: Laundry.

Other: Purser's safe.

Access for the Disabled The ship is not recommended for the disabled or for those in poor health.

Sun Line Cruises

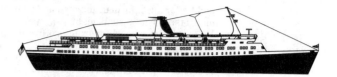

Ship   TSS *Stella Solaris*

Evaluation   In winter, Sun Line specializes in long cruises offering unusual itineraries normally available only on much more expensive ships: This line pioneered cruises along the Amazon River and to Carnival in Rio. In summer, the *Solaris* tours the Greek Islands. Though fares are relatively low, the *Solaris* is—in almost every other way—a traditional, mainstream cruise ship. Not surprisingly, ports are the main focus, and a fair amount of the on-board activities are geared toward excursions, as through lectures.

Though recently Amazon cruises have been attracting the younger set, most passengers are older than on other ships, most likely because of the time and money required for long cruises. Occasionally, one or two older gentlemen travel with the ship as guests to partner single ladies for dancing, dining, bridge games, and other social activities. Sun Line also adds some genteel touches likely to appeal to older passengers. Catholic Mass is celebrated every morning, the Jewish Sabbath every Friday evening, and a Protestant service every Sunday. Passengers can leave their shoes for the steward to polish and return by morning. Nearly half of those who sail on Sun Line are repeat passengers.

Activities   Expert lecturers from North American universities and prominent research societies conduct a shipboard "Enrichment Program," with talks covering local ports, history, art, stargazing (an astronomer accompanies every cruise), wildlife, and other subjects. Of particular note are talks by Captain Loren McIntyre, credited with discovering the source of the Amazon, who helped Sun Line pioneer Amazon cruising in 1983. Traditional activities, such as bingo, card and board games, and trivia contests, as well as classes in bridge, arts and crafts, cooking, wine tasting, and ballroom and Greek dancing, are also offered.

Dining   Dinner is served at two assigned seatings (6:30 and 8:30). The cuisine is essentially Continental, with a Greek specialty featured at lunch and ice-cream sundaes of a different type each day. The wine list is eclectic, ranging from very modest Italian vintages to expensive Bordeaux. Low-sodium, low-cholesterol,

---

Chart Symbols. *The following symbols are used in the cabin charts that accompany each ship's evaluation.* **D:** *Double bed;* **K:** *King-size bed;* **Q:** *Queen-size bed;* **T:** *Twin bed;* **U/L:** *Upper and lower berths;* ●: *All cabins have this facility;* ○: *No cabins have this facility;* ◑: *Some cabins have this facility*

and low-fat selections are available at every meal. Other dietary requests should be made in writing two weeks before sailing. One formal evening is held on seven-day cruises, three to four on cruises longer than 12 days. Men should wear a jacket and tie for all "informal" dinners, and women a cocktail dress or pantsuit. On "casual" nights, sportswear is sufficient. The Lido café serves early morning coffee and pastries, a buffet breakfast, mid-morning bouillon, and a buffet lunch. Self-serve coffee and iced tea are available at all times. Room service is available 24 hours from a limited menu.

Entertainment In addition to nightly variety shows, Sun Line offers piano music, cabarets, dance bands, late-night disco, masquerade parties, and passenger talent shows. Local performers are often brought on board to perform. Greek Night is an exuberant celebration of Sun Line's heritage that includes dancing, ethnic food, bouzouki music, singing, more dancing, and plenty of toasts with ouzo or wine. Movie lovers have a choice of an afternoon or an evening screening. After the evening show, the orchestra gets a good crowd in the lounge for ballroom dancing until midnight, after which night owls flock to the disco.

Service and Tipping Sun Line is proud of the way it treats the crew and points out that the *Solaris* was the first ship to provide most of the same cabin facilities for crew as for passengers. Some crew members have been with the company for more than 30 years; others inherited their positions from their fathers. As a result, the service is personable and efficient. Tips are pooled among the crew according to the rules of the Greek Stewards' Union; tip $7 or $8 per passenger per diem. Passengers are asked not to tip individual crew members except the beautician, barber, and masseuse.

For More Information Sun Line Cruises (1 Rockefeller Plaza, Suite 315, New York, NY 10020, tel. 800/872–6400 or 800/368–3888 in Canada).

TSS Stella Solaris

Specifications

Type of ship: Mainstream	*Passengers:* 620
Type of cruise: Traditional/senior	*Crew:* 310 (Greek)
	Officers: Greek
Size: Small (18,000 tons)	*Passenger/crew ratio:* 2 to 1
Number of cabins: 329	*Year built:* 1973
Outside cabins: 76%	

Itinerary **Fall:** Greek Isles. **Winter:** Two 15-day cruises along the Amazon River leave Manaus, calling at various Amazon ports and along the east coast of South America. A 14-day Christmas/New Year's loop leaves Fort Lauderdale, calling at St. Thomas/St. John, St. Maarten/St. Martin, the Netherland Antilles, Caracas/La Guaira, and Limón (Costa Rica). Three 12-day loops leave Galveston, Texas, calling at Ocho Rios (Jamaica), Cristóbal (Panama Canal Zone), along the Canal, the San Blas Islands (near Panama), Limón, and Cozumel/Playa del Carmen. **Spring–Summer:** Greek Isles.

Port tax: $65–$180 per passenger.

Overview The attractive *Solaris,* which previously sailed as the French Line's *Cambodge,* has curving lines, teak decks, and hardwood railings. A large ship with relatively few passengers, it has an open, airy feeling and an extremely friendly atmosphere. One crowded spot is the swimming pool, shaped in a figure 8 and designed to resist wave action. Throughout the cruise, get-to-gethers are scheduled to unite passengers who have interests other than tanning and swimming. With its oversize theater and closed-circuit TV network, the ship is ideal for meetings and conventions.

Although you won't find the sophistication of a luxury vessel or the glitz of a high-energy party ship, the *Solaris* is ideal for vacationers who want to do nothing more than relax amid friendly surroundings on the way to some truly unusual ports. There's plenty to do, but unwilling passengers are never coerced into sessions of arts and crafts and bingo.

Cabins and Rates

	Beds	Phone	TV	Sitting Area	Fridge	Tub	Per Diem
Deluxe Suite	D or T	●	●	●	○	●	$312–$519
Superior Outside	T	●	○	○	○	●	$231–$394
Standard Outside	T	●	○	○	○	○	$217–$344
Superior Inside	T	●	○	○	○	○	$207–$334
Standard Inside	T	●	○	○	○	○	$138–$264

Most cabins are generously apportioned, and many can be connected as adjoining staterooms. Each is equipped with a lockable drawer for valuables. Suites on the Boat Deck (category 1) look out onto a public promenade. In most cases, each has a large walk-in closet and a sitting area with coffee table, sofa, and chairs. Superior Inside and Standard Outside cabins have upper berths for third and fourth passengers. A third passenger may also be accommodated in a sofabed in the Deluxe Suites.

Outlet voltage: 110 AC.

Single supplement: 150%–200% of double-occupancy rate. Same-sex singles can be matched in a cabin; each pays the double-occupancy rate.

Discounts: A third or fourth passenger in a cabin pays the minimum fare for the cruise. Discounts are usually offered during the Christmas cruise; for example, a third or fourth person pays just $100 for the entire cruise. You get a discount for arranging your own airfare, and a 10%–35% discount for early booking. Special incentives are offered to repeat passengers on selected dates. Children 2–12 sharing a cabin with two adults pay 50% of the minimum fare for the cruise. Children under two pay $35 per diem.

Sports and Fitness   **Health club:** Fitness equipment, sauna, massage.

Walking/jogging: Unobstructed circuit on Boat Deck (7 laps=1 mile).

Other sports: Aerobics, table tennis, shuffleboard, pool.

Facilities   **Public rooms:** Four bars, three entertainment lounges, card room, cinema, disco, library/writing room, Lido, slot machines, blackjack tables.

Shops: Gift shop, beauty salon/barber.

Health care: Doctor and two nurses on call.

Child care: Playroom, youth programs with counselors when demand warrants it. Baby-sitting arranged privately with crew member.

Services: Full-service laundry, pressing service, photographer, film processing, shoe shines.

Other: Alcoholics Anonymous.

Access for the Disabled Access is quite limited generally, though all public areas except the disco are wheelchair-accessible. No cabin is specially equipped, and cabin and bathroom entrances have raised thresholds. Bathroom entries are 21½″ wide. Any passenger confined to a wheelchair must be accompanied by an able-bodied passenger.

Windstar Cruises

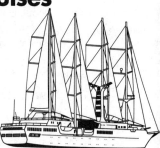

Ships *Wind Spirit*
Wind Star

Evaluation Few modern vessels capture the imagination the way the small Windstar ships do. These graceful ships—each powered by six enormous, computer-controlled sails—represent a true marriage of the new with the old. With 21,500 square feet of canvas, the sails are usually sufficient to power the ships, although they are sometimes assisted by diesel engines. More so than any other cruise ships, the *Wind Star* and *Wind Spirit* capture the feeling of really being at sea. These are sailing ships, not floating resorts.

This does not mean that passengers sleep in hammocks strung up in the hold. Windstar cruises are among the most luxurious around. Life on board is unabashedly sybaritic, attracting a sophisticated crowd happy to sacrifice bingo and masquerade parties for the attractions of remote islands and water sports. Surprisingly, the daily rates are little more than those charged on the large, upscale cruise ships. A third ship, the *Wind Song*, sails out of Tahiti.

Activities Shipboard life is unregimented and unstructured. No group activities are held; passengers pursue their own interests. Water-sports equipment can be used right off a swimming platform lowered from the stern. There's a small casino on board.

Dining Windstar's food is among the best served by any cruise line. Dinner is open seating, and passengers can wander in any time between 8 and 10. Elaborate formal wear is not considered appropriate, although men generally wear a jacket and tie. Breakfast and lunch are served in the glass-enclosed Veranda Lounge. Special dietary requests should be made four weeks before sailing. Other food service includes early morning coffee and croissants, plus afternoon tea. Limited room service is available 24 hours a day, for Continental breakfast or canapés and beverages,

Entertainment The little entertainment that is planned is strictly low-key. Every evening the ship's band or local musicians play in the lounge; there is also a piano bar and nightly dancing. The li-

Chart Symbols. *The following symbols are used in the cabin charts that accompany each ship's evaluation.* **D:** *Double bed;* **K:** *King-size bed;* **Q:** *Queen-size bed;* **T:** *Twin bed;* **U/L:** *Upper and lower berths;* ●: *All cabins have this facility;* ○: *No cabins have this facility;* ◑: *Some cabins have this facility*

brary has a selection of videotapes for use in the cabins. When the ship is in port, many passengers go ashore to sample the local nightlife.

Service and Tipping Service is comprehensive, competent, and designed to create an elite and privileged ambience. Tipping is not expected.

For More Information Windstar Cruises (300 Elliott Ave. W, Seattle, WA 98119, tel. 800/258-7245).

Wind Spirit and Wind Star

Specifications *Type of ship:* Luxury/ specialty
Type of cruise: Sail-powered/excursion
Size: Very small (5,350 tons)
Number of cabins: 74
Outside cabins: 100%

Passengers: 148
Crew: 91 (European)
Officers: Norwegian
Passenger/crew ratio: 1.6 to 1
Year built: 1988/1986

Itinerary **Early Fall:** Outside Western Hemisphere. **Late Fall–Winter:**
Wind Star Two alternating seven-day loops, which may be combined, leave Barbados, calling at Castries (St. Lucia), Iles des Saintes (Guadeloupe), St. Maarten/St. Martin, St. Barts, and St. Kitts; or at Tobago Cays (British Virgin Islands), Grenada, Carriacou and Bequia (Grenadines), Marigot Bay (St. Lucia), and Martinique. Longer cruises are available over Christmas and New Year's. **Spring–Summer:** Outside Western Hemisphere.

Port tax: $99 per passenger.

Wind Spirit **Early Fall:** Outside Western Hemisphere. **Late Fall–Winter:** Seven- day loops out of St. Thomas call at St. Barts, Nevis, St. Kitts, Virgin Gorda, Peter Island, Tortola, and Jost Van Dyke. **Spring–summer:** Outside Western Hemisphere.

Port tax: $99 per passenger.

Overview Inspired by the great sailing ships of a bygone era, Windstar's vessels are white, long, and lean, with bow masts and brass-rimmed portholes. To satisfy international safety regulations, the hulls are steel, not wood; the interiors, however, glow with wood paneling and teak trim—a look rare among modern cruise ships. Instead of the chrome-and-glass banisters so popular on other ships, Windstar vessels feature white-painted iron banisters with teak handrails. Although the ships are narrow—a necessity for sail-powered vessels—the interior is unusually spacious, mainly because there are so few passengers. The sense of space is heightened by huge glass windows that allow plenty of light into the public rooms.

Cabins and Rates

	Beds	Phone	TV	Sitting Area	Fridge	Tub	Per Diem
Suite/Cabin	T/Q	●	●	●	●	○	$368–$410

Windstar cabins represent the height of yachting luxury. All are outside suites with stocked refrigerators, sitting areas, safes, and VCRs. The larger Owner's Cabin (107) costs 30% more.

Outlet voltage: 110 AC.

Single supplement: 150% of double-occupancy rate; 200% for Owner's Suite.

Discounts: A third passenger in a cabin pays $1,100 for seven-day cruises. A child under 12 sharing a cabin with two adults pays the third-passenger rate. Airfare is not included in rates.

Sports and Fitness   **Health club:** Exercise equipment, sauna, massage.

Walking/jogging: Unobstructed circuit of ship is usually too crowded for fitness walks.

Other sports: Exercise classes, sailing, scuba diving (for certified divers), skeet shooting, snorkeling, volleyball, waterskiing, windsurfing, swimming platform, pool.

Facilities   **Public rooms:** Two bars, entertainment lounge, small casino (slots and blackjack), disco, library (including videotapes), piano bar.

Shops: Boutique, sports shop, hairstylist.

Health care: Doctor on call.

Child care: Bringing children on board is discouraged; no provisions are made for them.

Services: Full-service laundry.

Other: Underwater cameras available.

Access for the Disabled   No provisions are made to accommodate passengers in wheelchairs, and the lack of an elevator makes moving through the ship almost impossible for them. Tenders used to transport passengers from ship to shore are not designed to handle wheelchairs.

World Explorer Cruises

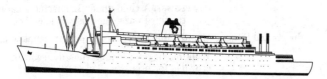

Ship SS *Universe*

Evaluation If you're intellectually inclined and willing to forgo some traditional comforts of cruise-ship life, then an Alaskan cruise on the *Universe* might be for you. If, on the other hand, you sleep through music recitals or cringe at the idea of a lecture on Eskimo art, take another ship. World Explorer specializes in low-cost educational and cultural cruises of Alaska, and they are superb. When you sail on the *Universe*, you can expect to learn more about Alaska and see more of the ports than on any traditional cruise to that region. For a certain type of passenger, no other Alaska cruise compares.

The *Universe* is really a floating campus that opens to the public during summer vacation. The rest of the year, the University of Pittsburgh offers two accredited "Semesters at Sea" that take students around the world. In summer, tourists take over the ship's closet-size cabins and bare-bones facilities. On a *Universe* cruise, the emphasis is clearly on Alaska.

Activities Days at sea and mornings en route to a port are packed with classes, slide presentations, videotape demonstrations, and educational films. Four or five experts each give a series of lectures on subjects ranging from Alaskan anthropology to history, glaciers, whales, and oceanography. College or tenure credit is offered at an extra fee to those who write a paper during the cruise. Much time is spent observing passing scenery and wildlife, but bridge, board games, and jigsaw puzzles are popular pastimes, too. The ship also offers a selection of first-run movies, bingo, trivia contests, and competitions.

Dining Seafood is purchased fresh in Alaska, but the food preparation on the *Universe* is adequate at best. Unfortunately, the kitchen staff seem to abide by the philosophy "Eat to live, rather than live to eat." Lunch and dinner are served at two assigned seatings. A classical guitarist or string quartet often plays during dinner, typically scheduled for 6 and 7:45 seatings. Breakfast is open seating. Make special diets requests in writing 30 days prior to sailing (no kosher available). Two semiformal evenings are held each cruise.

Chart Symbols. *The following symbols are used in the cabin charts that accompany each ship's evaluation.* **D:** *Double bed;* **K:** *King-size bed;* **Q:** *Queen-size bed;* **T:** *Twin bed;* **U/L:** *Upper and lower berths;* **●:** *All cabins have this facility;* **○:** *No cabins have this facility;* **◑:** *Some cabins have this facility*

Continental breakfast, light lunch, afternoon tea, and late-night snacks are served buffet-style on the enclosed Promenade Deck. The food selection tends to be skimpy, however. Self-serve coffee and tea are available at all times, but there is no room service.

Entertainment Lecturers become the entertainment on these cruises. Otherwise, you'll enjoy string quartets, a harp-and-dulcimer duo, and classical guitarists, along with dancing, passenger talent competitions, and costume shows.

Service and Tipping Crew members are friendly, but service is only slightly better than that found in any university cafeteria. There is no room service, not even coffee in the morning. Tip the room steward and the waiter $2.50 each per passenger per diem.

For More Information World Explorer Cruises (555 Montgomery St., San Francisco, CA 94111, tel. 800/854–3835). Adults may audit the floating university during the school year for about $10,000. Students pay $8,500–$9,500. For information on admission and possible grants or student loans, contact Semester at Sea/I.S.E. (University of Pittsburgh, 2E Forbes Quadrangle, Pittsburgh, PA 15260, tel. 412/648–7490 or 800/854–0195).

SS Universe

Specifications

Type of ship: Specialty	*Passengers:* 500
Type of cruise: Cultural	*Crew:* 220 (Chinese,
Size: Small (18,100 tons)	Filipino, American)
Number of cabins: 314	*Officers:* Chinese
Outside cabins: 43%	*Passenger/crew ratio:* 2.3 to 1
	Year built: 1954

Itinerary **Fall–Spring:** Not open to public. **Summer:** Fourteen-day loops leave Vancouver every other Sunday, calling at Wrangell, Juneau, Skagway, and Haines, Glacier Bay National Park, Hubbard Glacier, Valdez, Anchorage/Seward, Sitka, Ketchikan, and Victoria (British Columbia).

Port tax: $99 per passenger.

Overview The *Universe* is an inelegant ship that began as a freighter in 1953 and was subsequently transformed into the transatlantic liner *Atlantic.* Though cabins lack character and size, public areas and decks are spacious and classrooms are well laid out. The Commodore Lounge—the site of most lectures and evening shows, and the ship's largest bar—fills to standing room during lectures, which are also broadcast on closed-circuit TVs throughout the room and to the nonsmokers' Alyeska Lounge and the smokers' Denali Lounge. Smaller classrooms double as meeting rooms and a youth center (with its own video system).

The enclosed promenade is the ship's main artery, where large picture windows provide wonderful views of the Alaskan scenery and wildlife. Bridge players who would rather not be distracted by the scenery move inside to the cozy Mandarin Lounge, more like a living room. The stern lounge and bar on the Boat Deck is an excellent spot for socializing, reading, or having a nightcap. On the Sun Deck are two other very popular hubs of activity: the 12,000-volume library and the laundromat. You'd be surprised: Folding underwear while watching glaciers come into view can be a real life-affirming experience.

Cabins and Rates

	Beds	Phone	TV	Sitting Area	Fridge	Tub	Per Diem
Deluxe Stateroom	T	O	O	O	O	●	$264–$285
Stateroom	T	O	O	O	O	O	$249–$271
Outside Double	T or U/L	O	O	O	O	O	$192–$264
Inside Double	T or U/L	O	O	O	O	O	$150–$207
Outside Single	T	O	O	O	O	O	$243–$264
Inside Single	T	O	O	O	O	O	$193–$207

The cabins are tiny, the towels the size of postage stamps. Steel lockers replace closets. In Inside Doubles with upper and lower berths, two passengers dressing simultaneously can quickly degenerate into a game of Twister. Staterooms on the Boat Deck look onto a promenade.

Outlet voltage: 110 AC.

Single supplement: 200% of double-occupancy rate.

Discounts: A third or fourth passenger in a cabin pays $57 per diem. Vancouver airport transfers are complimentary; Seattle airport transfers cost $33 one-way per passenger. Airfare is not included in rates.

Sports and Fitness **Health club:** Weights, stationary bikes, rowing machines, massage.

Walking/jogging: Unobstructed circuit (cutting through interior hall) on enclosed Promenade Deck (12 laps=1 mile).

Other sports: Aerobics, table tennis.

Facilities **Public rooms:** Two bars, six lounges, extensive library, cinema/theater.

Shops: Gift shop, beauty salon/barber.

Health care: Doctor on call.

Child care: Playroom, children's program.

Services: Laundry service, laundromat.

Other: Safe-deposit boxes.

Access for the Disabled Some doorways have raised thresholds. The elevator doesn't reach the Main Deck cabins or the Coral Deck, where the cinema and beauty salon are located. Nevertheless, World Explorer welcomes disabled passengers when accompanied by an able-bodied companion.

4 Ports of Call

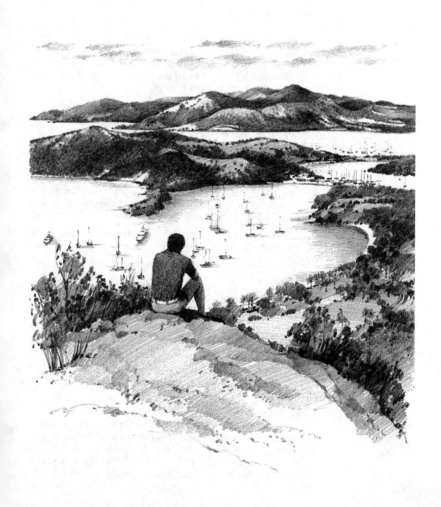

Ports of Embarkation

Most cruises to the Caribbean, the Bahamas, and the eastern
coasts of Mexico and South America leave from one of Florida's
three main ports: **Miami, Fort Lauderdale,** and **Port Canaveral.**
Less frequently, they originate in **Galveston,** in **New Orleans,**
or from a Caribbean island such as **Puerto Rico** or **Aruba.**
Cruises to the Mexican Riviera often leave from **Los Angeles,**
and typical Alaskan trips originate in **Vancouver** or **San Francisco.** Most cruises to Bermuda originate in **New York.** You'll
have to fly to **Honolulu** for most Hawaiian cruises and to **South
America, Australia,** or New Zealand for Antarctica cruises.

Cruise lines offer transportation from the airport to most passengers who have purchased fly/cruise packages or transfer
vouchers, although disabled travelers should check to see what
special provisions are available to them (For more information
about reaching your ship, *see* Arriving and Departing in Chapter 1.)

East Coast Ports

Fort Lauderdale Also known as Port Everglades, Florida's Fort Lauderdale
cruise port is the second largest in the world after Miami's—
and aiming to become the largest. The port is right in the middle of downtown Fort Lauderdale, but it's so spread out that
you need a car or taxi to get around.

Long-Term Parking A 2,500-space parking garage and street-level parking are
quite close to the terminals; free shuttles are available to those
lots farther away. The cost is $6 per day.

From the Airport The port is five to 10 minutes from Fort Lauderdale–Hollywood International Airport, depending on traffic. Take U.S. 1
north; at the first right, watch for signs to Port Everglades.

By Taxi: Taxis are metered, and a ride from the airport to the
ships costs about $6. Taxis circle the airport and meet all cruise
ships at the docks.

By Bus: Cruise-ship buses meet flights when they have been
notified that a transfer passenger is on board.

Miami The Port of Miami is on Dodge Island, across from the downtown area via a five-lane bridge. Just before the bridge on the
mainland is the large and attractive Bayside Marketplace,
whose waterfront ambience, two stories of shops and restaurants, and street entertainers provide a pleasant alternative to
the cruise terminals if you arrive before boarding begins. Free
shuttle buses are available to Bayside from the cruise terminals.

Long-Term Parking Street-level lots are right in front of the cruise terminals. Just
leave your luggage with a porter, tip him, and park. The cost is
$6 per day.

From the Airport Miami International Airport is a 20- to 30-minute drive from
the port. From the airport, take State Route 836 east until it
becomes I–395; take the south exit for Biscayne Boulevard, go
six blocks, then make a left turn at N.E. 5th Street. This will
have you going east on Port Boulevard. Cross the bridge and
follow the signs for your ship. The scene at the airport is hectic.

American Express offers Travelers Cheques built for two.

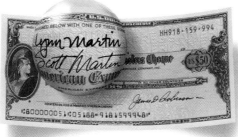

American Express® Cheques *for Two*. The first Travelers Cheques that allow either of you to use them because both of you have signed them. And only one of you needs to be present to purchase them.

Cheques *for Two* are accepted anywhere regular American Express Travelers Cheques are, which is just about everywhere. So stop by your bank, AAA* or any American Express Travel Service Office and ask for Cheques *for Two*.

AMERICAN EXPRESS Travelers Cheques

© 1993 American Express Travel Related Services Company, Inc. *Available at participating clubs.

Rediscover the most exciting and exotic country in the world... America.

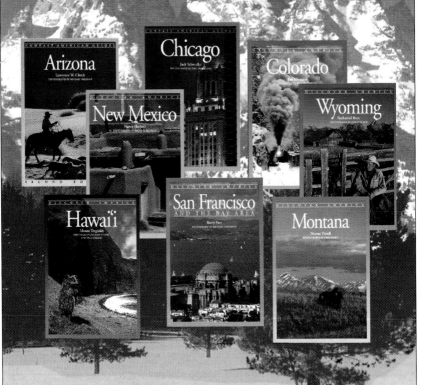

From Fodor's — Comprehensive, literate and beautifully illustrated guides to the individual cities and states of the United States and Canada, Compass American Guides are unparalleled in their cultural, historical and informational scope.

"Wickedly stylish writing." — *Chicago Sun-Times*
"Exceptional color photos." — *Atlanta Constitution*

$16.95, at bookstores everywhere, or call 1-800-533-6478

COMPASS AMERICAN GUIDES

Fodor's

Be sure that your bags are in the right pickup spot for your ship.

By Taxi: Taxis are numerous and can be hailed just about anywhere in the airport. The flat rate to the Port of Miami is $14 for up to five people. Limousines are available for $5.50 per person.

By Bus: Charter buses from all major cruise lines meet all major incoming flights. Even if you haven't purchased a transfer or aren't on a fly/cruise program, ask the person in charge of the bus for a ride to your ship.

New York City Though still less than charming, New York's Hudson River docks, on Manhattan's west-side waterfront, have been cleaned up considerably in recent years. If you're early and don't want to spend the wait exploring your own ship, walk over to neighboring Pier 86 to the *Intrepid* Sea-Air-Space Museum, where you can view a battleship, an aircraft carrier (with a variety of planes), and a submarine.

Long-Term Parking Outdoor long-term parking is available on the fenced-in top level of the pier for $15.50 per day.

From the Airport La Guardia, Newark, and Kennedy airports are not too far from Manhattan, but with traffic it can take you an hour and a half to get to the docks in a taxi. Pier porters expect a tip, even if they carry your bags only a few feet.

By Taxi: Taxis are metered and plentiful, and line up in front of every airline terminal. Unfortunately, given the traffic congestion, the following times and costs for taxi rides from the three airports are broad approximations only. Your ride could easily be longer and cost more. From **JFK,** a cab ride takes about one hour and costs about $45. From **La Guardia,** figure at least 40 minutes and a $35 fare. From **Newark International Airport,** a cab ride might take 45 minutes and cost about $50; however, the meters click away in traffic, so always budget double the expected fare for your taxi ride. Passengers pay for all bridge and tunnel tolls. Tip 15%.

Arriving by Bus Some cruise lines arrange free or very reasonably priced bus service from East Coast towns and cities, which is very convenient because your luggage is taken care of.

Port Canaveral Near the Kennedy Space Center and Cocoa Beach, Florida's Port Canaveral is currently used by very few cruise ships. The terminals are not yet as efficient at processing passengers as those at Miami and Fort Lauderdale, and a sense of confusion prevails during the busiest check-in periods.

The highway to Disney World from the east coast starts at nearby Cocoa Beach. For those passengers with a long wait before check-in, Cocoa Beach has superb beaches and numerous gourmet restaurants.

Long-Term Parking An outdoor long-term parking lot is directly outside the terminal and costs $5 per day ($9 per cruise for Premier's Disney cruise passengers).

From the Airport The Orlando airport is 45 minutes away. Go east on 528 Bee Line until the highway ends, then make a left into the port. Highway signs are easy to follow.

By Taxi: Taxi rates are exorbitant. Try taking the $18-per-person **Cocoa Beach Shuttle** (tel. 800/633–0427) bus instead, but call first to make a reservation.

West Coast Ports

Los Angeles The World Cruise Center in San Pedro has consolidated the old Port of Los Angeles cruise facilities into one modern center. Porters expect to be tipped.

A free shuttle bus runs from the World Cruise Center to Ports O' Call Village, a shopping center with a rustic seaside motif, about a half-mile away; to downtown San Pedro; and to the Cabrillo Marine Museum. Turn left out of the center for a quarter-mile stroll to the L.A. Maritime Museum.

A car-rental agency is right across the street from the World Cruise Center, or you can call another from pay phones in the terminal. Downtown Los Angeles is 25 miles north via the Harbor Freeway (Rte. 110).

Long-Term Parking Outdoor long-term parking is a five-minute walk from the terminals; a free shuttle bus also serves the area. Parking is $5 per day.

From the Airport Most passengers arriving by air use Los Angeles International Airport (LAX), about 20 miles from the cruise-ship docks; the trip can take 20 minutes to 1½ hours, depending on traffic. Long Beach airport is only about 12 miles away, but rather small. John Wayne/Orange County Airport is 45 minutes to an hour away by car.

By Taxi: Taxis are metered, and the ride from LAX will cost at least $40. Several shuttle services run vans between LAX and the cruise port for about $21 per person or about $50 for up to four people; they are boarded curbside at the airport but don't run in the evening. Families may find it cheaper to rent a car than to take a taxi or shuttle.

San Francisco The entire dock area of San Francisco is a tourist neighborhood of entertainment, shops, and restaurants called the Embarcadero Center. There's plenty to see and do within easy walking distance of the cruise terminals. With your back to the cruise pier, turn right to get to Fisherman's Wharf, Ghirardelli Square, and the Maritime Museum. If you don't want to walk, the No. 32 bus travels along the Embarcadero. You can also pick up a ferry to Alcatraz at Pier 41.

From the Airport San Francisco International Airport, one of the busiest in the country, is about 14 miles from the cruise pier.

By Taxi: From the airport to the cruise pier it's about $25–$35 and takes 25–30 minutes depending upon traffic.

By Bus: Less expensive (about $8 per person) shuttle buses can be picked up curbside at the airport, but they take longer. Make sure the shuttle will drop you off at the cruise pier.

Vancouver Many travelers consider British Columbia's Vancouver one of the most beautiful cities in the world, so it is only appropriate that its pier is also one of the most convenient and attractive. Right on the downtown waterfront, the pier is part of a building complex that sports a rooftop of dramatic sails and a convention center, hotel, shopping area, and restaurants. Porters are courteous and taxis plentiful.

If you are early, consider visiting historic Gastown just a couple of blocks away (to the left if you have your back to the water).

Long-Term Parking **Imperial Parking** (tel. 604/681–7311) offers long-term parking for about $35 for seven days. Another company is **Citipark** (tel. 604/681–8306). However, you must arrive two to four hours prior to departure time, and advance reservations are strongly recommended.

From the Airport Vancouver International Airport is approximately 11 miles away, but the road weaves through residential neighborhoods instead of highways. Returning American citizens can pre-clear U.S. Customs right in the Canadian terminal.

By Taxi: A taxi from the airport costs about $25 and takes about 25 minutes.

By Bus: Airport Express provides fast, frequent bus service between the airport and the pier for about $8.25 one way, $14 round-trip. However, it isn't nearly as convenient as using the cruise line's bus-transfer service, which may be taken from the Vancouver or Seattle airport and includes baggage transfers from cabin to airplane check-in. If you are booked on a Seattle flight, Quick Shuttle makes the four- to five-hour bus trip (in season) for about $35 one way, $70 round-trip; disembark at the Sandman Inn, about eight blocks from the port.

Going Ashore

Unless they're on a "cruise to nowhere," almost all ships call at one or more ports during a cruise. These stops can last a few hours or a few days. Even on short stopovers, however, passengers will have time to explore the port town, do some shopping, or head for the beaches. The myriad islands of the Caribbean are the most popular cruise destinations, and their proximity to one another allows ships to make several port calls in a week. Other popular destinations are Alaska, the Bahamas, Bermuda, the Mexican Riviera, the Panama Canal, and—to a lesser degree—South America, Antarctica, Hawaii, and the northeastern United States and Canada.

Itineraries are mapped out months in advance, but weather or political unrest can force last-minute changes. If a particular destination is important to you, check with a travel agent or the cruise line before booking: Though a change or itinerary may occur at the last minute, the cruise line may know, based on political circumstances, several months in advance that a destination is questionable.

Disembarking

When your ship arrives in a port, it either ties up alongside a dock or anchors out in a harbor. If the ship is docked, passengers just walk down the gangway to go ashore. Docking makes it easy to go back and forth between the shore and the ship.

If your ship anchors in the harbor, however, you will have to take a small boat—called a launch or tender—to get ashore. Tenders are a nuisance. Because they're difficult to board, disabled passengers may not be able to visit certain ports. The larger the ship, the more likely it is to use tenders. It is usually possible to learn before booking a cruise whether the ship will dock or anchor at its ports of call.

Before anyone is allowed to walk down the gangway or board a tender, the ship must first be cleared for landing. Immigration and customs officials board the vessel to examine passports and sort through red tape. Unless you're disembarking permanently, you'll be spared this procedure, although it may be more than an hour before you're actually allowed ashore. You will be issued a boarding pass, which you must have with you to get back onboard.

Port Stays

Most vessels spend the morning and afternoon in port; others may linger longer. In ports that have a vibrant nightlife, like San Juan or Nassau, many ships stay until midnight or overnight. Estimated times of arrival and departure in each port are provided in the cruise lines' brochures. Bermuda cruises are an interesting exception: Vessels stay in port for one to five days, acting more as floating hotels than ships.

Currency Passengers can change money at the ship's purser's office or ashore. It is inadvisable, however, to change large amounts of dollars into the local currency. At most cruise destinations, the dollar is welcome, and it can be difficult to change local money back into dollars. At the most, change a few dollars for public transportation, telephones, or museum passes. (*See* Before You Go in Chapter 1.)

Shore Excursions With the exception of a handful of cruise lines that include shore excursions in their basic ticket price, almost all ships sell these tours at extra cost. Shore excursions usually follow well-established formulas, although the quality of the tours varies enormously. Information about the shore excursions offered by a ship is sent to passengers before the cruise. Depending upon availability, shore excursions can be booked from the time you first reserve your cruise until right before the excursion begins.

If a shore excursion offered by the ship is fully booked, you might be able to purchase the same tour from a local vendor—and often at a better price. Tourist information offices, usually located on or near the pier, can tell you about local attractions and all the tours, including some not offered by the ships. Free maps are often available, too. Otherwise, local tourist hotels and many shopping districts have tour brokers with whom passengers can arrange a packaged tour.

Bus Tours The most common shore excursion is a bus tour—usually the best, fastest, and most economical way to see a port and environs. A good bus tour gives a sampling of the most noteworthy historical and cultural points of interest, as well as some of the local color. Passengers spend plenty of time in the bus, with a few stops for brief tours, photo opportunities, souvenir shopping, and sometimes lunch. Everything is strictly scheduled, with a limited amount of time spent at any one sight.

As a rule, few bus tours of the Mexican Riviera can be recommended. The tour from Martinique's Fort-de-France to St. Pierre, however, is a fascinating, though lengthy, trip to a part of the island that would otherwise be hard to reach, unless you rented a car and braved the local roads yourself.

A variation of the typical city or island bus tour is the cultural tour. In the few ports with archaeological sites, good museums, and authentic villages, some of these tours are interesting and well organized. Unfortunately, many ports that have no such attractions merely invent them.

If you're feeling adventurous, renting a car with a few friends will almost always save you money, and you can spend as long as you'd like wherever you'd like. However, this is a risky undertaking: If you get lost or for any other reason are late returning to the ship, you'll have to find a way to reach the next port on your own.

Boat Tours The typical **harbor boat tour** sails past small islands and waterfront sights where large cruise ships can't go; it may be combined with a bus tour or a stopover for lunch at a resort hotel. These tours usually don't provide music or entertainment. In some regions, especially Alaska, the boat tour focuses on an aspect of nature, such as whales, glaciers, or eagles. A variation of the harbor boat tour is a circumnavigation of the island or a cruise to a nearby island.

In stark contrast to the sedate harbor tours are **party boats** or **booze cruises.** Party boats are noisy, boisterous, and fun. Most boats have an open bar or a free rum punch, and a local mariachi band or rock group. Depending on the boat, which can range from a barge to a trimaran, it may even have a dance floor. Many booze cruises combine a beach party with the boat excursion. A **sunset sail** on a catamaran or trimaran can be a romantic, relaxing excursion. However, don't confuse a sunset sail with a sunset booze cruise; they are entirely different experiences.

Glass-bottom boats are small vessels with a panel of glass set into the bottom through which passengers sitting on benches view the underwater life. Although the tours are worthwhile for those who do not snorkel or dive, the sea life seen from such boats is often sparse and colorless. Nighttime tours are usually better, because the underwater lights attract fish from the reef.

A more exciting option is a **submarine tour.** (The submarine does not usually dive deep, and a surface boat accompanies it at all times.) Large windows give an excellent view of coral and marine life. The pilot points out unusual fish; display charts help with identification. Some submarine tours have scuba divers outside feeding and frolicking with the fish.

Aerial Tours Helicopter or small-plane tours tend to be short and expensive, but the view they provide is spectacular. This is especially true in Alaska, where the aircraft flies over, or even lands on, glaciers. Before booking a helicopter ride, find out if the helicopter holds three or four passengers. In a four-passenger aircraft, one person has to sit in the middle seat and won't be able to see properly out the windows.

Beach Parties Beach parties come in two types. The first centers on a barbecue on an isolated island or on a private beach to which all tour passengers are invited. These beach barbecues offer a host of activities, such as limbo contests, volleyball, swimming, and snorkeling. Although the barbecue and the games are free, passengers must pay for soft drinks and alcoholic beverages, as well as for rentals of snorkels and other water-sports equipment.

The second kind of beach party is sold as a shore excursion, with a tremendous difference in quality between what the various ships offer. Before signing up for a beach tour, make sure you know exactly what you're getting for your money. For instance, are lunch and drinks included? Are there changing rooms, lockers, and toilets? Are beach towels, chaises, and umbrellas provided, and is the use of sports equipment included in the price?

Nightclub Tours A variation on the daytime bus tours, with a drink or two and sometimes dinner thrown in, these are offered in ports where ships stay late or overnight. Although some nightclub tours are quite good (San Juan's is notable), more often than not the entertainment is amateurish.

Participant Sports You can arrange to participate in a variety of sporting activities during your stopover. If the ship doesn't offer an excursion, the shore-excursion director can usually make arrangements. Time limits obviously put some restrictions on what sports passengers can pursue, but port visits can mean a whole lot more than a bus tour and a shopping spree.

One of the best ways to experience Alaska is hiking through the wilderness or canoeing in the many bays and waterways. White-water rafting is available at some ports, but charter-boat fishing is offered everywhere. Many cruise ships offer fishing excursions.

In Mexico, the Caribbean, Bermuda, and the Bahamas, the emphasis is on water sports. Some beach excursions offered by ships include waterskiing, windsurfing, parasailing, and snorkeling. These activities can also usually be found on any beach that fronts a large resort hotel.

Almost every tropical port has several scuba-diving operators offering instruction and dives over coral reefs or wrecks. Though fishing-charter boats can easily be hired, take the excursions offered by your ship, if possible, since Mexican and Caribbean charters can rarely be guaranteed to get passengers back to the ship before it sails.

Golf and tennis are the most popular land sports in these regions. If the ship does not offer an excursion, the shore-excursion directors may, for a fee, arrange guest passes at private golf and tennis clubs, including some very exclusive ones. It may also be possible for the pro at your home club to arrange a guest pass. Golf equipment can usually be rented. Some ships have specific cruises that focus on tennis and/or golf, including on-board instruction, "19th-hole" parties, and celebrity pros. Ask a travel agent or the cruise lines about the dates for these sports-theme cruises.

Shopping Shopping is now a legendary sport among cruise passengers attracted by the heady perfume of duty-free merchandise. In reality, many of the typical consumer items, including electronics, jewelry, and liquor, carry price tags equivalent to those found at home. Throw in the labor of hauling these goods around with you, and you may come out a loser. Some bargains can be found, however. If you know what you want to buy, check its price at home first. (*See* Arriving and Departing in Chapter 1.)

In South America, Mexico, and certain areas of the Caribbean, shoppers are expected to haggle. The price first asked by most salespeople is about 50% more than the article's true value.

Before arrival at a port, cruise directors give a shopping talk. Although passengers can learn a great deal about the merchandise offered in a port, they should beware of endorsements of particular stores. Cruise directors often receive commissions from these stores to promote their wares.

Credit Cards The following credit card abbreviations are used: AE, American Express; D, Discover; DC, Diner's Club; MC, MasterCard; V, Visa.

Staying on Board

Many passengers prefer not to go ashore at all. Depending on the ship and the port, shore visits can be frenzied affairs, involving long lines and crowded towns. Life on board, however, can be at its most relaxing when the ship is in port. Comparatively few people stay on board, and passengers are left to their own devices. Operation of the ship's casino and many of the organized activities are suspended, although the bars and restaurants remain open. During port calls, meals are often open-seating.

Returning to the Ship

Cruise lines are strict about sailing times, which are posted at the gangway and elsewhere as well as announced in the daily activities sheets. Be certain to be back on board at least a half-hour before the announced sailing time or you may be stranded. If you are on a shore excursion that was sold by the cruise line, however, the captain will wait for your group before casting off. If the ship must leave without you, the cruise company will fly you, at its expense, to the next port. That is one reason many passengers prefer ship-packaged tours.

If you are not on one of the ship's tours and the ship does sail without you, immediately contact the cruise line's port representative, whose name and phone number are often listed on the daily activities sheets. You may be able to hitch a ride on a pilot boat, though that is unlikely. Passengers who miss the boat must pay their own way to the next port of call.

Alaska

"Cruise everywhere else in the world before visiting Alaska," experienced passengers often advise, "because once you've seen Alaska, everything else pales by comparison."

Detached from the contiguous United States, Alaska has Canada and Russia as its nearest neighbors, and some localities are closer to Japan than to Juneau, the state capital. But more than scale and geography set Alaska apart from the rest of North America: Alaska is youth, energy, space, and wilderness. The sense of excitement and adventure is palpable from the moment you step ashore in a misty port, where dramatic mountains tower over narrow streets and humanity is dwarfed by the power of nature.

On a wilderness trail in Chugach State Park, view mountain sheep and moose just 10 miles from downtown Anchorage, Alaska's largest city. Wander in hushed awe through the haunting totem-pole park outside Ketchikan, where sea breezes wind through a grove of Tlingit carved poles and ancient spruce trees.

Gliding through Glacier Bay National Park, watch from the ship rails as huge slabs of ice break away from a glacier, sounding like gunshots, and tumble into the bay, creating waves that rock the vessel. Harbor seals and their pups ride the ice floes like stowaways on a raft while passengers cool their cocktails with slivers of glacial ice created millions of years ago.

Alaskans are proud of their heritage and offer visitors ample opportunity to see and learn about totem poles, traditional dances, and modern artist colonies. In the Southeastern Panhandle, where Tlingit Indians are the predominant Native American community, bookstores offer a great selection of literature on the land's Native American and Russian heritage.

Alaskan cruises focus chiefly on the panhandle, though some venture into the south-central Gulf of Alaska. Though most cruise ships sail the Inside Passage—the protected waterway between Vancouver and Skagway, which connects scores of remote islands with the mainland—for part of their itinerary, the ports of embarkation and debarkation define the type of cruise offered. Sailings from San Francisco and Los Angeles spend a few days at sea before reaching Alaska. Loops to and from Vancouver are cruise-only and sail entirely within the Inside Passage. Cruises that start or end in Anchorage, or its port cities of Seward and Whittier, allow the option of spending additional time exploring inland.

Who *wouldn't* be enraptured by an Alaskan cruise! Teeming with wildlife, glaciers, snowcapped mountains, historical sites, and pioneer spirit, Alaska is the hottest cruise destination in the world.

When to Go The Alaska cruise season is short but growing longer. Cruise lines now schedule first sailings in mid-May and final sailings in late September. May and June are the driest cruise months. At least two cruise lines price sailings by five "seasons," with spring and fall departures least expensive and midsummer sailings most costly. Virtually every line offers "early booking discounts" to passengers on deposit in advance. Some lines pro-

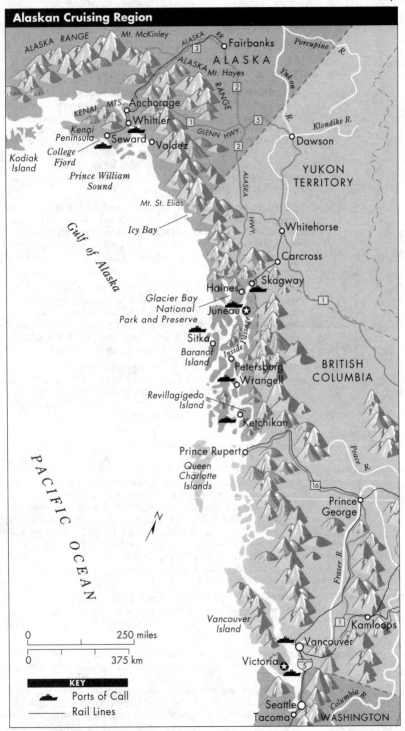

Alaskan Cruising Region

274

ALASKA RANGE
Mt. McKinley
ALASKA RR.
Porcupine R.
Fairbanks
ALASKA
ALASKA RANGE
Mt. Hayes
3
2
ALASKA
Yukon R.
Klondike R.
KENAI MTS.
Anchorage
Whittier
1
GLENN HWY.
5
Kenai Peninsula
Seward
Valdez
2
Dawson
College Fjord
YUKON TERRITORY
Kodiak Island
Prince William Sound
Mt. St. Elias
ALASKA HWY.
Gulf of Alaska
Icy Bay
Whitehorse
Carcross
Skagway
Haines
1
Glacier Bay National Park and Preserve
Juneau
Sitka
Inside Passage
BRITISH COLUMBIA
Baranof Island
Petersburg
Wrangell
Revillagigedo Island
Ketchikan
Prince Rupert
Queen Charlotte Islands
Peace R.
PACIFIC OCEAN
16
Prince George
N
Fraser R.
Vancouver Island
1
Kamloops
Vancouver
Victoria
5
Columbia R.
Seattle
Tacoma
WASHINGTON

0   250 miles
0   375 km

KEY
⛴ Ports of Call
— Rail Lines

mote early- and late-season cruises with special-interest themes, such as photography and natural history.

Shore Excursions
Aerial Tours Anyone unwilling to hike or boat in the backcountry should take at least one helicopter or small-plane tour to see the state in its full glory. The aircraft fly over glaciers and waterways; the best helicopter tours actually land on a glacier and let passengers out for a walk.

Fishing The prospect of bringing a lunker king salmon or a rainbow trout to net is the reason many people choose an Alaskan cruise. Every ship offers optional fishing excursions on charter boats.

Hiking Trekking through woods and mountains and along the beaches is southeastern Alaska's unofficial main pastime. Some trails are abandoned mining roads; others are natural routes or game trails that meander over ridges, through forests, and alongside streams and glaciers. Many ships offer hiking excursions, but every port is within easy access of at least some hiking. Trails go through real wilderness, so check with local park rangers or tourist offices for current conditions, and leave your intended itinerary with someone on the ship.

Salmon Bake Alaska is famous for outdoor salmon barbecues, called salmon bakes. Fresh fish is grilled on an open fire and served with plenty of fixings. Quality varies, so ask locals for advice on which bake to attend. Juneau's Gold Creek salmon bake is a good choice.

Whale-Watching Whale are plentiful in these waters, and several small-boat excursions offer excellent opportunities to see them up close. The captains of these craft keep in contact and let one another know when a whale pod is near.

Shopping Alaskan Native American handicrafts range from Tlingit totem poles—a few inches high to several feet tall—to Athabascan beaded slippers. Tlingit, Inuit, and Aleut wall masks, dance rattles, baskets, and beaded items in traditional designs can be found at gift shops up and down the coast. To ensure authenticity, buy items tagged with the state-approved AUTHENTIC NATIVE HANDCRAFT FROM ALASKA "Silverhand" label. Or buy at Saxman Village outside Ketchikan or similar Native American–run shops. Better prices are had the farther you go to the north and away from the coast.

Salmon—smoked, canned, or fresh—is another popular item. Most towns have a local company that packs and ships local seafood.

Dining Not surprisingly, seafood dominates most menus. In summer, king salmon, halibut, king crab, cod, and prawns are usually fresh. Restaurants are uniformly informal; clean jeans and windbreakers are the norm.

Category	Cost*
Expensive	over $40
Moderate	$20–$40
Inexpensive	under $20

*per person, excluding drinks, service, and sales tax

Anchorage

A local newspaper columnist once dubbed Anchorage "a city too obviously on the make to ever be accepted in polite society." And for all its cosmopolitan trappings, this city of 225,000 does maintain something of an opportunistic, pioneer spirit. Its inhabitants, whose average age is just 28, hustle for their living in the banking, transportation, and communications fields.

Superficially, Anchorage looks like any other western American city, but sled-dog races are as popular here as baseball is in California, and moose occasionally roam along city bike trails. This is basically a modern, relatively unattractive city, but the Chugach Mountains form a striking backdrop, and spectacular Alaskan wilderness is out the back door.

Anchorage took shape with the construction of the federally built Alaska Railroad (completed in 1923), and traces of the city's railroad heritage remain. With the tracks laid, the town's pioneer forefathers actively sought expansion by hook and—not infrequently—by crook. City fathers, many of whom are still alive, delight in telling how they tricked a visiting U.S. congressman into dedicating the site for a federal hospital that had not yet been approved.

Boom and bust periods followed major events: an influx of military bases during World War II; a massive buildup of Arctic missile-warning stations during the Cold War; and most recently, the discovery of oil at Prudhoe Bay and the construction of the trans-Alaska pipeline.

Anchorage today is the only true metropolis among Alaskan cities. New attractions are the art deco–style Fourth Avenue Theater, reopened nearly 50 years after its debut. And at Ship Creek, where Anchorage was first settled, a new waterfront tourism complex is planned, including a planetarium and aquarium.

Cruise ships visiting Anchorage either dock right in town or at Seward or Whittier—port cities on the east coast of the Kenai Peninsula—from which passengers must travel an hour by bus or train to Anchorage (*see* Seward and Whittier, *below*).

Shore Excursions For Anchorage's shore excursions, *see* sections on Seward and Whittier, *below.*

Getting Around The municipal **People Mover** (tel. 907/343–6543) bus system
By Bus covers the whole Anchorage bowl. It's not convenient for short downtown trips but can be used for visits to outlying areas. The central depot is at 6th Avenue and G Street. The fare is $1.

By Taxi Prices for taxis start at $2 for pick-up and $1.50 for each mile. Most people in Anchorage telephone for a cab, although it is not uncommon to hail one. Contact **Alaska Cab** (tel. 907/563–5353), **Checker Cab** (tel. 907/276–1234), and **Yellow Cab** (tel. 907/272–2422).

Exploring *Numbers in the margin correspond to numbered points of in-*
Anchorage *terest on the Downtown Anchorage map.*

The downtown is easily toured on foot in three to four hours, longer if you really browse. Start at the **Log Cabin Visitor Information Center** at the corner of 4th Avenue and F Street. A marker in front shows the mileage to various world cities.

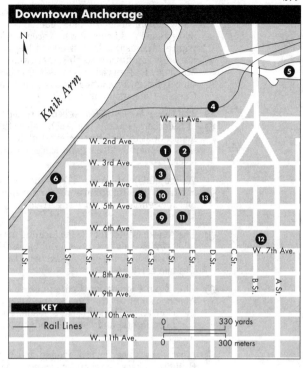

Downtown Anchorage

Fourth Avenue sustained heavy damage in the 1964 earthquake. The businesses on this block withstood the destruction,
but those a block east, where the McDonald's now stands, fell
into the ground as the earth under them slid toward Ship
Creek.

The **Old City Hall** is to the east, beside the visitor center. It was
built in 1936. The marble sculpture out front is a monument to
William Seward, the secretary of state who engineered the
purchase of Alaska from Russia.

Catercornered from the visitor center at 4th Avenue and F
Street is the **Alaska Public Lands Information Center.** The center has displays about Alaska's national parks, forests, and
wildlife refuges and shows films highlighting different parts of
the state.

Walk north (downhill) on F Street to 2nd Avenue. The houses
in this neighborhood are original town-site homes built by the
Alaska Engineering Commission, which built the Alaska Railroad early this century. A plaque by each house tells its history.

Turn east (right) on 2nd Avenue and head 1½ blocks to the
stairway leading downhill to the **Alaska Railroad depot.** Outside are totem poles and a 1907 locomotive. A monument here
relates the history of the railroad.

Just north of the depot, **Ship Creek** tumbles into Cook Inlet.
Salmon run up this creek all summer; they are visible from the
nearby viewing platform.

The paved walking and cycling coastal trail, which runs along the water for about 12 miles, can be reached by returning to 2nd Avenue and heading west three blocks to the marked entrance. Mt. Susitna (known as the Sleeping Lady) is the prominent low mountain to the northwest. To her north, Mt. McKinley is often visible. On the left is Resolution Park, a cantilevered viewing platform above the trail, dominated by the Captain Cook monument.

6
7 The **Oscar Anderson House** is next to the trail at the north end of **Elderberry Park.** It was Anchorage's first permanent frame house, built in 1915 by tent-city butcher Anderson. Tours are free. The park is also a good place to watch for whales off the coast.

8 Walk uphill on 5th Avenue from the park and continue east to H Street. The **Imaginarium** (725 5th Ave., tel. 907/276–3179), an experiential museum with a great shop, is a fun stop for kids and adults.

9 The **Alaska Center for the Performing Arts** (6th Ave. and G St., tel. 907/263–2900) occupies a full block. This is one of several major civic buildings planned during the oil boom of the late '70s and early '80s.

10 The **Egan Convention Center,** across 5th Avenue from the Alaska Center for the Performing Arts, was also built during the boom days. The lobby has a beaded curtain that evokes the northern lights, and several modern Native Alaskan sculptures.

11 Across the street at 5th Avenue and E Street, the **Kimball Building** houses two shops operated by Anchorage old-timers. Kimball's Dry Goods has been in this location for more than 60 years. Next door the Gold Pan sells coffee, tea, Russian goods, and native art and artifacts.

12 The **Anchorage Museum of History and Art** occupies the whole block at 6th Avenue and A Street. The entrance is on 7th Avenue. It houses a fine collection of historical and contemporary Alaskan art, displays on Alaskan history, and a special section for children.

13 Head back downtown on A Street to 5th Avenue. Turn left and go three blocks to D Street. One block down on the right, the white-turreted **Wendler Building** is embraced by a newer brick building. Moved to this site from its original home at 4th Avenue and I Street, the Wendler was built in 1915 and once housed a popular restaurant and, for a time, a ladies-only bar. It now houses an international import store on the ground floor.

Shopping The **Alaska Native Arts and Crafts Association** (333 W. 4th Ave., tel. 907/274–2932) sells items from all native Alaskan groups and carries the work of the best-known carvers, silversmiths, and beadworkers, as well as unknown artists. The best buys on native Alaskan artists' work are found at the **Alaska Native Medical Center** gift shop (3rd Ave. and Gambell St., tel. 907/257–1150, open weekdays 10–2, also 11–2 the first Saturday of each month). The **Stonington Gallery** (415 F St., tel. 907/272–1489) carries the work of better-known Alaskan artists, both native and non-native.

Sports *Canoeing/* *Kayaking*	Local lakes and lagoons, such as Westchester Lagoon, Goose Lake, and Jewel Lake, offer good boating. Some are stocked with fish as well. Rental boats are available from **Adventures and Delights** (between 4th and 5th Aves. on K St., tel. 907/276–8282) and from **Recreational Equipment Inc.** (1200 W. Northern Lights Rd., tel. 907/272–4565).
Jogging/ *Walking*	The coastal trail (*see* Exploring Anchorage, *above*) and other trails in Anchorage are used by runners and walkers. The trail from Westchester Lagoon at the end of 15th Avenue runs 2 miles to Earthquake Park and, beyond that, 7 miles out to Kincaid Park.
Dining	**The Club Paris.** It's dark and smoky up front in the bar, where for decades old-time Anchorage folks have met for a drink and a chat. Halibut and fried prawns are available, but the star attractions are the big, tender, flavorful steaks. No vegetables are served here except huge baked potatoes with optional cheddar cheese sauce. If you forget to make a reservation, have a drink at the bar and order the hors d'oeuvres tray—a sampler of steak, cheese, and prawns that could be a meal for two people. *417 W. 5th Ave., tel. 907/277–6332. Reserve early that day. AE, D, DC, MC, V. Moderate.* **Sack's Café.** This cool, modern café offers light New American food. The chefs use trendy ingredients like chèvre and interesting combinations of ethnic cuisines, such as pasta with a Mexican mole sauce. The large salads make light meals. Desserts include a decadent chocolate gâteau. *625 W. 5th Ave., tel. 907/276–3546. AE, MC, V. Moderate.* **The Lucky Wishbone.** At this old Anchorage eatery, where old-timers sit around the brightly lit Formica tables and waitresses never seem to have a bad day, great fried chicken is the fare. Order all white meat, with just the wishbone and no ribs, or try the livers or gizzards. *1033 E. 5th Ave., tel. 907/272–3454. No credit cards. Closed Sun. Inexpensive.*

Juneau

Juneau owes its origins to a trio of colorful characters: two pioneers, Joe Juneau and Dick Harris, and a Tlingit chief named Kowee, who discovered rich reserves of gold in the stream that now runs through the middle of town. That was in 1880, and shortly after the discovery a modest stampede led to the formation of first a camp, then a town, then the Alaska district (now state) capital.

For nearly 60 years after Juneau's founding, gold remained the mainstay of the economy. In its heyday, the Alaska Juneau gold mine was the biggest low-grade-ore mine in the world. Then, during World War II, the government decided it needed Juneau's manpower for the war effort, and the mines ceased operations. After the war, mining failed to start up again, and government became the city's principal employer.

Juneau is a charming, cosmopolitan frontier town. It's easy to navigate, has one of the best museums in Alaska, is surrounded by beautiful wilderness, and has a glacier in its backyard. To capture the true frontier ambience, stop by the Red Dog Saloon and the Alaskan Hotel. Both are on the main shopping drag, just a quick walk from the cruise ship pier.

Shore Excursions *Not all excursions are offered by all cruise lines. All times and prices are approximate. Unless otherwise noted, children's prices are for those 12 and under.*

Adventure **Mendenhall River Float Trip:** A rafting trip down the Mendenhall River passes through some stretches of gentle rapids. Experienced oarsmen row the rafts; rubber boots, ponchos, and life jackets are provided. The minimum age is six. An excellent first rafting experience for those in good health. Great fun. *3¹/2 hrs. Cost: $75–$89 adults, $48–$55 children.*

Mendenhall Glacier Helicopter Ride: One of the best helicopter glacier tours, including a landing on an ice field for a walk on the glacier. Boots and rain gear provided. *2 hrs. Cost: $130–$140.*

Cultural **Gold Panning and Gold Mine Tour:** Pan for gold with a prospector guide and tour the entrance of the Alaska Juneau mine. *1¹/2 hrs. Cost: $25–30 adults, $17–$19 children.*

Dining with a Difference **Gold Creek Salmon Bake:** An all-you-can-eat outdoor meal, featuring Alaska king salmon barbecued over an open alderwood fire. After dinner, walk in the woods, explore an abandoned mine, or pan for gold. *1¹/2 hrs. Cost: $20–$22 adults, $12 children.*

Taku Glacier Lodge Wilderness Salmon Bake: Fly over the Juneau Ice Field to Taku Glacier Lodge. Dine on barbecued salmon, then explore the virgin rain forest or enjoy the lodge. Expensive, but consistently gets rave reviews. *2¹/2–3 hrs. Cost: $130–$154.*

Scenic **Mendenhall Glacier and Hatchery Tour:** A bus tour to the "drive-in" glacier, just 13 miles from downtown Juneau, with a narrated city tour. Includes a visit to Juneau's newest attraction, the Gastineau Salmon Hatchery. *2¹/2–3¹/2 hrs. Cost: $26–$30 adults, $13–$15 children.*

Getting Around Passengers come ashore at **Marine Park,** where a small visitor kiosk at the downtown end of the docks is filled with tour brochures, bus schedules, and maps (open daily 9 AM–6 PM). With your back to the water, walk away from the kiosk toward the street and you'll be downtown.

By Taxi Taxis wait for cruise-ship passengers at Marine Park. There are no standard rates; they must be negotiated. If you need to, call **Taku Glacier Cab Co.** (tel. 907/586–2121); rates begin at $1.75 for pick-up, and $1.50 per mile.

Exploring Juneau *Numbers in the margin correspond to numbered points of interest on the Juneau map.*

❶ Begin at the visitor information kiosk at **Marine Park,** then head east a block to South Franklin Street. Buildings here and on Front Street are among the oldest and most interesting in the city. Many reflect the architecture of the '20s and '30s; some are even older.

The small **Alaskan Hotel** at 167 South Franklin Street was called "a pocket edition of the best hotels on the Pacific Coast" when it opened in 1913. Owners Mike and Betty Adams have restored the building with period trappings. The barroom's massive, mirrored oak bar, accented by Tiffany lamps and panels, is a particular delight.

Just down the street at No. 278 is the **Red Dog Saloon.** Less genteel than the Alaskan Hotel, with sawdust-covered floor

Alaska State Capitol, **2**

Alaska State
Museum, **13**

Centennial Hall, **14**

City Museum, **7**

Evergreen
Cemetery, **9**

Federal Building and
Post Office, **11**

Governor's House, **8**

House of
Wickersham, **5**

Juneau-Harris
Monument, **12**

Marine Park, **1**

Monument to
Chief Kowee, **10**

St. Nicholas Russian
Orthodox Church, **3**

State Office
Building, **6**

Totem pole, **4**

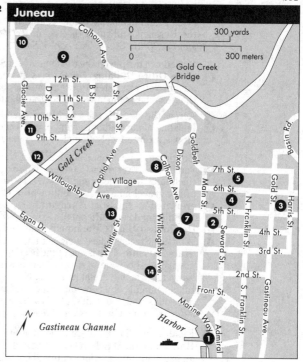

and stuffed bears and big-game heads mounted on the walls,
this is Alaska's most famous saloon.

Also on South Franklin Street is the **Alaska Steam Laundry
Building,** a 1901 structure with a windowed turret. It now
houses a coffeehouse, a film processing service, and other
stores. Across the street, the equally venerable **Senate Building Mall** contains one of the two Juneau Christmas Stores, a
children's shop, and a place to buy Russian icons.

Head uphill on Franklin and turn left onto 4th Street; at the
corner of Seward Street is the **Alaska State Capitol,** constructed in 1930, with pillars of southeastern Alaska marble.
The structure now houses the governor's offices and other
state agencies, and the state legislature meets here four
months each year. *Tel. 907/465–2479. Tours daily 8:30–5.*

Uphill again and to the east on Fifth Street is little **St. Nicholas
Russian Orthodox Church,** built in 1894 and the oldest Russian
church in Alaska. *Donation requested. Open daily in summer,
but hours vary. Check at the visitors' kiosk.*

At the top of Seward Street, between 5th and 6th streets,
stands a **totem pole** that is one of Juneau's finest; it tells a sym-
bolic story of Alaska. Walk up the hill to the totem pole and
continue up the stairs to 7th Street, where you'll find the **House
of Wickersham,** the onetime residence of James Wickersham,
a pioneer judge and delegate to Congress. The 1899 home is
now part of the Alaska state park system. Memorabilia from
the judge's travels range from rare Native American basketry

and ivory carvings to historic photos, 47 diaries, and a Chickering grand piano that came "round the horn" to Alaska while the Russians still ruled the region. *Tel. 907/586–9001. Admission: $2. Tours Sun.–Fri. noon–5, Sat. 10–2.*

Back down the hill on the west end of 4th Street, you'll pass the
6 **State Office Building.** On Fridays at noon in the four-story atrium you can listen to organ music played on a grand old theater pipe organ, a veteran of the silent-movie era.

7 Across the street is the **City Museum** and another totem pole.
8 Heading along Calhoun Avenue, you'll come to the **Governor's House,** a three-level colonial-style home completed in 1912.

Continuing on Calhoun Avenue, past the Gold Creek bridge,
9 you'll reach **Evergreen Cemetery,** where many Juneau pioneers (including Joe Juneau and Dick Harris) are buried. At the end
10 of the gravel lane is the **monument to Chief Kowee,** who was
11 cremated on this spot. Turn left here, walk past the **Federal Building and Post Office** at 9th Street and Glacier Avenue, past
12 the **Juneau-Harris Monument** near Gold Creek, then on to
13 Whittier Street, where a right turn takes you to the **Alaska State Museum.** This is one of the best museums in Alaska, and you'll probably want to spend at least an hour looking at exhibits on natural and social histories, Native Alaskan art and artifacts, mining, and contemporary art. Check out the gift shop for books and souvenirs. *395 Whittier St., tel. 907/465–2901. Admission: $2. Open weekdays 9–6, weekends 10–6.*

14 Finally, on Willoughby Avenue at Egan Drive is **Centennial Hall,** where the U.S. Forest Service and U.S. Park Service have an excellent information center. *Tel. 907/586–8751. Open daily 8–5.*

Shopping South Franklin Street is filled with shops; their main virtue is that they are close to the ship. The variety of merchandise is good (especially the hand-knit sweaters); prices are moderate to expensive.

Upstairs in the Senate Building Mall on South Franklin Street is the **Russian Shop** (tel. 907/586–2778), a repository of icons, samovars, lacquered boxes, nesting dolls, and other items that reflect Alaska's 18th- and 19th-century Russian heritage. One side of the shop is devoted to Norwegian wares, including traditional Norwegian wool sweaters. Across the way is an Irish shop.

Knowledgeable locals frequent the **Rie Munoz Gallery** (233 S. Franklin St., tel. 907/586–2112) for fine art. Munoz is one of Alaska's favorite artists, and her stylized, colorful design technique is much copied. Other artists' works are also on sale, including wood-block prints by nationally known artist Dale DeArmond.

Sports Contact **Beartrack Charters** (800 F St., Juneau, tel. 907/586–
Fishing 6945), **Gustavus Inn** (Box 60, Gustavus, tel. 907/697–2254), or **Juneau Sportfishing** (76 Degan Dr., Suite 230, Juneau, tel. 907/586–1887).

Hiking Surrounded by the 1,500-square-mile Juneau Icefield and the Tongass National Forest, Juneau is a hiker's paradise. For trail maps, information, and advice, stop at the visitor kiosk in Marine Park or, even better, **Centennial Hall** on Willoughby at Egan Drive. **Parks and Recreation/Juneau** (155 S. Seward St., tel. 907/586–5226) sponsors an open Wednesday-morning group hike.

Alaska Rainforest Tours (369 S. Franklin St., tel. 907/463–3466) offers guided hikes through Tongass National Forest. Backpacks and rain gear are provided. Tours are limited in size, so call before leaving home.

Mendenhall Glacier is only 13 miles from downtown, and you can walk right up to it. The bus ($1.25) that stops at South Franklin Street can take you within 1¼ miles of the Mendenhall visitor center. Plan on three or four hours total if you take the bus, including sightseeing.

Kayaking **Alaska Discovery** (234 Gold St., tel. 907/463–5500) offers escorted day tours for $95 per person, or you can rent your own for $40–$75 a day.

Dining **The Silver Bow Inn.** The ground floor of this little hotel houses one of Juneau's best restaurants. The dining room is furnished with mismatched antiques from the city's early days, and there's limited seating outdoors. Local fish is a specialty. Try the halibut in lemon garlic sauce, seafood gumbo, blackened meats and fish, and rich desserts. The wine list is extensive. *120 2nd St., tel. 907/586–4146. AE, D, MC, V. Moderate.*

The Fiddlehead. This is probably Juneau's favorite restaurant, a delightful place of light wood, softly patterned wallpaper, stained glass, hanging plants, and historic photos. Food is healthy, generously served, and *different.* How about a light dinner of black beans and rice? Or pasta Greta Garbo (locally smoked salmon tossed with fettuccine in cream sauce). The homemade bread is laudable. *429 W. Willoughby Ave., tel. 907/586–3150. Reservations advised. AE, D, MC, V. Inexpensive–Moderate.*

Ketchikan

Ketchikan sits at the base of 3,000-foot Deer Mountain. Until miners and fishermen settled here in the 1880s, the mouth of Ketchikan Creek was a summer fishing camp for Tlingit Indians. Today commercial and recreational fishing are still important to the area.

Ketchikan is Alaska's totem pole port: At the nearby Tlingit village of Saxman, 2½ miles south of downtown, there is a major totem park and residents still practice traditional carving techniques. The Ketchikan Visitors Bureau on the dock can supply information on getting to Saxman on your own, or you can take a ship-organized tour. Another outdoor totem display is at Totem Bight State Historical Park, a coastal rain forest 10 miles north of town.

Ketchikan is easy to explore, with walking-tour signs and lots of interesting places just a short stroll from the docks. It is also very wet—average annual precipitation is more than 150 inches.

Shore Excursions *Not all excursions are offered by all cruise lines. All times and prices are approximate. Unless otherwise noted, children's prices are for those 12 and under.*

Adventure **Misty Fjords Flightseeing:** Aerial views of granite cliffs rising 4,000 feet from the sea, waterfalls, rain forests, and wildlife. A landing on a high wilderness lake is the highlight. *1¹/₂–2¹/₂ hrs. Cost: $130–$144.*

Mountain Lake Canoeing: Paddle across a mountain lake in oversize canoes and see eagles roosting in the trees. Some tours include a guided nature hike and/or a snack of local foods, such as smoked salmon. Rubber boots, poncho, and life jacket are provided. *3–3¹/₂ hrs. Cost: $60–$67 adults, $38–$43 children.*

Cultural **Totem Bight Tour:** A look at Ketchikan's historical culture, focusing on Tlingit totem poles in Totem Bight State Historical Park. Guides interpret the myths and symbols in the traditional carvings. You'll also visit a salmon hatchery. *2¹/₂–3¹/₂ hrs. Cost: $22–$30 adults, $15 children.*

Scenic **Ketchikan Harbor & Fishing Industry:** A cruise around the harbor, viewing fishing boats and crews at work. A tour of a processing plant lets you sample various seafood products, which are for sale. Another similar excursion covers the same attractions on a walking tour. *1¹/₂–2 hrs. Cost: $40 adults, $20 children.*

Getting Around On the docks that line Front Street, near the Mission Street intersection, is the Ketchikan Visitors Bureau office, where brochures, maps (including a free historic-walking-tour map), and other information are available. Ketchikan is very manageable on foot.

By Taxi Metered taxis meet the ship right on the docks and also wait across the street. Rates are $2.10 for pick-up, 23¢ each ¹/₁₀ mile.

Exploring Ketchikan *Numbers in the margin correspond to numbered points of interest on the Ketchikan map.*

❶ From the **Ketchikan Visitors Bureau** on the dock, head up Mission Street, past the Trading Post and post office, and make a
❷ left on Bawden Street. On your left is **St. John's Church and Seamen's Center.** The 1903 church structure is the oldest house of worship in Ketchikan; its interior was formed from red cedar cut in the sawmill in Saxman. The Seamen's Center, next to the church, was built as a hospital in 1904.

❸ Turn right on Dock Street to reach the **Tongass Historical Museum and Totem Pole,** where you can learn about the early days of fishing and mining. *Dock and Bawden Sts. Admission: $1; free on Sun. Open May 15–Sept., daily 8–5.*

Continue north on Bawden, turn right onto Park Avenue, and
❹ see **Grant Street Trestle,** constructed in 1908. Virtually all of Ketchikan's walkways and streets were once wood trestles, but only this one remains. Get out your camera and set it for fast
❺ speed at the **Salmon Falls** and **Fish Ladder** just off Park Avenue. When the salmon start running in midsummer, thousands of fish literally leap the falls (or take the easier ladder) to spawn
❻ in Ketchikan Creek upstream. At **City Park** you can see small ponds that were once holding areas for the area's first hatchery
❼ that ran from 1923 to 1928. The modern **Deer Mountain Hatchery** now disperses tens of thousands of salmon annually
❽ into local waters. Also at the park is the **Totem Heritage Center and Nature Path,** where you can view authentic examples of carvers' art. *Admission: $2; free on Sun. Open May 15–Sept., daily 8–5.*

Continuing south on Deermont Street, then turning left onto
❾ Stedman Street, you pass a colorful wall mural called ***Return***

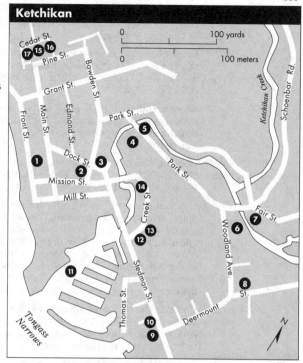

Ketchikan

of the Eagle. It was created by 25 Native American artists on the walls of the Robertson Building of the Ketchikan campus, University of Alaska–Southeast. Sharing space with the university is the **Ketchikan Indian Corporation,** site of a former Bureau of Indian Affairs school.

Next comes Thomas Street, built in 1913 as part of the New England Fish Company cannery, and **Thomas Basin.** One of four harbors in Ketchikan, the basin is home to a wide variety of pleasure and fishing boats.

Return to Stedman Street and head north to **Creek Street,** formerly Ketchikan's infamous red-light district. Today, its small houses, built on stilts over the creek, have been restored as trendy shops. The street's most famous brothel, **Dolly's House** (admission $2.50), has been preserved as a museum, complete with furnishings and a short history of the life and times of Ketchikan's best-known madam. There's more good salmon viewing in season at the **Creek Street Footbridge.**

If you're into steep street climbing, head left on Mission Street, then right up Main Street past the fire department to the **Kyan Totem Pole,** a replica of an 1880s original that once stood near St. John's Church. Nearby is **Monrean House,** a 1904 structure on the National Register of Historic Places, and a **scenic lookout** onto City Float boat basin and the waters of Tongass Narrows.

Shopping The **Saxman Village** gift shop has some superb handcrafted Tlingit merchandise, along with cheaper mass-produced souvenirs. Because artists are local, prices for Native American crafts are better here than at any other ports, and comparable to those in the interior.

Creek Street has several attractive boutiques with a variety of merchandise. At **Parnassus Bookstore** (28 Creek St., tel. 907/225–7690), coffee and pastries are served amid an eclectic collection of books.

Scanlon Gallery (310 Mission St., tel. 907/225–4730) handles not only major Alaskan artists and local talent, but also traditional and contemporary native art, soapstone, bronze, and walrus ivory.

Sports
Fishing

Contact **Chinook Charters** (428 Tower Rd., Ketchikan, tel. 907/225–9225) or **Tchaika Fishing Guide Service** (Box 1197, Ward Cove, tel. 907/247–8526).

Hiking

Check at the tourist information building on the dock for trail maps, advice, and information. If you're a tough hiker with sturdy shoes, the 3-mile trail from downtown (starting at the end of Fair Street) to the top of **Deer Mountain** will repay your effort with a spectacular panorama of the city below and the wilderness behind. **Ward Cove** recreation area, about 6 miles north of town, offers easier hiking along lakes and streams and beneath towering spruce and hemlock trees.

Kayaking and
Canoeing

Contact **Alaska Travel Adventures** (9085 Glacier Highway S, Juneau, tel. 907/789–0052) for a Native American canoe excursion on Connel Lake north of town; smoked fish and other native delights are part of the experience.

The **Ketchikan Parks and Recreation Department** (360 Main St., tel. 907/228–6650) rents canoes. **Southeast Exposure** (507 Stedman St., tel. 907/225–8829) offers kayak rentals, instruction, and tours.

Dining

Annabelle's Keg and Chowder House. Located in Gillmore's Hotel, this popular seafood restaurant takes you back to the '20s. The walls are covered with photos and paintings depicting the Ketchikan of years past. Specials include smoked salmon and clams on the half-shell. *326 Front St., tel. 907/225–6009. AE, D, DC, MC, V. Moderate–Expensive.*

Seward

On the southeastern coast of the Kenai Peninsula, Seward is surrounded by four major federal land holdings—**Chugach National Forest, Kenai Wildlife Refuge, Kenai Fjords National Park,** and the **Alaska Maritime National Refuge.** The entire area is breathtaking, and you should not miss it in your haste to get to Anchorage.

Seward was founded in 1903, at the time that planning for the railroad to Alaska's interior began. The tidal wave that followed the 1964 earthquake devastated the town, but fortunately, most residents saw the harbor drain almost entirely, knew the wave would follow, and ran to high ground. Since then the town has relied heavily on commercial fishing, and its harbor is important for shipping coal to the Orient.

If you're in Seward on the Fourth of July, stick around for the insane Mt. Marathon foot race, 3,000 feet straight uphill from downtown.

Shore Excursions *Not all excursions are offered by all cruise lines. All times and prices are approximate. Unless otherwise noted, children's prices are for those 12 and under.*

Aerial Tour **Mt. McKinley Flightseeing:** From Anchorage, fly to Denali National Park (filled with bears, wolves, caribou, and moose) to see North America's highest peak. The trip is often canceled due to cloudiness. *1¹/₂ hrs. Cost: $280.*

Adventure **Kenai Flightseeing:** A bush plane flight over the Harding Ice Field and through the Kenai fjords provides views of calving glaciers. *1¹/₂ hrs. Cost: $112.*

Fishing for Salmon and Halibut: Sail 40 miles outside Seward in search of fish weighing up to 250 pounds each. Tackle and bait included, licenses and butchering available. Maximum six participants. *8 hrs. Cost: $125.*

Cultural **Anchorage Overland Tour:** Part of this all-day bus trip runs along beautiful Turnagain Arm to Anchorage, where there's a brief orientation tour, then free time. This is a long journey to what most passengers consider an uninspiring city. *8 hrs. Cost: $85 adults, $43 children.*

Scenic **Kenai Fjords Lunch Cruise:** Narrated tour of Resurrection Bay aboard heated 100-foot vessel. All-you-can-eat seafood buffet. *3¹/₂–4 hrs. Cost: $65.*

Portage Glacier and the Kenai Mountains by Motorcoach: The drive along Turnagain Arm to Portage Glacier is one of Alaska's most beautiful. *5¹/₂ hrs. Cost: $65 adults, $33 children.*

Seward, Exit Glacier, and Sled Dog Demonstration: National park rangers provide information on the glacier and fjords that form part of the Kenai Fjords National Park. Passengers can walk right up to Exit Glacier. A stop at an Alaskan sled-dog training center follows. *3 hrs. Cost: $30 adults, $15 children.*

Getting Around Cruise ships dock within a half-mile of downtown. Turn left as you leave the ship. The **Kenai Fjords National Park visitor center** (tel. 907/224–3175) is within walking distance: Turn left as you leave the pier, left again onto 4th Avenue, and the center is two blocks ahead. The **Chugach National Forest Ranger District Information Center** (tel. 907/224–3374) is at 334 4th Avenue.

By Bus Public bus routes include stops timed to meet ships.

By Taxi Call a taxi from the pay phones at the dock (tel. 907/224–5000, $1.50 pick-up, $1.25 per mile; or tel. 907/224–5555, $2 point-to-point in town, 75¢ each additional mile).

Exploring Seward Seward offers little to compare with the splendors of its surroundings. Most passengers either head into Anchorage or explore the federal parks of the Kenai Peninsula. Don't miss the fjords in **Resurrection Bay,** with their bird rookeries and sea-lion colonies.

Shopping **The Alaska Shop** (210 4th Ave., tel. 907/224–5420) has a variety of merchandise, including gifts, books, magazines, and a mini grocery store. **The Treasure Chest** (Small Boat Harbor, tel. 907/224–8087) specializes in hand-painted and unusual T-shirts. **Bardarson Studio** (Small Boat Harbor, tel. 907/224–5448) has local Alaskan art—originals and reproductions—as well as imported goods.

Sports The Seward Jackpot Halibut Tournament runs through July,
Fishing and the Seward Silver Salmon Derby is in August. For fishing,
sightseeing, and drop-off/pick-up tours, contact **Fish House**
(Box 1209, Seward 99664, tel. 800/257–7760 or 800/478–8007 in
AK), Seward's oldest operator; **Kenai Fjords Tours** (Box 1889,
Seward 99664, tel. 907/224–8068), which has four charter boats
for sightseeing; and **Mariah Charters** (3812 Katmai Circle, An-
chorage 99517, tel. 907/224–8623 or 907/243–1238).

Hiking The Mt. Marathon trail starts at the west end of Lowell Street,
but it's practically straight uphill. Few areas in the world are
as rich in hiking possibilities as the **Kenai Peninsula.** The hard
part is getting there from the ship. One way is to go with a tour
group specializing in hiking. **Alaska Treks-n-Voyages** (Small
Boat Harbor, tel. 907/224–3960) can arrange hiking and glacier
treks, as well as kayak tours and rentals.

Dining **Harbor Dinner Club & Lounge.** The halibut is great at this little
house downtown, set back from the street. Try a halibut burger
with homemade french fries. *5th Ave., tel. 907/224–3012. MC, V.
Inexpensive–Moderate.*

Sitka

For centuries before the 18th-century arrival of the Russians,
Sitka was the home of the Tlingit nation. But Sitka's beauty,
mild climate, and economic potential caught the attention of
outsiders. Russian Territorial Governor Alexander Baranof
saw in the island's massive timbered forests raw materials for
shipbuilding, and its location suited trading routes to California, Hawaii, and the Orient. In 1799 Baranof established an
outpost that he called Redoubt St. Michael, 6 miles north of the
present town, and moved a large number of his Russian and
Aleut fur hunters there from their former base on Kodiak Island.

Though the Tlingits attacked Baranof's people and burned his
buildings in 1802, Baranof returned in 1804 with a formidable
force, including shipboard cannons. He attacked the Tlingits
at their fort near Indian River (site of the present-day 105-acre
Sitka National Historical Park) and drove them to the other
side of the island. Eventually, the capital of Russian America
was shifted to Sitka from Kodiak.

Under Baranof and succeeding managers, the Russian-American Company and the town prospered, becoming known as "the
Paris of the Pacific." Besides the fur trade, the community
boasted a major shipbuilding and repair facility, sawmills,
forges, and a salmon saltery, and even initiated an ice industry.

Shore Excursions *Not all excursions are offered by all cruise lines. All times and
prices are approximate. Unless otherwise noted, children's
prices are for those 12 and under.*

Adventure **Yacht and Raft Adventure:** A yacht takes you around Sitka's
islands, offering good views of whales, porpoises, and sea lions.
After transferring to motorized rafts, passengers get a closer
look at St. Lazaria National Bird and Wildlife Sanctuary. *3¹/₂–4
hrs. Cost: $80–$93 adults, $50–$57 children. Minimum age is 4.*

Cultural **Sitka Drive:** A tour of Sitka stops at the Sheldon Jackson Museum, Castle Hill, Centennial Hall, and St. Michael's Cathedral. Some tours include a performance by the New Archangel

Russian Dancers. *2¹/₂–3¹/₂ hrs Cost: $24–$36 adults, $13–$18 children.*

Nature **Eagle Hospital:** Visit the Alaska Raptor Rehabilitation Center, where injured birds of prey are nursed back to health. *1¹/₂–2 hrs. Cost: $20–$23 adults, $10.75 children. Minimum age is 6.*

Getting Around You'll come ashore near the Centennial Building, with its big Tlingit war canoe. Inside is the Sitka Visitors Bureau (tel. 907/747–5940), plus a small museum and the auditorium where the New Archangel Dancers perform. Pick up maps, brochures, and information here. In Sitka, good walkers can stretch their sea legs and see everything any guided tour of the city will offer.

By Taxi Taxis meet the cruise ships, but if none is around, call 907/747–8888 or 907/747–5001. A ride downtown costs about $2.50. A 30-minute taxi tour costs $20 per carload, an hour tour costs $44. Pay phones are in the Centennial Building and across the way in the Bayview Trading Company.

Exploring Sitka *Numbers in the margin correspond to numbered points of interest on the Sitka map.*

❶ Begin at the Sitka Visitors Bureau, in the **Centennial Building**
❷ (*see above*). To get a feel for the town, head for **Castle Hill,** which overlooks Crescent Bay, the John O'Connell Bridge to Japonski Island, and a profusion of other islands and rocks. A path and steps beside the post office take you to the top. A succession of residences for Russian managers was located on this lofty promontory. The last one, Baranof's Castle, burned in 1894. Atop the hill are old Russian cannons and the flagpole where, on October 18, 1867, the czarist Russian standard was lowered and the Stars and Stripes raised. Here also the first 49-star U.S. flag was flown on January 3, 1959, signifying Alaska's statehood.

❸ The large four-story, red-roofed structure with the imposing 14-foot statue in front is the **Sitka State Pioneers' Home,** built in 1934 as the first of several state-run retirement homes and medical-care facilities. The statue, symbolizing Alaska's frontier sourdough (as the locals are nicknamed) spirit, was modeled after an authentic pioneer, William "Skagway Bill" Fonda. It portrays a determined prospector with pack, pick, rifle, and supplies, headed for gold country.

Across the street in **Totem Square** are three old anchors found in local waters and believed to be from 19th-century British ships. Notice the double-headed eagle of czarist Russia on the park's totem pole.

❹ **St. Michael's Cathedral,** on Lincoln Street, had its origins in a frame-covered log structure built in the 1840s. In 1966 the church burned in a fire that swept through the business district. Using original blueprints, an almost-exact replica of St. Michael's was built and dedicated in 1976. *Tel. 907/747–8120. $1 donation requested. Open daily 9–3.*

❺ ❻ Near the Pioneers' Home on either side of Marine Street is a replica of an old **Russian blockhouse** and the **Russian cemetery.** The old headstones and crosses of the Russian Orthodox faith make this a striking sight.

❼ The **Russian Bishop's House** also stands on Lincoln Street. Constructed by the Russian-American Company for Bishop

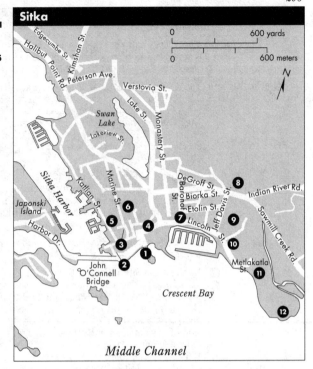

Innocent Veniaminov in 1842 and restored as a unit of Sitka National Historical Park, this is one of the few remaining Russian log homes in Alaska. *Admission free. Open daily 8–5.*

❽ Farther north and east, on Sawmill Creek Road, is the **Sitka National Cemetery,** where Civil War and World War II dead are buried alongside many other notable Alaskans.

Return to Lincoln Street and head southeast, keeping the cathedral to your back and the water to your right. A 15- to 20-
❾ minute walk will lead you to the campus of **Sheldon Jackson College,** founded in 1878.

❿ On campus, the octagonal **Sheldon Jackson Museum,** built in 1895, contains priceless Native American items collected by Dr. Sheldon Jackson in the remote regions of Alaska. Carved masks, Chilkat Indian blankets, dogsleds, kayaks—even the helmet worn by Chief Katlean during the 1804 battle between the Sitka Tlingits and the Russians—are displayed here. Allow an hour at the museum. *Tel. 907/747–8981. Admission: $2 adults. Open daily 8–5.*

⓫ **Sitka National Historical Park's visitor center** is a short walk farther along Lincoln Street. Audiovisual programs and exhibits including Native American and Russian artifacts give an overview of southeast Alaskan cultures, both old and new. Native American artists and craftspeople are on hand to demonstrate and interpret traditional crafts of the Tlingit people. A self-guiding trail (maps available at the visitor center) to the
⓬ site of the **Tlingit Fort** passes by some of the most skillfully carved totem poles in the state; some of the 15 poles date back

more than eight decades. *Tel. 907/747–6281. Admission free. Open daily 8–5.*

Shopping Shopping in Sitka is limited, though the town has its share of souvenir shops. Other ports offer a better selection of merchandise.

At the **Sitka National Historical Park Visitor Center,** you can purchase interesting booklets on interpreting totem poles and other Tlingit art. A few stores, such as the **Russian-American Company** (407 Lincoln St., tel. 907/747–6228) and the **New Archangel Trading Co.** (335 Harbor Dr., across from the Centennial Building, tel. 907/747–8181), sell Russian items, including the popular *matruchka* nesting dolls.

Sports Fishing is excellent here, and this is a good port from which to *Fishing* set off on a charter. Contact **Steller Charters** (2810 Sawmill Creek Rd., Sitka 99835, tel. 907/747–6711). See the information desk in the Centennial Building for a list of other charter operators.

Hiking Hiking in the area is very civilized. From the Centennial Building, turn right onto Harbor Drive, then right again onto Lincoln Street for **Sitka National Historical Park**'s well-marked trails, which rival those at Ketchikan for drama. Even inexperienced hikers enjoy the stroll through the glades, along the coast, across Indian River, to Tlingit Fort.

Kayaking **Baidarka Boats** (201 Lincoln St., Room 201, Sitka, tel. 907/747–8996) rents sea kayaks and offers guided trips in the island-strewn waters around Sitka.

Dining **Channel Club.** This is Sitka's best gourmet restaurant—a five-time winner of the Silver Spoon award from the Gourmet Club of America. Halibut cheeks are a favorite, and the recipe for the steak's delicious seasoning is a closely held secret. Decor is nautical, with glass fishing balls, whale baleen, and Alaska pictures on the walls. *Mile 3.5 on Halibut Point Rd., tel. 907/747–9916. AE, DC, MC, V. Moderate–Expensive.*

Skagway

The early gold-rush days of Alaska, when dreamers and hooligans descended on the Yukon via the murderous White Pass, are preserved in Skagway. Now a part of the Klondike Gold Rush National Historical Park, downtown Skagway was once the picturesque but violent gateway for the frenzied stampede to the interior gold fields.

Local park rangers and residents now interpret and re-create that remarkable era for visitors. Old false-front stores, saloons, brothels, and wood sidewalks have been completely restored. You'll be regaled with tall tales of con artists, golden-hearted "ladies," stampeders, and newsmen. Such colorful characters as outlaw Jefferson "Soapy" Smith and his gang earned the town a reputation so bad that, by the spring of 1898, the superintendent of the Northwest Royal Mounted Police had labeled Skagway "little better than a hell on earth." But Soapy was killed in a duel with surveyor Frank Reid, and soon a civilizing influence, in the form of churches and family life, prevailed. When the gold played out just a few years later, the town of 20,000 dwindled to its current population of 700.

Shore Excursions *Not all excursions are offered by all cruise lines. All times and prices are approximate. Unless otherwise noted, children's prices are for those 12 and under.*

Aerial Tours **Chilkat Bald Eagles Preserve Flightseeing and Float Trip:** Glide over ice fields and Glacier Bay on a one-hour flight, then land in Haines. The tour continues with a float trip through Eagle Preserve, which boasts the world's largest concentration of bald eagles. *5¹/₂ hrs. Cost: $185–$197. Minimum age: 7.*

Gold Rush Helicopter Tour: Fly over the Chilkoot Gold Rush Trail into a remote mountain valley for a landing on a glacier. Special boots are provided for walking on the glacier. *1¹/₂ hrs Cost: $130–$140.*

Cultural **City and Historical Tour:** A drive, accompanied by historical narrative, wends through town to the Gold Rush Cemetery and Reid Falls. The Skagway Streetcar Company conducts this tour in vintage 1930s limos. *2 hrs. Cost: $36 adults, $18 children.*

Madam Jan's Gold-Panning Camp: Restored gold-rush community at the foot of the White Pass trail. Pan for gold and keep what you find. *2¹/₂ hrs. Cost: $38 adults, $19 children.*

Entertainment **Days of '98 Revue:** Dance-hall girls, play-money gambling, and a historic melodrama about gold-rush Skagway. Usually combined with an excursion to the White Pass summit, a gold-panning camp, or a city tour. *2¹/₂–3¹/₂ hrs Cost: $32–$50 adults, $21–$24 children.*

Scenic **Carcross Excursion:** A bus tour takes you along the Klondike Highway into Canada, past mountains, lakes, and canyons. A stop in Carcross, Yukon, includes a lunch of Yukon stew, sourdough rolls, and hot coffee, followed by a museum visit. *5–6 hrs. Cost: $70 adults, $35 children.*

Burro Creek Homestead: Cruise the historic Skagway waterfront to a family-run hatchery set in a modern-day, log-cabin homestead. Also view the famed White and Chilkoot passes, plus the gold-rush ghost town of Dyea. *2¹/₂–3 hrs. Cost: $60 adults, $22–$30 children.*

White Pass and Yukon Railroad: The 20-mile trip in vintage railroad cars, on narrow-gauge tracks built to serve the Yukon gold fields, runs past the infamous White Pass, skims along the edge of granite cliffs, crosses a 215-foot-high steel cantilever bridge over Dead Horse Gulch, climbs to a 2,865-foot elevation at White Pass Summit, and zigzags through dramatic scenery—including the actual Trail of '98, worn into the mountainside a century ago. A must for railroad buffs; great for children. *3 hrs. Cost: $72–$78 adults, $36–$39 children.*

Getting Around The cruise-ship docks are a short stroll from the beginning of Broadway and downtown Skagway. Since Broadway is the main road, and the only artery that concerns most tourists, you don't need a taxi. Horse-drawn surreys, antique buses, and modern vans leave from the pier for tours, or you can walk the half-block to downtown, where you can pick up a tour later.

Exploring Skagway *Numbers in the margin correspond to numbered points of interest on the Skagway map.*

Skagway is perhaps the most manageable port in Alaska for exploring by foot. Just walk up and down Broadway, detouring here and there into the side streets.

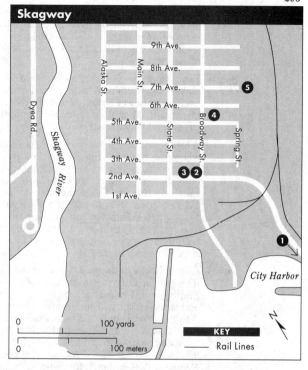

Arctic Brotherhood
Hall, **2**
Cruise ship dock, **1**
Eagles Hall, **4**
Soapy's Parlor, **3**
Trail of '98 Museum, **5**

❶ From the **cruise ship dock** you can see the large yellow-and-red
White Pass & Yukon Railroad Depot, now the **National Park
Service Visitor Center** (tel. 907/983–2921). This should be your
first stop: View an excellent photographic exhibit and superb
documentary films, pick up a free map, or ask the rangers for
information on safe and interesting hiking trails.

Across the street is a robust and friendly bar, the **Red Onion
Saloon,** where a lady-of-the-evening mannequin peers down
from the former second-floor brothel. A couple of doors up is
❷ the **Arctic Brotherhood Hall,** with its curious driftwood-mosaic
facade. Around the corner is a tiny, almost inconsequential
❸ shack that was **Soapy's Parlor,** but it is rarely open to tourists.

You'll find down-home sourdough cooking at the **Golden North
Hotel** and a rip-roaring revue, "Skagway in the Days of '98," at
❹ the **Eagles Hall.** Keep an eye out for the humorous architectural details and advertising irreverence that mark the Skagway spirit.

Turn right onto 7th Avenue and walk about two blocks to City
❺ Hall, where the **Trail of '98 Museum** is located. Here you will
find interesting facts about the real lives of the people who settled here at the turn of the century.

Shopping Broadway is filled with somewhat overpriced curio shops, although some merchandise is unusual. **David Present's Gallery**
(tel. 907/983–2873) has outstanding but pricey art by Alaskan
artists. **Dedman's Photo Shop** (tel. 907/983–2353) has been a
Skagway institution since the early days; here you'll find un-

usual historical photos, guidebooks, and old-fashioned newspapers. **Kirmse's** (tel. 907/983–2822) has a large selection of expensive, inexpensive, and downright tacky souvenirs. On display is the world's largest, heaviest, and most valuable gold-nugget watch chain.

Sports Real wilderness is within a stone's throw of the docks, which
Hiking makes this an excellent hiking port. Try the short jaunt to beautiful **Upper Dewey Lake**. Start at the corner of 4th and Spring, go toward the mountain, cross the footbridge over Pullen Creek, and follow the trail.

A less strenuous hike is the trip through **Gold Rush Cemetery**, where the epitaphs offer strange but lively bits of social commentary. To get there, keep walking up Broadway, turn left onto 8th Avenue, then right onto State Street. Go through the railroad yards and follow the signs to the cemetery, which is 1½ miles, or a 30- to 45-minute walk, from town. To reach 300-foot-high **Reid Falls**, continue through the cemetery for ¼ mile. The National Park Service Center (tel. 907/983–2921) offers trail maps, advice, and the helpful brochure *Skagway Gold Rush Cemetery Guide*.

Dining **Golden North Restaurant.** To eat in the Golden North Hotel's dining room is to return to the days of gold-rush con man Soapy Smith, heroic Frank Reid, and scores of pioneers, stampeders, and dance-hall girls. The decor is authentic and has been tastefully restored. Popular choices include sourdough pancakes for breakfast; soup, salad bar, and sandwiches for lunch; salmon or other seafood for dinner. *3rd Ave. and Broadway, tel. 907/983–2294. AE, MC, V. Inexpensive–Moderate.*
Prospector's Sourdough Restaurant. "Sourdough" is the nickname for locals, who often outnumber the tourists here. Breakfast specialties are hotcakes and snow-crab omelets. *4th Ave. and Broadway, tel. 907/983–2865. AE, DC, MC, V. Inexpensive.*

Victoria, British Columbia

Though Victoria is not in Alaska, it is a port of call for several Alaskan cruises. Rudyard Kipling described Victoria as comprising the best of Bournemouth (a British seaside resort) arranged "around the Bay of Naples." Today the city is a mix of stately buildings and tourist tack. Flower baskets hang from lampposts, shops sell Harris tweed and Irish linen, locals play cricket and croquet, and visitors sightsee aboard red double-decker buses or horse-drawn carriages.

Shore Excursions *Not all excursions are offered by all cruise lines. All times and prices are approximate. Unless otherwise noted, children's prices are for those 12 and under.*

Cultural **City Drive and Craigdarrock Castle:** Drive through residential areas and tour of the castle. *2½ hrs. Cost: $16 adults, $8 children.*

Grand City Drive and Afternoon High Tea: A drive through downtown, past Craigdarrock castle and residential areas, finishing with a British-style high tea at a hotel. *2½ hrs. Cost: $25 adults, $20 children.*

Short City Tour and Butchart Gardens: Drive through key places of interest, like the city center and residential areas, on the way to Butchart Gardens—a must for garden aficionados. *3¹/2 hrs. Cost: $28 adults, $14 children.*

Getting Around Cruise ships dock at Odgen Point, about seven minutes by taxi from the Inner Harbour. Metered taxis meet the ship. Rates are $2.15 for pick-up, $1.30 per kilometer (Canadian dollars). The tourist-information office is at 812 Wharf Street (tel. 604/382–2127), in front of the Empress Hotel, in the middle of the Inner Harbour.

Most points of interest are within walking distance of the Empress. For those that aren't, the public bus system is excellent. Pick up route maps and schedules at the tourist information office.

Exploring Victoria, British Columbia *Numbers in the margin correspond to numbered points of interest on the Inner Harbour, Victoria, map.*

Victoria's heart is the **Inner Harbour,** always bustling with ferries, seaplanes, and yachts from all over the world. The ivy-covered **Empress Hotel** (721 Government St., tel. 604/384–8111), with its well-groomed gardens, is the dowager of Victoria. High tea in this little patch of England is a local ritual: Recline in deep armchairs and nibble on scones or crumpets with honey, butter, jam, and clotted cream while sipping blended tea.

❷ The **Crystal Gardens,** across Douglas Street from the hotel, were built in 1925 under a glass roof as a public saltwater swimming pool. They have been renovated into a tropical conservatory and aviary, with flamingos, parrots, fountains, and waterfalls. Tea is on from 2 to 5 under garden umbrellas on the Upper Terrace overlooking the lush, indoor jungle.

❸ Nearby **Thunderbird Park** claims the world's finest collection of colorful totem poles and a ceremonial longhouse (a communal dwelling).

❹ Next to the park is **Helmcken House,** the province's oldest residence, which has a display of antique medical instruments. *10 Elliot St. Sq., tel. 604/387–4697. Admission: $3.25 adults, $2.25 senior citizens, $1.25 children 6–12. Open Thurs.–Mon. 11–5.*

❺ Next door is the superb **Royal British Columbia Museum.** Plan to spend at least an hour there. *675 Belleville St., tel. 604/387–3014. Admission: $5 adults, $3 senior citizens and children 13–18, $2 children 6–12. Open daily 10–5:30.*

❻ Across Government Street are the stately, neo-Gothic **British Columbia Parliament Buildings,** constructed of local stone and wood and opened in 1898. At night the harbor is brilliantly lit with thousands of electric lights, like a fairy-tale castle.

❼ Down Government Street a short way is the **Emily Carr House,** the beautifully restored residence of the famous early 20th-century painter. Prints by Carr, who was a member of the "Canadian Group of Seven," adorn the walls. *207 Government St., tel. 604/387–4697. Admission: $3.25 adults, $2.25 senior citizens, $1.25 children 6–12. Open Thurs.–Mon. 11–5.*

❽ The **Pacific Underseas Gardens,** beside the Blackball Ferry terminal, is a natural aquarium with more than 5,000 species from the area. You actually descend beneath the water for a live scuba show with Armstrong, the Pacific octopus. *490 Belleville St., opposite Parliament Bldgs., tel. 604/382–5717. Admission:*

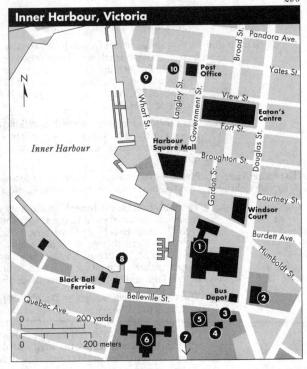

Bastion Square, **9**

British Columbia
Parliament
Buildings, **6**

Crystal Gardens, **2**

Emily Carr House, **7**

Empress Hotel, **1**

Helmcken House, **4**

Maritime Museum
of B.C., **10**

Pacific Underseas
Gardens, **8**

Royal British
Columbia Museum, **5**

Thunderbird Park, **3**

Inner Harbour, Victoria

Pandora Ave.

Broad St.

Yates St.

Post Office

View St.

Eaton's Centre

Fort St.

Wharf St.

Langley St.

Government St.

Inner Harbour

Harbour Square Mall

Broughton St.

Douglas St.

Gordon St.

Courtney St.

Windsor Court

Burdett Ave.

Humboldt St.

Black Ball Ferries

Belleville St.

Bus Depot

Quebec Ave.

0   200 yards

0   200 meters

$6 adults, $5.50 senior citizens, $4.50 children 12–17, $2.75 children under 12. Open 9–9.

Just a short walk from the Inner Harbour is **Bastion Square,**
off Government Street between Yates and Fort streets, at the
foot of View Street. Established in 1843 as the original site of
Ft. Victoria, it now boasts several restored buildings open for
viewing. The old courthouse is now the **Maritime Museum of
B.C.** It has a collection of maritime artifacts—including a 38-
foot Indian dugout canoe and the 20-foot ketch *Trekka,* which
has sailed around the world—as well as a Captain Cook gallery.
*28 Bastion Sq., tel. 604/385–4222. Admission: $5 adults, $3 chil-
dren 12–17, $2 children 6–11. Open daily 9–6:30.*

Take a taxi or drive to **Butchart Gardens.** These 35 acres in a
city of gardens rank among the most beautiful gardens in the
world. *14 mi north of Victoria on Hwy. 17, tel. 604/652–5256.
Admission: $3 adults, $2 children 13–17, $1 children 5–12.*

Shopping Save your receipts to receive a VAT tax refund from the Canadian government when you leave Canada; ask for a form at
customs. Victoria stores specializing in English imports are
plentiful, though Canadian-made goods are usually a better
buy for foreigners. Look for Hudson's Bay Co. blankets and
other woolens. From the Empress Hotel walk along Government Street to reach **George Straith Ltd., Piccadilly Shoppe
British Woolens,** and **Sasquach Trading Company,** all of which
sell high-quality woolen clothing.

Turn right onto Fort Street and walk 4 blocks to **Antique Row,** between Blanchard and Cook streets. **The Connoisseurs Shop** and **David Robinson, Ltd.** offer a wide variety of 18th-century pieces.

Dining   **Bengal Lounge.** Buffet lunches in the elegant Empress Hotel include curries with extensive condiment trays of coconuts, nuts, cool *raita* (yogurt with mint or cucumber), and chutney. Popular with cabinet ministers and bureaucrats, the Bengal Lounge offers splendid garden views. *721 Government St., tel. 604/384–8111. AE, D, DC, MC, V. Moderate.*

La Ville d'Is. This cozy and friendly seafood house, run by Brittany native Michel Duteau, is one of the best bargains in Victoria. Although seafood, like *perche de la Nouvelle Aelande* (orange roughie in Muscadet with herbs), is the chef's strong suit, rabbit, lamb, and beef tenderloin are also available. The wine list is limited but imaginative. On warm days there's seating outside. *26 Bastion Sq., tel. 604/388–9414. Reservations advised. AE, MC, V. Lunch 11:30–2 Mon.–Sat., dinner 5:30–10 Mon.–Sat. Closed Sun. Moderate.*

Whittier

Whittier, on the east coast of the Kenai Peninsula, is the main access port connecting Prince William Sound to south-central Alaska. It was built in World War II as a military port—chosen because its ubiquitous cloud cover provided safety from air raids. On sunny days Whittier is gorgeous, but these are rare.

Ships and state ferries call at Passage Canal, across from the Kittiwake rookery and next to the small boat harbor. Upon arrival, cruise ship passengers in buses are loaded directly onto Alaska Railroad trains for the short ride to Portage, where the railroad meets the Seward Highway. It's another 50 miles to Anchorage along Turnagain Arm, named by Captain James Cook for its huge tides, which forced him back in his search for a northwest passage. Look for beluga whales in the inlet and Dall sheep on the rocks above the road just past the little Native American settlement. The drive along Turnagain Arm is one of the most beautiful in the world.

Those who remain in Whittier for the day will find a few blocks of warehouses, a railway, and a marina, smack in the middle of breathtaking Prince William Sound.

Shore Excursions   *Not all excursions are offered by all cruise lines. All times and prices are approximate. Unless otherwise noted, children's prices are for those 12 and under.*

Cultural   **Anchorage City Tour:** After a constricting ride in a bus loaded onto a freight train, passengers stay in the bus to see a typical western American city. The native Alaskan displays at the Anchorage Museum of History and Art make the trip worthwhile. *3¹/₂ hrs Cost: $23 adults, $11.50 children.*

Scenic   **College Glaciers Catamaran:** See 26 glaciers in Prince William Sound, where whales and other wildlife can often be spotted. Exquisite scenery makes this the best tour from Whittier. *6 hrs. Cost: $119.*

Antarctica

Antarctica is bigger than the continental United States, drier than the Sahara, colder than Siberia, and less populated than the Arabian Empty Quarter. Of all the fresh water in the world, 60% is locked in Antarctica's ice, which in places is more than 10 times thicker than the Empire State Building is tall.

First visited by only a handful of hearty whalers and intrepid explorers, Antarctica has been almost exclusively the domain of research scientists. Its purity and distance from civilization make it an ideal laboratory in which to study many problems that plague the rest of the planet.

In the late 1950s, a small company that specialized in adventure vacations began offering cruises to Antarctica. Although only a few ships followed over the next quarter-century, a sudden surge of interest in travel to Antarctica recently has produced a flood of inquiries and bookings. This year at least six ships will be steaming south during the brief austral summer, carrying an estimated 8,000 passengers.

Cruising to Antarctica requires a certain temperament and a moderate level of physical fitness. It involves a small degree of inconvenience, discomfort, and even risk. Because there are no tenders, landing wharfs, or tour buses on the continent, getting from the ship to land means bundling up in bulky jackets and life preservers, climbing into small rubberized boats called Zodiacs, maneuvering in as close to the shore as possible, and, quite often, wading through the shallow surf. Then the only way to get inland to the research stations or penguin rookeries is by walking, sometimes miles, up rocky beaches or uneven ice surfaces. While all ships carry doctors and nurses, the nearest hospital is several thousand miles away.

Since the weather conditions in Antarctica are so unpredictable, itineraries are extremely flexible and more than usually subject to last-minute changes. Heavy seas may prevent your ship from landing at a particular research station, and floating ice may cut a half-day tour into an hour stop. So, regardless of what the brochures promise, about the only certainties are the dates you will start and complete your cruise.

Catching your ship entails flying great distances to ports in either South America, New Zealand, or Australia. Flights are expensive and often arduous; it can take more than 24 hours to get to your initial departure point. For a cruise to the Antarctic Peninsula, you must fly first to either Santiago, Chile, or Buenos Aires, Argentina, and you'll usually be put up in a hotel overnight. To save you money, some cruise companies book charters or flights from Miami on relatively unknown airlines. If given a choice, spend the extra couple hundred dollars and opt for a scheduled flight on **Varig, Lan Chile, Aerolinas Argentinas,** or another major carrier; some smaller carriers give poor service or fail to leave on time. The day after your initial flight, you'll be chartered to a small airport in Tierra del Fuego, and then bused three to five hours to your final destination. The charters used to fly directly to the ships, but since a 1991 plane crash in Puerto Williams, most cruise companies have chosen safety over convenience. If your cruise leaves from Christchurch, New Zealand, or Hobart in Tasmania, Australia, you probably won't run into this problem.

When to Go Cruise ships visit Antarctica only from early December to mid-February—the austral summer. The best time is between mid-December and mid-January, when the weather is mildest and the wildlife most active.

What to Bring Packing for Antarctica is quite different from preparing for any other cruise. Forget about elegance and formality, although you may wish to take a sports jacket and tie or a simple all-purpose dress for the captain's informal get-together.

The most common mistake in packing for an Antarctic cruise is bringing gear designed for sub-zero temperatures. While it gets as cold as –100°F in the dead of winter (July and August), the median coastal temperatures in December and January average 35°F–55°F. The cruise lines supply recommended packing lists, as well as a bulky red parka that will provide your primary protection. Waterproof pullover pants and waterproof boots at least 12 inches high are necessities. You'll also want a good pair of binoculars, a 35mm camera with telephoto and wide-angle lenses, and lots of color film—remember, it's illegal to take a single stone, bone, feather, or artifact as a souvenir.

It's a nice idea to bring small gifts for the scientists and other workers in the research stations: recent magazines, books, candy, and fresh fruit. Iron-on fabric patches from your home town or travels are also appreciated.

Currency Since there are practically no stores or shops in Antarctica, you won't need much money there. Some of the research stations sell sweatshirts and T-shirts with Antarctica logos, decorative patches that can be sewn or ironed onto your parka, and postcards with Antarctic postmarks that you can mail to friends or relatives (the mail goes out with your ship and can take days, weeks, or months to be delivered). You can pay for these in U.S. dollars. In some places the merchandise is available only to station personnel, who will sometimes barter with you for books, magazines, and patches.

Passports and Visas No one visiting or living in Antarctica needs any kind of documents, but to get there, you will have to fly through Argentina, Chile, Australia, or New Zealand, all of which require passports and visas from U.S., Canadian, and British citizens.

Shore Excursions *Not all excursions are offered by all cruise lines. All times and prices are approximate.*

The only stops in Antarctica are at the research stations of various nations, historic huts built by explorers from the heroic era early in the century, and the penguin rookeries and other places of interest to naturalists. Keep in mind that it is never known where a ship will be allowed to stop. Weather conditions as well as the needs and desires of the research station personnel will dictate your itinerary.

Research Stations If you do visit a research station, you may or may not be invited into the common room, may or may not be able to buy a souvenir postcard or patch, and may or may not meet with scientists who speak English. Also, because of the dramatic increase in tourists, many stations have cut back, not only on the number of cruise ships permitted to visit, but on the areas open to visitors. Be prepared for cancellations or substitutions—the sta-

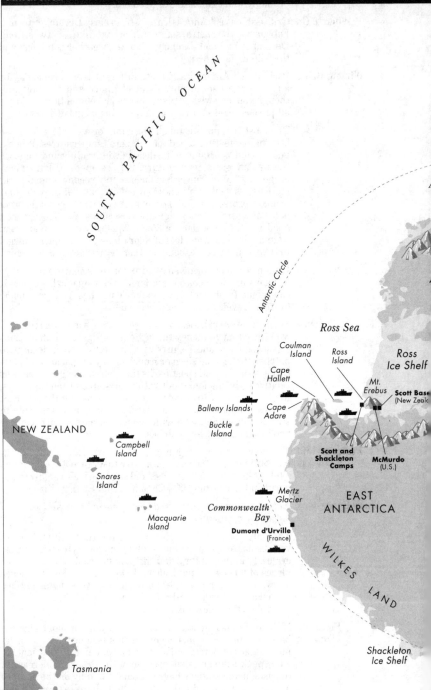

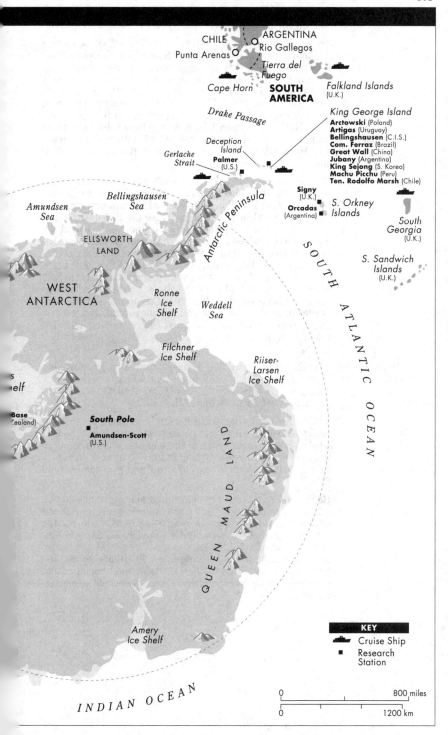

CHILE **ARGENTINA**
Punta Arenas ○ ○ Rio Gallegos
Tierra del Fuego
Cape Horn **SOUTH AMERICA**
Falkland Islands (U.K.)

Drake Passage

King George Island
Arctowski (Poland)
Artigas (Uruguay)
Bellingshausen (C.I.S.)
Com. Ferraz (Brazil)
Great Wall (China)
Jubany (Argentina)
King Sejong (S. Korea)
Machu Picchu (Peru)
Ten. Rodolfo Marsh (Chile)

Gerlache Strait
Deception Island
Palmer (U.S.)

Signy (U.K.)
Orcadas (Argentina)
S. Orkney Islands

South Georgia (U.K.)

Amundsen Sea
Bellingshausen Sea
ELLSWORTH LAND
Antarctic Peninsula

S. Sandwich Islands (U.K.)

S O U T H   A T L A N T I C   O C E A N

WEST ANTARCTICA
Ronne Ice Shelf
Weddell Sea
Filchner Ice Shelf
Riiser-Larsen Ice Shelf

...s ...elf
...Base ...ealand)

South Pole ■
Amundsen-Scott (U.S.)

Q U E E N   M A U D   L A N D

Amery Ice Shelf

KEY
⛴ Cruise Ship
■ Research Station

0 ———— 800 miles
0 ———— 1200 km

INDIAN OCEAN

tions try to accommodate, but with such a short research season, it's not always possible. Each visit to a station is different.

Those traveling from Australia or New Zealand will be visiting the area known as the Ross Sea. Here is New Zealand's **Scott Base,** which has a souvenir shop that takes credit cards, U.S. currency, and New Zealand currency. Also in this area is **McMurdo Station,** a U.S. base with a Navy PX that also sells souvenirs (because it's a PX, the merchandise is cheaper here). Ships traveling through these waters may visit **Cape Adare, Cape Hallett, Coulman Island,** or the **Shackelton and Scott huts,** as well as **Mt. Erebus. Dumont d'Urville,** a French base, and **Mertz Glacier** and **Commonwealth Bay** are less-visited stops.

If you come from South America, you'll explore the area known as the Antarctic Peninsula, home to **Palmer Station,** a U.S. base with a PX; **Gonzalez Videla Station,** or **Esperanza;** and the nine bases on King George Island, including the Polish **Arctowski.** Your ship may also stop at **Deception Island, Nelson Island,** the **South Georgia Islands,** or the **South Orkney Islands.** Some adventure ships stop at the **Falkland Islands,** one of the most remote and forbidding inhabited places on Earth. Argentina calls these islands the Malvenas and went to war with Britain in 1982 in an unsuccessful attempt to seize sovereignty; who owns them is still a hot issue in this part of the world. You may visit Port Stanley, the Falklands' picturesque capital, which seems like a transplanted north Scotland village; or New Island, a 7-mile rock that is home to several species of penguin and albatross.

Penguins and Other Wildlife You will see lots of wildlife, especially penguins, seals, whales, sea lions, and birds. Unlike in most other parts of the world, wild creatures here have no fear of people, but it's illegal to get closer than within 15–30 feet of the animals.

Zodiacs are used to get you ashore, take you on tours through bays filled with ice floes and icebergs, and bring you to pods of whales. Sitting on the edge of these crafts, you are bound to get wet—sometimes everything in the Zodiac gets drenched. Be sure to pack plastic Ziploc bags to protect your cameras and film.

Before you go ashore, the ship's naturalists give orientation talks. Don't miss these: You'll learn where it is safe to walk and what areas you should avoid, as well as where best to see the wildlife. If you follow the naturalists' guidelines, hiking in Antarctica is an exciting, invigorating adventure. If you ignore their warnings, it can be dangerous. There are no marked trails, so be sure not to wander off alone, and remember that distances can be deceiving here. Gauge your abilities conservatively.

The Bahamas

The Bahamas is an archipelago of more than 700 islands that begins in the Atlantic Ocean off the coast of Florida and stretches in a great southeasterly arc for more than 750 miles to the Caribbean Sea. Each island is bordered by soft, white-sand beaches lined with whispering casuarinas and swaying palms. Offshore, the islands are fringed by coral reefs and surrounded by a palette of blue and green waters of unbelievable clarity.

Fewer than 250,000 people live in the Bahamas, most of them in the two major urban resort centers of Nassau and Freeport. The Bahamas are becoming increasingly popular as a cruise destination; three- and four-day cruises from Florida to Nassau and Freeport are a big hit among young and budget-conscious travelers. New cruise destinations have been opened up by Premier Cruise Lines in the Abaco chain, attracting passengers who want to see the "untouched" Bahamas.

In fact, many cruise lines now offer a beach party or barbecue at one of several isolated Bahamian islands. For some, these excursions are the highlight of a cruise. One of the best such destinations is Blue Lagoon Island (also called Sale Cay). It is used by Dolphin Cruises and Premier Cruise Lines, as well as by a private tour company in Nassau.

When to Go Winter, from mid-December through April, is the traditional high season. However, Bahamas cruises are offered all year, and the weather remains consistently mild, in the 70s and 80s. The Goombay Summer, from June through August, is filled with social, cultural, and sporting events. June through October is the rainy season, and humidity is high.

Currency The Bahamian dollar is held at par with the U.S. dollar, and the two currencies are used interchangeably. Be sure to request U.S. dollars and coins when you receive change, however. Traveler's checks and major credit cards are accepted by most fine restaurants and stores.

Passports and Visas U.S., Canadian, and British citizens do not need passports or visas if they have proof of citizenship; however, a passport is preferable.

Telephones and Mail Long-distance connections are good. Hotels will add a service charge; public telephone centers are a better bet. The operator will place your call at regular international rates. Credit-card and collect calls can be made from most public phones. Airmail rates to the United States and Canada are 45¢ for first-class letters and 40¢ for postcards.

Shore Excursions Many ships offer excursions to one of the Bahamas' four casinos, which offer round-the-clock gaming action, bars, restaurants, and entertainment, including elaborate floor shows and topless revues. Some ships stay overnight in Freeport or Nassau.

In addition, many ships offer shopping excursions. Both Freeport and Nassau have a host of malls and stores (*see below*). Water sports are a major draw, and most ships offer snorkeling or boat trips to outlying islands, as well as fishing.

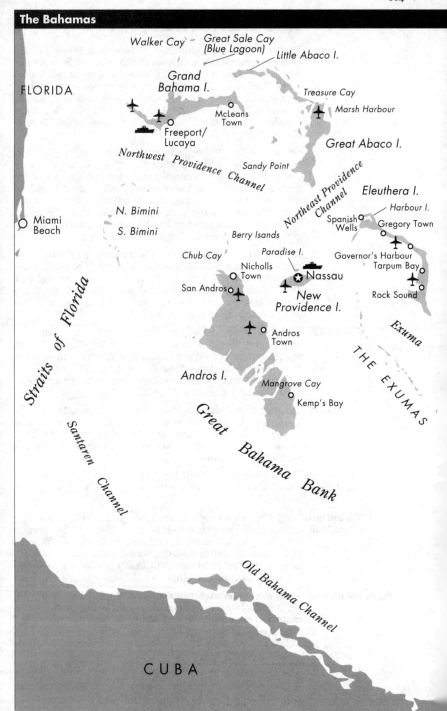

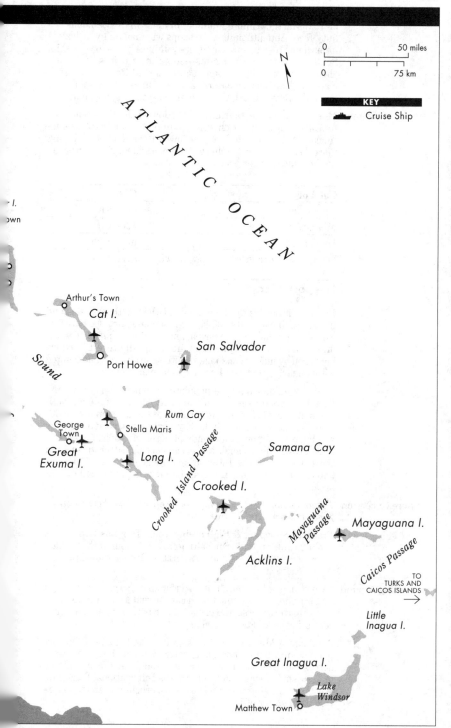

ATLANTIC OCEAN

0   50 miles
0   75 km

KEY
Cruise Ship

Arthur's Town
Cat I.
Port Howe
San Salvador
Sound
Rum Cay
George Town
Stella Maris
Great Exuma I.
Long I.
Crooked Island Passage
Samana Cay
Crooked I.
Mayaguana Passage
Mayaguana I.
Acklins I.
Caicos Passage
TO TURKS AND CAICOS ISLANDS →
Little Inagua I.
Great Inagua I.
Lake Windsor
Matthew Town

Shopping Unlike some of the Caribbean destinations, such as St. Thomas and St. Martin, a limited number of items in the Bahamas are duty-free. And although some shops will mail bulky or fragile items home to you, no one delivers your purchases to your ship. Still, you may find bargains—sometimes prices 30%–50% cheaper than at home—on such imported items as crystal, watches, cameras, sweaters, and perfumes. Most shops are open Monday–Saturday 9–5; some close at noon on Thursday.

Dining Most Bahamian restaurants have adopted the European custom of adding a service charge to your bill—usually 15%, sometimes as little as 10%. Use your own discretion about tipping more. Where no service charge has been added, give a tip based on the quality of service.

Category	Cost*
Expensive	over $30
Moderate	$20–$30
Inexpensive	under $20

per person, excluding drinks, service, and sales tax

Freeport/Lucaya

Freeport is on Grand Bahama Island, the fourth largest island in the archipelago. Its 530-square-mile interior is heavily forested with palmetto, casuarina, and Caribbean pines. The 96-mile southern coastline is made up of sheltered harbors bordered by miles of unspoiled white-sand beaches and fringed with a nearly unbroken line of spectacular reefs.

Virtually unknown and unpopulated a generation ago, Grand Bahama was developed in the early 1950s. Modern, well-planned Freeport is the centerpiece of the development, with its boulevards and shops linked by a palm-lined road to Lucaya, a suburb set among thousands of acres of tropical greenery that sprawls along canals and ocean beach. Scattered here and there are hotels, the International Bazaar, four golf courses, two casinos, and Port Lucaya, the new shopping mall/tourist area.

Shore Excursion *The following excursion may not be offered by all cruise lines. Time and price are approximate.*

Freeport Shopping & Sightseeing Tour: This bus trip covers about 26 miles round-trip, halting for a half-hour at the Garden of the Groves, with a shopping stop at the International Bazaar. *3 hrs. Cost: $12.*

Getting Around Everything in Freeport/Lucaya is far apart, so you need to sign up for a shore excursion, take a cab, or rent a car or moped. To make matters worse, the cruise-ship harbor is in an industrial center in the middle of nowhere.

A Bahamas Ministry of Tourism office is at the port, but depending on where your ship is berthed, it may be a short walk across the parking lot or a long hike. You'll also find a Ministry of Tourism Information Center at the International Bazaar on West Sunrise Highway. Pick up maps, brochures, and information from either office.

By Bus Once you get within the Freeport/Lucaya area, scheduled buses cover most of the region, including some outlying villages. Check with the tourism office for schedules and routes.

By Car Car rentals average $48–$85 daily, and a significant deposit is required. Contact **Avis** (tel. 809/352–7666), **Hertz** (tel. 809/352–9250), or **National** (tel. 809/352–9308).

By Moped Rental mopeds and bicycles are available dockside and at several resorts on the island. Rates for bicycles start at about $10 per day, with a $50 deposit; motor scooters average about $30–$40 per day with a $50–$100 deposit. Helmets are mandatory.

By Taxi Metered taxis meet all the incoming cruise ships. A taxi tour costs $12–$18 an hour, but rates for longer trips are negotiable. Always settle the fare in advance. Taxis are also available in most major tourist areas. Try **Freeport Taxi Company** (809/352–6666).

Exploring Freeport/Lucaya *Numbers in the margin correspond to numbered points of interest on the Freeport/Lucaya map.*

You will enjoy driving or riding around Freeport/Lucaya as long as you remember to drive on the left. Broad, landscaped "dual carriageways"—British for highways—and tree-lined streets wind through parks, past lovely homes, and along lush green fairways.

❶ A enormously popular attraction is the **International Bazaar and Strawmarket,** a vast array of shops and markets on West
❷ Sunrise Highway (*see* Shopping, *below*). Next door is the **Bahama Princess Resort & Casino.**

From here, travel east by car to the first traffic circle and turn
❸ left onto the Mall. This will take you to **Churchill Square** and the Freeport town center, where residents shop and tend to business. If you're hungry, **Mum's Coffee Shop and Bakery,** at 7 Yellow Pine Street, has delicious homemade breads, soups, and sandwiches. Head north on the Mall to Settler's Way East,
❹ then turn right and follow the tree-lined highway to the **Rand Memorial Nature Center.** The 100-acre park, composed of natural woodland, preserves more than 400 indigenous varieties of subtropical plants, trees, and flowers. It is also a sanctuary for thousands of native and migratory birds. A mile of well-marked nature trails leads to a 30-foot waterfall. Guided walks are conducted by the resident naturalists.

Leaving the nature center, continue east on Settler's Way, then
❺ turn south (right) onto West Beach Road to the **Garden of the Groves.** The park features some 5,000 varieties of rare and familiar subtropical and tropical trees, shrubs, plants, and flowers. Well-marked paths lead past clearly identified plants, a fern gully and grotto, and a tiny, stone interdenominational chapel.

From here, head for the sea, then turn right onto Royal Palm
❻ Way and drive until you come to the **Underwater Explorers Society** (UNEXSO). In 1987 five wild bottle-nosed dolphins were brought to Lucaya and trained to interact with people. As the dolphins cavort in the water, swimmers and snorkelers dive in with them, and the dolphins seem to love it. You can join the dolphins in their pool for $59.

❼ Almost next door is **Port Lucaya,** the new marketplace on the waterfront. About 85 shops, boutiques, restaurants, and

Freeport/Lucaya

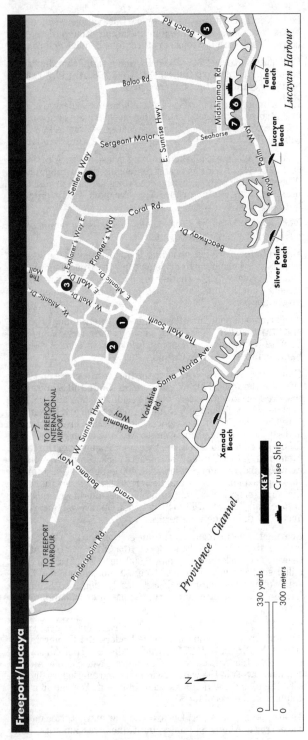

N

TO FREEPORT
INTERNATIONAL
AIRPORT

TO FREEPORT
HARBOUR

Pinderspoint Rd.

Grand Bahama Way

Bahama Way

W. Sunrise Hwy.

Yorkshire Rd.

Santa Maria Ave.

The Mall South

W. Atlantic Dr.

The Mall

W. Mall Dr.

E. Mall Dr.

E. Atlantic Dr.

Explorer's Way E.

Pioneer's Way

Coral Rd.

Settlers Way

Sergeant Major

E. Sunrise Hwy.

Balao Rd.

W. Beach Rd.

Midshipman Rd.

Seahorse

Royal Palm

Beachway Dr.

Xanadu Beach

Silver Point Beach

Lucayan Beach

Taino Beach

Providence Channel

Lucayan Harbour

KEY

Cruise Ship

0 ___ 330 yards
0 ___ 300 meters

Bahama Princess
Resort & Casino, **2**
Churchill Square, **3**
Garden of the
Groves, **5**
International Bazaar
and Strawmarket, **1**

Port Lucaya, **7**
Rand Memorial Nature
Center, **4**
Underwater Explorers
Society (UNEXSO), **6**

lounges are housed in low-rise colonial-style buildings. The complex overlooks Lucayan Harbour, with a 50-slip marina that moors *El Galleon*, a replica of a 16th-century Spanish galleon, offering day and dinner cruises.

Shopping   The **International Bazaar and Strawmarket** is on West Sunrise Highway, next to the Princess Casino. You enter through the 35-foot red-lacquer Torii Gate, traditional symbol of welcome in Japan. Within the bazaar are a straw market and exotic shops with merchandise from around the world. Most are priced at 20%–40% below U.S. *retail* prices, which means that they may or may not be a bargain when compared with prices in discount stores at home. A dozen countries are represented in the 10-acre bazaar, with nearly a hundred shops. The vendors in the straw market expect you to haggle over the price, but don't bargain in the stores. For a less touristy experience, go to **Churchill Square** and the Freeport town center. An open-air produce market offers mangoes, papayas, and other fruit for snacking as you walk. **Port Lucaya** is an attractive waterfront complex with 85 shops, boutiques, restaurants, and lounges.

Sports   Contact **Lucayan Harbour Marina** (tel. 809/373–8888), **Run-**
Fishing   **ning Mon Marina** (tel. 809/352–6834), or **Xanadu Beach Hotel Marina** (tel. 809/352–6782).

Golf   Grand Bahama's three championship 18-hole courses are among the best in the Caribbean: **Bahamas Princess Golf Courses** (tel. 809/352–6721), **Fortune Hills Golf & Country Club** (tel. 809/373–4500), and **Lucayan Golf & Country Club** (tel. 809/373–1066). Fees range from $18 to $70 for 18 holes and from $10 to $45 for nine.

Water Sports   Several hotels offer windsurfing and parasailing rentals. For instruction and equipment, contact **Atlantik Beach Hotel** (tel. 809/373–1444). One of the most famous scuba schools and NAUI centers in the world is the **Underwater Explorers Society** (UNEXSO), adjacent to Port Lucaya. Beginners can learn to dive for $79, which includes three hours of professional instruction in the club's training pools, and a shallow reef dive. For experienced divers, there are three trips daily (tel. 809/373–1244, or write to UNEXSO, Box F-2433, Freeport, Grand Bahama).

Dining   **The Pub on the Mall.** Opposite the International Bazaar, this splendid English pub has authentic atmosphere and decor. The Prince of Wales Lounge serves good fish and chips, and steak-and-kidney pie. Bass ale is on tap. Baron's Hall serves superb dinners at night—try the coquilles St. Jacques, Cornish game hen, or roast beef with Yorkshire pudding. *At Ranfurly Circus, tel. 809/352–5110. AE, MC, V. Moderate.*
Pusser's Co. Store and Pub. Fashioned after an old Welsh pub, this amiable establishment overlooking Port Lucaya is part bar, part restaurant, and part maritime museum. It has a nautical decor with antique copper measuring cups and Tiffany lamps suspended from the wood-beam ceiling. Locals swap tall tales and island gossip with tourists over rum-based Pusser's Painkillers. Solid English fare is favored: shepherd's pie, fisherman's pie, steak-and-ale pie. *Port Lucaya Marketplace, tel. 809/373–8450. AE, MC, V. Inexpensive.*

Nassau

The 17th-century town of Nassau, the capital of the Bahamas, has witnessed Spanish invasions and hosted pirates, who made it their headquarters for raids along the Spanish Main. The new American Navy seized Ft. Montagu here in 1776, when they won a victory without firing a shot.

The cultural and ethnic heritage of old Nassau includes the southern charm of British loyalists from the Carolinas, the African tribal traditions of freed slaves, and a bawdy history of blockade-running during the Civil War and rum-running in the Roaring Twenties. Over it all is a subtle layer of civility and sophistication, derived from three centuries of British rule.

Reminders of the island's British heritage are everywhere in Nassau. Court justices sport wigs and scarlet robes. The police wear colonial garb: starched white jackets, red-striped navy trousers, tropical pith helmets. Traffic keeps to the left, and the language has a British-colonial lilt, softened by a slight drawl.

Much of the Caribbean's charm lies here in old Nassau: the colorful harbor ship market, with out-island sloops hauling in the day's fish and conch, and stalls selling tropical fruit and exotic vegetables. Elsewhere on the island, however, are glittering resorts, casinos, and beaches that are just a short taxi or ferry ride from the Nassau cruise-ship docks.

Shore Excursions *Not all excursions are offered by all cruise lines. Times and prices are approximate.*

Boats and Beaches **Catamaran Cruise:** Cruise the waters and the islands around Nassau with a calypso band accompaniment. Stop at a beach for swimming and sunbathing; drinks and snacks are for sale, and there are changing facilities. *3 hrs. Cost: $15.*

Snorkeling Adventure: The Bahamas is an underwater wonderland. On this tour you can learn to snorkel, then join an escorted tour or set off on your own. *2¹/₂–3 hrs. Cost: $20–$25.*

Entertainment **Casino Show:** At a casino see a show-girl revue, with time for gambling. A free drink is included. Stay as late as you wish. *Cost: $35.*

Drumbeat Club: A native show with island entertainers. A free drink is included. *2 hrs. Cost: $20–$25.*

Scenic **Nassau and Ardastra Gardens:** Stop at the touristy gardens to see flamingos march on command, all synchronized to music. Then visit Ft. Charlotte, Ft. Fincastle, and the Queen's Staircase. *2¹/₂ hrs. Cost: $25.*

Nassau and Paradise Island: Stop at Ft. Fincastle and the Queen's Staircase, then continue on to Paradise Island for an overview tour. *2 hrs. Cost: $13.*

Coral World: The visit to the marine park with its underwater observatory is excellent if you have never been snorkeling or scuba diving in the region. Budget about three hours, but you can stay as long as you want—the ferry back to the cruise-ship docks leaves every half-hour. *Cost: $15 ($18 with ferry transfers).*

On Your Own   If your ship doesn't have an out-island beach party planned for the cruise, you may wish to join one in Nassau. It is for many the best way to experience the Bahamas. Excellent tours are offered on the **MV *Calypso*** (tel. 809/763–3577) and *El Bucanero II* (tel. 809/393–8772).

Getting Around   The cruise-ship docks in Nassau are right in the center of town. Just walk away from the pier and within a block you'll be in the middle of the main shopping district.

By Carriage   Across from the docks, along Rawson Square, are surreys drawn by straw-hatted horses, which will take you through the old city and past some of the nearby historic sites. The cost is $10 for two for 45 minutes, but verify prices before getting on.

By Car   Car-rental rates range from $45 to $129 a day; a substantial deposit is required. Contact **Avis** (tel. 809/327–7121), **Budget** (tel. 809/327–7405), **Hertz** (tel. 809/327–6866), or **National** (tel. 809/327–7301).

By Ferry   A ferry commutes between the dock area and Paradise Island. Another goes to Coral World.

By Moped   Mopeds and bicycles are available for rent at several resorts on the island. Rates for bicycles average $20 per day, with a $40 deposit; motor scooters average $14 per half-day, $28 per day, with a $50 deposit. Helmets are mandatory.

By Tour Car   As you disembark from your ship you will find a row of taxis and luxurious air-conditioned limousines. The latter are Nassau's fleet of tour cars, useful and comfortable for a guided tour of the island. A two-hour city tour should cost about $20 per person; negotiate for shorter or longer trips and settle on a rate before getting in.

Exploring Nassau   *Numbers in the margin correspond to numbered points of interest on the Nassau map.*

The **Ministry of Tourism Information Centre** (tel. 809/328–7810), in Rawson Square, right at the entrance to the docks, is well stocked with brochures, maps, and expert advice. You can join a free one-hour walking tour conducted by well-trained guides on most days, call for hours.

❶ Within **Rawson Square** are benches and the Sands Fountain. Take the small pathway through the square to the bust of Sir Milo Butler, the first Bahamian governor-general of the Bahamas.

❷ Directly across Bay Street from Rawson Square is **Parliament Square.** Dating from the early 1800s and patterned after southern U.S. colonial architecture, this cluster of yellow colonnaded buildings with green shutters is striking. In the center of the square is a statue of the young Queen Victoria, and the **Bahamas House of Parliament.**

❸ At the head of Elizabeth Avenue is the **Queen's Staircase,** a famous Nassau landmark. Its 66 steps, hewn from the coral limestone cliff by slaves in 1793, were designed to provide a direct route between town and **Ft. Fincastle** at the top of the hill. The staircase was named more than a hundred years later, in honor of the 66 years of Queen Victoria's reign.

❹ Climb the staircase to reach **Ft. Fincastle.** The fort, shaped like the bow of a ship, was built in the early 1790s. It never fired a shot in anger but served as a lookout and signal tower. For a

312

Nassau

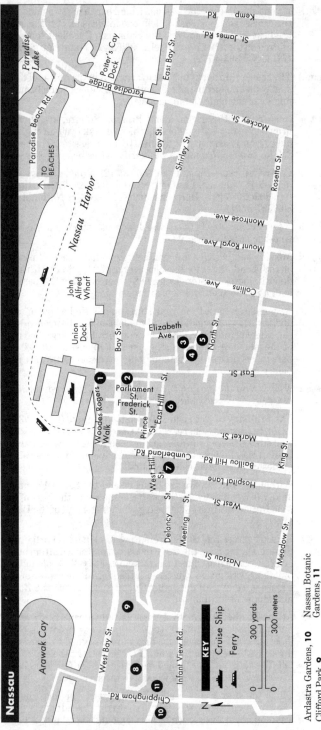

Ardastra Gardens, **10**
Clifford Park, **9**
Ft. Charlotte, **8**
Ft. Fincastle, **4**
Graycliff, **7**
Gregory Arch, **6**

Nassau Botanic
Gardens, **11**
Parliament Square, **2**
Queen's Staircase, **3**
Rawson Square, **1**
Water Tower, **5**

really spectacular view of the island of New Providence, climb
⑤ (or ride the elevator) to the top of the nearby **Water Tower.**
Rising to 126 feet, more than 200 feet above sea level, the tower
is the highest point on the island.

Continue down Parliament Street, by the post office, toward
the harbor to **Green Shutters,** a charming Bahamian house
from 1865, converted into an English-style pub.

Back toward the pier on East Hill Street, you'll see historic
mansions. Just beyond the **Bank House,** on the north side of
the street, is a broad flight of stairs that leads down to Prince
Street. Here are two historic churches, **St. Andrew's Kirk, Pres-
byterian** (1810) and **Trinity Methodist** (1866). Continue west
along Prince Street. As you pass Market Street look up the hill
⑥ for a good view of **Gregory Arch,** the picturesque entrance to
Grant's Town. Known as the "over-the-hill" section of Nassau,
Grant's Town was laid out in the 1820s by Governor Lewis
Grant as a settlement for freed slaves.

On Duke Street, follow the high Government House wall
around the corner to Baillou (pronounced "blue") Hill Road.
⑦ Take West Hill Street; across Baillou Hill is the **Graycliff** hotel,
a superb example of Georgian colonial architecture, dating
from the mid-1700s, that now houses a gourmet restaurant.

⑧ Next, visit the most interesting fort on the island, **Ft. Charlotte,**
built in the late 18th century and replete with a waterless moat,
drawbridge, ramparts, and dungeons. Lord Dunmore, the
builder, named the massive structure in honor of George III's
wife. At the time, some called it Dunmore's Folly because of the
staggering expense of building it—eight times more than originally planned. (Dunmore's superiors in London were less than
ecstatic when they saw the bills, but he managed to survive
unscathed.) Ironically, no shots were ever fired in anger from
the fort. Ft. Charlotte is located at the top of a hill and commands a fine view of Nassau Harbor and Arawak Cay, a small
man-made island that holds huge storage tanks of fresh water
barged in from Andros Island. *Off W. Bay St. at Chippingham
Rd., tel. 809/322–7500. Admission free. Local guides conduct
tours Mon.–Sat. 8:30–4.*

⑨ At the foot of Ft. Charlotte lies **Clifford Park,** where colorful
Independence Day ceremonies are held on July 10. The park
has a large reviewing ground, grandstands, and playing fields,
where you can watch the local soccer, rugby, field hockey, and
cricket teams in action.

⑩ A block farther west, on Chippingham Road, are the **Ardastra
Gardens,** with 5 acres of tropical greenery and flowering
shrubs, an aviary of rare tropical birds, and exotic animals from
different parts of the world. The gardens are renowned for the
parade of pink, spindly legged, marching flamingos that performs daily at 11, 2, and 4. The flamingo, by the way, is the
national bird of the Bahamas. *Near Ft. Charlotte, off Chippingham Rd., tel. 809/323–5806. Admission: $7.50 adults, $3.75 children under 10. Open daily 9–5.*

⑪ Across the street is the **Nassau Botanic Gardens,** which has 18
acres featuring 600 species of flowering trees and shrubs; two
freshwater ponds with lilies, water plants, and tropical fish;
and a small cactus garden that ends in grotto. The many trails
wandering through the gardens are perfect for leisurely

strolls. *Near Ft. Charlotte, off Chippingham Rd., tel. 809/323–5975. Admission: $1 adults, 50¢ children. Open daily 8–4:30.*

Shopping Most of the stores are clustered along an eight-block stretch of Bay Street in old Nassau or spill over onto a few side streets downtown. Savings on many big-ticket items average 20%–50% over prices in retail stores in the United States and Canada. In fact, *Forbes* magazine once claimed that the two cities in the world with the best buys on wristwatches were Hong Kong and Nassau. Most stores are open Monday–Saturday 9–5; some close at noon on Thursday. The straw market is open seven days a week. Most shops accept major credit cards.

Sports Contact **Nassau Harbour Club** (tel. 809/393–0771) or **Nassau**
Fishing **Yacht Haven** (tel. 809/393–8173).

Golf Three excellent 18-hole championship courses are open to the public: **Carnival's Crystal Palace Golf Course,** with 18 holes, restaurant, and pro shop (opposite the Wyndham Ambassador Hotel, tel. 809/327–6000 or 800/222–7466 in the U.S.); **Paradise Island Golf Club,** with 18 holes, restaurant, and pro shop (eastern end of Paradise Island, tel. 809/363–3925 or 800/321–3000 in the U.S.); and **Ramada Inn Beach Resort and Country Club,** with 18 holes, bars, restaurant, and pro shop (adjacent to Divi Bahamas Beach Resort, tel. 809/362–4391 or 800/228–9898 in the U.S.). Fees are $50–$70 for 18 holes.

Water Sports Windsurfing is available at a variety of hotels for $17 an hour. Parasailing is offered by several hotels along the shore of Cable Beach and Paradise Island, costing about $35 for a 3-mile run, which lasts five to seven minutes. Offshore on the reefs surrounding the island are many excellent dive sites. The following offer one or more dive trips daily: **Stuart Cove's Nassau Undersea Adventures** (tel. 809/362–4171) and **Sun Divers Ltd.** (tel. 809/322–3301).

Beaches **Paradise Beach,** the Bahamas' most famous beach, stretches for more than a mile on the western end of Paradise Island. The $3 admission includes a welcome drink, towels, and use of changing rooms and locker. **Caves Beach,** on West Bay Street beyond the Cable Beach hotels, features a series of caves reputed to have been pirates' hideaways. **Ft. Montagu Beach,** on East Bay Street, is a popular gathering place for Bahamians, especially on Saturday. The beach bar serves juicy burgers and frosty beers, and you can buy lunch from a local vendor "cooking out." **Goodman's Bay,** on West Bay Street just before the Cable Beach hotel strip, is popular with Bahamians for picnics and cookouts on weekends and holidays.

Dining **Graycliff.** Situated in a magnificent 200-year-old colonial mansion, Graycliff is filled with antiques and English country-house charm. The outstanding Continental and Bahamian menu includes beluga caviar, grouper *au poivre vert,* and chateaubriand, with elegant pastries and flaming coffees for dessert. The wine cellar is excellent. *West Hill St., across from Government House, tel. 809/322–2796 or 800/633–7411. Reservations required. Jacket required. AE, DC, MC, V. Expensive.*
The Shoal and Lounge. Saturday mornings at 9 you'll find hordes of jolly Bahamians digging into boiled fish and johnny-cake, the marvelous specialty of the house. A bowl of this peppery local dish, filled with chunks of boiled potatoes, onions, and grouper, may keep you coming back to this dimly lit, basic, and off-the-tourist-beat "ma's kitchen," where standard Nas-

sau dishes, including peas 'n' rice and cracked conch, are served. If it suits you, you'll find native mutton here, too, which is sometimes hard to find locally. *Nassau St., tel. 809/323–4400. No reservations. Dress: casual. AE.*

Nightlife Some ships stay late into the night or until the next day so that passengers can enjoy Nassau's nightlife. You'll find nonstop entertainment nightly along Cable Beach and on Paradise Island. All the larger hotels offer lounges with island combos for listening or dancing, and restaurants with soft guitar or piano background music.

Casinos The three casinos on New Providence Island—**Carnival's Crystal Palace Casino, Paradise Island Resort and Casino,** and **Ramada Inn Casino**—open early in the day, remain active into the wee hours of the morning, and offer Continental gambling and a variety of other entertainment. Visitors must be 18 or older to enter a casino, 21 or older to gamble.

Discos **Club Waterloo** (tel. 809/393–1108) on East Bay Street is one of Nassau's most swinging night spots. Also hot is the **Palace Theatre** (tel. 809/327–6200), at the Crystal Palace, but you'll have to meet the dress code to dance within its elegant black marble confines. Disco and rock can be heard nightly at **Club Pastiche** (tel. 809/363–3000), at the Paradise Island Resort and Casino.

Local Entertainment The **Drumbeat Club** (tel. 809/322–4233) on West Bay Street, just up from the Best Western British Colonial Hotel, features the legendary Peanuts Taylor, still alive and well and beating away at those tom-toms; his band and gyrating dancers put on two shows nightly at 8:30 and 10:30.

Bermuda

Blessed with fabulous beaches and surrounded by a turquoise sea, Britain's oldest colony and most famous resort island lies isolated in the Atlantic Ocean, more than 500 miles from Cape Hatteras, North Carolina, the nearest point on the U.S. mainland. Although it looks like one island, Bermuda actually consists of about 150 islands—the seven largest connected by bridges and causeways—all arranged in the shape of a giant fishhook. Bermuda, which is 22 square miles, is never more than 2 miles wide. The islands are surrounded by coral reefs that offer not only protection from Atlantic storms but wonderful scuba diving as well.

Bermuda's residents are known as "onions"—after the sweet, succulent Bermuda onion that was their livelihood a century ago. Their homes, whose addresses are unusual names rather than numbers, are studies in color—pink and yellow, lime and turquoise—all topped with sparkling white roofs that funnel rainwater into cisterns. (The islands have no freshwater supply of their own.)

Bermuda was stumbled upon accidentally by Spaniard Juan de Bermudez in 1503. In 1609 the British ship *Sea Venture,* commanded by Sir George Somers and on its way to Jamestown, Virginia, struck one of the reefs that surround the islands. Although it received bad press in Shakespeare's *The Tempest,* Bermuda has thrived and is now home to 58,460 residents.

In spite of its proximity to the American mainland, Bermuda has maintained a distinctly British visage. Cricket and pubs, for instance, are very much a part of Bermudian life. Today, Bermudians are protective of their country, and change is not undertaken lightly. To avoid road congestion and air pollution, the number of cars is limited to one per residential household. There are no rental cars, so most visitors buzz around the island on mopeds.

Proper dress is stressed on Bermuda. Tourists in short shorts are frowned upon, and bathing suits are unacceptable away from the beach. Bare feet and hair curlers are not acceptable in public, nor is appearing without a shirt or in just a bathing-suit top.

Bermuda has long been a favorite destination of cruise lines, and it is usually a cruise's only port of call. Most ships make seven-day loops from New York, with four days spent at sea and three days tied up in port. Three Bermuda harbors serve cruise ships: Hamilton, St. George's or the Royal Duckyard. Concerned about overcrowding, the Bermudian government limits the number of regular cruise ship visits to four per week, none on weekends.

The traditional port is Hamilton, Bermuda's most commercialized area; if you want to shop until you drop, this centrally located capital is the proper port for you. Passengers whose ships tie up at St. George's walk off the vessel into Bermuda's equivalent of Colonial Williamsburg. If you enjoy history, you'll prefer St. George's, which has its share of stores, too. The West End dock is the farthest from the major sights, but nothing in Bermuda is far away, and it takes almost no time to cross the island in a taxi or on a moped.

317

Bermuda

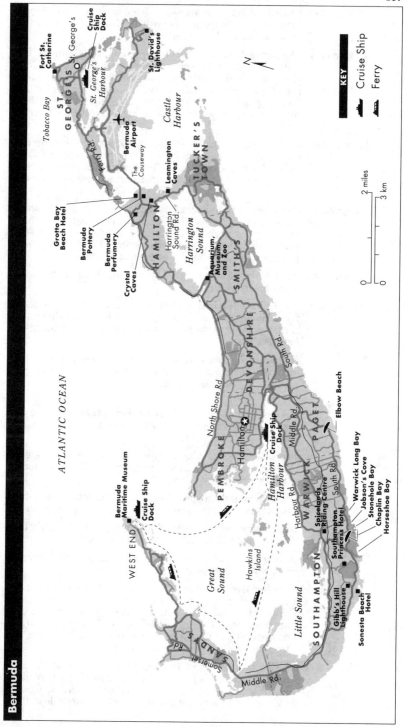

ATLANTIC OCEAN

Bermuda Maritime Museum

WEST END

Cruise Ship Dock

Great Sound

Hawkins Island

Little Sound

SANDY'S

Somerset Rd.

Middle Rd.

Gibb's Hill Lighthouse

Sonesta Beach Hotel

SOUTHAMPTON

Southampton Princess Hotel

Spicelands Riding Centre

Harbour Rd.

Middle Rd.

South Rd.

WARWICK

Warwick Long Bay

Jobson's Cove

Stonehole Bay

Chaplin Bay

Horseshoe Bay

Hamilton Harbour

Cruise Ship Dock

Hamilton

PEMBROKE

North Shore Rd.

Middle Rd.

DEVONSHIRE

South Rd.

PAGET

Elbow Beach

SMITH'S

Aquarium, Museum, and Zoo

Harrington Sound

Harrington Sound Rd.

TUCKER'S TOWN

HAMILTON

Crystal Caves

Bermuda Perfumery

Bermuda Pottery

Grotto Bay Beach Hotel

Leamington Caves

Castle Harbour

The Causeway

Bermuda Airport

Ferry Rd.

Tobacco Bay

ST. GEORGE'S

Fort St. Catherine

St. George's

St. George's Harbour

Cruise Ship Dock

St. David's Lighthouse

N

KEY
Cruise Ship
Ferry

0   2 miles
0   3 km

When to Go Cruises to Bermuda are scheduled only from April through October, when temperatures are in the 70s and 80s. One or two ships sail here in November.

Currency The Bermuda dollar (BD$) is pegged on a par with the U.S. dollar, so there is no need to change your U.S. dollars. Most shops take credit cards, but many hotels and restaurants do not. U.S. traveler's checks, however, are widely accepted. Ask for change in U.S. dollars and coins; all shopkeepers have them. All other currencies must be exchanged at banks for local tender.

Passports and Visas U.S. citizens need proof of citizenship. A passport is preferable, but a stamped birth certificate or voter registration card with photo ID are also acceptable. You must also have a return or ongoing ticket. Canadian and British citizens need a valid passport.

Telephones and Mail Calling home from Bermuda is as easy as from any city in the United States, and public phones can be found everywhere, including the docks. Federal Express can provide two-day package service to the United States. First-class airmail postage stamps are 60¢ for letters and postcards.

Shore Excursions *Not all excursions are offered by all cruise lines. All times and prices are approximate.*

Boats and Beaches **South Shore Beaches:** Sightseeing along the South Road allows for an hour to swim at Horseshoe Bay Beach. Wet bathing suits are not allowed on the bus, but there are changing facilities. *4 hrs. Cost: $28.*

Helmut Diving: Walk on the bottom of the sea, play with fish, and learn about coral, all without getting your hair wet. Helmets cover your head and feed you air from the surface. *3¹/₂ hrs. Cost: $40.*

Bermuda Glass-Bottom Boat Cruise: A tame but pleasant cruise through the harbor and over reefs. You can feed the fish from the boat. *2 hrs. Cost: $24.*

Snorkeling Tour: Equipment, lessons, and underwater guided tour are included. Underwater cameras are available for an extra charge. *3³/₄ hrs. Cost: $35.*

Coral Reef and Calypso Cruise: A glass-bottom party boat provides rum swizzles and island music. *2¹/₂ hrs. Cost: $30.*

Reef Roamer Island Party: A beach party includes snorkeling, dancing, and rum swizzles. *3¹/₂ hrs. Cost: $36.*

Sailing Cruise: It's relaxing, romantic, and quiet, and there's a short stop for a swim. *3 hrs. Cost: $34.*

Cultural and Scenic **West End Highlight Tour:** Visit the Island Pottery, Art Centre, Crafts Market, Maritime Museum, Heydon Trust Chapel, and Gibb's Hill Lighthouse during a drive through Somerset. This tour is a must if you are docked in Hamilton or St. George's and wouldn't go to the West End on your own. *4 hrs. Cost: $29 (depending on where you are docked).*

St. George's Highlight Tour: A quick overview of the area around St. George's includes Ft. St. Catherine, Ft. William, Gates Fort, the Unfinished Church, Somers Garden, Tobacco Bay, and the government housing complex. The guide is informative and will point out the popular shopping areas. *2 hrs. Cost: $50 (depending on where you are docked).*

Bermuda's Attractions Tour: Visit Leamington or Crystal Caves, the aquarium, and the zoo. Then see perfume made from flowers at the Bermuda Perfumery. *4 hrs. Cost: $27.*

Entertainment **Clayhouse Inn:** A popular song-and-dance show. Two free drinks are included. *Cost: $35.*

Hamilton Princess Revue: A salute to famous female performers such as Ella Fitzgerald and Anita Baker. Includes two free drinks. *4 hrs. Cost: $44.*

Getting Around The Bermuda Department of Tourism maintains an information booth in the Hamilton cruise-ship terminal; on King's Square in St. George's; in Hamilton on 8 Front Street and at the Royal Naval Dockyard in the West End. Cars cannot be rented in Bermuda.

By Bus Buses are a good way to get around, although some stop running in the evening. The pink-and-blue buses are easy to spot, especially along the principal route between Hamilton and St. George. Most operate about every 15–25 minutes except on weekends. Bermuda is divided into 14 zones of about 2 miles each. The adult fare for traveling within the first three zones is $1.50; a longer ride is $3. Booklets of tickets and tokens are sold at a discount at the central bus terminal and in many hotels. Bus stops are marked by green-and-white-striped posts, and passengers must have the correct change. The central bus terminal is next to City Hall on Washington Street in Hamilton.

By Carriage Horse-drawn carriages line up along Front Street in Hamilton, near the cruise-ship terminal. They can be hired by the half-hour or hour. The fee for a one-horse carriage is $15 for the first half-hour, $10 for each additional half-hour. For a two-horse carriage, it's $20 for the first half-hour, $15 for each additional half-hour.

By Ferry If your ship is tied up at the Royal Naval Dockyard, the ferry to Hamilton is the easiest and most pleasant way to get to the capital. Other ferries connect various points throughout the harbor. Mopeds and bicycles can be taken aboard the West End ferries only. One-way fare is $1.50–$3, with an extra $3 for mopeds.

By Moped Most visitors to Bermuda drive around on mopeds. However, be careful: The number of accidents is considerable. Mopeds can be rented all over the island at a daily rate of about $25. Riders are required to wear a strapped helmet. Gas stations are open Monday–Saturday 7 AM–7 PM. Stop by the tourist information office to pick up a map for the Railway Trail, which is especially fun on a moped.

By Taxi Taxis are plentiful and meet every ship. The blue flag signifies that the driver has passed a written examination to qualify as a guide. The drivers of these blue-flag taxis do not charge more than other taxi drivers. Taxis are metered, but a 25% surcharge is added between 10 PM and 6 AM. Taxis can be hired at $20 per hour (three-hour minimum) for up to six per car.

Exploring Hamilton *Numbers in the margin correspond to numbered points of interest on the Hamilton map.*

320

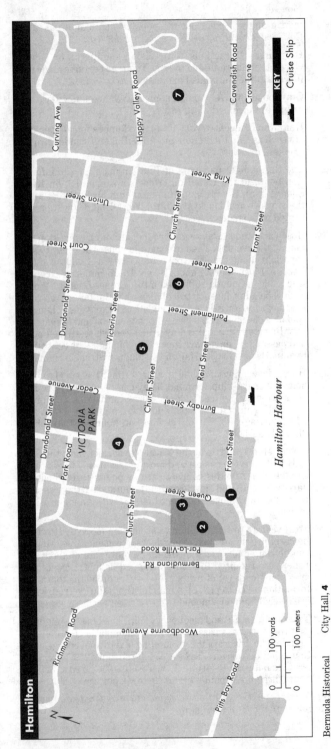

Hamilton

Bermuda Historical
Society Museum and
Bermuda Library, **3**
Birdcage, **1**
Cathedral of the Most
Holy Trinity, **5**

City Hall, **4**
Ft. Hamilton, **7**
Par-la-Ville Park, **2**
Sessions House, **6**

KEY

Cruise Ship

When you walk off the ship in Hamilton, you are right in the middle of the capital of Bermuda. Walk out onto Front Street, where the most famous and prestigious of Bermuda's stores are located. In the middle of Front Street at Queen Street is

❶ the **Birdcage,** where a policeman sometimes directs traffic.
❷ Turn right onto Queen Street. On your left is **Par-la-Ville Park,** once the private garden of William B. Perot, Bermuda's first postmaster and the creator of the famous 1848 Perot Stamp. The huge rubber tree was planted by Perot in 1847. In front of

❸ the park are the two-room **Bermuda Historical Society Museum and Bermuda Library,** housed in what used to be Perot's home. *Open Mon.–Sat. 9:30–12:30 and 2–4.*

Continue up Queen Street and turn right onto Church Street.
❹ The large building to the left is **City Hall,** a handsome modern structure with a traditional Bermudian feeling and a weather vane in the shape of the *Sea Venture.* The second-floor East Wing houses the Bermuda National Gallery, which opened in March 1992 with permanent displays of Old Masters and Bermudian artists, as well as traveling exhibits. The second-floor West Wing is home to the Bermuda Society of Arts Gallery (admission free; open weekdays 10:30–4:30, Sat. 9–noon), with changing exhibits of local and foreign painters and photographers. City Hall is also home to a theater in which many of the Bermuda Festival events are mounted. *Admission to Bermuda National Gallery: $3 adults, $2.50 senior citizens, children under 17 free. Open Mon.–Sat. 10–4, Sun. 12:30–4.*

❺ On the next block of Church Street is Bermuda's **Cathedral of the Most Holy Trinity,** dedicated in 1894. Commonly called the Bermuda Cathedral, it was built mainly from native limestone; decorative touches are of marble, granite, and English oak.

❻ Turning right down Parliament Street you will see **Sessions House** on the left. In this building, with its pink Italianate towers, the House of Assembly meets upstairs under the portraits of King George III and Queen Charlotte. The Speaker of the House, as well as the Supreme Court chief justice and barristers, all wear the traditional English wig and black robes. Climb up to the visitor galleries in the upper floors. *Admission free. Open weekdays 9–5.*

Walk back to Church Street and turn right onto it, then turn left onto King Street. Here you can walk or ride the steep incline up to Happy Valley Road, then continue into **Ft. Hamilton**
❼ for a spectacular panoramic view of the city and harbor. Visitors approach the main gate over a moat—now dry and filled with exotic plants—which can be reached from the fort's underground galleries. On the upper level, now a grassy slope filled with park benches, the Royal Arms of Queen Victoria are emblazoned on the main armaments. *Admission free. Open weekdays 9:30–5.*

Exploring St. George's *Numbers in the margin correspond to numbered points of interest on the St. George's map.*

❶❷ Cruise ships tie up at either **Ordance Island** or **Penno's Wharf** two blocks away. Over the bridge from the island is **King's Square,** the heart of St. George's, where replicas of the **stocks and pillory** that stood on the site 300 years ago are on display. Another 17th-century form of punishment was the **ducking stool,** one of which can be seen on Ordnance Island.

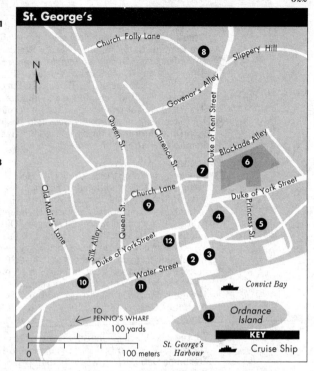

St. George's

322

3 The beautifully restored **Town Hall** follows the lines of the original building that was erected in 1782 and is still in use as the town's administrative headquarters. "The Bermuda Journey" multimedia show presented here depicts Bermuda's past and present. *Admission to Town Hall free. Open Mon.–Sat. 9–4. "Bermuda Journey" admission: $2.50 adults, $1.75 children under 12, $2 senior citizens.*

4 Northeast of Town Hall is **Bridge House,** an 18th-century home that belongs to the National Trust and now houses an art gallery. From there, walk east on York Street, then turn right on
5 Princess Street for the **Old State House,** Bermuda's oldest surviving building. The first building on the island constructed entirely of native limestone, the State House was built in the Italianate style because Governor Butler believed Bermuda to be on the same latitude as Italy. *Admission free. Open Wed. 10–4.*

Heading back up Princess Street, you'll come to York Street
6 and the entrance to **Somers Garden,** created out of a former
7 swampland. On Kent Street is the **Historical Society,** a museum, set in a 1725 home, that shows how Bermudians lived more than
8 two centuries ago. Continue up the hill to the **Unfinished Church.** It was begun in 1874 as a replacement for St. Peter's Church, but work was abandoned in 1899 so that the funds could be used to rebuild the church in Hamilton, which had been destroyed by fire. In 1992, the church was acquired by the Bermuda National Trust, which will stabilize and preserve

it; it may eventually be used as a backdrop for theatrical productions.

9 Walk west on Governor's Alley, turn left onto Clarence Street, then right onto Church Street. Here is the churchyard of **St. Peter's,** the site of the oldest Anglican church in the Western Hemisphere. The tombstones offer a fascinating lesson in social history.

West of St. Peter's are two interesting lanes leading down to York Street. Silk Alley, also called Petticoat Lane, got its name in 1834 when two newly emancipated slave girls walked down the street with their new, rustling silk petticoats. The other is called Old Maid's Lane because some spinsters lived along here a century ago.

10 Head toward the harbor and you will come to Water Street, boasting one of the town's most historic homes. When the **President Henry Tucker House** was built in 1711, it was not hanging over the street, as it is today, but faced a broad expanse of lawn that went down to the harbor. The house was acquired in 1775 by Henry Tucker, who was president of the town council during the American Revolution and whose family was divided over the conflict. *Admission: $3. Open weekdays 10–5.*

11 Across the street is the **Carriage Museum,** where you can spend an hour admiring the custom-built vehicles that traveled along the island's roads before the automobile arrived in 1946. *Admission free. Open weekdays 10–4.*

12 Back along Water Street is the post office, facing King's Square. The pink structure on the corner of the block is the **Confederate Museum** and site of the old Globe Hotel. During the U.S. Civil War, this part of the island sided with the southern Confederates for economic reasons. The town of St. George became the focus of gun-running between the Southern United States and Europe. *Admission: $3. Open Mon.–Sat. 10–5.*

Exploring the Until the mid-1950s the West End was a working dockyard of
West End the British Royal Navy, which still keeps a presence here. The area is now a shopping/sightseeing minivillage for tourists.

The **Maritime Museum,** in the inner fortifications of the Royal Naval Dockyard is the most spectacular of the restored buildings and presents exhibits of Bermuda's seagoing history.

A self-guided tour of the indoor/outdoor museum starts in the **Queen's Exhibition Hall,** originally built in 1850 to store gunpowder, and continues to the gun emplacements that surround the dockyard. Exhibits in the museum's several buildings include relics from shipwrecks, ship models, Bermuda Fitted Dinghies, SCUBA-diving equipment, a Treasure House, and an Age of Discovery Exhibit, which was unveiled by Diego Colón in October 1992. *Admission: $6 adults, $2 children under 12. Open daily 10–4:30.*

Across the street from the Maritime Museum, the old Cooperage now houses the **Neptune Cinema,** which shows first-run films from the United States and Europe, and the Frog & Onion Pub (*See* Dining, below). *Admission: $2.50 adults, $1.50 children.*

The **Crafts Market,** in the adjacent Bermuda Arts Centre, displays local crafts in informal stalls. The Dockyard also has two nightclubs, branches of stores in Hamilton, and stalls selling ice cream and pizza. In the nearby village of Somerset are more restaurants and branch shops of the main department stores in Hamilton.

Shopping There is no sales tax in Bermuda—the price you see is what you pay. This is a place to shop for luxury items, and topping the list of good buys are cashmere sweaters, bone china, Irish linens, Scottish tweeds, perfumes, and liquor. Local handicrafts include pottery, cedar ware, and paintings by local artists.

Hamilton The majority of stores are located on Front Street and in the arcades of Reid Street. Bermuda's top three department stores, all located on Front Street, Hamilton, are **H.A.&E. Smith's, A.S. Cooper,** and **Trimingham's.** Each is a full-service department store, with good buys in cashmere and woolens. Smith's is arguably the best men's clothier in Bermuda.

Archie Brown & Son, on Front Street, carries higher-priced cashmere sweaters, while several outlets of **The English Shop** stock some of Britain's finest woolens, particularly men's sports coats.

Fine jewelry and gems can be found in **Solomon's** (17 Front St.), and at several locations of **Crisson's** and of **Astwood-Dickinson.** The best for fine china is **William Bluck & Co.** on both Front and Reid Streets.

St. George's **Frangipani** is one of St. George's best shops, selling clothes from Greece, Hawaii, and Bali; the cotton sweaters from Greece are a must. On Somers Wharf, off Water Street, **The Cow Polly** has reasonable buys in cashmeres and **Constable's of Bermuda** has heavy Icelandic woolens in smoky colors.

Sports Fishing is excellent in Bermuda, with numerous boats going
Fishing out from just about every marina on the island. Do some comparison shopping at the tourist information office or booth. Or contact the **Bermuda Charter Fishing Boat Association** (tel. 809/292–6246), the **Bermuda Sport Fishing Association** (tel. 809/295–2370), or **St. George's Game Fishing & Cruising Association** (tel. 809/297–1622).

Golf Bermuda has eight golf courses; some require an introduction.

Horseback Riding The "breakfast rides" at the **Spicelands Riding Centre** (tel. 809/238–8212), on Middle Road in Warwick, are an invigorating way to start a Bermuda day. Reservations are a must. Riders should wear sneakers or boots; hats are provided.

Water Sports Bermuda's clear waters are perfect for scuba diving, helmet diving, and snorkeling. Check at the tourist information booth or office about which operators are offering dives and snorkel tours. Excellent programs are offered at **Southampton Princess, Sonesta Beach Hotel,** and **Grotto Bay Hotel.**

The tourist submarine *Enterprise* (tel. 809/234–3547), which operates out of Dockyard, takes passengers for a look at the coral reefs of the Sea Gardens.

Waterskiing is allowed only in certain protected waters, and by law can be offered only by licensed skippers. **Bermuda Waterskiing** (Grotto Bay Beach Hotel, tel. 809/293–3328) and **Bermuda Waterski Centre** (Robinson's Marina, Somerset, tel. 809/234–3354) both offer lessons and outings.

Windsurfers should contact **Mangrove Marina Ltd.** (Mangrove Bay, Somerset, tel. 809/234–0914), **Salt Kettle Boat Rentals Ltd.** in Paget Parish (tel. 809/236–4863 or 809/236–3612), and **South Side Scuba Water Sports** (Grotto Bay Beach Hotel and Marriott's Castle Harbour Resort, tel. 809/293–2915). Board rental is $15 an hour; 1½-hour lessons are $50.

Beaches Bermuda has some of the most beautiful beaches in the world. The cream of the crop are along the south shore from Southampton to Tucker's Town: **Horseshoe Bay, Chaplin Bay, Stonehole Bay, Jobson's Cove, Warwick Long Bay,** and **Elbow Beach.** Some are long sweeps of unbroken pink sand; others are divided by low coral cliffs into protected little coves. All are easily accessible by bicycle, moped, or taxi.

Dining Many restaurants require gentlemen to wear a jacket and tie, and women to be appropriately dressed. When the gratuity is not included in the bill, an overall tip of 10%–15% is the accepted amount. Reservations are recommended for most restaurants.

Category	Cost*
Very Expensive	over $40
Expensive	$30–$40
Moderate	$20–$30
Inexpensive	under $20

per person, excluding drinks, service, and sales tax

Fourways Inn. At the very top of fine dining in Bermuda is this gourmet restaurant in an 18th-century Georgian home. The menu is impressive; specialties include fresh mussels simmered in white wine and cream, fresh veal sautéed in lemon butter, Caesar salad, and strawberry soufflé. The wine list is excellent. A gourmet brunch is offered on Sunday. *Paget, tel. 809/236–6517. Reservations suggested. Gratuity added to the bill. AE, MC, V. Very Expensive.*

Once Upon a Table. Many locals consider this the finest restaurant on Bermuda. In an 18th-century home, dinner becomes theater, with costumes and setting creating a sense of a bygone era. Rack of lamb, roast duckling, and pork are served on elegant china. *Serpentine Rd., Hamilton, tel. 809/295–8585. Reservations recommended. Jacket and tie required. Dinner only. AE, DC, MC, V. Very Expensive.*

Pub on the Square. Smack on King's Square in St. George, this British-style pub is nothing fancy but offers cool draft beer, juicy hamburgers, and fish and chips. *King's Sq., St. George, tel. 809/297–1522. AE, MC, V. Moderate.*

Frog & Onion. An instant hit with locals when it opened in 1992, this pub-style eatery is housed in one of Dockyard's restored 19th-century buildings. Despite its cavernous size and soaring ceilings, the restaurant manages a cozy ambience, thanks in part to subdued lighting. Seafood and pub-grub are recommended over the steak offerings. *Cooperage Building, Dockyard, tel. 809/234–2900. Reservations required. MC, V. Moderate.*

Caribbean

Nowhere in the world are conditions better suited for cruising than in the ever-warm, treasure-filled Caribbean Sea, which attains incomparable shades of blue. Tiny island nations, within easy sailing distance of one another, form a chain of tropical enchantment that curves from Cuba in the north all the way down to the coast of Venezuela. There is far more to life here than sand and coconuts, however. The islands are vastly different, with their own cultures, topographies, and languages. Colonialism has left its mark, and the presence of the Spanish, French, Dutch, Danish, and British is still felt. Slavery, too, has left its cultural legacy, blending African overtones into the colonial/Indian amalgam. The one constant, however, is the weather. Despite the islands' southerly position, the climate is surprisingly gentle, due in large part to the cooling influence of the trade winds.

The Caribbean is made up of the Greater Antilles and the Lesser Antilles. The former consists of those islands closest to the United States: Cuba, Jamaica, Hispaniola (Haiti and the Dominican Republic), and Puerto Rico. (The Cayman Islands lie south of Cuba.) The Lesser Antilles, including the Virgin, Windward, and Leeward islands and others, are greater in number but smaller in size, and constitute the southern half of the Caribbean chain. Most cruise lines include Caracas, Venezuela, and the east coast of Mexico in their Caribbean itineraries as well.

More cruise ships ply these waters than any others in the world. In peak season, it is not uncommon for several ships to disgorge thousands of passengers into a small town on the same day—a phenomenon not always enjoyed by locals.

Despite some overcrowding, however, the plethora of cruise ships in the area also allows you to pick and choose the one with the itinerary that best suits you. Whether it's shopping or scuba diving, fishing or sunbathing, you're sure to find the Caribbean cruise of your dreams.

When to Go Average year-round temperatures throughout the Caribbean are 78°F–85°F, with a low of 65 and a high of 95; downtown shopping areas seem *always* to be unbearably hot. High season runs from December 15 to April 14; during this most fashionable, most expensive, and most crowded time to go, reservations up to a year in advance are necessary for many ships. For some, a summer visit may be even better: Temperatures are virtually the same as in winter (even cooler on average than in parts of the U.S. mainland), island flora is at its height, and the water is smoother and clearer. Some tourist facilities close down in summer, however, and many ships move to Europe, Alaska, or the northeastern United States.

Hurricane season runs from August through October. Although cruise ships stay well out of the way of these storms, they can affect the weather throughout the Caribbean for days, and damage to ports can force last-minute itinerary changes.

Currency Currencies vary throughout the islands, but U.S. dollars are widely accepted. Don't bother changing more than a few dollars into local currency for phone calls, tips, and taxis.

Passports and Visas In general, American citizens need only proof of identity and nationality (two pieces of I.D., including a passport) to travel through the Caribbean; British travelers need a passport. For island specifics, *see* individual port sections, *below*.

Shore Excursions Typically, these include a bus tour of the island or town, a visit to a local beach or liquor factory, boat trips, snorkeling or diving, and charter fishing. As far as island tours go, it's always safest to take a ship-arranged excursion, but it's almost never cheapest, and you sacrifice enjoying your own space, your own pace, and the joys of venturing off the beaten path.

If you seek adventure, find a knowledgeable taxi driver or tour operator—they're usually within a stone's throw of the pier— and wander around on your own. A group of four to six people will find this option more economical and practical than will a single person or a couple.

Renting a car is also a good option on many islands—again, the more people, the better the deal. But get a good island map before you set off, and be sure to find out how long it will take you to get around. The boat will leave without you unless you're on a ship-arranged tour.

Conditions are ideal for water sports of all kinds, and excursions offering scuba diving, snorkeling, windsurfing, sailing, waterskiing, and fishing abound. Your shore-excursion director can also arrange these activities for you individually if no formal excursion is offered.

Many ships give beach parties on a private island or an isolated beach in the Bahamas, the Grenadines, or (depending on the current political climate) Haiti. These parties are either included in your fare, with snorkeling gear and other water-sports equipment extra, or offered as an optional tour for which you pay. Rarely do these excursions exceed your expectations—they're sure to deliver fun in the sun, but don't expect a private beach party to be the highlight of any worthwhile cruise.

Golf and tennis are popular draws on shore, and several ships offer special packages. Most golf courses rent clubs.

Dining Cuisine on these islands is hard to classify. The region's history as a colonial battleground and ethnic melting pot creates plenty of variety. The gourmet French delicacies of Martinique, for example, are far removed from the hearty Spanish casseroles of Puerto Rico and even further from the pungent curries of Trinidad.

The one quality that defines most Caribbean cooking is its essential spiciness. Seafood is naturally quite popular. Some of it is even unique to the region, such as Caribbean lobster: Clawless and tougher than other types, it is more like crawfish than Maine lobster. And no island menu is complete without at least a half-dozen dishes featuring conch, a mollusk biologically similar to escargots that is served in the form of chowder, fritters, salad, and cocktail. Dress is generally casual—though in Caracas men should not wear shorts.

The Caribbean

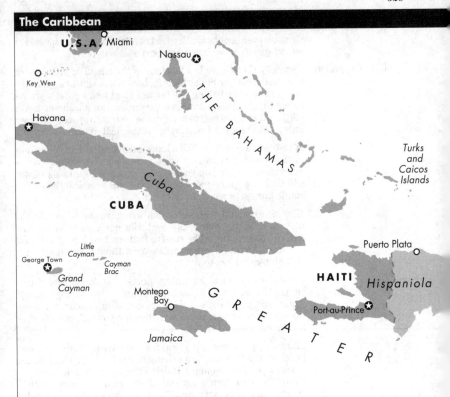

U.S.A. Miami

Key West

Nassau

THE BAHAMAS

Turks and Caicos Islands

Havana

Cuba

CUBA

Little Cayman

George Town

Cayman Brac

Grand Cayman

Montego Bay

GREATER

Jamaica

Puerto Plata

HAITI

Hispaniola

Port-au-Prince

Caribbean

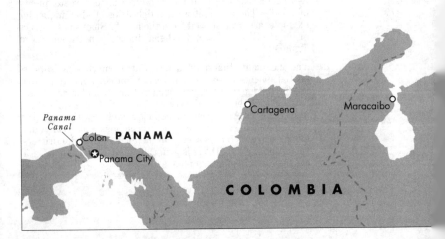

Panama Canal

Colon

PANAMA

Panama City

Cartagena

Maracaibo

COLOMBIA

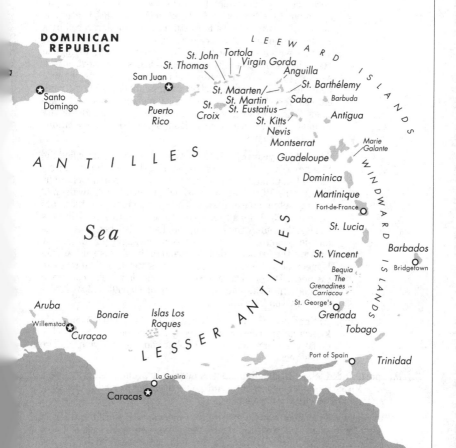

Category	Cost*
Expensive	over $25
Moderate	$15–$25
Inexpensive	under $15

per person for a three-course meal, excluding drinks, service, and sales tax

Antigua

Some say Antigua has so many beaches that you could visit a different one every day for a year. Most have snow-white sand, and many are backed by lavish resorts offering sailing, diving, windsurfing, and snorkeling.

The larger of the British Leeward Islands, Antigua was the headquarters from which Lord Horatio Nelson made his forays against the French and pirates in the late 18th century. A decidedly British atmosphere still prevails, underscored by a collection of pubs that will raise the spirits of every Anglophile. Visitors with a taste for history will want to explore English Harbour and its carefully restored Nelson's Dockyard, as well as tour an 18th-century Royal Naval base, old forts, historic churches, and tiny villages. Hikers can wander through a tropical rain forest lush with pineapples, banana trees, and mangoes. Those of an archaeological bent will head for the megaliths of Greencastle to seek out some of the 30 excavations of ancient Indian sites.

About 4,000 years ago Antigua was home to a people called the Siboney. They disappeared mysteriously, and the island remained uninhabited for about 1,000 years. When Columbus sighted the 108-square-mile island in 1493, the Arawaks had already set up housekeeping. The English moved in 130 years later, in 1623. Then a sequence of bloody battles involving the Caribs, the Dutch, the French, and the English began. Africans had been captured as slaves to work the sugar plantations by the time the French ceded the island to the English in 1667. On November 1, 1981, Antigua, with its sister island 30 miles to the north, Barbuda, achieved full independence. The combined population of the two islands is about 90,000—only 1,200 of whom live on Barbuda.

Currency Antigua uses the Eastern Caribbean (E.C.) dollar, commonly known as beewees. Figure about E.C. $2.60 to U.S. $1. U.S. dollars are generally accepted, but you may get your change in beewees.

Passports and Visas U.S. and Canadian citizens need only proof of identity, but a passport is preferred. A driver's license is not sufficient. British citizens need a passport.

Telephones and Mail The phone system in Antigua is notorious. If possible, call from your next port. In an emergency you can make calls at Cable & Wireless (WI) Ltd., 42–44 St. Mary's Street, St. John's; and at Nelson's Dockyard, English Harbour. AT&T's USADIRECT is available from only a few designated telephones, such as those at the cruise terminal at St. John's, English Harbour Marina, the Pineapple Beach Club, and the Sugar Mill Hotel. New public telephones accept a phone card (purchased at post offices) that, acting like a prepaid credit card, permits local and international calls. Airmail letters to North America cost E.C. 60¢; postcards, E.C. 40¢. The post office is at the foot of High Street in St. John's.

Shore Excursions *Not all excursions listed are offered by all cruise lines. All times and prices are approximate.*

Jolly Roger Cruise: A boat/beach party includes snorkeling near an old shipwreck, a limbo contest, and a free open bar. Tends to be rather raucous and boozy. *3 hrs. Cost: $24–$38. Some ships offer a 5-hr. lunch cruise: $55.*

Nelson's Dockyard and Clarence House: Driving through Antigua's lush countryside, you will visit the 18th-century residence of the duke of Clarence. Then visit Nelson's Dockyard, a gem of Georgian British maritime architecture and a must for history buffs and Anglophiles. *3 hrs. Cost: $22–$28.*

If you want to feel like Indiana Jones, opt for a tour with **Tropikelly** (tel. 809/461–0383). You'll be given an insider's look at the whole island by four-wheel-drive, complete with deserted plantation houses, rain forest trails, ruined sugar mills and forts, and even a picnic lunch with drinks. The highlight is the luxuriant tropical forest around the island's highest point, Boggy Peak. *Cost: $55.*

Getting Around Though some ships dock at the deep-water harbor in downtown St. John's, most use the town's Heritage Quay, a multimillion-dollar complex with shops, condominiums, a casino, and a food court. Most St. John's attractions are an easy walk from Heritage Quay. A tourist information booth is in the main docking building.

By Bus Avoid public buses. They're unreliable and hard to find.

By Car To rent a car, you'll need a valid driver's license and a temporary permit, which is available through the rental agent for $12. Rentals average about $35–$50 per day, with unlimited mileage. *Driving is on the left,* and Antiguan roads are generally unmarked and full of potholes. Rental agencies are on High Street in St. John's, or they can be called from the terminal. Contact **Antours** (tel. 809/462–4788), **Budget** (tel. 809/462–3009 or 800/527–0700), **Carib Car Rentals** (tel. 809/462–2062), or **National** (tel. 809/462–2113 or 800/468–0008), all in St. John's.

By Taxi Taxis meet every cruise ship. They are unmetered; fares are fixed, and drivers are required to carry a rate card. A 10% tip is expected. All taxi drivers double as guides, and you can arrange an island tour for about $20 an hour. The most reliable and informed driver-guides are at **Capital Car Rental** (High St., St. John's, tel. 809/462–0863).

Exploring Antigua *Numbers in the margin correspond to numbered points of interest on the Antigua map.*

Ships dock at **Heritage Quay.** To the south, **Redcliffe Quay** is an attractive waterfront marketplace with shops, restaurants, and boutiques. Long ago, Africans were held on this site prior to being sold as slaves. At the far south end of town, where Market Street forks into Valley and All Saints roads, locals jam the marketplace every Friday and Saturday to buy and sell fruits, vegetables, fish, and spices. Be sure to ask before you aim a camera, and expect the subject of your shot to ask for a tip.

332

Antigua

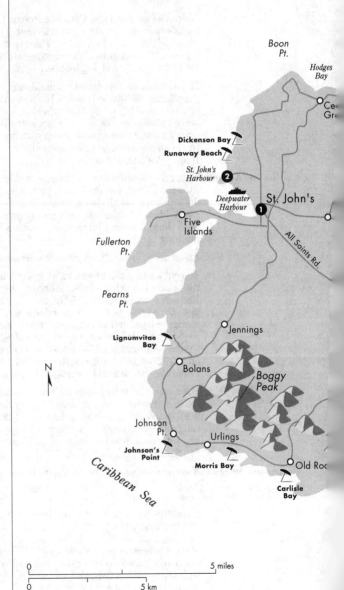

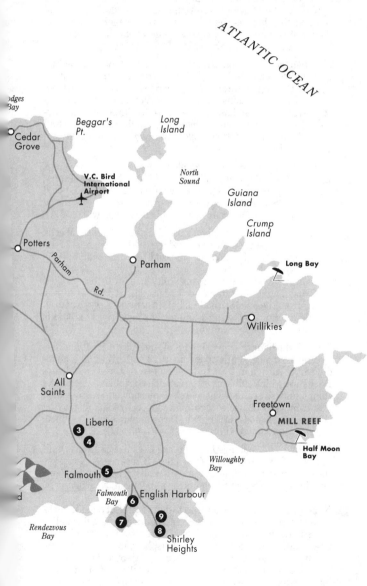

ATLANTIC OCEAN

odges
Bay

Cedar
Grove

Beggar's
Pt.

Long
Island

V.C. Bird
International
Airport

North
Sound

Guiana
Island

Crump
Island

Long Bay

Potters

Parham

Parham

Rd.

Willikies

All
Saints

Freetown

MILL REEF

Liberta

③
④

Half Moon
Bay

Falmouth ⑤

Falmouth
Bay

English Harbour

⑥

Willoughby
Bay

⑨

⑦

⑧

Rendezvous
Bay

Shirley
Heights

Guadeloupe Passage

KEY

Cruise Ship

❶ It's an eight-block trek from Heritage Quay to the older part of **St. John's,** home to about 40,000 people (nearly half the island's population). The city has seen better days, but it's currently receiving a face-lift, and there are some notable sights. Before you set out on your walk, stop at the **Tourist Bureau** in the main building of Heritage Quay for maps and information.

If you've a serious interest in archaeology, see the historical displays at the **Museum of Antigua and Barbuda.** The colonial building that houses the museum is the former courthouse, which dates from 1750. *Church and Market Sts. Admission free. Open weekdays 8:30–4, Sat. 10–1.*

Walk two blocks east on Church Street to **St. John's Cathedral.** The Anglican church sits on a hilltop, surrounded by its churchyard. At the south gate are figures said to have been taken from one of Napoleon's ships. A previous structure on this site was destroyed by an earthquake in 1843, so the interior of the current church is completely encased in pitch pine to forestall heavy damage from future quakes. *Between Long and Newcastle Sts. Admission free.*

❷ A favorite car excursion is to follow Fort Road northwest out of town. After 2 miles you'll come to the ruins of **Ft. James,** named for King James II. If you continue on this road, you'll arrive at **Dickenson Bay,** with its string of smart, expensive resorts on one of the many beautiful beaches you will pass.

❸ Eight miles south of St. John's on All Saints Road is **Liberta,** one of the first settlements founded by freed slaves. East of the **❹** village, on Monk's Hill, are the ruins of **Ft. George,** built in 1669.

❺ **Falmouth,** 1½ miles farther south, sits on a lovely bay, backed by former sugar plantations and sugar mills. **St. Paul's Church,** dating from the late 18th and early 19th centuries, was a church for the military in Nelson's time; it has been restored and is now used for Sunday worship.

❻ **English Harbour,** the most famous of Antigua's attractions, lies on the coast just south of Falmouth. The Royal Navy aban-**❼** doned the station in 1889, but it has been restored as **Nelson's Dockyard,** which epitomizes the colonial Caribbean. Within the compound are crafts shops, hotels, a marina, and restaurants. The **Admiral's House Museum** has several rooms displaying ship models, a model of English Harbour, and various artifacts from Nelson's days. *Admission: $2 per vehicle. Open daily 8–6.*

On a ridge overlooking the dockyard is **Clarence House,** built in 1787 and once the home of the duke of Clarence. As you leave the dockyard, turn right at the crossroads in English Harbour **❽** and drive up to **Shirley Heights** for a spectacular harbor view.

❾ Nearby, the **Dows Hill Interpretation Center** opened in 1993, chronicling the island's history and culture from Amerindian times to the present. A highlight of the center is its multimedia presentation in which illuminated displays, incorporating lifelike figures and colorful tableaux, are presented with running commentary, television, and music—resulting in a cheery, if bland, portrait of Antiguan life. *Admission: E.C. $15. Open daily 9–5.*

Shopping   **Redcliffe Quay** and **Heritage Quay** are waterfront markets with boutiques, restaurants, and snack bars. The main tourist shops in St. John's are along **St. Mary's, High,** and **Long streets.** In general, shops are open Monday–Saturday 8:30–noon and 1–4; some shops close for the day at noon on Thursday and Saturday. The duty-free shops of Heritage Quay cater to tourists and often have more flexible hours; however, the price of real estate here boosts the price of merchandise, so you may find better deals at Redcliffe Quay. In downtown St. John's, hand-printed fabrics with original designs by George Kelsick are at **Kel-Print** (St. Mary's St.). Also on St. Mary's Street, **The Map Shop** has a wonderful collection of antique maps and nautical books and charts, and **Coco Shop** sells Sea Island cotton designs, Daks clothing, and Liberty of London fabrics. **The Cigar Shop** (Heritage Quay) has Cuban cigars.

At Redcliffe Quay: Antiguan pottery is sold in **The Pottery Shop.** For batiks, sarongs, and swimwear, try **A Thousand Flowers. Things Antiguan** is a source for local crafts. **Karibbean Kids** has great gifts for the younger set, and **Windjammer Clothing** sells nautically inspired attire for men and women. For cooling down, **Ye Olde Coffee Shop** serves ice cream in an 1881 building. Off the little grassy square where Africans were once penned is **Bona,** which has fine Italian china.

Sports You'll find an 18-hole course at **Cedar Valley Golf Club** (tel.
Golf 809/462–0161) and a nine-hole course at **Half Moon Bay Hotel** (tel. 809/460–4300).

Scuba Diving Antigua has plenty of wrecks, reefs, and marine life. Contact **Dive Antigua** (tel. 809/462–3483) or **Aquanaut Dive Center** (tel. 809/462–3483). **Dockyard Divers** (St. Johns, tel. 809/464–8591), run by British ex–merchant seaman Captain A. G. Finchman, is one of the oldest and most reputable diving and snorkeling outfits on the island.

Beaches Antigua's 366 beaches are public, and many are dotted with resorts that provide water-sports equipment rentals and a place to grab a cool drink. Since most hotels have taxi stands, you can get back to the ship easily. The following are just a few excellent possibilities: **Carlisle Bay,** where the Atlantic meets the Caribbean Sea, is a long, snow-white beach over which the Curtain Bluff resort sits. A large coconut grove adds to its tropical beauty. **Dickenson Bay** has a lengthy stretch of powder-soft white sand and a host of hotels that cater to water-sports enthusiasts. **Half Moon Bay,** a three-quarter-mile crescent of shell-pink sand, is a great place for snorkeling and windsurfing. The Half Moon Bay hotel will let you borrow gear with a refundable deposit. **Johnsons Point** is a deliciously deserted beach of bleached white sand on the southwest coast.

Dining *In restaurants a 10% service charge is usually added to the bill.*

Jumby Bay. This 300-acre private island retreat can be reached by traveling 30 minutes by cab from St. John's and then 15 minutes on the launch. A limited number of lunch and dinner reservations are accepted. An extensive buffet luncheon with complimentary wine and launch service is $55 per person. The dinner menu continually changes, but you might find sautéed breast of chicken filled with wild mushrooms, Mediterranean seafood terrine sprinkled with saffron, or a soufflé of scallops with basil purée. *Tel. 809/462–6000. Reservations required. Closed Sept.–Oct. AE, MC, V. Expensive.*

The Admiral's Inn. Known simply as "The Ad" to yachtsmen around the world, this historic inn in the heart of English Harbour is a must for Anglophiles and mariners. Dine on curried conch, fresh snapper with lime, or lobster thermidor while taking in the splendid harbor views. *Nelson's Dockyard, tel. 809/460–1027. Reservations required. AE, MC, V. Moderate.*

Coconut Grove. There are few more pleasant eateries on the island than this waterfront spot at the Siboney Beach Club. With the coconut palms growing up through the roof and the waves lapping on the white coral sand a few feet away, you'll feel as though you're in the South Seas. The Trinidad-born chef makes good use of local produce, though the menu is mainstream European. *Dickenson Bay, tel. 809/462–1538. Reservations advised. MC, V. Moderate.*

Shirley Heights Lookout. This restaurant is in part of an 18th-century fortification; the view of English Harbour below is breathtaking. The breezy pub downstairs opens onto the lookout point, and upstairs is a cozy, bright room with hardwood floors and beam ceilings. Pub offerings include burgers, sandwiches, and barbecue, while the upstairs room serves such fare as pumpkin soup and lobster in lime sauce. *Shirley Heights, tel. 809/463–1785. Reservations required in season. AE, MC, V. Moderate.*

Aruba

Though the "A" in the ABC (Aruba, Bonaire, Curaçao) Islands is small—only 19.6 miles long and 6 miles at its widest—the island's national anthem proclaims "the greatness of our people is their great cordiality," and this is no exaggeration. Once a member of the Netherlands Antilles, Aruba became independent within the Netherlands in 1986, with its own royally appointed governor, a democratic government, and a 21-member elected parliament. Long secure in a solid economy, with good education, housing, and health care, the island's population of about 70,000 regards tourists as welcome guests and treats them accordingly. Waiters serve you with smiles and solid eye contact. English is spoken everywhere. Aruba has recently seen a huge boom in cruise traffic and is now the home base to Seawind's *Seawind Crown* and Dolphin's *Oceanbreeze.*

The island's distinctive beauty lies in the stark contrast between the sea and the countryside: rocky deserts, cactus jungles, secluded coves, and aquamarine panoramas with crashing waves.

Currency Arubans accept U.S. dollars, so you've no need to exchange money, except for pocket change for cigarettes, bus fare, or pay phones. Local currency is the Aruban florin (AFl). At press time, U.S. $1 will get you AFl 1.77 cash, or AFl 1.79 in traveler's checks. Note that the Netherlands Antilles florin used in Bonaire and Curaçao is not accepted on Aruba.

Passports and Visas U.S. and Canadian residents need only proof of identity—a valid passport, original birth certificate, naturalization certificate, green card, valid nonquota immigration visa, or valid voter registration card. Other foreigners must have a valid passport.

Telephones and Mail International calls are placed at the Government Long Distance Office, which is in the post office in Oranjestad. To reach the United States, dial 011, area code, and the local number. An airmail letter from Aruba to anywhere in the world costs AFl 1, a postcard AFl .70.

Shore Excursions *Not all shore excursions listed are offered by all cruise lines. All times and prices are approximate.*

Boats and Beaches **Atlantis Submarines** (Seaport Village Marina, tel. 297/8–36090) operates a 65-foot modern, air-conditioned sub that takes 46 passengers 50–90 feet below the surface along Aruba's Barcadera Reef. *50 minutes. Cost: $68.*

Glass-Bottom Boat Tour: A 60-passenger vessel (some with cash bar) allows you to view Aruba's extensive underwater life. *2 hrs. Cost: $21.*

Trimaran Sailing Booze Cruise: This cruise has an open bar serving rum punch, fruit punch, and soft drinks. *2 hrs. Cost: $29.*

Snorkeling Beach Party: Boat to a beach where equipment and instruction are provided. *3–4 hrs. Cost: $25–$40.*

Cultural **Aruba Town and Countryside Drive:** A comprehensive town-and-country bus tour. When the bus sets off to return to the ship, passengers may choose to stay in town, on the beach, or at the casino, returning to the pier by taxi. *3 hrs. Cost: $19.*

Getting Around Ships tie up at the Aruba Port Authority cruise terminal; inside is a tourist information booth. From here, you're a five-minute walk from various shopping districts and downtown Oranjestad.

By Bus Buses run hourly between the beach hotels and Oranjestad. They also stop across the street from the terminal on L.G. Smith Boulevard. The fare is $1.50, exact change.

By Car It's easy to rent a car, jeep, or motorbike in Aruba, and most roads are in excellent condition. Contact **Avis** (tel. 297/8–28787), **Budget** (tel. 297/8–28600), or **Hertz** (tel. 297/8–24400).

By Taxi A dispatch office is located at Alhambra Bazaar and Casino (tel. 297/8–22116). Taxis can also be flagged down on the street. Because taxis have no meters, rates are fixed but should be confirmed before you get in. All drivers have participated in the government's Tourism Awareness Programs and have received a Tourism Guide Certificate. An hour tour of the island by taxi will cost about $30 for up to four people.

Exploring Aruba *Numbers in the margin correspond to numbered points of interest on the Aruba map.*

❶ Aruba's charming capital, **Oranjestad,** is best explored on foot. From the terminal walk up Shuttestraat from where it meets the boulevard to the traffic circle. Bear left, then turn right on Kazernestraat. Continue until you get to Caya G.F. Betico Croes, Oranjestad's main shopping street.

If you're interested in Dutch architecture, walk back to the corner of Oude School Straat and go three blocks south (toward the harbor) to Wilhelminastraat, where some of the buildings date back to Oranjestad's 1790 founding. Walk west and you'll pass old homes, a government building, and the Protestant church. When you reach Shuttestraat again, turn left and go one block south to Zoutmanstraat. The small **Archaeology Museum** here has two rooms of Indian artifacts, farm and domes-

Aruba

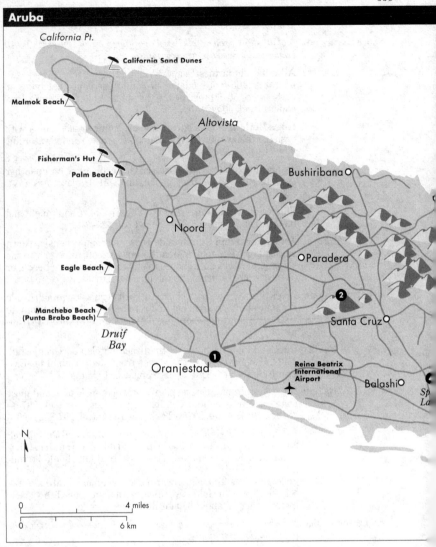

California Pt.

California Sand Dunes

Malmok Beach

Altovista

Fisherman's Hut

Palm Beach

Bushiribana○

○Noord

○Paradera

Eagle Beach

❷

Manchebo Beach
(Punta Brabo Beach)

Santa Cruz○

*Druif
Bay*

❶

Oranjestad

Reina Beatrix
International
Airport

Balashi○

N

0 _____ 4 miles

0 _____ 6 km

Balashi Gold
Mine, **4**
Frenchman's Pass, **3**
Hooiberg (Haystack
Hill), **2**
Oranjestad, **1**
San Nicolas, **6**
Spanish Lagoon, **5**

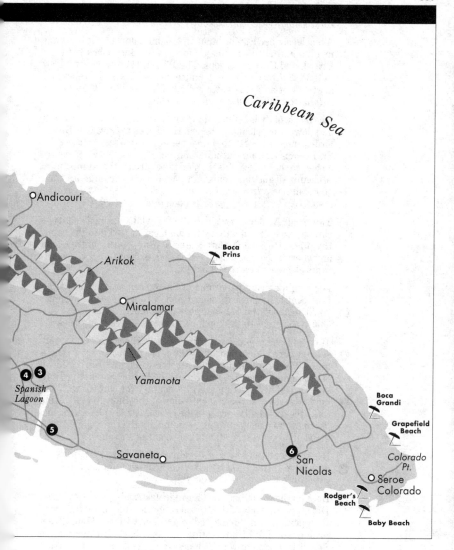

tic utensils, and skeletons. *Zoutmanstraat 1, tel. 297/8–28979. Admission free. Open weekdays 8–noon and 1:30–4:30.*

A block east lies **Ft. Zoutman,** the island's oldest building, built in 1796 and used as a major fortress in skirmishes between British and Curaçao troops. The Willem III tower was added in 1868. The fort's Historicalmuseum displays island relics and artifacts in an 18th-century Aruban house. *Tel. 297/8–26099. Admission: $1. Open weekdays 9–noon and 1–4.*

One block south is **Wilhelmina Park,** a small grove of palm trees and flowers overlooking the sea. Head back to Caya G.F. Betico Croes and turn north to the corner of Hendrikstraat to see the **St. Francis Roman Catholic Church.** The post office is cater-corner to the church. Just behind the church is the **Numismatic Museum,** displaying coins and paper money from more than 400 countries. *Iraussquinplein 2–A, tel. 297/8–28831. Admission free. Open weekdays 8:30–noon and 1:30–4:30.*

The "real" Aruba—or what's left of its wild, untamed beauty— can be experienced only by taking a car or taxi into the countryside. (Be aware that there are no public bathrooms anywhere once you leave Oranjestad, except in a few restaurants elsewhere on the island.)

For a shimmering panorama of blue-green sea, drive east on L.G. Smith Boulevard toward San Nicolas. Past the airport, ❷ you'll soon see the 541-foot peak of **Hooiberg** (Haystack Hill). Climb 562 steps to the top for an impressive view of the city.

Turn left where you see the drive-in theater. At the first inter- ❸ section, turn right, then follow the curve to the right to **Frenchman's Pass,** a dark, luscious stretch of highway arbored by overhanging trees. Legend claims the French and native Indians warred here during the 17th century for control of the island. ❹ Nearby are the cement ruins of the **Balashi Gold Mine** (take the dirt road veering to the right), a lovely place to picnic, listen to the parakeets, and contemplate the towering cacti. A gnarled divi-divi tree stands guard at the entrance.

Backtrack all the way to the main road (back past the drive-in) ❺ and drive through the area called **Spanish Lagoon,** where pirates once hid to repair their ships.

❻ Back on the main road, visit **San Nicolas,** Aruba's oldest village. During the heyday of the Exxon refineries, the town was a bustling port; now it's dedicated to tourism, with the Main Street promenade full of interesting kiosks. **Charlie's Bar** on Main Street is a popular tourist lunch spot, good for both gawking at the thousands of license plates, old credit cards, baseball pennants, and hardhats covering every inch of the walls and ceiling, and for gorging on "jumbo and dumbo" shrimp.

Shopping Caya G.F. Betico Croes in Oranjestad is Aruba's chief shopping street. The stores are full of Dutch porcelains and figurines, as befits the island's Netherlands heritage. Also consider the Dutch cheeses (you are allowed to bring up to one pound of hard cheese through U.S. Customs), hand-embroidered linens, and any product made from the native plant aloe vera, such as sunburn cream, face masks, and skin fresheners. There is no sales tax, and Arubans consider it rude to haggle.

Artesania Arubiano (L.G. Smith Blvd. 47, next to the Aruba Tourism Authority) has charming home-crafted pottery and

folk objets d'art. **Aruba Trading Company** (Caya G.F. Betico
Croes 14) offers brand names at 30% discounts offers 30% discounts on brand-name perfumes and cosmetics (first floor),
jewelry (second floor), men's and women's clothes, and liqueurs. **Gandleman's Jewelers** (Caya G.F. Betico Croes 5–A)
sells jewelry, including a full line of watches.

Sports Contact **De Palm Tours** (L.G. Smith Blvd. 142, Oranjestad, tel.
Fishing 297/8–24400).

Golf The **Aruba Golf Club** (Golfweg 82, near San Nicolas, tel. 297/8–
42006) has a nine-hole course with 25 sand traps, roaming
goats, and lots of cacti. Greens fees are $7.50 for nine holes, $10
for 18. Golf carts and clubs can be rented.

Hiking **De Palm Tours** (tel. 297/8–24400) offers a guided three-hour
trip to remote sites of unusual natural beauty accessible only
on foot. The fee is $25 per person, including refreshments and
transportation; a minimum of four people is required.

Horseback Riding At **Rancho El Paso** (tel. 297/8–23310), one-hour jaunts ($15)
take you through countryside flanked by cacti, divi-divi trees,
and aloe vera plants; two-hour trips ($30) go to the beach as
well. Wear lots of sunblock.

Water Sports **De Palm Tours** (L.G. Smith Blvd. 142, Box 656, Oranjestad, tel.
297/8–24400) has a near monopoly on all water sports, including
equipment and instruction for scuba, snorkeling, and windsurfing. **Pelican Watersports** (Box 1193, Oranjestad, tel. 297/8–
31228) offers water-sports packages, including snorkeling,
sailing, windsurfing, fishing, and scuba.

Beaches Beaches in Aruba are not only beautiful but clean. On the north
side the water is too choppy for swimming, but the views are
great. The following are among the finer beaches. Once named
by the *Miami Herald* as one of the 10 best beaches in the world,
Palm Beach—which stretches behind the Americana, Aruba,
Concorde, Aruba Palm Beach, and Holiday Inn hotels—is the
center of Aruban tourism, offering the best in swimming, sailing, and fishing. In high season, however, it's packed.
Manchebo Beach, by the Manchebo Beach Resort, is an im-
pressively wide stretch of white powder. Aruba's unofficial topless beach, it is known locally as Punta Brabo Beach. On the
island's eastern tip, tiny **Baby Beach** is as placid as a wading
pool and only four to five feet deep—perfect for tots and bad
swimmers. Thatched shaded areas are available. **Malmok
Beach,** considered one of Aruba's finest spots for shelling and
windsurfing, has a wreck of the German ship %-2>*Antilla* just
off its coast.

Dining *Restaurants usually add a 15% service charge.*

Bali Floating Restaurant. Floating in an Oriental houseboat in
Oranjestad's harbor, the Bali has some of the best Indonesian
food on the island. Service is terminally slow but well-meaning.
L.G. Smith Blvd., tel. 297/8–22131. AE, MC, V. Moderate.
La Paloma. "The Dove" has an air of low-key loveliness with
no gimmicks, and it's usually packed. The restaurant has its
own fishing boat, ensuring freshness. Try conch stew with *pan
bati* (pancake-like bread), and fried bananas. Minestrone is a
house specialty. *Noord 39, tel. 297/8–62770. AE, MC, V. Closed
Tues. Inexpensive.*

Barbados

Barbados has a life of its own that goes on long after the passengers have packed up their suntan oil and returned to their ships. A resort island since the 1700s, Barbados has slowly cultivated a civilized attitude toward and services for tourists. Since the government is stable, the difference between the haves and have-nots is less marked than on other islands, and visitors are neither fawned upon nor resented for their assumed wealth. Unemployment hovers around 20%, however, so this could conceivably change.

Barbadian beaches are all public and lovely. The Atlantic surf pounds the gigantic boulders along the rugged east coast, where the Bajans themselves have their vacation homes. The northeast is dominated by rolling hills and valleys covered by acres of impenetrable sugarcane. Elsewhere on the island, which is linked by almost 900 miles of good roads, are historic plantations, stalactite-studded caves, a wildlife preserve, and the Andromeda Gardens, an attractive small tropical garden.

Barbados retains a British accent. Afternoon tea is habitual, cricket is the national sport, and the tradition of dressing for dinner is firmly entrenched. A daytime stroll in a swimsuit is as inappropriate in Bridgetown as it would be on New York's Fifth Avenue. The atmosphere is hardly stuffy, however, and you can be assured that no one and nothing will arrive on time.

Currency One Barbados dollar (BDS$) equals about U.S. 50¢. Both currencies and the Canadian dollar are accepted everywhere on the island. Always ask in which currency prices are quoted.

Passports and Visas American and Canadian citizens need proof of citizenship. A U.S. passport or original birth certificate and photo ID are acceptable. British citizens need a valid passport.

Telephones and Mail Public phones are at the docks. Use the same dialing procedure as in the United States, or dial for assistance for collect and credit-card calls. Airmail letters to the United States or Canada cost BDS 95¢ per half-ounce; airmail postcards cost BDS 65¢.

Shore Excursions *Not all shore excursions listed are offered by all cruise lines. Times and prices are approximate.*

Boats and Beaches **Atlantis Submarine:** An excursion on a real submarine for an exciting view of Aruba's profuse marine life. For non–scuba divers, this trip to the depths is a thrilling experience. *1¹/₂ hrs. Cost: $70.*

Jolly Roger Pirate Tour: Fun Cruise (tel. 809/436–6424 or 809/429–4545) offers a sailboat cruise down the west coast to Holetown, with a beach party. Rum punch, beer, and soft drinks are included. *4 hrs. Cost: $50–$55.*

Carlisle Bay Centre: Most cruise ships organize transportation to and from the beach here, which features changing facilities, safe-deposit boxes, a restaurant, gift shops, and water-sports facilities.

Cultural **Barbados Island Tour:** A comprehensive bus tour around the island may include a brief tour of Bridgetown. *3 hrs.*

Scenic **Harrison's Cave:** A bus tour (tel. 809/438–6640) into the center of the island, where passengers board an electric tram into an underground cave. At the lowest point, a 40-foot waterfall plunges into a deep pool. *3 hrs.*

Getting Around Bridgetown Harbour, where ships dock, is on the northwest side of Carlisle Bay. Go straight ahead to reach Bridgetown. The interesting areas start about 400 yards away from the dock. There's a tourist information desk at the pier.

By Bus The bus system is good, connecting Bridgetown with all parts of the island, but the buses can be crowded and late. Fare is BDS$1.50 wherever you go.

By Car Barbados is a pleasure by car, provided you take the time to study a good map and don't mind asking directions. Unfortunately for North Americans, driving is on the left; this is not a pleasure. You'll need an international driver's license to rent a car; get one at the rental agency for $5 with your valid home license. Contact **National** (tel. 809/426–0603) or **P&S Car Rentals** (tel. 809/424–2052). Daily prices start at $45 to $55 per day.

By Taxi Taxis may be rented at the pier or major hotels, or can be called. Drivers accept U.S. dollars and expect a 10% tip.

Exploring Barbados *Numbers in the margin correspond to numbered points of interest on the Barbados map.*

Bridgetown At the center of the bustling city of **Bridgetown** is **Trafalgar Square,** with its monument to Lord Nelson that predates its London counterpart by about two decades. Also here are a war memorial and a three-dolphin fountain commemorating the advent of running water in Barbados in 1865.

To get to Trafalgar Square from the docks, walk straight as far as you can, then follow the **Careenage,** a narrow strip of sea that made early Bridgetown a natural harbor. Here, working schooners were careened (turned on their sides) to be scraped of barnacles and repainted. Today, the Careenage serves mainly as a berth for fiberglass pleasure yachts. Spanning it are the **Chamberlain Bridge** and the **Charles O'Neal Bridge;** both lead south to the **Fairchild Market.** Saturday is market day at the Fairchild and at the **Cheapside Market** (at the northwest end of Lower Broad Street, across from St. Mary's Church Square).

The principal shopping area is **Broad Street,** which leads west from Trafalgar Square past the **House of Assembly** and **Legislative Council Buildings.** These Victorian Gothic structures, like so many smaller buildings in Bridgetown, stand beside a growing number of modern office buildings and shops.

East of the square is **St. Michael's Cathedral,** where George Washington is said to have worshiped on his only visit outside the United States. The structure was nearly a century old when he visited in 1751; destroyed by hurricanes, it was rebuilt in 1780, then again in 1831. Farther east, in **Queen's Park,** is an immense baobab tree more than 10 centuries old. The historic **Queen's Park House,** former home of the commander of the British troops, has been converted into a theater and a restaurant. The park is a long walk from Trafalgar Square; consider a taxi. *Open daily 9–5.*

About a mile south of Bridgetown on Highway 7, housed in what used to be a military prison, the **Barbados Museum** has artifacts and mementos of military history and everyday life in the 19th century; wildlife and natural history exhibits; a well-

Barbados

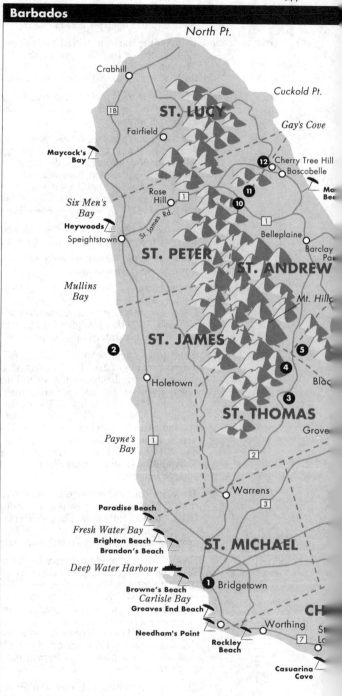

North Pt.

Crabhill

Cuckold Pt.

ST. LUCY

Gay's Cove

1B

Fairfield

Maycock's Bay

12 Cherry Tree Hill
Boscobelle

**Mo
Bea**

Rose
Hill 1

11

*Six Men's
Bay*

10

1

Heywoods

St. James Rd.

Belleplaine

Speightstown

ST. PETER

Barclay
Par

ST. ANDREW

*Mullins
Bay*

Mt. Hillc

ST. JAMES

6

2

5

4

Holetown

Blac

3

ST. THOMAS

Grove

*Payne's
Bay* 1

2

Warrens

3

Paradise Beach

Fresh Water Bay

Brighton Beach
Brandon's Beach

ST. MICHAEL

Deep Water Harbour

1 Bridgetown

CH

Browne's Beach
Carlisle Bay
Greaves End Beach

Worthing

S
Lo

Needham's Point

7

**Rockley
Beach**

**Casuarina
Cove**

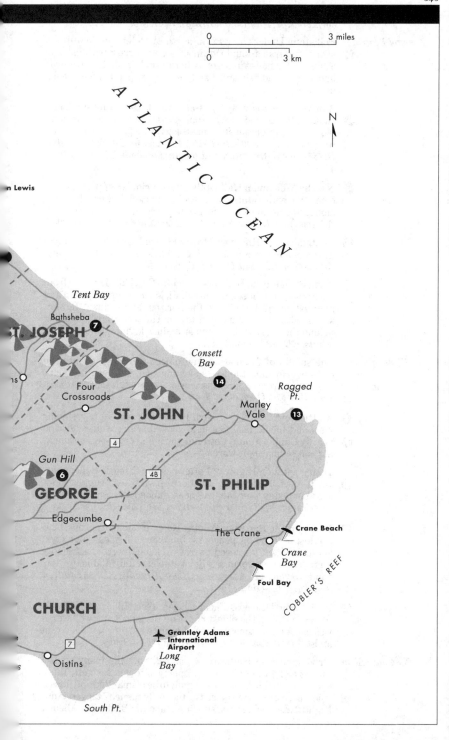

0 [_____] 3 miles
0 [_____] 3 km

N

A T L A N T I C   O C E A N

n Lewis

Tent Bay

Bathsheba
ST. JOSEPH **7**

ns

Four
Crossroads

*Consett
Bay*

14

*Ragged
Pt.*

Marley
Vale
13

ST. JOHN

[4]

[4B]

Gun Hill
6

GEORGE

ST. PHILIP

Edgecumbe

The Crane **Crane Beach**

*Crane
Bay*

Foul Bay

COBBLER'S REEF

CHURCH

[7]

Oistins

✈ **Grantley Adams
International
Airport**
*Long
Bay*

South Pt.

stocked gift shop; and a good café. *Garrison Savannah, tel. 809/427–0201. Admission: BDS$7. Open Mon.–Sat. 10–6.*

Central Barbados **Folkstone Underwater Park,** north of Holetown, features a ❷ snorkeling trail around Dottin's Reef, with glass-bottom boats available for nonswimmers. A barge sunk in shallow water is home to myriad fish, and it and the reef are popular with scuba divers.

A drive along Highway 2 passes several interesting sights, in- ❸ cluding **Harrison's Cave.** The pale-gold limestone caverns, complete with subterranean streams and waterfalls, can be toured by tram. *Tel. 809/438–6640. Admission: BDS$15 adults, BDS$7.50 children. Reservations recommended. Open daily 9– 4.*

❹ Nearby **Welchman Hall Gully** offers a similar opportunity to commune with nature, with acres of labeled flowers, the occasional green monkey, and great peace and quiet. *[Hwy. 2] Admission: BDS$5 adults, BDS$2.50 children. Open daily 9–5.*

❺ Continue along Highway 2 to the **Flower Forest,** 8 acres of fragrant bushes, canna and ginger lilies, and puffball trees. *Admission: BDS$10. Open daily 9–5.*

❻ From Bridgetown, Highway 4 leads to **Gun Hill.** The view from here is so pretty it seems unreal. Fields in shades of green and gold extend all the way to the horizon, and brilliant flowers surround a picturesque gun tower. The white limestone lion behind the garrison is a famous landmark. *Admission: BDS$5 adults, BDS$2.50 children.*

Eastern Shore/ The small but fascinating **Andromeda Gardens,** set into the *North-Central* cliffs overlooking the sea, holds unusual and beautiful plant *Barbados* specimens from around the world. *Tel. 809/433–9261. Admis-* ❼ *sion: BDS$10. Open daily 9–5.*

❽ A little north of the gardens, **Barclay's Park** offers a similar view and picnic facilities in a wooded seafront area. At the ❾ nearby **Chalky Mount Potteries** you'll find craftspersons making and selling their wares.

Taking a left on Highway 1 after passing through Belleplaine, ❿ you'll reach **Farley Hill,** a national park whose rugged landscape explains why this has been dubbed the Scotland area. *Admission: BDS$2 per car; walkers free. Open daily 8:30–6.*

⓫ Nearby is the **Barbados Wildlife Reserve,** home to herons, land turtles, screeching peacocks, innumerable green monkeys, geese, brilliantly colored parrots, a kangaroo, and a friendly otter. The fauna roam freely, so step carefully and keep your hands to yourself. *Admission: BDS$10 adults, BDS$5 children under 12. Open daily 10–5.*

⓬ Back toward the coast, near Cherry Tree Hill, is **St. Nicholas Abbey** (c. 1650), the oldest house on the island and well worth visiting for its stone and wood architecture in the Jacobean style. *Admission: $2.50. Open weekdays 10–3:30.*

The South Shore Driving east on Highways 4 and 4B, note the many **chattel houses** along the route; the property of tenant farmers, these ever-expandable houses were built to be dismantled and moved ⓭ when necessary. On the coast, the aptly named **Ragged Point Lighthouse** is where the sun first shines on Barbados. About 4 miles to the northwest of the lighthouse, in the eastern corner of St. John Parish, the coral-stone buildings and serenely beautiful grounds of **Codrington Theological College,** founded in 1748, stand on a cliff overlooking Consett Bay.

Shopping Most stores are located on Broad Street, Bridgetown; they are usually open weekdays 8–4 and Saturday 8–1. At Bridgetown's **Pelican Village Handicrafts Center** (tel. 809/426–1966), on the Princess Alice Highway near the Cheapside Market, you can watch goods and crafts being made before you purchase them; rugs and mats are good buys. For antiques and fine memorabilia, try **Greenwich House Antiques** (tel. 809/432–1169), in Greenwich Village, Trents Hill, St. James Parish; and **Antiquaria** (tel. 809/426–0635), on St. Michael's Row next to the Anglican cathedral in Bridgetown. Exclusive designs in "wearable art" by Carol Cadogan are available at **Cotton Days Designs** in Rose Cottage, opposite St. Patrick's Cathedral in Bridgetown (Lower Bay St., tel. 809/427–7191), and on the wharf in Bridgetown.

Sports Contact **Blue Jay Charters** (tel. 809/422–2098) for information
Fishing on fishing charters.

Golf Three courses—at **Sandy Lane Club** (18 holes), **Rockley Resort** (nine holes), and **Heywoods** (nine holes)—are open to the public.

Horseback Riding Try **Valley Hill Stables** (Christ Church, tel. 809/423–6180).

Water Sports Waterskiing, snorkeling, and parasailing are available on most beaches of St. James and Christ Church parishes. Windsurfing is best learned on the south coast at **Barbados Windsurfing Club Hotel** (Maxwell, Christ Church Parish, tel. 809/428–9095). For scuba divers, Barbados is a rich and varied underwater destination. Two good dive shops are **The Dive Shop Ltd.** (Grand Barbados Beach Resort, [where; ditto next] tel. 809/426–9947) and **Dive Boat Safari** (Barbados Hilton, tel. 809/427–4350).

Beaches The west coast has the stunning coves and white-sand beaches dear to the hearts of postcard publishers, plus calm, clear water for snorkeling, scuba diving, and swimming. While beaches here are seldom crowded, the west coast is not the place to find isolation. Good spots for swimming include **Paradise Beach,** just off the Paradise Village & Beach Hotel; **Brandon's Beach,** a 10-minute walk south; **Browne's Beach** in Bridgetown; and **Greave's End Beach,** south of Bridgetown at Aquatic Gap. If you don't mind a short drive along Highway 7, the **Crane Beach Hotel,** where the Atlantic meets the Caribbean, is a great find. Waves pound in, but a reef makes it safe for good swimmers and the sands are golden. For refreshment, there's the hotel's dining room on the cliff above.

Dining *A 5% tax and 10% service charge are added to most restaurant bills. When no service charge is added, tip waiters 10%–15%.*

Ocean House. With so many dining choices in Barbados, finding a restaurant with its own special character isn't easy. Ocean House has happily resolved this dilemma. At this throwback to the mid-1930s, you can enjoy the comforts of colonial wicker chairs, fresh flowers, and the sea lapping the nearby shore. Traditional Bajan dishes include. *Hastings, Christ Church Parish, tel. 809/427–7821. Reservations advised. AE, MC, V. Moderate.*

Caracas/La Guaira, Venezuela

The busy harbor of La Guaira is the port for nearby Caracas, the capital of Venezuela. Most passengers go directly from the dock into air-conditioned excursion buses for the 15-mile (45-minute) drive into the big city. La Guaira itself, though steeped in history, is a little dangerous these days. If you're going to stick around town, bring your friends but not your valuables.

Caracas is a bustling, multiethnic, cosmopolitan city of 6 million people. It isn't the safest spot in the world, especially with the recent political unrest that saw several violent and failed coup attempts late in 1992. Be aware that some cruise lines canceled their visits to Caracas in 1993.

Still, this is a fascinating city and a truly unique Caribbean cruise stop. Few passengers consider it their favorite call, but most are glad for having had a chance to wander, however briefly, through the capital of a South American country. Unless you want to stick out like a sore thumb, and a rather rude one at that, men should wear long slacks and women should wear slacks or a short-sleeve dress—poor or rich, everyone tries to be chic.

Due to its rapid growth, Caracas is a hodgepodge of styles. Many of the buildings, such as **Centro Banaven,** a black, glass-sided box, display innovative touches; but there is also a healthy share of neoclassical buildings, like the 19th-century Capitol and the 20th-century Fine Arts Museum, as well as heavier, neogothic structures. Nothing, however, compares with the charming colonial dwellings of La Guaira.

Currency The monetary unit is the bolivar (Bs). At press time the dollar exchange stood Bs 84 on the free market. Store owners prefer U.S. dollars, however, and may even give you a discount for paying in greenbacks.

Passports and Visas You will need a passport and a tourist card, which should be issued by your cruise line. If you don't receive a card with your tickets, check with your travel agent or the cruise line.

Telephones and Mail Direct dialing is possible to major cities abroad from most exchanges in Caracas. To call the United States, dial 001, then the area code and telephone number. For operator-assisted international calls, dial 122. AT&T now offers a collect-call service to the United States: Dialing 800/11120 connects you directly with an English-speaking operator. Airmail letters to North America cost Bs 40, postcards Bs 25. The "Expreso Internacional" service is worth the extra Bs 15.

Shore Excursions *Not all shore excursions listed are offered by all cruise lines. All times and prices are approximate.*

Angel Falls and Canaima Lagoon: A jet ride carries you into the lush jungle interior and over Angel Falls—at 3,212 feet, the world's highest waterfall. After landing, you travel by canoe to a resort jungle camp to see another waterfall and the rich vegetation up close. Lunch is followed by a swim in a lagoon, with enough time to hike and explore. Not all ships offer this unforgettable tour. If yours doesn't, ask your shore-excursion director if it can be arranged for you. *9 hrs. Cost: $200.*

Caracas: A half- or full-day bus tour to see the main attractions of Caracas. Lunch may be included. *5–7 hrs. Cost: $25–$30.*

Getting Around   In Caracas the efficient Metro runs east–west, from Palo Verde
By Subway   to Propatria and from Silencio to Caricuao. Fares are from Bs
12 to Bs 18. Air-conditioned cars on rubber wheels whiz a million passengers daily. It is such a pleasant ride that some city-tour shore excursions include a jaunt on the subway as a highlight.

By Taxi   Taxis are plentiful, inexpensive, and usually metered. A cab ride from La Guaira to Caracas costs about $30.

Exploring La Guaira   If you don't want to take off for Caracas, you might enjoy walking around La Guaira. **Plaza Vargas,** with its statue of José Maria Vargas, a Guaireño who was Venezuela's third president, is a good place to begin exploring. The plaza is bounded by Calle Bolívar, running between the shore road and the mountain. Lined by the cool and cavernous warehouses of another century's trade and by one- and two-story houses with their colonial windows and red-tile roofs, the street funnels the sea breezes like voices from a more gracious age.

One of the most important old buildings in La Guaira is **Casa Guipuzcoana,** on the main shore road. Built in 1734, it was the colony's largest civic structure, housing first the Basque company that held a trading monopoly for 50 years, then the customs office. Restored as a cultural center, it is now the Vargas District Town Hall.

Behind the Casa is the **Boulton Museum,** a tall house with an ample wood balcony. Inside is a treasury of paintings, maps, documents, pistols, and other miscellany collected by the family of John Boulton, occupants of the house for more than 140 years. An Englishman who came to Venezuela in 1826 at age 20, Boulton soon became a leading exporter and importer. *Tel. 031/25921. Open Tues.–Fri. 9:30–1 and 3–6, weekends 9–1.*

Exploring Caracas   *Numbers in the margin correspond to numbered points of interest on the Caracas map.*

Caracas is a complicated city; a car or taxi is necessary, except in the downtown area. The city has spread east and west from
1 its historic center, **Plaza Bolívar.** The old Cathedral, Town Council, and Foreign Ministry (or Casa Amarilla) all face Plaza Bolívar, a pleasant shady square with benches, pigeons, and the fine equestrian statue of Simón Bolívar, who was born only a
2 block away. Nearby also are the **Capitol,** the presidential offices
3 4 in **Miraflores Palace,** and the twin towers of the **Simón Bolívar Center** in El Silencio.

Now replacing the twin towers as the symbol of modern Cara-
5 cas is the concrete **Parque Central,** with its two 56-story skyscrapers. Built over 16 years, the office and apartment complex was finished in 1986. Designed for 10,000 people, with seven condominiums and two towers, Parque Central encompasses not only shops, supermarkets, and restaurants, but also schools, a swimming pool, a convention center, a hotel, the **Museum of Contemporary Art,** the **Children's Museum,** and the **Corporación de Turismo** (tourist-board offices). A pedestrian
6 bridge links Parque Central to the **Museum of Natural Science,**
7 8 the **Museum of Fine Arts,** and **Los Caobos Park.** Beyond this bower of mahogany trees, once a coffee plantation, lies the cir-
9 cular fountain of **Plaza Venezuela.**

350

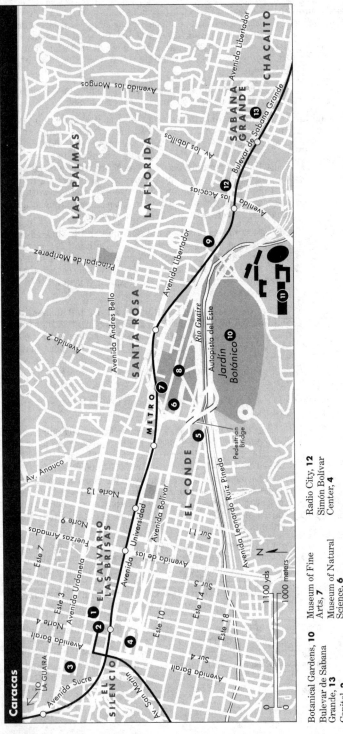

Caracas

Botanical Gardens, **10**
Bulevar de Sabana
Grande, **13**
Capitol, **2**
City University
campus, **11**
Los Caobos Park, **8**
Miraflores Palace, **3**

Museum of Fine
Arts, **7**
Museum of Natural
Science, **6**
Parque Central, **5**
Plaza Bolívar, **1**
Plaza Venezuela, **9**

Radio City, **12**
Simón Bolívar
Center, **4**

Across the *autopista* (highway) from Plaza Venezuela are the
❿ ⓫ **Botanical Gardens** and the **City University campus.** Here, art
was conceived as an organic part of architecture by master
designer Carlos Raúl Villanueva. In courtyards and buildings
are a stained-glass wall by Fernand Léger, murals by Léger
and Mateo Manaure, sculptures by Antoine Pevsner, Jean Arp,
and Henry Laurens, and in the **Aula Magna Auditorium,** acous-
tic "clouds" by Alexander Calder.

The great fountain with colored lights in Plaza Venezuela is
part of the urban renewal undertaken by the **Caracas Metro.**
The modern and handsome subway with its elegant French
cars covers 21 kilometers between Propatria in the west and
Palo Verde in the east. The Metro is changing the face of Caracas. When entire avenues were torn up, architects and land-
scapers converted the commercial high street of Sabana
Grande into a pedestrian boulevard of shops, popular sidewalk
cafés, potted plants, and chess tables. Cars are banned be-
⓬ tween the **Radio City** theater and Chacaito, the pedestrian mall
⓭ popularly known as the **Bulevar de Sabana Grande.** People of
all ages and nationalities come to savor the best cappuccino and
conversation in town, from midday to midnight. "Meet you at
the Gran Café" is how dates often start in Caracas.

Shopping Many of Caracas's sophisticated shops are in modern com-
plexes known as *centros commerciales,* less stocked with imports than formerly, since devaluation has put foreign goods
beyond most local shoppers' purses. Caracus is a buyer's market for fine clothing, tailored suits, elegant shoes, leather
goods, and jewelry.

For wholesale jewelry go to **Edificio La Francia,** whose nine
floors off Plaza Bolívar hold some 80 gold workshops and gem
traders; profit margins are low, so buys are attractive. Since
alluvial gold is found in Venezuela, nuggets of *cochanos* are
made into pendants, rings, and bracelets. Expert gold designer
Panchita Labady, who originated the popular gold orchid earrings and pins, works in a small shop at No. 98 Calle Real de
Sabana Grande, opposite Avenida Los Jabillos (tel. 02/712016).

Devil's masks are much sought after for colorful souvenirs.
Used in ritual dances marking the Corpus Christi festival (usually in early June), they are made of brightly painted papier-
mâché. A good place to find these and other uniquely Venezuelan things is **El Taller de La Esquina,** Nivel Galeria, in the Paseo
Las Mercedes shopping center. Explore other *artesania* shops
in Paseo Las Mercedes.

Dining *There is a 10% service charge in Venezuelan restaurants, and it
is customary to tip the waiter another 10%.*

Dama Antañona. Set in a charming 150-year-old house, this
downtown restaurant offers typical Venezuelan fare, including
a Sunday *criollo* breakfast of fried yucca, ham, eggs, black
beans, and juice. *No. 14 Jesuitas a Maturin, tel. 02/563–5639.
Moderate.*
Doña Arepota. This typical Venezuelan restaurant with sidewalk tables specializes in *arepas*—hot corn flatcakes served
with a choice of fillings, from white cheese to shrimp and avocado. *Arepas* are best accompanied by tropical fruit juice. *Edificio Doral, Av. Mexico at Bellas Artes Metro station near the
Hilton, no phone. Open 24 hours. Inexpensive.*

Cozumel, Mexico

Sun-saturated Cozumel, its ivory beaches fringed with coral reefs, fulfills the tourist's vision of a tropical Caribbean island. More Mexican than Cancún and far less developed, Cozumel surpasses its better-known, fancier neighbor to the north in several ways. It has more—and lovelier—secluded beaches, superior diving and snorkeling, more authentically Mexican cuisine, and a greater diversity of handicrafts at better prices.

A cruise ship may anchor for one day off Cozumel and offer excursions to nearby **Playa del Carmen,** the **Yucatán Peninsula,** and **Cancún,** or it may stay in the area for two days, anchoring off Cozumel for one day and off Playa del Carmen for the other.

Life on this flat jungle island centers on **San Miguel,** where the cruise ships dock. Most of the salespeople speak English, and the duty-free shops stay open as long as a ship is anchored offshore. With the world-renowned **Palancar Reef** nearby, San Miguel is also a favorite among divers.

Playa del Carmen, across the water on the Yucatán Peninsula, is a ferry ride away. From there, tours leave for the nearby Mayan ruins of **Tulum, Cobá,** and **Chichén Itzá,** or the resort town of Cancún.

Currency Although U.S. dollars are widely accepted, local currency is the Mexican peso (P$). If you plan to take the ferry or go exploring on your own, you'll want some pesos in hand. Since 1988, the government has worked to reduce inflation and slowly devalue the peso against the dollar. At press time, the rate was about P$3.20 to U.S. $1. (In January 1993, Mexico created the "new peso," knocking three zeros off the old unit.)

Passports and Visas U.S. and Canadian citizens need only proof of citizenship (a passport is best) and a Mexican tourist card, which the cruise line will provide. All British subjects require a passport and a Mexican tourist card.

Telephones and Mail The telephone service from Cozumel is not very good. It's best to call home from another port. Hotels in Cancún can help you place a long-distance call, but expect to pay a hefty service charge. Though postal rates are quite low in Mexico, service is notoriously slow. Postcards to the United States cost P$2; to Britain, P$1.20. Letters (up to 10 grams) cost P$1.50 to the United States and P$1.70 to Britain.

Shore Excursions *Not all shore excursions listed are offered by all cruise lines. All times and prices are approximate.*

Archaeological **Tulum Ruins and Xel-ha Lagoon:** The tour of this superbly preserved ancient Mayan city perched on the cliffs above a beautiful beach is conducted by an English-speaking guide. A box lunch is usually included. A stop is made for a swim in the glass-clear waters of Xel-ha. The tour leaves from Playa del Carmen. *6 hrs. Cost: $50.*

Chichén Itzá: This incredible and awe-inspiring ruin of a great Mayan city is a 45-minute flight from Cozumel (bus tours are also available; the ride, which leaves from Playa del Carmen, takes four hours one way. A box lunch is included. *Full day. Cost: $130.*

Cobá Jungle Hike: Still mostly covered by dense jungle, this archaeological site may prove to be the Yucatán's most exciting yet. Cobá may be the largest Mayan city ever discovered. The tour is an exotic and romantic evocation of what archaeology is all about. Good walking shoes are a must. A box lunch is provided. *5 hrs. Cost: $55.*

Boats and Beaches **Glass-Bottom Party Boat:** A glass-bottom catamaran with an open bar takes passengers to a beach party for swimming, sunbathing, and games. *4 hrs. Cost: $23.*

Snorkeling: This region has been acknowledged by experts from Jacques Cousteau to *Skin Diver Magazine* as one of the top diving destinations in the world. If your ship offers a snorkeling tour, take it. Equipment and lessons are included. *2 hrs. Cost: $30.*

City Tour **Cancún City/Shopping:** This bus tour from Playa del Carmen to the resort town of Cancún briefly covers the history of the area, but is centered on providing shopping opportunities in the hotel zone. A Mexican buffet lunch and folkloric show are usually included. Mediocre. *5 hrs. Cost: $30.*

Entertainment **Mexican Fiesta Show:** A folkloric show with live music at a Cozumel hotel includes two drinks. *1¹/₄ hrs. Cost: $25.*

Getting Around A tourist information booth is on the main Cozumel pier by the Plaza del Sol (open daily 8 AM–1 PM). The main office is on the second floor of the crafts mall on the east end of the plaza. *Tel. 987/2–0972. Open weekdays 9–2.*

By Ferry To get to Playa del Carmen from Cozumel, you can take a ferry or a water-jet trimaran from the downtown pier. It costs about $6 for a one-way trip and takes 40–60 minutes. *Do not miss the return ferry.*

By Car or Moped Mopeds are great fun, and you can circumnavigate the island on one tank of gas. Be careful not to get stranded—the only gas station is at the corner of Avenida Juárez and Avenida 30 (open 7 AM–midnight). Wear a helmet and be careful: Accidents are frequent on Cozumel. Four-wheel drive is recommended if you're planning to explore the many dirt roads around the island. For two- or four-wheel rentals, contact **Avis** (Calle 20, tel. 987/2–1923), **Budget** (Av. 5 and Calle 2 N, tel. 987/2–0903), **Fiesta Cozumel** (Hotel Mesón San Miguel, tel. 987/2–1389), or **Hertz** (Av. Juárez and Calle 10, tel. 987/2–2136). Rates start at about $50 per day.

By Taxi Taxis are ubiquitous. Stands are on Avenida Melgar, just north of the main pier, and in front of all the major hotels.

Exploring Cozumel San Miguel is tiny—you cannot get lost—and best explored on foot. The main attractions are the small eateries and shops that line the streets. Activity centers on the ferry and the main square, where the locals congregate in the evenings. The lovely **Museo de Cozumel,** with exhibits devoted to the island environment and to the ecosystem of the surrounding reefs and water, is on the main coastal drag, near the ferry dock. On the second floor are displays on Mayan and colonial life and on modern-day Cozumel. *Av. Melgar and Calle 4 N. Admission: $2. Open Sun.–Fri. 10–6.*

If you have wheels, head south out of town on Avenida Melgar; after 6½ miles your first stop will be the **Chankanaab Lagoon and Park.** The natural aquarium has been designated an underwater preserve for more than 50 species of tropical fish, as well as crustaceans and coral. Snorkeling and scuba equipment can be rented, and instruction and professional guides are available, along with gift shops, snack bars, and a restaurant (open 10–5) serving fresh seafood. *Admission: $4. Open daily 9–5.*

Shopping San Miguel's biggest industry—even bigger than diving—is selling souvenirs and crafts to cruise-ship passengers. The primary items are ceramics, onyx, brass, wood carvings, reproductions of Mayan artifacts, shells, silver, gold, sportswear, T-shirts, perfume, and liquor. Almost all stores take U.S. dollars.

The shopping district centers on the Plaza del Sol and extends out along Avenida Melgar and Avenida 5 S and N. The east side of the plaza is occupied by the **Plaza del Sol Mall.** Here is one of the finest crafts stores, **La Piñata,** and Cozumel's high-fashion store, the **Emma B. Boutique.** Another shop with an excellent selection of crafts is **Los Cinco Soles,** on Avenida Melgar near Calle 4 N. The most bizarre store on the island is the **Cozumel Flea Market,** on Avenida 5 N between Calles 2 and 4, which sells reproductions of erotic Mayan figurines, antique masks, rare coins, and Xtabentún, the local anise-and-honey liqueur. Down the street at Avenida 5 N #14, **Arte Na Balam** sells high-quality Mayan reproductions, jewelry, and batik clothing. For atmosphere, fresh fruit, and other foods, go to the **Municipal Market** at Avenida 25 S and Calle Salas.

Sports Contact **Yucab Reef Diving and Fishing Center** (Cozumel, tel.
Fishing 987/2–4110) or **Club Naútico Cozumel** (Cozumel, tel. 987/2–0118 or 800/253–9701 in the U.S.)

Scuba Diving and Cozumel is famous for its reefs. The most accessible are those
Snorkeling just off the **Chankanaab Lagoon and Pak,** where you can dive or snorkel just off the beach; nearby scuba shops rent equipment and offer instruction. Another great dive site is **La Ceiba Reef,** in the waters off La Ceiba and Sol Caribe hotels. Here lies the wreckage of a sunken airplane that was blown up for a Mexican disaster movie. Cozumel's dive shops include **Aqua Safari** (Av. Melgar 39A, tel. 987/2–0101), **Blue Angel** (Hotel Villablanca, tel. 987/2–1631), **Dive Paradise** (Av. Melgar 601, tel. 987/2–1007), and **Fantasia Divers** (Av. 25 off Adolfo Rosado Salas, tel. 987/2–2840).

Dining *Although it is not common in Mexico, a 10%–15% service charge may be added to the bill. Otherwise, a 10%–20% tip is customary.*

Carlos'n'Charlies. The local branch of the popular Mexican chain, this second-floor waterfront restaurant is decorated with oddball T-shirts and even has its own volleyball court. It's also been known to host its share of wild drinking contests. Food is American-style ribs, tacos, nachos, quesedillas, and fajitas. *Av. Rafael Melgar, between Calles 2 and 4N, tel. 987/2–0191. MC, V. Moderate.*

Rincón Maya. This is the top place on the island for Yucatan cuisine and a popular spot with locals and divers. Lobster and fresh fish *a la plancha* (grilled) and *poc chuc* (marinated grilled pork) are among the excellent dishes. The decor is festive; a colorful mural, hats, and fans adorn the walls. *Av. 5A S and Calle 3 S. No credit cards. Moderate. No lunch.*

El Foco. This *taquería* serves tacos and quesadillas, but you can also order ribs and steak. Come for lots of beer and the funky atmosphere. *Av. 5 S/Calle 13. MC, V. Inexpensive.*

Curaçao

Try to be on deck as your ship sails into Curaçao. The tiny Queen Emma Floating Bridge swings aside to open the narrow channel. Pastel gingerbread buildings on shore look like doll-houses, especially from the perspective of a large cruise ship. Although the gabled roofs and red tiles show a Dutch influence, the riotous colors of the facades are peculiar to Curaçao. It is said that white gave the first governor of Curaçao migraines, so all the houses were painted in colors.

Thirty-five miles north of Venezuela and 42 miles east of Aruba, Curaçao is, at 180 square miles, the largest of the Netherlands Antilles. While always sunny, it is never stiflingly hot here, due to the cooling influence of the trade winds. Water sports attract enthusiasts from all over the world, and the reef diving is excellent.

History books still don't agree as to whether Alonzo de Ojeda or Amerigo Vespucci discovered Curaçao, only that it happened around 1499. In 1634 the Dutch came and promptly shipped off the Spanish settlers and the few remaining Indians to Venezuela. To defend itself against French and British invasions, the city built massive ramparts, many of which now house unusual restaurants and hotels.

Today, Curaçao's population, which comprises more than 50 nationalities, is one of the best educated in the Caribbean. The island is known for its religious tolerance, and tourists are warmly welcomed, almost never pestered by vendors and shopkeepers.

Currency U.S. dollars are fine, so don't worry about exchanging money, except for pay phones or soda machines. The local currency is the guilder or florin, indicated by "fl" or "NAf" on price tags. The official rate of exchange at press time was NAf 1.79 to U.S. $1.

Passports and Visas U.S. and Canadian citizens need only proof of citizenship and a photo ID. British citizens must have a passport.

Telephones and Mail The telephone system is reliable. Dialing to the United States is exactly the same as dialing long distance within the United States. To air-mail a letter to anywhere in the world costs NAf 1.25; a postcard costs NAf .70.

Shore Excursions *The following excursions may not be offered by all cruise lines. Times and prices are approximate. Check with your travel agent or cruise director.*

Island Tour: A bus tour covers most of the important sites near town, including at least one restored plantation house, a distillery where Curaçao liqueur is made and sold, and the Seaquarium. *2¹/₂–3 hrs. Cost: $24–$28.*

Country Drive: This is a good tour if you'd like to see Westpunt and Mt. Christoffel but don't want to risk driving an hour there yourself. Other stops are the Museum of Natural History, Boca Tabla, and Knip Beach. *3¹/₂ hrs. Cost: $25.*

Getting Around Willemstad is small and navigable on foot; you needn't spend more than two or three hours wandering around here. English, Spanish, and Dutch are widely spoken. The city is divided by the narrow Santa Anna Bay into the Punda, where the main

Curaçao

North
Point

Westpunt

Westpunt

❷ Christoffel
Park
○ Savonet

❸
Mt. Christoffel
○ San Hyronimo

Knip Bay

Jeremi
Bay

Barber

○ Ascencion

Santa Cruz

Santa Marta Bay

San Juan Bay

**Curaçao
International
Airport**

St. Willibrordus
Port Marie Bay
Boca
St. Marie

Daaibooi Bay

Bullen
Bay

St. Michiel ○

St. Michiel Bay
Blauw Bay

Pis

N

0 ——————— 10 miles
0 ——————— 15 km

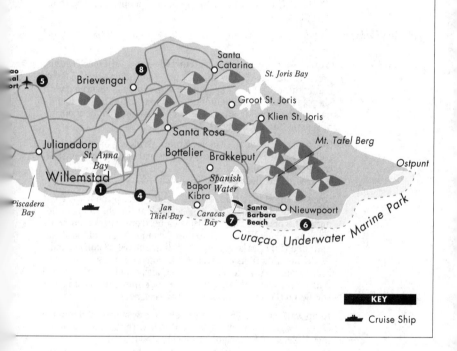

Caribbean Sea

Curaçao International Airport

Brievengat

Santa Catarina

St. Joris Bay

Groot St. Joris

Klien St. Joris

Mt. Tafel Berg

Ostpunt

Julianadorp

St. Anna Bay

Santa Rosa

Bottelier

Brakkeput

Willemstad

Spanish Water

Bapor Kibra

Piscadera Bay

Jan Thiel Bay

Caracas Bay

Santa Barbara Beach

Nieuwpoort

Curaçao Underwater Marine Park

KEY

⛴ Cruise Ship

shopping district is, and the Otrobanda, where the cruise ships dock. You can cross from the Otrobanda to the Punda in one of three ways: Walk across the Queen Emma Pontoon Bridge; ride the free ferry, which runs when the bridge swings open (at least 30 times a day) to let seagoing vessels pass; or take a cab across the Julianna Bridge (about $7).

By Car To rent a car, call **Avis** (tel. 599/9–681163), **Budget** (tel. 599/9–683420), or **National** (tel. 599/9–683489). All you'll need is a valid U.S. or Canadian driver's license.

By Moped Rentals are available right at the pier. If you want to explore farther into the countryside, mopeds are a viable alternative to tours.

By Taxi Taxi drivers have an official tariff chart, but confirm the price before getting in. Taxis meet every cruise ship, and they can be picked up at hotels. Otherwise, call **Central Dispatch** (tel. 599/9–616711). A taxi tour for up to four people will cost about $20–$25 an hour.

Exploring Curaçao *Numbers in the margin correspond to numbered points of interest on the Curaçao map.*

Willemstad A quick tour of downtown **Willemstad** covers a six-block radius.
❶ Santa Anna Bay divides the city into the Punda and the Otrabanda (literally, the "other side"). The Punda is crammed with shops, restaurants, monuments, and markets. The Otrabanda has narrow winding streets full of homes notable for their gables and Dutch-influenced designs.

Start your tour at the **Queen Emma Bridge,** which the locals call the Lady. The toll to cross the original bridge, built in 1888, was 2¢ per person if wearing shoes and free if barefoot. Today it's free, regardless of what is on your feet.

Once on the Punda side, turn left and walk up the waterfront along **Handelskade** to take a closer look at the charming buildings. The original red roof tiles came from Europe on trade ships as ballast. Walk down to the corner at the end of the street and turn right at the customs building onto Sha Caprileskade. At the bustling **floating market** that convenes here each morning, dozens of Venezuelan schooners arrive laden with tropical fruits and vegetables. Any produce bought at the market should be thoroughly washed before eating.

Keep walking down Sha Caprileskade toward the Wilhelmina Drawbridge, which connects the Punda with the once-flourishing district of **Scharloo.** The early Jewish merchants built stately homes in Scharloo; it is now a red-light district. At the bridge turn right and walk down Columbusstraat to the **Mikveh Israel-Emmanuel Synagogue,** founded in 1651 and the oldest temple still in use in the Western Hemisphere. It draws 20,000 visitors a year. Enter through the gates around the corner on Hanchi Snoa. A museum in the back displays Jewish antiques and fine Judaica. *Hanchi Snoa 29, tel. 599/9–611067. Small donation expected. Open weekdays 9–11:45, 2:30–5.*

Continue along Columbusstraat till you reach the courthouse, with its stately balustrade, and the impressive Georgian facade of the Bank of Boston. The statue keeping watch over **Wilhelminaplein** is of Queen Wilhelmina, a popular monarch of the Netherlands who gave up her throne to her daughter Juliana after her Golden Jubilee in 1948.

Turn right at Breedestraat and go down toward the Pontoon Bridge, turning left at the waterfront. At the foot of the bridge are the mustard-color walls of **Ft. Amsterdam;** take a few steps through the archway and enter another century. In the 1700s the structure was actually the center of the city and the most important fort on the island. Now it houses the governor's residence, the Fort Church, the ministry, and several other government offices.

Western Curaçao The road that leads through the village of Soto to the northwest tip of the island winds through landscape that Georgia O'Keeffe might have painted—towering cacti, flamboyant dried shrubbery, aluminum-roofed houses. In these parts you'll see fishermen hauling in their nets, women pounding cornmeal, and donkeys blocking traffic. Landhouses—large estate homes, most of which are closed to the public—can often be glimpsed from the road.

❷
❸ Past **Boca Tabla,** where the sea has carved a magnificent grotto, is **Christoffel Park.** It's a good hour from Willemstad (so watch your time) but worth a visit. This fantastic 4,450-acre garden and wildlife preserve with Mt. Christoffel at its center consists of three former plantations. As you drive through the park, watch for tiny deer, goats, and other small wildlife that might suddenly dart in front of your car. If you skip everything else on the island, it's possible to drive to the park and climb 1,230-foot Mt. Christoffel, which takes two to three strenuous hours. The island panorama you get from the peak is amazing—on a clear day you can even see the mountain ranges of Venezuela, Bonaire, and Aruba. *Savonet, tel. 599/9–640363. Admission: $5 adults, $3 children. Open Mon.–Sat. 8–5, Sun. 8–3.*

Eastern Curaçao At the **Curaçao Seaquarium,** more than 400 varieties of exotic
❹ fish and vegetation are displayed. Outside is a 495-yard- long artificial beach of white sand, well-suited to novice swimmers and children. *Tel. 599/9–616666. Admission: $6 adults, $3 children. Open daily 9 AM–10 PM.*

❺ Near the airport is the island's newest attraction, **Hato Caves,** where you can take an hour-long guided tour into various chambers containing water pools, a voodoo chamber, fruit bats' sleeping quarters, and Curaçao Falls—where a stream of silver joins a stream of gold. Hidden lights illuminate the limestone formations and gravel walkways. This is one of the better Caribbean caves open to the public. *Tel. 599/9–680378. Admission: $4.25 adults, $2.75 children. Open Tues.–Sun. 10–5.*

❻ **Curaçao Underwater Park** (*see* Sports, *below*) is the best spot for snorkeling—though the seabed is sadly litter-strewn in places. The park stretches along the southern shore from the Princess Beach Hotel in Willemstad to the eastern tip of the island.

Along the southern shore, you'll pass several private yacht clubs that attract sports anglers from all over the world for international tournaments. Stop at **Santa Barbara Beach,** especially on Sundays, when the atmosphere approaches party
❼ time. **Caracas Bay,** off Bapor Kibra, is a popular dive site, with a sunken ship so close to the surface that even snorkelers can balance their flippers on the helm.

8 A 10-minute drive northeast of Willemstad is **Arawak Clay Products** (tel. 599/3–77658), whose factory showroom of native crafts is open 7:30–5. You can buy a variety of tiles, plates, pots, and tiny landhouse replicas. Tour operators usually stop here.

Shopping Curaçao has some of the best shops in the Caribbean, but in many cases the prices are no lower than in U.S. discount stores. Hours are usually Monday–Saturday 8–noon and 2–6. Most shops are within the six-block area of Willemstad described above. The main shopping streets are **Heerenstraat, Breedestraat,** and **Madurostraat.** The hippest shopping area lies under the **Waterfort arches,** along with a variety of restaurants and bars.

Check out **Bamali** (tel. 599/9–612258) for Indonesian batik clothing and leather, and **The African Queen** (tel. 599/9–612682), an exotic bazaar of fine African jewelry, batik clothes, and Kenyan pocketbooks handmade of coconut husk and sisal. On the ritzy end, **Spritzer & Fuhrmann** (Gomezplein 1, tel. 599/9–612600), the top jeweler in the Netherlands Antilles, carries gold, watches, crystal, diamonds, emeralds, and china. **Fundason Obra di Man** (Bargestraat 57, tel. 599/9–612413) sells native crafts and curios. Try **New Amsterdam** (Gomezplein 14, tel. 599/9–613823) for hand-embroidered tablecloths, napkins, and pillowcases.

Sports **Christoffel Park** (*see* Exploring Curaçao, *above*) has a number
Hiking of challenging trails.

Scuba Diving and The **Curaçao Underwater Park** (tel. 599/9–78344) is about
Snorkeling 12½ miles of untouched coral reef that have been granted national park status. Mooring buoys mark the most interesting dive sites. If your cruise ship doesn't arrange diving or snorkeling, contact **Curaçao Seascape** (tel. 599/9–625000, ext. 177), **Peter Hughes Diving** (tel. 599/9–614944, ext. 5047), or **Underwater Curaçao** (tel. 599/9–618131).

Beaches Curaçao doesn't have long, powdery stretches of sand. Instead you'll discover the joy of inlets: tiny bays marked by craggy cliffs, exotic trees, and scads of interesting pebbles. **Westpunt,** on the northwest tip of the island, is rocky with very little sand, but shady in the morning and with a bay view worth the one-hour trip. On Sunday watch the divers jump from the high cliff.

Knip Bay has two parts: Groot (Big) Knip and Kleine (Little) Knip. Both have alluring white sand, and Kleine Knip is shaded by (highly poisonous) manchineel trees. Take the road to the Knip Landhouse, then turn right; signs will direct you. **Blauwbaai** (Blue Bay)—one of the largest, most spectacular beaches on Curaçao—offers plenty of white sand and shade, as well as showers and changing facilities. Admission is about $2.50 per car. Take the road that leads past the Holiday Beach Hotel north toward Julianadrop, and follow the sign to Blauwbaai and San Michiel.

Dining *Restaurants usually add a 10%–15% service charge to the bill.*

Bistro Le Clochard. This romantic gem is built into the 18th-century Rif Fort and is suffused with the cool, dark atmosphere of ages past. The use of fresh ingredients in consistently well-prepared French and Swiss dishes makes dining a dream. Try the fresh fish platters or the tender veal in mushroom sauce. Save room for the chocolate mousse. *On the Otrabanda Rif*

Fort, tel. 599/9–625666. Reservations required. AE, DC, MC, V. Closed Sun. off-season; no lunch Sat. Expensive.

Jaanchi Christiaan's Restaurant. Tour buses stop regularly at this open-air restaurant for lunch and for weird-sounding but mouth-watering native dishes. The main-course specialty is a hefty platter of fresh fish, potatoes, and vegetables. *Westpunt 15, tel. 599/9–640126. AE, DC, MC, V. Inexpensive.*

Grand Cayman

The largest and most populous of the Cayman Islands, Grand Cayman is one of the hottest tourist destinations in the Caribbean, largely because it doesn't suffer from the ailments afflicting many larger ports: panhandlers, hasslers, and crime. Instead, the Cayman economy is a study in stability, and residents are renowned for their courteous behavior. Though cacti and scrub fill the dusty landscape, Grand Cayman is a diver's paradise, with translucent waters and a colorful variety of marine life protected by the government. The island is also famous for the 544 offshore banks in George Town; not surprisingly, the standard of living is high and nothing is cheap.

Currency The U.S. dollar is accepted everywhere. The Cayman Island dollar (C.I.$) is worth about U.S. $1.25. Prices are often quoted in Cayman dollars, so make sure you know which currency you're dealing with.

Passports and Visas Passports are not required for U.S. or Canadian citizens, but you must have proof of citizenship. British and Commonwealth subjects do not need a visa but must carry a passport.

Telephones and Mail Phone service is better here than on most islands. Calling the United States is the same as calling long distance in the States. Stamps are available at the main post office in downtown George Town (open weekdays 8:30–4). Sending a postcard to the United States, Canada, elsewhere in the Caribbean, or Central America costs C.I. 10¢; an airmail letter, C.I. 25¢ per half-ounce. To Europe, rates are C.I. 15¢ for a postcard and C.I. 50¢ per half- ounce for airmail letters.

Shore Excursions *Not all shore excursions listed are offered by all cruise lines. All times and prices are approximate.*

Beaches and Boats **Kon-Tiki Cruise:** A booze cruise on a glass-bottom raft takes you to a beach party. Unlimited rum punch, calypso music, snorkeling, and limbo contests are available, as is a souvenir shop. *2¹/₂ hrs.. Cost: $27.*

Snorkeling Adventure: The most memorable sights on the island are underwater. A boat trip to one or two snorkeling sites—Sting Ray City is highly recommended—offers lessons for novices, good adventure for experienced snorkelers. *2 hrs. Cost: $25–$26.*

Atlantis **Submarine:** Take an excursion on a real submarine for an exciting view of Grand Cayman's profuse marine life. *1 hr. Cost: $48.*

Cultural **Island Sightseeing and Turtle Farm:** Bus tour includes a visit to the Green Sea Turtle Farm, a stop at the village of Hell (to have postcards canceled from Hell), and a stop at Seven Mile Beach. *2 hrs. Cost: $15.*

Getting Around Ships anchor in George Town harbor and tender you onto Harbour Drive. The main office of the Department of Tourism is located in the Harbour Center (N. Church St., tel. 809/949–0623). There is also an information booth in the George Town Craft Market on Cardinal Avenue (tel. 809/949–8342).

By Bicycle or Moped There isn't enough to see to warrant renting a car, but the island does have its share of agencies that rent mopeds, bikes, and motorcycles. Contact **Caribbean Motors** (tel. 809/949–4051 or 809/947–4466), **Cayman Cycle** (tel. 809/947–4020), **Honda** (tel. 809/947–4466), and **Soto Scooters** (tel. 809/947–4652).

By Taxi Taxis offer island-wide service. Fares are determined by an elaborate rate structure set by the government, and although it may seem expensive, cabbies rarely try to rip off tourists. Ask to see the chart if you want to double-check the quoted fare.

Exploring Grand Cayman **George Town** is small enough to explore on foot. When you disembark on the **cruise-ship landing dock,** you will be on Harbour Drive. To your left, across the street, is the small but fascinating **National Museum,** well worth visiting. *Tel. 809/949–8368. Admission: C.I. $5. Open Mon.–Sat. 9:30–4:30.*

On the other side of the street is the entrance to **Cardinal Avenue,** the main shopping street. On Cardinal Avenue is the **General Post Office,** built in 1939, with strands of decorative colored lights and about 2,000 private mailboxes (island mail is not delivered). Behind that is **Elizabethan Square,** a complex that houses clothing and souvenir stores.

At the corner of Fort and Edward streets, notice the small **clock tower** dedicated to Britain's King George V and the huge fig tree pruned into an umbrella shape. Turn left onto **Fort Street,** a main shopping street, with a row of jewelry stores featuring black coral products, and walk toward the water. On the waterfront along North Church Street, notice part of the original wall of the old **Ft. George,** which is now being restored.

Rent a moped or hire a taxi to get to the **Cayman Maritime and Treasure Museum,** located in front of the Hyatt Hotel, and a real find. Dioramas show how Caymanians became seafarers, boat builders, and turtle breeders. Owned by a professional treasure-salvaging firm, the museum displays a lot of artifacts from shipwrecks. A shop offers excellent buys on authentic ancient coins and jewelry. *West Bay Rd., tel. 809/947–5033. Admission: $5. Open Mon.–Sat. 9–4:30.*

The **Turtle Farm** is the most popular attraction on the island. Here you'll see turtles of all ages, from day-old hatchlings to huge 600-pounders that can live to be 100. In the adjoining café, sample turtle soup or turtle sandwiches. *West Bay Rd., tel. 809/949–3893. Admission: $5 adults, $2.50 children 6–12. Open daily 9–5.*

Shopping Turtle and black-coral products are banned in the United States. **Fort Street** and **Cardinal Avenue** are the main shopping streets in George Town. On Cardinal Avenue is **Kirk Freeport Plaza,** with lots of jewelry shops; the **George Town Craft Market;** a tourist information office; and **Native Taste,** a café with outdoor tables. On South Church Street and in the Hyatt Hotel, **Pure Art** (tel. 809/949–4433) features the work of local artists.

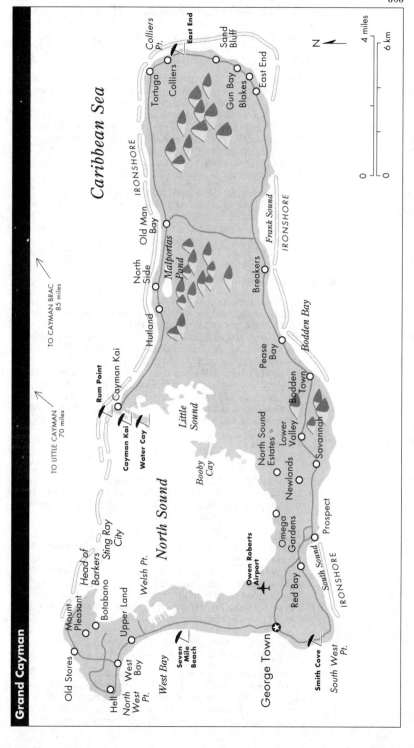

Grand Cayman

Caribbean Sea

TO CAYMAN BRAC
85 miles

TO LITTLE CAYMAN
70 miles

Colliers Pt.
East End
Sand Bluff
Tortuga
Colliers
Gun Bay
Blakes
East End

N

4 miles

6 km

IRONSHORE

Old Man Bay

Malportas Pond

North Side

Frank Sound

IRONSHORE

Hutland

Breakers

Bodden Bay

Pease Bay

Rum Point

Cayman Kai

Cayman Kai

Water Cay

Bodden Town

Little Sound

Bodden Town

Savannah

North Sound Estates

Lower Valley

Newlands

Mount Pleasant

Head of Barkers

Sting Ray City

Botabano

Upper Land

Welsh Pt.

North Sound

Booby Cay

Omega Gardens

Prospect

Old Stores

West Bay

North West Pt.

Hell

Seven Mile Beach

Owen Roberts Airport

Red Bay

South Sound

IRONSHORE

George Town

Smith Cove

South West Pt.

Sports For fishing enthusiasts, Cayman waters have plenty to offer in
Fishing the form of blue and white marlin, yellowfin tuna, sailfish, dolphin fish, bonefish, and wahoo. If your ship does not offer a
fishing excursion, about 25 boats are available for charter; try
Charter Boat Hg. (tel. 809/947–4340).

Scuba Diving The island's most impressive sights are under water. Snor-
and Snorkeling keling, diving, and glass-bottom-boat and submarine rides can
be arranged at major aquatic shops. Contact **Bob Soto's Diving
Ltd.** (tel. 809/947–4631), **Don Foster's Dive Grand Cayman** (tel.
809/949–5679 or 809/947–5732), and *Atlantis* **submarine** (tel.
809/949–7700). The best snorkeling is off the **Ironshore reef**
(south of George Town on the west coast) and in the reef-pro-
tected shallows of the north and south coasts, where coral and
fish are much more varied and abundant.

Beaches The west coast, the island's most developed area, is where
you'll find the famous **Seven Mile Beach.** The white powdery
beach is free of both litter and peddlers, but it is also Grand
Cayman's busiest vacation center, and most of the island's accommodations, restaurants, and shopping centers are located
along this strip. The Holiday Inn rents Aqua Trikes, Paddle
Cats, and Banana Rides.

Dining *Many restaurants add a 10%–15% service charge.*

Lantana's. Alfred Schrock, longtime chef at the top-rated
Wharf Restaurant, now serves his own excellent American
Southwestern cuisine at lunch and dinner. The decor is as
imaginative and authentic as the food, and both are top quality.
*Caribbean Club, West Bay Rd., George Town, tel. 809/947–5595.
Reservations required. AE, MC, V. Expensive.*
White Hall Bay. This restaurant, with a tin roof and a front-
porch view of the bay, features West Indian fare, including tur-
tle stew, salt beef and beans, and pepperpot stew. Dessert
specials are yam cake and coconut cream pie. *N. Church St.,
George Town, tel. 809/949–8670. No credit cards. Inexpensive.*

Grenada

The aroma of cinnamon and nutmeg, mace and cocoa, fill the
air and all memories of Grenada (pronounced Gruh-NAY-da).
Only 21 miles long and 12 miles wide, Grenada is a tropical gem
of lush pine forests, green hillsides, white beaches, secluded
coves, and the startling colors of exotic flowers.

Until 1983, when the U.S.–Eastern Caribbean invasion of
Grenada catapulted this little nation into the headlines, it was
a relatively obscure island providing a quiet hideaway for
lovers of fishing, snorkeling, or simply lazing in the sun. Today
Grenada is back to normal, a safe and secure vacation spot with
enough good shopping, restaurants, and pubs to make it a regular port of call. But expansion to accommodate the increased
tourist trade is controlled: No building can stand taller than a
coconut palm, and new construction on the beaches must be at
least 165 feet back from the high-water mark. As a result,
Grenada remains the archetypal Caribbean island.

Currency Grenada uses the Eastern Caribbean (E.C.) dollar. At press
time, the exchange rate was E.C. $2.60 to U.S. $1. Always ask
which currency is referred to when asking prices—unless otherwise noted, prices quoted here are in U.S. dollars, which are
readily and happily accepted, but U.S.-denominated change is

not so easy to come by. At the very least, exchange enough cash for cab fare.

Passports and Visas Passports are not required of U.S., Canadian, or British citizens if they have two proofs of citizenship.

Telephones and Mail Follow the Carenage away from the ships, past the Tourist Bureau to Hughes Street. There you'll find the **Overseas Telephone building.** Airmail rates for letters to the States and Canada are E.C. 75¢ for a half-ounce letter and E.C. 35¢ for a postcard.

Shore Excursions *Not all excursions listed are offered by all cruise lines. All times and prices are approximate.*

Beaches **Rhum Runner Cruise Tour:** Hop on a glass-bottom boat where a party's going on. Sip on unlimited rum punch and soda while you watch fish and coral glow beneath your feet. Stops on the beach for sunbathing and snorkeling are included. *3 hrs. Cost: $25 ($32 for snorkeling gear).*

Scenic **Island Tour:** A ride through the countryside to see a nutmeg station, the sugar belt, residential areas, and Grand Anse Beach. *3 hrs. Cost: $20–$25.*

Getting Around Ships call at St. George's. The center of cruise-ship activity is the Carenage, a horseshoe-shaped inner harbor. The Tourist Bureau has an information office at the pier, just before the spice and souvenir market. For $1 you can take a water taxi from one end of the Carenage to the other; water taxis are also the quickest and cheapest way to get to most beaches. The capital can be toured easily on foot if you don't mind a few hills.

By Bus Minivans ply the winding road between St. George's and Grand Anse Beach. Hail one anywhere along the way, pay E.C. $1, and hold onto your hat.

By Car If you want to venture outside St. George's, hiring a taxi or arranging a guided tour is more sensible than renting a car, unless you're well versed in driving on the *left side* of these hairy roads and willing to pay at least $45 per day rental, plus about $11 for a local license. You'll also need a valid driver's license. In St. George's, contact **Avis** at Spice Island Rentals (Paddock and Lagoon Rds., tel. 809/440–3936 or 809/444–4563), **David's** (Church St., tel. 809/440–2399), or **McIntyre Brothers** (Young St., tel. 809/440–2044).

By Taxi Taxis are plentiful, and rates are posted at the pier on the Carenage. For trips outside St. George's, you'll be charged E.C. $4 a mile for the first ten miles, and E.C. $3 a mile thereafter. Fare from the pier to Grand Anse is about E.C. $7.

Exploring Grenada *Numbers in the margin correspond to numbered points of interest on the Grenada map.*

St. George's **St. George's** is one of the most picturesque and truly West Indian towns in the Caribbean. Pastel warehouses cling to the curving shore along the horseshoe-shaped Carenage; rainbow-colored houses rise above it and disappear into the green hills. You can walk the town in about two hours.

Follow the curve of the **Carenage** past the public library, a spice and souvenir market, the **Grenada Tourist Office,** and some restaurants. If you're too tired to walk up the steep hill, the fastest way from the Carenage to the Esplanade is through the **Sendall Tunnel.**

Grenada (and Carriacou)

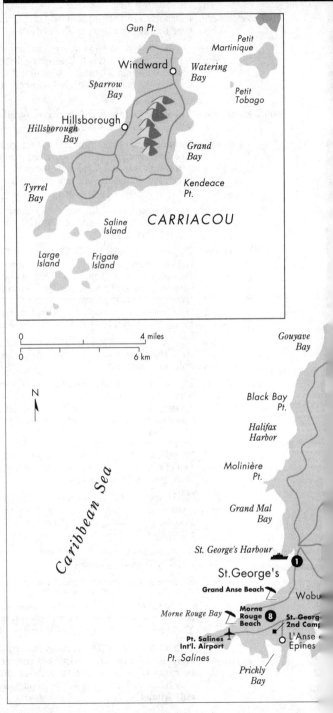

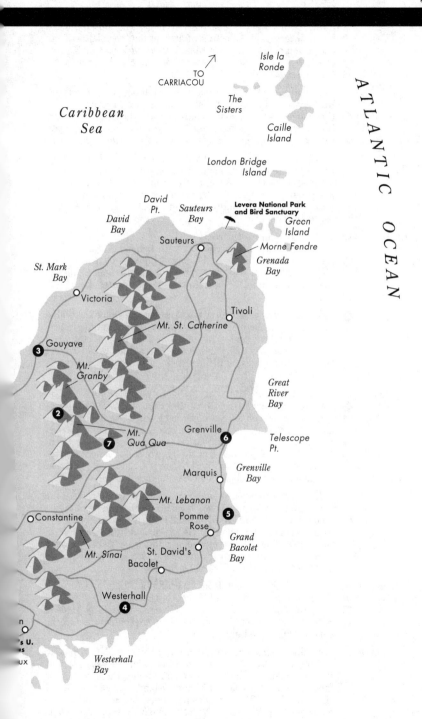

Isle la Ronde

TO CARRIACOU

The Sisters

Caribbean Sea

Caille Island

London Bridge Island

ATLANTIC OCEAN

David Pt.

Sauteurs Bay

Levera National Park and Bird Sanctuary

Green Island

David Bay

Sauteurs

Morne Fendre

Grenada Bay

St. Mark Bay

Victoria

Tivoli

Mt. St. Catherine

Gouyave

Mt. Granby

Great River Bay

Grenville

Mt. Qua Qua

Telescope Pt.

Marquis

Grenville Bay

Mt. Lebanon

Constantine

Pomme Rose

Grand Bacolet Bay

Mt. Sinai

St. David's

Bacolet

Westerhall

Westerhall Bay

The **Grenada National Museum** is across from the cruise ships docks, on the west side of the Carenege. The museum has a small, interesting collection of ancient and colonial artifacts and recent political memorabilia. *Young and Monckton Sts., tel. 809/440-3725. Admission: $1 adults, 50¢ children under 18. Open weekdays 9-4:30, Sat. 10-1:30.*

Continue along Young Street, turning left onto Church Street. **Ft. George,** built by the French in 1708, rises above the point that separates the harbor from the ocean. The inner courtyard is now the police headquarters, but the outer courtyard is open to visitors. *Admission free. Open daily during daylight hours.*

Head up Bruce Street and you'll reach the **Esplanade**—the thoroughfare that runs along the ocean side of town and has a number of fine stores. A right onto Granby Street leads to **Market Square,** which comes alive every Saturday from 6 AM to 4 PM with vendors selling baskets and fresh produce, including exotic tropical fruit.

The West Coast The coast road north from St. George's winds past soaring mountains and valleys covered with banana and breadfruit **②** trees, palms, bamboo, and tropical flowers. **Concord Falls,** about 8 miles out, is a great spot for hiking—about 2 miles to the main falls, another hour to the second spectacular waterfall.

❸ Continuing north to the town of **Gouyave,** the **Dougaldston Estate** has a spice factory where you can see cocoa, nutmeg, mace, cloves, cinnamon, and other spices in their natural state, laid out on giant trays to dry in the sun. Old women walk barefoot through the spices, shuffling them so they dry evenly. *No phone. Admission free. Open weekdays 9-4.*

The East Coast **Westerhall,** a residential area about 5 miles southeast of St. **④** George's, is known for its beautiful villas, gardens, and pano- **❺** ramic views. From here, a dirt road leads north to **Grand Bacolet Bay,** a jagged peninsula on the Atlantic where the surf **❻** pounds against deserted beaches. Some miles north is **Grenville,** Granada's second-largest city, where schooners set sail for the outer islands. As in St. George's, Saturday is market day, and the town fills with locals shopping for the week.

Take the interior route back to town to fully appreciate the lush, mountainous nature of Grenada. In the middle of the island is **Grand Etang Lake National Park,** a bird sanctuary and **❼** forest reserve where you can fish, hike, and swim. The lake, in the crater of an extinct volcano, is a 13-acre glasslike expanse of cobalt-blue water. *Main Interior Rd., between Grenville and St. George's, tel. 809/442-7425. Open weekdays 8-4.*

Grand Anse/ Most of Grenada's hotels and nightlife are in Grand Anse or *South End* the adjacent community of L'Anse aux Epines. Here you'll find **❽** one of the two campuses of **St. George's University Medical School.** Chez Josephine, its unofficial beachfront cafeteria, serves drinks and light snacks.

Carriacou A number of smaller ships, such as those operated by Windstar, call at Carriacou, 16 miles north of Grenada; it is also reachable from Grenada by plane. At 13 square miles, the island is the largest among the chain of 32 small islands and cays known as the Grenadines. Other increasingly popular cruise ports in the chain are **Bequia** (near St. Vincent) and **Mayreau,** a tiny island of 182 residents, with no phones but some of the region's most beautiful beaches.

The colonial history of Carriacou (pronounced "Kair-ee-uh-kyoo") parallels Grenada's—the island's tiny size has restricted its role in the area's political history. Like Grenada, it is verdant and mountainous. A chain of hills cuts a wide swath through the center, from Gun Point in the north to Tyrrel Bay in the south. Its greatest assets to cruise passengers are its great water- sports opportunities.

Shopping Where Cross Street intersects with the Esplanade in St. George's is the **Yellow Poui Art Gallery** (tel. 809/444–3001), which exhibits and sells Caribbean art and antique engravings. Across from the gallery, on Cross Street, is a row of tiny shops selling similar goods, as well as such treats as guava jelly and coconut fudge. Six-packs of tiny hand-woven baskets lined with bay leaves and filled with spices (about $8) make good souvenirs. Stores are generally open weekdays 8–noon and 1–4, Saturday 8–noon; most are closed on Sunday, though many boutiques and vendors open if ships are in town.

The **Grand Anse Shopping Centre** has a supermarket/liquor store, a clothing store, a shoe store, and several small shops with good souvenirs and some luxury items. Prices are competitive with other Caribbean duty-free shops.

Sports **The Grenada Golf Club** (tel. 809/444–4128) in Grand Anse has
Golf an 18-hole golf course. Fees are $16 for 18 holes, $8 for nine holes.

Water Sports Major hotels on **Grand Anse Beach** have water-sports centers where you can rent small sailboats, Windsurfers, and Sunfish. For scuba diving, contact **Dive Grenada** at Grand Anse Beach's Ramada Renaissance (tel. 809/444–4372) or **Dive Silver Beach** on Carriacou (tel. 809/443–7337).

Beaches Grenada has about 80 miles of coastline, 65 bays, and 45 white-sand beaches, many with secluded coves. Beaches are public and within an easy cab ride of the harbor. **Grand Anse,** the most popular, is a gleaming 2-mile curve of sand and clear, gentle surf about a 10-minute taxi ride from St. George's. **Morne Rough Beach,** a little farther west, is less crowded and has a reef offshore that's terrific for snorkeling.

Dining *Some restaurants add a 10% service charge to your bill. If not, a 10%–15% gratuity should be added for a job well done.*

Canboulay. You'll have to hop a ride to Morne Rough Beach and trade in your cruise bermuda shorts for something a little more chic. But it's worth it for the best cuisine on the island and a drop-dead view of St. George's harbor at night. *Tel. 809/444–4401. Closed Sun.; no lunch Sat. AE, D, MC, V. Moderate.*
The Nutmeg. Fresh seafood like grilled turtle steaks, lobster, or shrimp is the specialty at this second-floor restaurant with a great view of the harbor. *The Carenage, St. George's, tel. 809/440–2539. AE, D, MC, V. Moderate.*
Rudolf's. This informal, publike place offers fine West Indian fare—such as crab back, *lambi* and delectable nutmeg ice cream—along with the best gossip on the island. *The Carenage, St. George's, tel. 809/440–2241. Closed Sun. No credit cards. Moderate.*

Guadeloupe

On a map, Guadeloupe looks like a giant butterfly resting on the sea between Antigua and Dominica. Its two wings—Basse-Terre and Grande-Terre—are the two largest islands in the 659-square-mile Guadeloupe archipelago. The Rivière Salée, a 4-mile seawater channel flowing between the Caribbean and the Atlantic, forms the "spine" of the butterfly. A drawbridge over the channel connects the two islands.

If you're seeking a resort atmosphere, casinos, and white sandy beaches, your target is Grande-Terre. Basse-Terre's Natural Park, laced with mountain trails and washed by waterfalls and rivers, is a 74,100-acre haven for hikers, nature lovers, and anyone yearning to peer into the steaming crater of an active volcano.

This port of call is one of the least touristy. Guadeloupeans welcome visitors, but their economy does not rely on tourism. Pointe-à-Pitre, the port city, comprises smart boutiques, wholesalers, sidewalk cafés, a throbbing meat and vegetable market, barred and broken-down buildings, little parks, and bazaarlike stores. Though not to everyone's liking, the city has more character than many other island ports, and the new cruise- ship terminal, Centre St-John Perse, is a convenient complex of shops and restaurants.

French is the official language, but most locals converse in Creole and may have trouble understanding your French. Be as patient as they must be when you're trying to decipher their English. Like other West Indians, many Guadeloupeans do not appreciate having their photographs taken. Always ask permission first, and don't take a refusal personally. Also, many locals take offense at short shorts or swimwear worn outside bathing areas.

Currency Legal tender is the French franc, composed of 100 centimes. At press time, U.S. $1 bought 5.1F.

Passports and Visas U.S. and Canadian citizens need only proof of citizenship, but a passport is best. British citizens need a valid passport.

Telephones and Mail To call the United States from Guadeloupe, dial 191, the area code, and the local number. For calls within Guadeloupe, dial the six-digit number. Postcards to the United States cost 3.50F; letters up to 20 grams, 4.40F. To Canada, the rate is 3.30F for postcards and letters.

Shore Excursions *The following excursion may not be offered by all cruise lines. Time and price are approximate.*

Pointe-à-Pitre/Island Drive: A half-day drive through the city into Grande-Terre covers various districts and residential areas, including a visit to Ft. Fleur d'Epée and a refreshment stop at a hotel. *3 hrs. Cost: $27.*

Getting Around Cruise ships dock at the Maritime Terminal of Centre St-John Perse in downtown Pointe-à-Pitre, about a block from the shopping district. To get to the tourist information office, walk left along the quay for about five minutes to the Place de la Victoire.

The official language is French. Waiters and waitresses often do not speak English, nor do people in the countryside. Some taxi drivers speak a little English. It is sensible to carry a postcard of the ship with the name of where it is docked written in French. This will come in handy in an emergency.

By Car Guadeloupe has 1,225 miles of excellent roads (marked as in Europe), and driving around Grande-Terre is relatively easy. Cars can be rented at **Avis** (tel. 590/82–33–47), **Budget** (tel. 590/82–95–58), **Hertz** (tel. 590/82–00–14), or **National-Europcar** (tel. 590/82–50–51).

By Taxi Taxi fares are regulated by the government and posted at taxi stands. If your French is good, you can call for a cab (tel. 590/82–15–09, 590/83–64–27, or 590/84–37–65). Many drivers own their own taxis and don't expect a tip; others expect about 10%. Before you agree to use a taxi driver as a guide, make sure you speak a common language.

By Moped Vespas can be rented at **Vespa Sun** in Pointe-à-Pitre (tel. 590/82–17–80).

Exploring *Numbers in the margin correspond to numbered points of in-*
Guadeloupe *terest on the Guadeloupe map.*

❶ **Pointe-à-Pitre,** a city of some 100,000 people, lies almost on the "backbone" of the butterfly, near the bridge that crosses the Salée River. Bustling and noisy, with its narrow streets, honking horns, and traffic jams, it is full of pulsing life. The most interesting area, with food and clothing stalls, markets, old shophouses, and modern buildings, is compact and easy to see on foot. Stop at the **Office of Tourism**—across the road at the top of the section of the harbor called La Darse and two blocks from your ship—to pick up maps and brochures.

Turn left out of the office, and walk one block along rue Schoelcher; turn right onto rue Achille René-Boisneuf. Two more blocks will bring you to the **Musée St-John Perse,** dedicated to the Guadeloupean poet who won the 1960 Nobel Prize in literature. Inside the restored colonial house is a complete collection of his poetry, as well as many of his personal effects. *Corner rue Noizières, tel. 590/90–01–92. Admission: 10F. Open weekdays 8–12:30 and 2:30–5:30, Sat. 8–12:30.*

You'll find the **Marketplace** by backtracking one block from the museum and turning right on rue Frébault. Located between rues St-John Perse, Frébault, Schoelcher, and Peynier, it's a cacophonous and colorful place where locals bargain for papayas, breadfruit, christophine, tomatoes, and a vivid assortment of other produce.

A left at the corner of rue Schoelcher onto rue Peynier leads to the **Musée Schoelcher,** which honors the memory of Victor Schoelcher, the 19th-century Alsatian abolitionist who fought slavery in the French West Indies. Exhibits trace his life and work. *24 rue Peynier, tel. 509/82–08–04. Admission: 5F. Open weekdays 9–noon and 2:30–5:30.*

Walk back three blocks along rue Peynier, past the market, to **Place de la Victoire.** Surrounded by wood buildings with balconies and shutters and lined by sidewalk cafés, the square was named in honor of Victor Hugues's 1794 victory over the British. The sandbox trees in the park are said to have been planted by Hugues the day after the victory. During the French Revolution a guillotine here lopped off the heads of many an aristocrat.

Guadeloupe

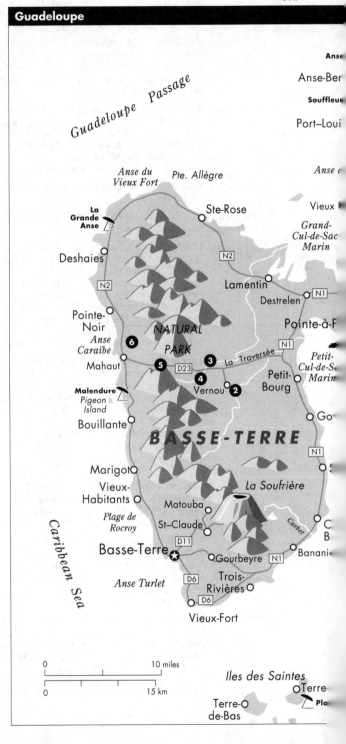

Guadeloupe Passage

Anse

Anse-Ber

Souffleu

Port–Loui

Anse

Anse du Vieux Fort   Pte. Allègre

Ste-Rose   Vieux

La Grande Anse   *Grand-Cul-de-Sac Marin*

Deshaies   `N2`

`N2`   Lamentin   `N1`

Destrelen

Pointe-à-F

Pointe-Noir   *NATURAL*

Anse Caraïbe   **6**   *PARK*   `N1`

5   `D23`   **3** La Traversée   *Petit-Cul-de-S Marin*

Mahaut   **4**

Vernou **2**   Petit-Bourg

Malendure *Pigeon Island*

Bouillante   Go

B A S S E - T E R R E   `N1`

Marigot

Vieux-Habitants   *La Soufrière*

Plage de Rocroy   Matouba

St–Claude   `D11`

Caribbean Sea   Basse-Terre ★   Gourbeyre `N1`   Banani

Trois-Rivières

Anse Turlet   `D6`

`D6`   Vieux-Fort

0   10 miles

0   15 km   *Iles des Saintes*   Terre

Terre-O de-Bas   Pl

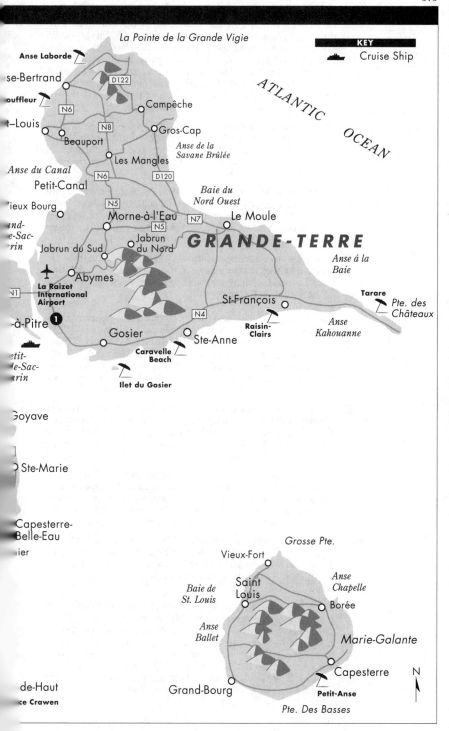

La Pointe de la Grande Vigie

Anse Laborde

se-Bertrand

ouffleur

t–Louis

Beauport

Campêche

Gros-Cap

Anse de la
Savane Brûlée

Les Mangles

Anse du Canal

Petit-Canal

ieux Bourg

nd-
e-Sac-
rin

Morne-à-l'Eau

Baie du
Nord Ouest

Le Moule

GRANDE-TERRE

Jabrun du Sud

Jabrun
du Nord

Anse á la
Baie

Abymes

La Raizet
International
Airport

Tarare

Pte. des
Châteaux

St-François

Anse
Kahouanne

-à-Pitre

etit-
e-Sac-
rin

Gosier

Ste-Anne

Raisin-
Clairs

Caravelle
Beach

Ilet du Gosier

Goyave

Ste-Marie

Capesterre-
Belle-Eau

ier

Grosse Pte.

Vieux-Fort

Baie de
St. Louis

Saint
Louis

Anse
Chapelle

Borée

Anse
Ballet

Marie-Galante

Capesterre

de-Haut

ce Crawen

Grand-Bourg

Petit-Anse

Pte. Des Basses

N

ATLANTIC OCEAN

KEY
Cruise Ship

D122

N6

N8

N6

D120

N5

N5

N7

N1

N4

Rue Duplessis runs between the southern edge of the park and **La Darse,** where fishing boats dock and motorboats depart for the choppy ride to the neighboring islands of Marie-Galante and Les Saintes. Walk north (away from the harbor) along rue Bebian, the western border of the square, and turn left onto rue Alexandre Isaac. There you'll see the imposing **Cathedral of St. Peter and St. Paul.** Earthquakes and hurricanes have wrought havoc on the 1847 church, now reinforced with iron ribs. Note the lovely stained-glass windows.

If you have transport, high adventure is to be had by driving across Basse-Terre, which swirls with mountain trails and lakes, waterfalls, and hot springs. Basse-Terre is the home of the Old Lady, as the Soufrière volcano is called, and of the capital, also called Basse-Terre.

Begin your tour by heading west from Pointe-à-Pitre on Route N1, crossing the Rivière Salée on the **pont de la Gabare** drawbridge. At the Destralen traffic circle turn left and drive 6 miles south through sweet-scented fields of sugarcane to the **Route de la Traversée** (D23), where you turn west.

Five miles from where you picked up D23, turn left at the junction and go a little over a mile south to **Vernou.** On a path that leads beyond the village through lush forest is a pretty waterfall at **Saut de la Lézarde.**

Back on La Traversée and 3 miles farther is **Cascade aux Ecrevisse,** where a marked trail leads to a splendid waterfall. Two miles farther is the **Parc Tropical de Bras-David,** where you can park and explore various nature trails. The **Maison de la Forêt** has displays on the park's flora, fauna, and topography, signposted in French. There are picnic tables. *Admission free. Open daily 9–5.*

Two and a half miles away are the two mountains known as **Les Mamelles** ("The Breasts"). The pass that runs between Les Mamelles to the south and a lesser mountain to the north offers a spectacular view. Trails ranging from easy to arduous lace the surrounding mountains.

You don't have to be much of a hiker to climb the stone steps leading from La Traversée to the **Zoological Park and Botanical Gardens.** Titi the raccoon is the mascot of the park, which also features cockatoos, iguanas, and turtles. *Tel. 590/98–83–52. Admission: 20F adults, 10F children. Open daily 9–5.*

Shopping For serious shopping in Pointe-à-Pitre, browse the boutiques and stores along **rue Schoelcher, rue Frébault,** and **rue Nozières.** The market square and stalls of **La Darse** are filled with mostly vegetables, fruits, and housewares, but you will find some straw hats and dolls.

There are some 80 shops at the cruise terminal, **Centre St-John Perse.** Many stores here offer a 20% discount on luxury items purchased with traveler's checks or major credit cards. You can find good buys on anything French—perfume, crystal, wine, cosmetics, and scarves. As for local handcrafted items, you'll see a lot of junk, but you can also find island dolls dressed in madras, finely woven straw baskets and hats, salako hats made of split bamboo, madras table linens, and wood carvings.

The following shops are all in Point-à-Pitre: For Baccarat, Lalique, Porcelaine de Paris, Limoges, and other upscale tableware, check **Selection** (rue Schoelcher), **A la Pensée** (44 rue Frébault, tel. 590/82–10–47), and **Rosebleu** (5 rue Frébault, tel. 590/82–93–44). Guadeloupe's exclusive purveyor of Orlane, Stendhal, and Germaine Monteil is **Vendômen** (8–10 rue Frébault, tel. 590/83–42–44). You'll find new designs in leather bags and belts at **Long Courrier** (18 rue Schoelcher, tel. 590/82–04–89). **Tim Tim** (16 rue Henri IV, tel. 590/83–48–71) is an upscale nostalgia shop with elegant (and expensive) antiques; be sure to see the museum-quality displays. For doudou dolls, straw hats, baskets, and madras table linens, try **Au Caraibe** (4 rue Frébault, no phone). The largest selection of perfumes is at **Phoenicia** (8 rue Frébault, tel. 590/82–25–75). You many also want to try **Au Bonheur des Dames** (49 rue Frébault, tel. 590/82–00–30).

Sports

Fishing Contact **Caraibe Peche** (Marina Bas-du-Fort, tel. 590/90–97–51), **Fishing Club Antilles** (Bouillante, tel. 590/98–78–10), or **Nautilus Club** (Bouillante, tel. 590/98–85–69).

Golf **Golf Municipal Saint-François** (St-François, tel. 590/88–41–87) has an 18-hole Robert Trent Jones course, an English-speaking pro, and electric carts for rent.

Hiking Basse-Terre's **Parc Tropical de Bras-David** is abundant with trails, many of which should be attempted only with an experienced guide. Trips for up to 12 people are arranged by **Organisation des Guides de Montagne de la Caraibe** (Maison Forestière, Matouba, tel. 590/80–05–79).

Horseback Riding Beach rides and picnics are available through **Le Criolo** (St-Felix, tel. 590/94–38–90) and **Le Relais du Moulin** (Châteaubrun, between Ste-Anne and St-François, tel. 590/88–23–96).

Water Sports Windsurfing, waterskiing, and sailing are available at almost all beachfront hotels. The main windsurfing center is at **UCPA** (tel. 590/88–64–80) in St-François. You can also rent equipment at **Holywind** (Résidence Canella Beach, Pointe de la Verdure, Gosier, tel. 590/90–44–84) and at the **Tropical Club Hotel** (tel. 590/93–97–97) at Le Moule, blessed with the constant Atlantic trade winds. **The Nautilus Club** (tel. 590/98–85–89) at Malendure Beach is one of the island's top scuba operations and offers glass-bottom-boat and snorkeling trips to **Pigeon Island,** just offshore—one of the best diving spots in the world.

Beaches Some of the island's best beaches of soft white sand lie on the south coast of Grande-Terre from Ste-Anne to Pointe des Châteaux. For a small fee, hotels allow nonguests to use changing facilities, towels, and beach chairs. **Caravelle Beach,** just outside Ste-Anne, has one of the longest and prettiest stretches of sand. Protected by reefs, it's a fine place for snorkeling, and water-sports equipment can be rented from Club Med, located at one end of the beach. **Raisin-Clairs,** just outside St-François, offers windsurfing, waterskiing, sailing, and other activities, with rentals arranged through the Meridien Hotel. **Tarare** is a secluded cove close to the tip of Pointe des Châteaux where locals tan in the buff. **La Grande Anse,** just outside Deshaies on the northwest coast of Basse-Terre, is a secluded beach of soft beige sand sheltered by palms. The waterfront Karacoli restaurant serves rum punch and Creole dishes.

Dining *Restaurants are legally required to include a 15% service charge in the menu price. No additional gratuity is necessary.*

Château de Feuilles. Located 15 kilometers from Le Moule on the Campêche road, between Gros Cap and Campêche, this restaurant is worth a special trip for lunch. Start with a swim in the pool, then indulge in one of the 20 fruit punches offered in this country setting. The menu may include goose rillettes, breaded conch, tuna carpaccio, or deep-sea fish *capitan* grilled with lime and green pepper. Try the pineapple flan for dessert. *Tel. 590/22–19–10. Reservations required. V. Expensive.*

La Canne à Sucre. This favorite over the years for its innovative Creole cuisine has the reputation for being the best (and most expensive) restaurant in Pointe-à-Pitre. In early 1991 the restaurant moved to a new two-story building at the corner of the harbor's breakwater, adjacent to the Centre St-John Perse. Fare at the main-floor Brasserie ranges from crayfish salad with smoked ham to skate in puff pastry with saffron sauce. Dining upstairs is more elaborate and twice as expensive. *Quai No. 1, Port Autonome, tel. 590/82–10–19. Reservations suggested. Jacket required upstairs. Restaurant closed Sun.*

La Maison de la Marie-Galante. More sophisticated than a café but not as pricey as Canne à Sucre, this restaurant has tables inside and on a patio. The menu ranges from roast pork and onion quiche to poached fish with a purée of aubergine. *16 bis Place de la Victoire, Point-à-Pitre, tel. 590/90–10–41. No credit cards. Moderate.*

Jamaica

The third-largest island in the Caribbean, the English-speaking nation of Jamaica enjoys a considerable self-sufficiency based on tourism, agriculture, and mining. Its physical attractions include jungle mountains, clear waterfalls, and unforgettable beaches, yet the country's greatest resource may be its people. Although 95% of Jamaicans trace their bloodlines to Africa, their national origins also lie in Great Britain, the Middle East, India, China, Germany, Portugal, and South America, as well as many other islands in the Caribbean. Their cultural life is a wealthy one; the music, art, and cuisine of Jamaica are vibrant with a spirit easy to sense but as hard to describe as the rhythms of reggae or the streetwise patois.

While most cruise ships dock at Ocho Rios, a growing number are using the city of Montego Bay (nicknamed "Mo Bay") as their Jamaican port of call. Where your cruise calls will determine how and what you will see. The town of Ocho Rios is close to the cruise port and not as busy as Montego Bay, 67 miles away, which is crowded with cars and locals running errands among the bustling shops and markets. The cruise port in Mo Bay is a $5 taxi ride from town.

Don't let Jamaica's beauty cause you to relax the good sense you would use in your own hometown. Resist the promise of adventure should any odd character offer to show you the "real" Jamaica. Jamaica *on* the beaten track is wonderful enough, so don't take chances by wandering too far off it.

Currency Currency exchange booths are set up on the docks at Montego Bay and Ocho Rios whenever a ship is there. The U.S. dollar is accepted virtually everywhere. Check the value of the JM$ on arrival—it fluctuates greatly; your change will be in local currency, don't get ripped off.

Passports and Visas Passports are not required of U.S. or Canadian citizens, but every visitor must have proof of citizenship. British visitors need passports but not visas.

Telephones and Mail Direct telephone, telegraph, telefax, and telex services are available in communication stations at the ports. Phones take phone cards, which are available from kiosks on variety shops. Airmail postage from Jamaica to the United States and Canada is JM $1.10 for letters, JM 90¢ for postcards.

Shore Excursions *Not all excursions are offered by all cruise lines. All times and prices are approximate.*

Boats and Beaches **Mystique Yacht Tour:** An elegant yacht party serves fresh island fruit, champagne, and Blue Mountain coffee. When the boat anchors, snorkel, swim, beachcomb, or climb Dunn's River Falls. *3 hrs. Cost: $55.*

Sundancer Yacht Cruise: A party cruise takes you to Dunn's River Falls for a climb up the falls or a swim on the beach. *3 hrs. Cost: $35.*

Scenic **Ocho Rios Highlights Tour including Dunn's River Falls:** A wet and fun climb up Dunn's River Falls, a tour of Shaw Park gardens, and a drive through Ocho Rios and Fern Gully, topped off with a shopping stop. *3¹/2 hrs.. Cost: $30.*

Prospect Plantation including Dunn's River Falls: Stopping at the falls only briefly, this tour goes to see the beautiful gardens of Prospect Plantation. *3¹/2 hrs. Cost: $30.*

Montego Bay Highlights & Rose Hall Great House: A general bus tour of the port includes a shopping stop at the crafts market and a tour of a beautiful 18th-century Rose Hall. *3 hrs. Cost: $35.*

Shopping A bus trip to more than 75 stores in three shopping areas. *3 hrs. Cost: $6.*

Getting Around Less than a mile from the Ocho Rios cruise-ship pier are the Taj Mahal Duty Free Shopping Center and the Ocean Village Shopping Center, where the Jamaica Tourist Board maintains an office (tel. 809/974–2582) but rarely answers its phones. Getting anywhere else in Ocho Rios will require a taxi.

There is one shopping center within walking distance of the Montego Bay docks. The Jamaica Tourist Board office is about 3½ miles away on Gloucester Avenue (tel. 809/952–4425).

Neither Ocho Rios nor Montego Bay is a walking port, and driving is not recommended for cruise passengers because renting a car tends to be a time-consuming hassle because you reserve a car and send a deposit *before* you reach Jamaica.

By Moped Mopeds are available for rent, but drive carefully: Jamaicans are not admired for their driving skills. Daily rates run from about $35. Deposits of $200 or more are required. Call **Motor Trails** (tel. 809/974–5058).

By Taxi Some of Jamaica's taxis are metered; rates are per car, not per passenger. Cabs can be summoned by phone or flagged down on the street. All licensed and properly insured taxis display red Public Passenger Vehicle (PPV) plates as well as regular plates. Licensed minivans also bear the red PPV plates. If you

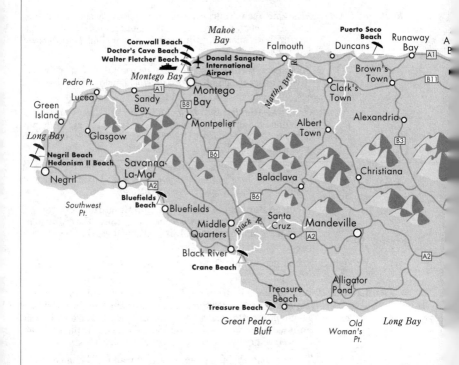

Mahoe
Bay

Puerto Seco Beach Runaway
Duncans Bay A

Falmouth

Cornwall Beach
Doctor's Cave Beach
Walter Fletcher Beach

Donald Sangster International Airport

Brown's Town

Pedro Pt.

Clark's Town

B11

Montego Bay

Lucea

Montego Bay

Green Island

Sandy Bay

B8

Martha Brae R.

Albert Town

Alexandria

Montpelier

B3

Long Bay

Glasgow

Negril Beach
Hedonism II Beach

B6

Savanna-La-Mar

Christiana

Balaclava

Negril

A2

Southwest Pt.

Bluefields Beach

Bluefields

Santa Cruz

Mandeville

B6

Middle Quarters

Black R.

Black River

A2

A2

Crane Beach

Alligator Pond

Treasure Beach

Great Pedro Bluff

Treasure Beach

Old Woman's Pt.

Long Bay

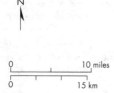

N

0   10 miles

0   15 km

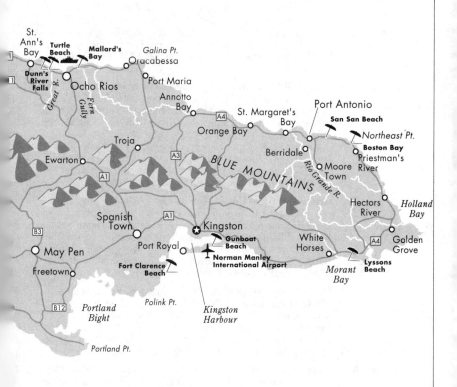

St.
Ann's
Bay **Turtle
Beach** **Mallard's
Bay** *Galina Pt.*
1 Oracabessa
1 **Dunn's
River
Falls** Ocho Rios Port Maria
Great R. Annotto
Fern Gully Bay A4 St. Margaret's Port Antonio
Orange Bay Bay **San San Beach**
Troja A3 Berridale *Northeast Pt.*
Ewarton BLUE MOUNTAINS Moore **Boston Bay**
A1 *Rio Grande R.* Town Priestman's
River
B3 Spanish Hectors *Holland
Town River Bay*
A1 Kingston
B3 Port Royal **Gunboat White A4 Golden
May Pen Beach** Horses Grove
Freetown Norman Manley **Fort Clarence International Airport** **Lyssons
Beach** *Morant Beach*
B12 *Portland Polink Pt. Kingston Bay*
Bight Harbour*

Portland Pt.

*Caribbean
Sea*

KEY
Cruise Ship

hire a taxi driver as a tour guide, be sure to agree on a price *before* the vehicle is put into gear.

Exploring Jamaica

Ocho Rios **Dunn's River Falls** is 600 feet of cold, clear mountain water splashing over a series of stone steps to the warm Caribbean. Don a swimsuit, climb the slippery steps, take the hand of the person ahead of you, and trust that the chain of hands and bodies leads to an experienced guide. The climb leaders are personable, reeling off bits of local lore while telling you where to step. Bring a towel and wear tennis shoes. *Tel. 809/974–2857. Admission: $3 adults, $1.50 children.*

The tour of **Prospect Plantation** is the best of several offerings that delve into the island's former agricultural lifestyle. It's not just for specialists; virtually everyone enjoys the beautiful views over the White River Gorge and the tour by jitney through a plantation with exotic fruits and tropical trees. Horseback riding through 1,000 acres is available, with one hour's notice, for about $20 per hour. *Tel. 809/974–2058. Admission: $7.50.*

Montego Bay **Rose Hall Great House,** perhaps the most impressive in the West Indies in the 1700s, enjoys its popularity less for its architecture than for the legend surrounding its second mistress. The story of Annie Palmer—credited with murdering three husbands and a plantation overseer who was her lover—is told in two novels sold everywhere in Jamaica: *The White Witch of Rose Hall* and *Jamaica Witch.* The great house is east of Montego Bay, across the highway from the Rose Hall resorts. *Tel. 809/953–2323. Admission: $10. Open daily 9–6:00.*

Greenwood Great House, 15 miles east of Montego Bay, has no spooky legend to titillate visitors, but it's much better than Rose Hall at evoking the atmosphere of life on a sugar plantation. Highlights of Greenwood include oil paintings of the family, china made especially for them by Wedgwood, a library filled with rare books, fine antique furniture, and a collection of exotic musical instruments. *Open daily 10–6.*

One of the most popular excursions in Jamaica is rafting on the **Martha Brae River,** (tel. 809/952–0889) a gentle waterway filled with the romance of a tropical wilderness. Wear your swimsuit for a plunge at the halfway point and pick a raft that has a comfortable cushion. Excursions on the **Lethe River** are offered by Mountain Valley Rafting (tel. 809/952–0527).

Shopping Jamaican crafts take the form of resort wear, hand-loomed fabrics, silk-screening, wood carvings, and paintings. Jamaican rum makes a great gift, as do Tia Maria (Jamaica's famous coffee liqueur) and Blue Mountain coffee. Cheap sandals are good buys. While workmanship and leather don't rival those found in Italy or Spain, neither do the prices (about $20 a pair).

Avoid the "craft" stalls in Mo Bay and Ocho Rios, which are filled with peddlers desperate to sell touristy straw hats, T-shirts, and cheap jewelry. If you're looking to spend money, head for **Overton Plaza, Westgate Plaza, Miranda Ridge Plaza,** or **St. James's Place Shopping Center,** all in Montego Bay, or **Coconut Grove** and **Island Plaza** in Ocho Rios.

For Jamaican and Haitian paintings, go to the **Gallery of West Indian Art** (1 Orange La., Montego Bay, tel. 809/952–4547). A corner of the gallery is devoted to hand-turned pottery and beautifully carved birds and jungle animals. Six miles east of the docks in Ocho Rios is **Harmony Hall** (tel. 809/975–4222), a huge house that has been converted into an art gallery, restaurant, and bar. Wares here include arts and crafts, carved items, ceramics, antiques, books, jewelry, fudge, spices, and Blue Mountain coffee.

Sports The best courses may be found at the **Half Moon Club** (tel.
Golf 809/953–2560), in Montego Bay, and **Runaway Bay** (tel. 809/973–2561) and **Upton** (tel. 809/974–2528) in Ocho Rios. Rates range from $25 to $50 for 18 holes at the Ocho Rios courses to $110 (with cart) at the Half Moon Club.

Horseback Riding **Chukka Cove** (St. Ann, tel. 809/972–2506), near Ocho Rios, is the best equestrian facility in the English-speaking Caribbean. Riding is also available at **Prospect Plantation** (between Negril and Green Island, tel. 809/974–2058) and **Rocky Point Stables** (Half Moon Club, Montego Bay, tel. 809/953–2286 or 809/957–4258).

Beaches **Doctor's Cave Beach** at Montego Bay is getting crowded, attracting Jamaicans and tourists alike. The 5-mile stretch of sugary sand has been spotlighted in so many travel articles and brochures that it's no secret to anyone anymore. Two other popular beaches near Montego Bay are **Cornwall Beach,** farther up the coast, which has food and drink options, and **Walter Fletcher Beach,** on the bay near the center of town. Fletcher offers protection from the surf on a windy day and has unusually calm waters for swimming. **Mallard's** is Ocho Rios's busiest beach; Jamaica Grande hotel and the Americana (Divi-Divi) hotels are both here, spilling out large convention groups at all hours of the day. **Turtle Beach** is the islanders' favorite place to swim in Ocho Rios.

Dining *Many restaurants add a 10% service charge to the bill. Otherwise, a tip of 10%–15% is customary.*

Sugar Mill. One of the finest restaurants in Jamaica, the Sugar Mill (formerly the Club House) serves seafood with flair on a terrace. Steak and lobster are usually offered in a pungent sauce that blends Dijon mustard with Jamaica's own Pickapeppa. *At Half Moon Golf Course, Montego Bay, tel. 809/953–2228. Reservations recommended (even for lunch). AE, DC, MC, V. Expensive.*
Almond Tree. This very popular restaurant offers Jamaican dishes enlivened by a European culinary tradition. The swinging rope chairs of the terrace bar and the tables perched above a lovely Caribbean cove are great fun. *83 Main St., Ocho Rios, tel. 809/974–2813. Reservations required. AE, DC, MC, V. Moderate–Expensive.*
Pork Pit. Enjoy Jamaica's fiery jerk pork at this open-air hangout. Plan to arrive around noon, when the first jerk is lifted from its bed of coals and pimiento wood. *Adjacent to Fantasy Resort, Montego Bay, tel. 809/952–1046. No reservations. No credit cards. Inexpensive.*

Martinique

One of the most beautiful islands in the Caribbean, Martinique is lush with wild orchids, frangipani, anthurium, jade vines, flamingo flowers, and hundreds of hibiscus varieties. Trees bend under the weight of tropical treats such as mangoes, papayas, bright red West Indian cherries, lemons, and limes.

Acres of banana plantations, pineapple fields, and waving sugarcane fill the horizon.

The towering mountains and verdant rain forest in the north lure hikers, while underwater sights and sunken treasures attract snorkelers and scuba divers. Martinique is also wonderful if your idea of exercise is turning over every 10 or 15 minutes to get an even tan, or if your adventuresome spirit is satisfied by a duty-free shop.

The largest of the Windward Islands, Martinique is 4,261 miles from Paris, but its spirit and language are decidedly French, with more than a soupçon of West Indian spice. Tangible, edible evidence of that fact is the island's cuisine, a superb blend of classic French and Creole dishes.

Fort-de-France, where ships call, is the capital, but at the turn of the 20th century, St-Pierre, farther up the coast, was Martinique's premier city. Then, in 1902, volcanic Mont Pelée blanketed the city in ash, killing all its residents—save for a condemned man in prison. Today, the ruins are a popular excursion for cruise passengers.

Currency Legal tender is the French franc, which consists of 100 centimes. At press time, the rate was 5.1F to U.S. $1. Dollars are accepted, but for convenience it's better to convert some money into francs.

Passports and Visas U.S. and Canadian citizens must have a passport or proof of citizenship. British citizens are required to have a passport.

Telephones and Mail It is not possible to make collect or credit-card calls from Martinique to the United States. There are no coin telephone booths on the island. If you must call home and can't wait until the ship reaches the next port, go to the post office and purchase a Telecarte, which looks like a credit card and is used in special booths marked TELECOM. Long-distance calls made with Telecartes are less costly than operator-assisted calls. Airmail letters to the United States are 4.40F for up to 20 grams; postcards, 3.50F.

Shore Excursions *Not all excursions are offered by all cruise lines. All times and prices are approximate.*

Kon Tiki Raft Tour: A booze cruise/beach party offers unlimited rum punch, a lively steel band, and limbo contests. *2¹/₂ hrs. Cost: $26–$29.*

Island Tour: A bus drive through the lush green mountains, past picturesque villages, to St-Pierre, with a stop at the museum there. This is one of the best island tours in the Caribbean, but a long time in a bus for a short visit to the museum. Wander beyond the museum if you have the time. *3 hrs. Cost: $24–$29.*

Getting Around By late 1993, a new pier at the north end of the Baie des Flamands will open. This will alleviate the previous inconvenience of ships anchoring offshore and tendering in or docking at the Maritime Terminal, which is a ways off from downtown Fort-de-France. The new pier will eventually have duty-free shops, but the town center is just a 10-minute walk. Also nearby is Quai Esnambuc, the terminal for ferries to Les Trois Islets, Anse-Mitan, and Anse-à-l'Ane. To get to the Maritime Terminal tourist information office, turn right and walk along the waterfront; there's another office at boulevard Alfassa (tel.

596/63–79–60). If your ship still docks at the old Maritime Terminal, a taxi is the only way to get to the Quai d'Esnambuc.

By Car Martinique has about 175 miles of well-paved roads marked with international road signs. Streets in Fort-de-France are narrow and clogged with traffic, country roads are mountainous with hairpin curves, and the Martiniquais drive with controlled abandon. If you drive in the country, be sure to pick up a map from the tourist office; an even better one is the *Carte Routière et Touristique*, available at any local bookstore.

For rental cars, contact **Avis** (tel. 596/70–11–60 or 800/331–1212), **Budget** (tel. 596/63–69–00 or 800/527–0700), **Europcar/National Car Rental** (tel. 596/51–20–33 or 800/328–4567), or **Hertz** (tel. 596/60–64–64 or 800/654–3131). Count on paying $60 a day, with unlimited mileage.

By Ferry Weather permitting, *vedettes* (ferries) operate daily between Fort-de-France and the marina Méridien, in Pointe du Bout, and between Fort-de-France and the beaches of Anse-Mitan and Anse-à-l'Ane. The Quai d'Esnambuc is the arrival and departure point in Fort-de-France. The one-way fare is 12F; round-trip, 20F.

By Taxi Taxi rates are regulated by the government; the minimum charge is 9.50F (about $1.80). Pick up cabs at taxi stands. Before you agree to use a taxi driver as a guide, check to make sure his English is good. For destinations beyond Fort-de-France, you will find taxis expensive and drivers keen to overcharge you.

Exploring Martinique *Numbers in the margin correspond to numbered points of interest on the Martinique map.*

Fort-de-France On the island's west coast, on the beautiful Baie des Flamands, **❶** lies the capital city of **Fort-de-France.** Its narrow streets and pastel buildings with ornate wrought-iron balconies are reminiscent of the French Quarter in New Orleans—though whereas New Orleans is flat, Fort-de-France is hilly.

Stop first at the **Office of Tourism,** which shares a building with Air France on boulevard Alfassa, right on the bay near the ferry landing. English-speaking staffers provide excellent free material, including detailed maps and the visitors' guides called *Martinique Info* and *Bienvenue en Martinique.*

Thus armed, walk across the street to **La Savane,** a 12½-acre landscaped park filled with gardens, tropical trees, fountains, and benches. It's a popular gathering place and the scene of promenades, parades, and impromptu soccer matches. Near the harbor is a **marketplace** where beads, baskets, pottery, and straw hats are sold.

On rue de la Liberté, which runs along the west side of La Savane, look for the main post office (between rue Blénac and rue Antoine Siger) and, across from it, the **Musée Départementale de Martinique.** Artifacts from the pre-Columbian Arawak and Carib periods include pottery, beads, and part of a skeleton that turned up during excavations in 1972. One exhibit examines the history of slavery; costumes, documents, furniture, and handicrafts from the island's colonial period are on display. *9 rue de la Liberté, tel. 596/71–57–05. Admission: 5F. Open weekdays 9–1 and 2–5, Sat. 9–noon.*

384

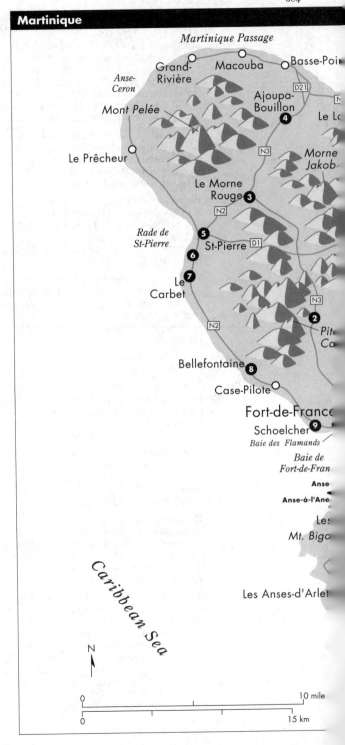

Martinique

Martinique Passage

Grand-Rivière
Macouba
Basse-Poi

Anse-Ceron

Ajoupa-Bouillon **4**

Le L

Mont Pelée

Le Prêcheur

N3

Morne Jakob

Le Morne Rouge **3**

N2

Rade de St-Pierre

5
St-Pierre D1

6

7

Le Carbet

N3

2

Pit Ca

Bellefontaine **8**

Case-Pilote

Fort-de-France
9
Schoelcher
Baie des Flamands

Baie de Fort-de-Fran

Anse

Anse-à-l'Ane

Les
Mt. Bigo

Caribbean Sea

Les Anses-d'Arlet

N

0   10 mile

0   15 km

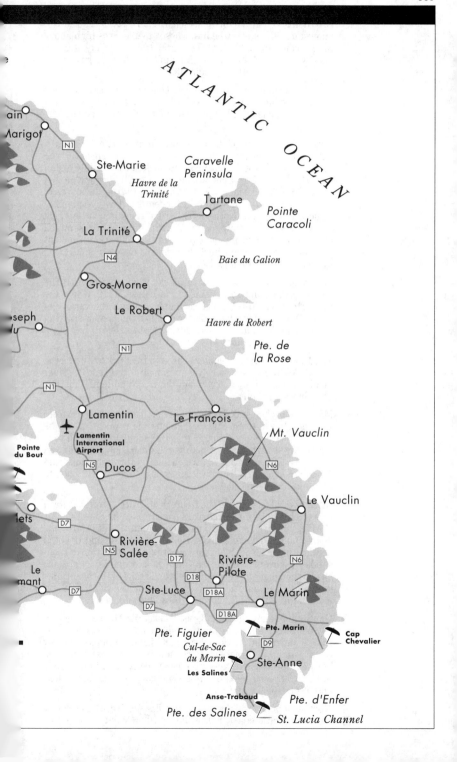

ATLANTIC OCEAN

ain
Marigot
N1
Ste-Marie
Caravelle Peninsula
Havre de la Trinité
Tartane
Pointe Caracoli
La Trinité
N4
Baie du Galion
Gros-Morne
Le Robert
Havre du Robert
Pte. de la Rose
N1
seph
lu
N1
Lamentin
Le François
Mt. Vauclin
Lamentin International Airport
N6
Pointe du Bout
N5
Ducos
Le Vauclin
lets
D7
N5
Rivière-Salée
D17
Rivière-Pilote
N6
Le
mant
D7
D18
Ste-Luce
D18A
Le Marin
D7
D18A
Pte. Marin
Cap Chevalier
Pte. Figuier
D9
Cul-de-Sac du Marin
Les Salines
Ste-Anne
Anse-Trabaud
Pte. d'Enfer
Pte. des Salines
St. Lucia Channel

386

Leave the museum and walk west (away from La Savane) on rue Blénac to rue Victor Schoelcher. There you'll see the Romanesque **St-Louis Cathedral,** whose steeple rises high above the surrounding buildings. The cathedral has lovely stained-glass windows. A number of Martinique's former governors are interred beneath the choir loft.

Rue Schoelcher runs through the center of the capital's primary **shopping district**—a six-block area bounded by rue de la République, rue de la Liberté, rue Victor Sévère, and rue Victor Hugo.

Three blocks north of the cathedral, up rue Schoelcher, turn right onto rue Perrinon and go one block. At the corner of rue de la Liberté is the **Bibliothèque Schoelcher,** the wildly elaborate Byzantine-Egyptian-Romanesque public library named after Victor Schoelcher, who led the fight to free the slaves in the French West Indies in the 19th century. The eye-popping structure was built for the 1889 Paris Exposition, after which it was dismantled, shipped to Martinique, and reassembled piece by piece on its present site. Inside is a collection of ancient documents recounting Fort-de-France's development. *Open weekdays 8:30–noon and 2:30–6, Sat. 8:30–noon.*

Follow rue Victor Sévère five blocks west, just beyond the Hôtel de Ville, and you'll come to Place José Marti, where the **Parc Floral et Culturel** will acquaint you with the variety of exotic flora on this island. There's also an aquarium showing native fish. *Sermac, tel. 596/71–66–25. Admission free. Open Mon.–Sat. 9–noon and 3–6.*

The Levassor River meanders through the park and joins the bay at **Pointe Simon,** where yachts can be chartered. The river divides the downtown area from the ritzy residential district of Didier in the hills.

The North Martinique's "must do" is the drive north along the coast from Fort-de-France to St-Pierre. The 40-mile round-trip can be done in an afternoon, although there is enough to see to fill your entire day at port. A nice way to see the lush island interior and St-Pierre is to take the N3, which snakes through dense rain forests, north to Le Morne Rouge; then take the N2 back to Fort-de-France via St-Pierre.

2 Along the N3 (also called the Route de la Trace), stop at **Balata** to see the **Balata Church,** an exact replica of Sacré-Coeur Basilica in Paris, and the **Jardin de Balata** (Balata Gardens). Jean-Phillipe Thoze, a professional landscaper and devoted horticulturalist, spent 20 years creating this collection of thousands of varieties of tropical flowers and plants. There are shaded benches where you can relax and take in the panoramic views of the mountains. *Rte. de Balata, tel. 596/72–58–82. Admission: 30F adults, 10F children. Open daily 9–5.*

3 Continuing north on the N3, you'll reach **Le Morne Rouge,** on the southern slopes of Mont Pelée. This town was, like St-Pierre, destroyed by the volcano and is now a popular resort town. Signs will direct you to the narrow road that takes you halfway up the mountain—you won't really have time to hike to the 4,600-foot peak, but this side trip gets you fairly close and offers spectacular views.

4 Northeast of here on the N3, a few miles south of **Basse-Pointe** on the Atlantic coast, is the flower-filled village of **Ajoupa-**

Bouillon. This 17th-century settlement in the midst of pineapple fields is a beautiful area, but skip it if you've never seen St-Pierre and are running out of time. From Le Morne Rouge, you'll need a good three hours to enjoy the coastal drive back to Fort-de-France.

❺ Take the N2 west a few miles to **St-Pierre,** the island's oldest city. It was once called the Paris of the West Indies, but Mont Pelée changed all that in the spring of 1902, when it began to rumble and spit steam. By the first week in May, all wildlife had wisely vacated the area, but city officials ignored the warnings, needing voters in town for an upcoming election. On the morning of May 8, the volcano erupted, belching forth a cloud of burning ash with temperatures above 3,600°F. Within three minutes, Mont Pelée had transformed St-Pierre into Martinique's Pompeii. The entire town was annihilated, its 30,000 inhabitants calcified. There was only one survivor: a prisoner named Siparis, who was saved by the thick walls of his underground cell. He was later pardoned and for some time afterward was a sideshow attraction at the Barnum & Bailey Circus.

You can wander through the site to see the ruins of the island's first church, built in 1640; the theater; the toppled statues; and Siparis's cell. While in St-Pierre, which now numbers only 6,000 residents, you might pick up some delicious French pastries to nibble on the way back after stopping in at the **Muséee Vulcanologique.** Established in 1932 by American volcanologist Franck Perret, the collection includes photographs of the old town, documents, and excavated relics, including molten glass, melted iron, and contorted clocks stopped at 8 AM, the time of the eruption. *Tel. 596/78–15–16. Admission: 5F adults, 1F children. Open daily 9–noon and 3–5.*

A short way south is **Anse-Turin,** where Paul Gauguin lived briefly in 1887 with his friend and fellow artist Charles Laval. **❻** The **Musée Gauguin** traces the history of the artist's Martinique connection through documents, letters, and reproductions of paintings he completed while on the island. *Tel. 596/77–22–66. Admission: 10F. Open daily 10–5.*

❼ Continuing down the coast, **Le Carbet** is where Columbus is believed to have landed on June 15, 1502. In 1635, Pierre Belain d'Esnambuc arrived here with the first French settlers. The **Zoo de Carbet** here features rare birds, snakes, wildcats, and caimans. *Admission: 20F adults, 10F children. Open daily 9–6.*

On your way back to port, you'll pass two of the island's more **❽** interesting towns. **Bellefontaine** is a small fishing village with pastel houses spilling down the hillsides and colorful boats bobbing in the water. Just north of Fort-de-France, **Schoelcher** is **❾** home of the University of the French West Indies and Guyana.

Shopping French products, such as perfume, wines and liquors, designer scarves, leather goods, and crystal, are all good buys in Fort-de-France. In addition, luxury goods are discounted 20% when paid for with traveler's checks or major credit cards. Look for Creole gold jewelry, white and dark rum, and handcrafted straw goods, pottery, and tapestries.

Small shops carrying luxury items proliferate around the cathedral in Fort-de-France, particularly on rue Victor Hugo, rue Moreau de Jones, rue Antoine Siger, and rue Lamartine. Look for Lalique, Limoges, and Baccarat at **Cadet Daniel** (72 rue

Antoine Siger, tel. 596/71–41–48) and at **Roger Albert** (7 rue Victor Hugo, tel. 596/71–71–71), which also sells perfume. An art gallery exhibiting local work is **Artibijoux** (89 rue Victor Hugo, tel. 596/63–10–62). A wide variety of dolls, straw goods, tapestries, and pottery is available at the **Caribbean Art Center** (Centre de Métiers Art, opposite the tourist office, Blvd. Alfassa, tel. 596/70–32–16).

In Pointe du Bout, a number of small, up-market resort boutiques cluster around the marina. **The Bleu Caraibe** (Arcades du PLM Marina, tel. 596/66–05–90) offers a fun assortment of beach and casual wear, as well as costume jewelry. You'll find an odd assortment of gifts and knickknacks in a tiny shop called L'Orchidée (Le Marina, tel. 596/66–07–73).

Sports Contact **Bathy's Club** (Hôtel Méridien, Anse-Mitan, tel.
Fishing 596/66–00–00).

Golf **Golf de l'Impératrice Joséphine** (tel. 96/68–32–81) has an 18-hole Robert Trent Jones course with an English-speaking pro, a pro shop, a bar, and a restaurant. Located at Trois-Ilets, a mile from the Pointe du Bout resort area and 18 miles from Fort-de-France, the club offers special greens fees for cruise-ship passengers.

Hiking **Parc Naturel Régional de la Martinique** (Caserne Bouille, Fort-de-France, tel. 596/73–19–30) organizes inexpensive guided hiking tours. Information is available at the island tourist office.

Horseback Riding Excursions and lessons are available at the **Black Horse Ranch** (near La Pagerie in Trois-Ilets, tel. 596/66–03–46), **La Cavale** (near Diamant on the road to the Novotel hotel, tel. 596/76–44–23), and **Ranch Jack** (near Anse-d'Arlets, tel. 596/68–63–97).

Water Sports Hobie Cats, Sunfish, and Sailfish can be rented by the hour from hotel beach shacks. If you're a member of a yacht club, show your club membership card and enjoy the facilities of **Club de la Voile de Fort-de-France** (Pointe Simon, tel. 596/70-26–63) and **Yacht Club de la Martinique** (Blvd. Chevalier, Ste-Marthe, tel. 596/63–26–76). To explore the old shipwrecks, coral gardens, and other undersea sites, you must have a medical certificate and insurance papers. Among the island's dive operators are **Bathy's Club** (Hotel Méridien, Anse-Mitan, tel. 596/66–00–00), **Carib Scuba Club** (Hôtel Latitude, north of Fort-de-France, tel. 596/78–08–08), and the **Sub Diamant Rock** (Diamant-Novotel, tel. 596/76–42–42).

Beaches Topless bathing is prevalent at the large resort hotels. Unless you're an expert swimmer, steer clear of the Atlantic waters, except in the area of Cap Chevalier and the Caravelle Peninsula. **Pointe du Bout** has small, white-sand beaches, most of which are commandeered by resort hotels. **Anse-Mitan,** south of Pointe du Bout, is a white-sand beach with superb snorkeling. **Anse-à-l'Ane** offers picnic tables and a nearby shell museum; bathers cool off in the bar of the Calalou Hotel. **Grande-Anse** is less crowded—the preferred beach among people who know the island well. **Les Salines** is the best of Martinique's beaches, whether you choose to be with other sun worshippers or to find your own quiet stretch of sand. However, it's an hour's drive from Fort-de-France and 5 miles beyond Ste-Anne.

Dining Martinique offers a chance to try French Creole cuisine, complemented by French wines better priced than in the United States. Some of the best eateries are tucked away in the countryside, and therein lies a problem of transportation and language barriers. Take along a phrase book or a translation of food terms used on the island. Some foods are specific to the islands, so even if you speak French you may have trouble.

All restaurants include a 15% service charge in their menu prices.

La Belle Epoque. The nine tables on the terrace of this turn-of-the-century house are much in demand. You can feast on duck fillet in mango sauce, hot spinach mousse, and veal kidneys. *Km 2.5, rue de Didier, Fort-de-France, tel. 596/64–47–98. Reservations and jacket required for dinner. DC, MC, V. Closed Sun., Mon. Expensive.*

Relais Caraibes. For a leisurely lunch, a magnificent view of Diamond Rock, and possibly a swim in the pool, head out to this tasteful restaurant and hotel. (A taxi will take you there for about 150F from Fort-de-France, less from Pointe du Bout.) Dishes include a half-lobster in two sauces, fresh-caught fish in a basil sauce, and fricassee of country shrimp. *Le Cherry (on the small road leading to the Diamant-Novotel), Le Diamant, tel. 596/76–44–65. No credit cards. Closed Mon. Expensive.*

Chez Gaston. The cozy upstairs dining room is very popular with local residents and features a Creole menu. The brochettes are especially recommended. Downstairs, snacks are served all day. *10 rue Felix Eboue, Fort-de-France, tel. 596/71–45–48. AE, MC, V. Inexpensive–Moderate.*

St. Croix

St. Croix is the largest of the three U.S. Virgin Islands that form the northern hook of the Lesser Antilles. Its position, 40 miles south of its sisters, unfortunately put the island in the path of 1989's Hurricane Hugo, which stalled over St. Croix for several hours, ripping the island to shreds with 150-mile-an-hour winds. Fortunately, evidence of Hugo's wrath is largely absent thanks to an immense clean-up over the past four years. Most shops, restaurants, and hotels are back and often in better shape than ever—rebuilt inside and out.

St. Croix remains quite beautiful and maintains a slow, quiet pace that is far more attractive than the hustle and bustle of St. Thomas. Christopher Columbus landed here in 1493, skirmishing briefly with the native Arawak Indians. Since then, the three U.S. Virgin Islands have played a colorful, if painful, role as pawns in the game of European colonialism. Theirs is a history of pirates and privateers, sugar plantations, slave trading, and slave revolt and liberation. Through it all, Denmark had staying power; from the 17th to the 19th century, Danes oversaw a plantation slave economy that produced molasses, rum, cotton, and tobacco. Many of the stones you see in buildings or tread on in the streets were once used as ballast on sailing ships, and the yellow fort of Christiansted is a reminder of the value once placed on this island treasure.

Currency The U.S. dollar is the official currency of St. Croix and all of the U.S. Virgin Islands.

Passports   U.S. and Canadian citizens need proof of citizenship; a passport
and Visas   is best. British citizens need a passport.

Telephones   Calling the mainland from St. Croix is as easy as calling within
and Mail   the United States. Local calls from a public phone cost 25¢ for
every five minutes. Postal rates are the same as elsewhere in
the States. Post offices are within walking distance of the piers
in Frederiksted and Christiansted.

Shore Excursions   Private tours of the **Cruzan Distillery,** the **Whim Greathouse** (a
beautiful plantation home dating back to the 1800s), and the **St.
George Village Botanical Gardens** can easily be arranged with
tour guides at the pier. Snorkeling along the underwater trail
of **Buck Island** is also available.

Getting Around   Smaller ships (less than 200 passengers) dock in Christiansted,
larger ones in Frederiksted. Information centers near both
piers offer phones and rest rooms. Both towns are easily explored on foot and offer nearby beaches.

By Car   Driving is on the left-hand side of the road, although steering
wheels are on the left-hand side of the car. In Hugo's aftermath,
all the roads have been resurfaced and many new sidewalks
have been built. Car rentals are available from **Avis** (tel.
809/778–9355), **Budget** (tel. 809/778–4663), and **Hertz** (tel.
809/778–1402), which are all near the Airport; **Caribbean Jeep
& Car** (on Hospital St., Frederiksted, tel. 809/773–4399); and
Olympic (Rte. 75 near Basin Triangle, tel. 809/773–2208). Rates
begin at about $35 daily.

By Taxi   Taxis of all shapes and sizes are available at the cruise pier and
at various shopping and resort areas; they also respond quickly
when telephoned. Taxis do not have meters, so you should
check the list of standard rates available from the visitor center
and settle the fare with your driver before you start. Taxi drivers are required to carry a copy of the official rates and must
show it to you when asked. Remember, too, that you can hail a
taxi that is already occupied. Drivers take multiple fares and
sometimes even trade passengers at midpoints. Try **St. Croix
Taxi Association** (tel. 809/778–1088) or **Antilles Taxi Service**
(tel. 809/773–5020).

Exploring St. Croix   *Numbers in the margin correspond to points of interest on the
St. Croix map.*

Most of this tour must be done by car, although Frederiksted
and Christiansted are best explored on foot. Next to the cruise-
❶ ship pier in **Frederiksted** is the restored **Ft. Frederik,** completed in the late 18th century. Here, in 1848, the slaves of the
Danish West Indies were freed by Governor Peter van Schol-
ten. Down Market Street is the **Market Place,** where you can
buy fresh fruit and vegetables early in the morning.

Around the corner on Prince Street is the **Old Danish School,**
designed in the 1830s and now part of the Ingeborg Nesbett
Clinic. **St. Paul's Episcopal Church,** a mixture of classic and
Gothic Revival architecture, is two blocks south on Prince
Street; it has survived several hurricanes since its construction
in 1812 and became Episcopal when the United States purchased the island in 1917. A few steps away, on King Cross
Street, is **Apothecary Hall,** which survived the great fire of
1878. Walk south and turn right on Queen Cross Street to the
Old Public Library, or **Bell House,** which now houses an arts-
and-crafts center and the **Dorsch Cultural Center** for the per-

forming arts. Back at the waterfront, walk up Strand Street to the **fish market.** By the cruise-ship pier is **Victoria House,** on your right. Once a private home and the town's best example of Victorian gingerbread architecture, it was heavily damaged by Hurricane Hugo but is currently undergoing renovation.

② Drive south from Frederiksted to the largest beach in the U.S. Virgin Islands, **Sandy Point.** This National Natural Landmark at the island's southwestern tip consists of a splendid stretch of sand (good for seashell collecting) and the **West End Salt Pond,** rife with mangroves and little blue herons. In the spring, large leatherback sea turtles clamber up the white sand to lay their eggs. You will also see brown pelicans.

③ Head up Centerline Road to the **Whim Greathouse.** The lovingly restored estate, with windmill, cookhouse, and other buildings, gives a real sense of what life was like for the owners of St. Croix's sugar plantations in the 1800s. The great house, with a singular oval shape and high ceilings, features antique furniture and utensils, as well as a major apothecary exhibit. Note the house's fresh and airy atmosphere—the waterless moat was used not for defense but for gathering cooling air.

④ A little farther along Centerline Road are the **St. George Village Botanical Gardens,** 17 lush and fragrant acres amid the ruins of a 19th-century sugarcane plantation village. Across **⑤** Centerline Road off Route 64 is the **Cruzan Distillery,** where rum is made with pure rainwater, making it (so it is said) superior to any other. Visitors are welcome for a tour and a free rum-laced drink (the concoction changes daily). If you hear a whoosh in your head, it's probably the air traffic at nearby Alexander Hamilton Airport—though it could just be the rum.

⑥ Turn left off Centerline Road onto Northside Road (Route 75), and continue into **Christiansted.** Dominated by its yellow fort, the town is well worth an hour of your time. Pick up a copy of the *Walking Tour Guide,* available all over town or at the visitor center at the pier.

⑦ Retrace your route along Northside Road to **Judith's Fancy,** on your right. Once home to the governor of the Knights of Malta, this old great house and tower are now in ruins. The "Judith" comes from the name of a woman buried on the property. From here you have a good view of **Salt River Bay,** where Columbus landed.

Continue west on Northside Road and then north on Route 80 toward the coast, pulling over at windy **Cane Bay.** This is one of St. Croix's best beaches for scuba diving; near the small stone jetty you may see a few wet-suited figures making their way to the "drop-off." (A bit farther out there is a steeper drop-off, to 12,000 feet.) Rising behind you is **Mt. Eagle,** at 1,165 feet St. Croix's highest peak.

⑧ Leaving Cane Bay and passing North Star Beach, follow the beautiful coast road to **Davis Bay,** both for the panoramic views of the sea along this winding corniche and for a glimpse of the striking setting of Carambola, a luxury resort. The road ends here, so backtrack to Route 69 and turn right. Turn right again onto Centerline Road and head for Frederiksted, then travel north on Route 63. The area north and east of town is **rain forest,** much of it private property but laced with roads open to the public. Just north of Frederiksted, turn right onto Route

St. Croix

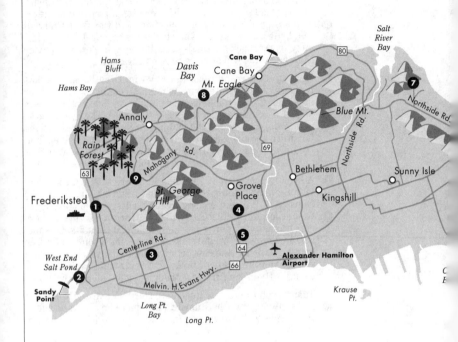

Salt River Bay

Hams Bluff

Hams Bay

Davis Bay

Cane Bay

Mt. Eagle

Blue Mt.

Northside Rd.

Annaly

Rain Forest

Mahogany Rd.

St. George Hill

Bethlehem

Sunny Isle

Frederiksted

Grove Place

Kingshill

Centerline Rd.

West End Salt Pond

Sandy Point

Melvin H. Evans Hwy.

Alexander Hamilton Airport

Krause Pt.

Long Pt. Bay

Long Pt.

Caribbean Sea

KEY

Cruise Ship

Christiansted, **6**
Cruzan Distillery, **5**
Davis Bay, **8**
Frederiksted, **1**
Judith's Fancy, **7**

St. Croix Leap, **9**
St. George Village Botanical Gardens, **4**
West End Salt Pond, **2**
Whim Greathouse, **3**

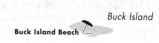

Buck Island

Buck Island Beach

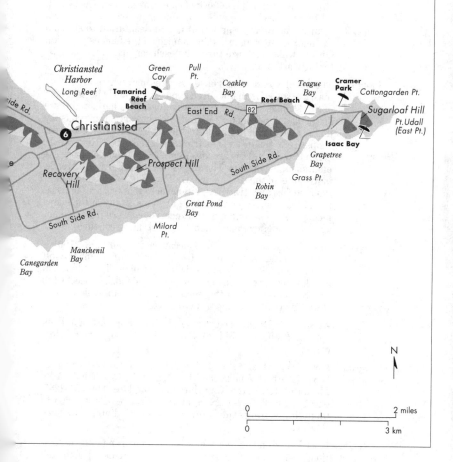

Christiansted
Harbor

Long Reef

Green
Cay

Pull
Pt.

Coakley
Bay

Teague
Bay

Cramer
Park

Cottongarden Pt.

 side Rd.

Tamarind
Reef
Beach

East End Rd.   82   Reef Beach

Sugarloaf Hill

Christiansted

6

Pt. Udall
(East Pt.)

Isaac Bay

Prospect Hill

South Side Rd.

Grapetree
Bay

Recovery
Hill

Grass Pt.

e

Robin
Bay

South Side Rd.

Great Pond
Bay

Milord
Pt.

Manchenil
Bay

Canegarden
Bay

N

0   2 miles

0   3 km

9 76, or **Mahogany Road** (the best of the roads in this area), and watch for the sign on the right to **St. Croix Leap,** where you can purchase handsome articles of mahogany, saman, or thibet wood carved by local artisans. You'll find the rain-forest air surprisingly cool.

Return west to the coast road (Route 63) and head north to **Sprat Hall Plantation,** owned and run for generations by the Hurd Family and famed for its home-cooked food. The beautiful great house is the oldest in the Virgin Islands. Pull up a chair at the breezy **Sprat Hall Beach Restaurant** to sip on a cooling soda or rum drink and munch on the famous pumpkin fritters while you gaze through beach sea-grapes at the glistening Caribbean.

Shopping Though St. Croix doesn't have nearly as many shops as St. Thomas, the selection of duty-free goods is still fairly large. Many of St. Thomas's leading shops have branches here, and there are plenty of independent merchants who carry items you may not be able to find in Charlotte Amalie. In **Christiansted,** most shops are in the historic district near the harbor. **King Street, Strand Street,** and the arcades that lead off them comprise the main shopping district. The longest arcade is **Caravelle Arcade,** in the hotel of the same name. **Gallows Bay,** just east of Christiansted, has an attractive boutique area that features unusual island-made silver jewelry and gift items. Many of the shops facing the cruise-ship pier in **Frederiksted** were heavily damaged during Hurricane Hugo, but most have reopened.

Sports
Golf The 18-hole course at **The Buccaneer** (tel. 809/773–2100) is close to Christiansted. More spectacular is the **Carambola Golf Course** (tel. 809/778–3800), designed by Robert Trent Jones, in a valley in the northwestern part of the island. The **Reef Club** (tel. 809/773–8844), in the northeast, has a nine-hole course. Rates for 18 holes range from $18 to $25.

Horseback Riding At Sprat Hall, near Frederiksted, **Jill's Equestrian Stables** (tel. 809/772–2880 or 809/772–2627) offer rides through the rain forest.

Scuba Diving and **Dive Experience** (tel. 809/773–3307), at Club Comanche in *Snorkeling* Christiansted, is one of the island's best dive specialists. **Mile Mark Charters** at the King Christian Hotel (tel. 809/773–2285, ext. 111, or 809/773–2628) offers a full range of water sports including sailing, snorkeling, and scuba diving. *Also see* Beaches, *below.*

Beaches **Buck Island** and its reef, which is under environmental protection, can be reached only by boat from Christiansted but is well worth a visit. The beach is beautiful, but its finest treasures are those you see when you plop off the boat and adjust your face mask, snorkel, and flippers. The waters are not always gentle at **Cane Bay,** a breezy north-shore beach, but the diving and snorkeling are wondrous, and there are never many people around. Less than 200 yards out is the drop-off, called Cane Bay Wall, or just swim straight out to see elkhorn and brain corals. **Sandy Point** (*see* Exploring St. Croix, *above*) boasts shallow, calm water that is ideal for swimming. Surprisingly, you don't see many people around. Also here is West End Salt Pond, prized by bird-watchers and environmentalists. **Tamarind Reef Beach** is a small but attractive beach with good snorkeling east of Christiansted. Green Cay and Buck Island seem smack in front of you and make the view arresting.

Dining   **Captain's Table.** Seafood is the forte at this pleasant courtyard restaurant—from shellfish appetizers to island conch, wahoo with white wine, shrimp Indonesian style, and bouillabaisse. You can also have steak or surf and turf. *Company St., Christiansted, tel. 809/773–2026. Reservations required. AE, MC, V. Expensive.*

Club Comanche. The atmosphere is very friendly and casual at this upstairs terrace restaurant, where the decor includes an outrigger canoe hanging from the ceiling. The varied menu includes some 15 appetizers, as well as such popular entrées as curry of beef fillet and stuffed shrimp Savannah. *Strand St., Christiansted, tel. 809/773–2665. Reservations advised. AE, MC, V. Moderate. Closed Sun.*

St. Lucia

Oval, lush St. Lucia—a ruggedly beautiful island, with towering mountains, green valleys, and acres of banana plantations—sits at the southern end of the Windward Islands. In addition to its beaches, it is distinguished by two special topographical features: the twin peaks of the Pitons (Petit and Gros), each soaring more than 2,400 feet, and Soufrière's bubbling sulfur springs, part of a low-lying volcano that erupted thousands of years ago, which attract visitors for their curative waters. Other attractions are the diving and, no less, the "liming"—the Caribbean term for hanging out.

Vendors and self-employed guides can be tenacious. If you do hire a guide, be sure the fee is clearly fixed up front. As a courtesy, you should always ask before taking an islander's picture, and be prepared to part with a few coins. In general, stick to established routes—St. Lucia is not immune to crime. The official language is English.

Currency   St. Lucia uses the Eastern Caribbean (E.C.) dollar. Figure about E.C. $2.60 to U.S. $1. U.S. dollars are widely accepted, but you'll usually get change in E.C. dollars. Major credit cards are widely accepted, as are traveler's checks.

Passports and   U.S., Canadian, and British citizens need proof of citizenship;
Visas   a passport is best.

Telephones   Long-distance connections from St. Lucia are excellent, and
and Mail   numbers can be dialed directly. International telephone and telex services are available at Pointe Seraphine, where ships dock. Postage for airmail letters to foreign countries is E.C. 95¢ for up to one ounce; postcards cost E.C. 65¢.

Shore Excursions   *Not all excursions listed are offered by all cruise lines. All times and prices are approximate.*

Boat and Beach   **Buccaneer Day Cruise:** A sailing ship offers a scenic tour of St. Lucia's west coast, passing Soufrière and the Pitons, then a sightseeing tour to the springs and volcano. A lunch stop and a visit to a beach for swimming and sunning are included. *6 hrs. Cost: $52.*

Scenic   **City Sightseeing and Beach:** Visit Bagshaw Studios for shopping and watch silk-screen artisans at work. Also included are a photo stop at Morne Fortune outlook, a visit to Pigeon Island National Park and its museum, and a stop at a beach for swimming and sunning. *3 hrs. Cost: $23.*

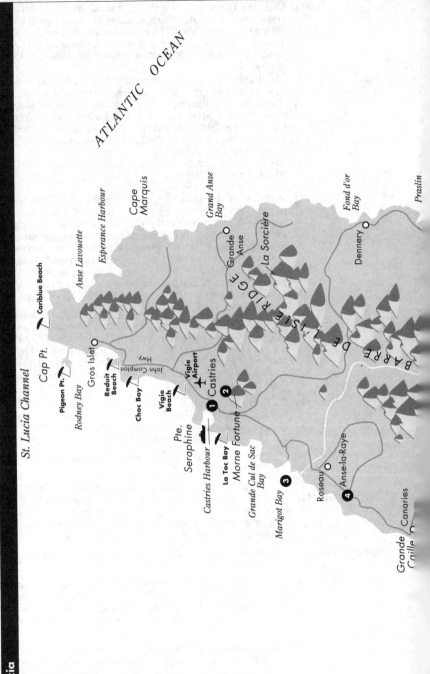

St. Lucia

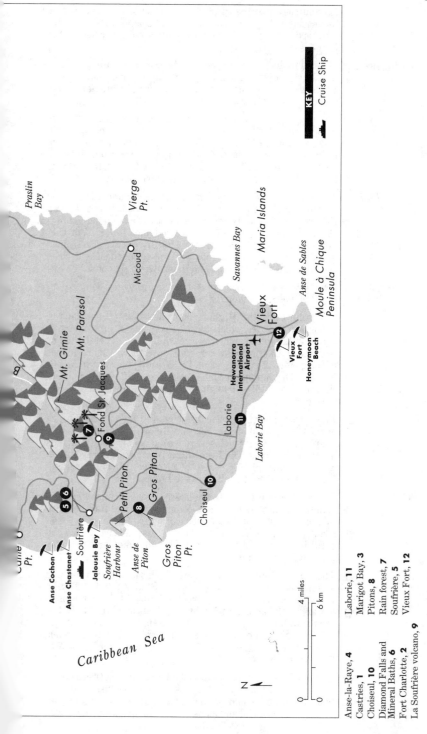

La Soufrière and the Pitons: A bus tour of the countryside, mountains, sulfur springs, volcano, and Diamond Baths. A buffet lunch accompanies this beautifully scenic overview of the island. *8 hrs. Cost: $43.*

Getting Around Most ships dock at the brand-new facilities at Pointe Seraphine in Castries, except for a couple of tiny vessels that sail into Soufrière. Tourist information offices are at Pointe Seraphine, and downtown Castries is a 20-minute walk away.

By Car Passengers are advised to rent a car or hire a taxi driver to explore the island. To rent, you have to buy a temporary St. Lucian license, which costs E.C. $40. Remember that driving is on the *left* side of the road. Rental agencies include **Avis** (tel. 809/452–2700), **Carib Touring Ltd.** (tel. 809/452–3184), **Dollar** (tel. 809/452–0994), and **National** (tel. 809/452–8028).

By Taxi Taxis are unmetered, and although the government has issued a list of suggested fares, they're not regulated. Negotiate with the driver before you depart, and be sure that you both understand whether the price you've agreed upon is in E.C. or U.S. dollars. Taxi drivers expect a 10% tip. Drivers are also trained guides; a taxi tour is a personalized way to see the island, costs about $20 an hour plus tip, and takes five to six hours.

Exploring *Numbers in the margin correspond to numbered points of in-*
St. Lucia *terest on the St. Lucia map.*

❶ The John Compton Highway connects Pointe Seraphine to downtown **Castries,** which doesn't really lend itself to an interesting walking tour. When you reach Bridge Street (by car or taxi), head east past **Government House,** the official residence of the governor-general of St. Lucia, until you come to **Morne Fortune.** Driving up the "hill of good fortune," you'll see beautiful tropical plants—frangipani, lilies, bougainvillea, hibiscus, oleander.

❷ **Ft. Charlotte** on the Morne was begun in 1764 by the French as the Citadelle du Morne Fortune. Before it was completed 20 years later, several battles were waged, and it changed hands a number of times. The **Inniskilling Monument** is a tribute to a famous battle of 1796, when the 27th Foot Royal Inniskilling Fusiliers wrested the hill from the French.

❸ The road from Castries to Soufrière travels through beautiful country. Near Roseau make a detour to **Marigot Bay,** a beautiful resort community where you can arrange to charter a boat,
❹ swim, or snorkel. The next village is **Anse-la-Raye,** with a colorful beach where fishing nets dry on poles and brightly painted fishing boats bob in the water.

❺ The town of **Soufrière,** which dates from the mid-18th century, was named after the nearby volcano. Stop at the new **Tourist Information Centre** on Bay Street (tel. 809/454–7419) for infor-
❻ mation on the area. At the **Diamond Falls and Mineral Baths,** see the waterfalls and gardens before slipping into your swimsuit for a dip in the steaming curative waters, fed by an underground flow from the volcano's sulfur springs. *Admission: E.C. $5. Open daily 9–5.*

❼ St. Lucia's dense tropical **rain forest** is east of Soufrière on the road to Fond St. Jacques; the trek through the lush landscape takes three hours, and you'll need a guide. The road south out of Soufrière is awful and leads up a steep hill, but if you perse-

8 vere, you'll be rewarded by the best land view of the **Pitons'** two pyramidal cones.

9 South of Soufrière, a left turn leads to **La Soufrière,** the drive-in volcano and its sulfur springs—more than 20 pools of black, belching, smelly sulfurous waters. Take the guided tour offered by the Tourist Board. *Admission: E.C. $5 (including tour). Open daily 9–5.*

Follow the road farther south past the coastal villages of
10 11 **Choiseul** and **Laborie.** An underground passage here leads from an old fort at Saphire to an opening at the sea. Drive now
12 along the south coast to **Vieux Fort,** St. Lucia's second-largest city. Drive out on the Moule-à-Chique Peninsula, the southernmost tip of the island. If you look north, you can see all of St. Lucia; if the day is especially clear, you can spot St. Vincent 21 miles to the south.

A good road leads from Vieux Fort through the Atlantic coast towns of Micoud and, a few miles farther north, Dennery. At Dennery, the road turns west and climbs across the Barre de l'Isle Ridge. This bumpy road will take you back to Castries.

Shopping Shopping on St. Lucia is low key, but the island's best-known products are the unique and attractive silk-screened and handprinted designs of **Bagshaw Studios.** In Soufrière, visit **Joyce Alexander's boutique** at the Humming Bird Beach Resort to see her batik designs. St. Lucia entered the duty-free market with the opening of **Pointe Seraphine,** a modern, Spanish-style complex by the harbor where 23 shops sell designer perfume, china and crystal, jewelry, watches, leather goods, liquor, and cigarettes; to get the duty-free reduction, you must show your boarding pass or cabin key. Castries has a number of shops, mostly on **Bridge Street** and **William Peter Boulevard,** that sell locally made souvenirs. At **Caribelle Batik** (Old Victoria Rd., The Morne, Castries, tel. 809/452–3785), visitors are welcome to watch artisans creating batik clothing and wall hangings. Trays, masks, and figures are carved from mahogany, red cedar, and eucalyptus trees in the studio adjacent to **Eudovic's** (Morne Fortune, 15 minutes south of Castries, tel. 809/452–2747).

Sports Contact **Captain Mike's** (tel. 809/452–0216) for information on
Fishing fishing charters.

Scuba Diving **Scuba St. Lucia** (tel. 809/454–7000) is a PADI five-star training facility that offers daily beach and boat dives, resort courses, underwater photography, and day trips. **Marigot Bay Resort** (tel. 809/453–4357) offers a full scuba program.

Beaches All of St. Lucia's beaches are public, and many are flanked by hotels where you can rent water-sports equipment and purchase refreshments. It is not advisable to swim along the east coast, because the Atlantic waters are rough. The most popular beaches are on the Caribbean side, north of Castries. **Anse Chastanet** is a gray-sand beach just north of Soufrière; with a backdrop of green hills, it has the island's best reefs for snorkeling and diving. **Vigie Beach** and **Choc Bay,** north of Castries harbor, have fine beige sand and calm waters.

Dining *Most restaurants add a 10% service charge to the bill.*

Rain. This restaurant in a Victorian building overlooking Castries's Columbus Square is usually crowded and the tables are too close together, but it's one of the island's best. Lunchtime offerings include Creole soup, crab farci, burgers, quiches, and salads; Creole chicken is a specialty. For dessert: old-fashioned, hand-cranked ice cream. *Tel. 809/452–3022. Reservations advised. AE, MC, V. Moderate.*

St. Martin/St. Maarten

St. Martin/St. Maarten: one tiny island, just 37 square miles, with two different accents, and ruled by two separate nations. Here French and Dutch have lived side by side for hundreds of years, and when you cross from one country to the next there are no border patrols, no customs. In fact, the only indication that you have crossed a border at all is a small sign and a change in road surface.

St. Martin/St. Maarten epitomizes tourist islands in the sun, where services are well developed but life remains distinctly Caribbean. The Dutch side is ideal for people who like plenty to do. The French side has more ambience, more fashionable shopping, more Continental flair, and topless (and nude) beaches. The combination of the two halves makes an almost ideal port. On the negative side, the island has been thoroughly discovered and completely developed. There is gambling, but table limits are so low that high rollers will have a better time gamboling on the beach. It can be fun to shop, and you'll find an occasional bargain, but many goods (particularly electronics) are cheaper in the United States.

Though Dutch is the official language of St. Maarten, and French of St. Martin, almost everyone speaks English. If you hear a language you can't quite place, it's Papiamento, a Spanish-based Creole.

Currency Legal tender on the Dutch side is the Netherlands Antilles florin (guilder), written NAf; on the French side, the French franc (F). In general, the exchange rate is about NAf 1.80 to U.S. $1, and 5F to U.S. $1. Dollars are accepted everywhere, however.

Passports and U.S. citizens need proof of citizenship; a passport is preferred. Visas British and Canadian citizens need valid passports.

Telephones Telephone communications, especially on the Dutch side, leave and Mail something to be desired. At the Landsradio in Philipsburg, St. Maarten, there are facilities for overseas calls and an AT&T USADIRECT telephone where you are directly in touch with an AT&T operator who will put through collect or credit-card calls. On the French side, it is not possible to make collect or credit-card calls to the States. There are no coin phones, so you need to go to the special desk at Marigot's post office on the French side and buy a Telecarte (it looks like a credit card) for use in public phones. A small kiosk by the tourist office accepts credit-card phone calls. (The operator assigns you a pin number.) Calls to the United States cost $4 per minute. A letter from the Dutch side to the United States and Canada costs NAf 1.30; postcards, NAf .60. From the French side, letters up to 20 grams cost 4.10F; postcards, 3.50F.

Shore Excursions *Not all excursions listed are offered by all cruise lines. All times and prices are approximate.*

Island Tour: A bus tour of the two countries includes a stop in French Marigot for sightseeing and shopping. *2¹/₂ hrs. Cost: $13–$24.*

Snorkel Tour: Take a boat to a beach where you will be taught how to snorkel, then given the choice of joining a snorkeling tour or setting off on your own. Refreshments may be served. *3 hrs. Cost: $27.*

Boat Tour: Take a cruise to the French side, with stops in Marigot and at a beach. Rum punch is usually included. *3¹/₂ hrs. Cost: $26.*

Getting Around Except for a few vessels that stop on the French side, all cruise ships anchor in the harbor of Philipsburg, the Dutch capital. Tenders ferry you to the Town Pier, in the middle of town, where taxis wait; next to the pier, on Wathey Square, is the **Tourist Bureau,** where you can pick up information and maps. If your ship takes you in to the marina rather than the Town Pier, you can walk to the road and turn left to reach town, a good 15 minutes away, or take a taxi. Plans to construct a new passenger terminal are on hold.

By Bus One of the island's best bargains, public buses cost from 80¢ to $2.30 and run frequently between 7 AM and 7 PM, from Philipsburg through Cole Bay to Marigot.

By Car The island roads are good, and it would be quite difficult to get lost. Also, because everything is within an easy drive of Philipsburg, this is an excellent port for renting a car. The cost is about $30 a day, plus collision insurance, with unlimited mileage. It's best to reserve a car before you leave home, especially at the height of the winter season. Contact **Avis** (tel. 800/331–1212), **Budget** (tel. 800/527–0700), **Hertz** (tel. 800/654–3131), or **National** (tel. 800/223–6472).

By Taxi Taxi rates are government-regulated, and authorized taxis display stickers of the St. Maarten Taxi Association. Taxis are also available at Marigot.

Exploring St. *Numbers in the margin correspond to numbered points of in-*
Martin/St. Maarten *terest on the St. Martin/St. Maarten map.*

❶ The Dutch capital of **Philipsburg,** which stretches about a mile along an isthmus between Great Bay and Salt Pond, is easily explored on foot. It has three parallel streets: Front Street, Back Street, and Pond Fill. Little lanes called *steegjes* connect Front Street (which has been recobbled and its pedestrian area widened) with Back Street, considerably less congested because it has fewer shops. Altogether, a walk from one end of downtown to the other takes a half-hour, even if you stop at a couple of stores.

Head first for **Wathey Square,** in the middle of the isthmus, which bustles with vendors, souvenir shops, and tourists. The streets to the right and left are lined with hotels, duty-free shops, restaurants, and cafés, most in West Indian cottages decorated in pastels with gingerbread trim. Narrow alleyways lead to arcades and flower-filled courtyards with yet more boutiques and eateries.

If you have use of a car, start at the west end of Front Street. The road (which becomes Sucker Garden Road) leads north along Salt Pond and begins to climb and curve just outside
❷ town. Take the first right to **Guana Bay Point,** from which you

St. Martin/St. Maarten

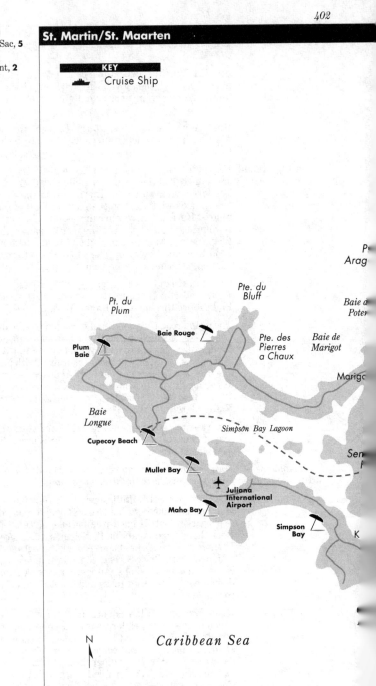

KEY

🚢 Cruise Ship

P·
Arag·

Pte. du
Bluff

Pt. du
Plum

Baie a
Poter

Baie Rouge

Pte. des
Pierres
a Chaux

Baie de
Marigot

**Plum
Baie**

Marigc

Baie
Longue

Simpson Bay Lagoon

Cupecoy Beach

Ser
I

Mullet Bay

✈ **Juliana
International
Airport**

Maho Bay

**Simpson
Bay**

K

N

Caribbean Sea

0   2 miles

0   3 km

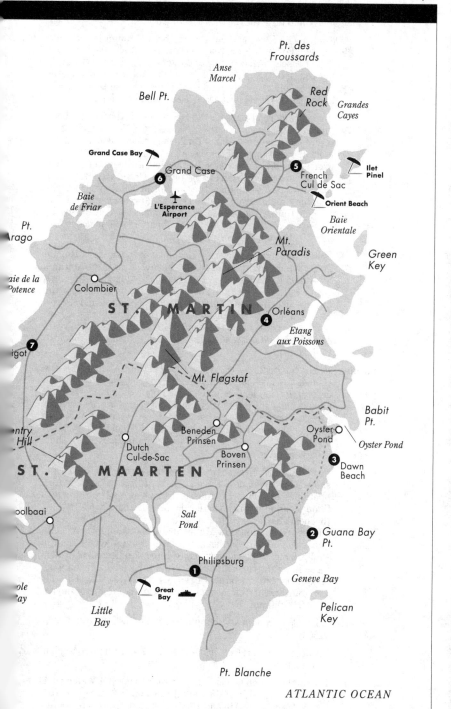

Pt. des Froussards

Anse Marcel

Bell Pt.

Red Rock

Grandes Cayes

Grand Case Bay

Grand Case

Ilet Pinel

Baie de Friar

⑥

✈ L'Esperance Airport

⑤ French Cul de Sac

Orient Beach

Pt. Arago

Baie Orientale

Green Key

aie de la Potence

Colombier

S T.   M A R T I N

Mt. Paradis

Orléans

④

Etang aux Poissons

⑦

igot

Mt. Flagstaf

Babit Pt.

entry Hill

Beneden Prinsen

Oyster Pond

Oyster Pond

S T.   M A A R T E N

Dutch Cul-de-Sac

Boven Prinsen

③ Dawn Beach

olbaai

Salt Pond

② Guana Bay Pt.

Philipsburg ①

Geneve Bay

ole ay

Great Bay 🚢

Pelican Key

Little Bay

Pt. Blanche

ATLANTIC OCEAN

get a splendid view of the island's east coast, tiny deserted islands, and little St. Barts in the distance.

❸ Sucker Garden Road continues north through spectacular scenery. Follow the dirt road to **Dawn Beach,** an excellent snorkeling beach, then continue to **Oyster Pond,** with an active sailing community. The rough, potholed road winds around the **❹** shore to join the main road at **Orléans.** This settlement, also known as the French Quarter, is the island's oldest.

A rough dirt road leads east to **Orient Beach,** the island's best-**❺** known nudist beach. North of Orléans is the **French Cul de Sac,** where you'll see nestled in the hills the French colonial mansion of St. Martin's mayor. From here the road swirls south through green hills and pastures, past flower-entwined stone fences. **❻** Past L'Esperance airport is the town of **Grand Case,** known as the "Restaurant Capital of the Caribbean." Scattered along its mile-long main street are more than 20 restaurants serving French, Italian, Indonesian, and Vietnamese fare, as well as the freshest seafood. At the Town Pier, vendors sell delicious barbecued chicken, beef on skewers, and other delicacies.

❼ Follow the signs south from Grand Case to rue de la République, which brings you to the French capital of **Marigot.** Marina Port La Royale is the shopping complex at the port; rue de la République and rue de la Liberté, which border the bay, are also filled with duty-free shops, boutiques, and bistros. The road south from Marigot leads to the official border, where a simple marker, placed here in 1948, commemorates 300 years of peaceful coexistence. This road will bring you back to Philipsburg.

Shopping   Prices can be 25%–50% below those in the United States and Canada for French perfume, liquor, cognac and fine liqueurs, crystal, linens, leather, and other luxury items. However, it pays to know the prices back home; not all goods are a bargain. Caveat emptor: While most merchants are reputable, there are occasional reports of inferior or fake merchandise passed off as the real thing. When vendors bargain excessively, their wares are often suspect.

In Philipsburg, **Front Street** is one long strip of boutiques and shops; **Old Street,** near the end of Front Street, has 22 stores, boutiques, and open-air cafés. At Philipsburg's **The Shipwreck Shop,** look for Caribelle batiks, hammocks, handmade jewelry, the local guava-berry liqueur, and herbs and spices. You'll find almost 100 boutiques in **Mullet** and **Maho** shopping plazas. In general, you will find smarter fashions in Marigot than in Philipsburg. In Marigot, wrought-iron balconies, colorful awnings, and gingerbread trim decorate the shops and tiny boutiques in the **Marina Port La Royale,** at the **Galerie Perigourdine,** and on the main streets, **rue de la Liberté** and **rue de la République.**

Sports   Contact **Wampum** at Bobby Marina, Philipsburg (tel. 599/5–
Fishing   22366).

Golf   **Mullet Bay Resort** (tel. 599/5–42081) has an 18-hole championship course.

Water Sports   Myriad boats can be rented at **Lagoon Cruises & Watersports** (tel. 599/5–52801, ext. 1873) and **Caribbean Watersports** (tel. 599/5–42801). NAUI- and PADI-certified dive centers offer scuba instruction, rentals, and trips. On the Dutch side, try

Tradewinds Dive Center (tel. 599/5–54387) and **St. Maarten Divers** (tel. 599/5–22446). On the French side, there's **Lou Scuba** (tel. 590/87–28–58) and **Blue Ocean** (tel. 509/87–89–73), both PADI-certified.

Beaches The island's 10 miles of beaches are all open to the public. Those occupied by resort properties charge a small fee (about $3) for changing facilities, and water-sports equipment can be rented at most hotels. Some of the 37 beaches are secluded; some are in the thick of things. Topless bathing is common on the French side. If you take a cab to a remote beach, be sure to arrange a specific time for the driver to return for you. Don't leave valuables unattended on the beach.

Baie Longue, the island's best beach, is a mile-long curve of white sand at the western tip offering excellent snorkeling and swimming but no facilities. **Cupecoy Beach** is a narrower, more secluded curve of white sand just south of Baie Longue near the border. There are no facilities, but a truck often pulls up with cold beer and sodas. Clothing becomes optional at the far end of the beach.

Dining *By law, restaurants on the French side figure a service charge into the menu prices, so no tips are expected. On the Dutch side, most restaurants add 10%–15% to the bill.*

Dutch Side **Chesterfield's.** Burgers and salads are served at lunch, but menus are more elaborate for dinner on this indoor/outdoor terrace overlooking the marina. Offerings include French onion soup, roast duckling with fresh pineapple and banana sauce, and chicken Cordon Bleu. The Mermaid Bar is popular with yachtsmen. *Great Bay Marina, Philipsburg, tel. 599/5–23484. AE, MC, V. Inexpensive–Moderate.*

Turtle Pier Bar and Restaurant. Chattering monkeys and squawking parrots greet you at the entrance to this classic Caribbean hangout, festooned with creeping vines and teetering over the lagoon. There are 200 animals in the zoo, but that's nothing compared to the menagerie at the bar during happy hour. Genial owners Sid and Lorraine Wathey have fashioned one of the funkiest, most endearing places in the Caribbean, with cheap beer on tap, huge American breakfasts, all-you-can-eat ribs for $9.95, and eclectic live music several nights a week. *Airport Rd., Philipsburg, tel. 599/5–52230. No credit cards. Inexpensive.*

French Side **Le Poisson d'Or.** At this posh and popular restaurant set in a stone house, the waters of the bay lap the 20-table terrace as you feast on hot foie gras salad in raspberry vinaigrette, smoked lobster boiled in tea with parsley cream sauce, or veal with Roquefort, hazelnut, and tarragon sauce. The young chef, François Julien, cooks with enthusiasm, but his cuisine must compete for attention with the striking setting. *Off rue d'Anguille, Marigot, tel. 590/87–72–45. Reservations recommended. AE, MC, V. No lunch in the off-season. Expensive.*

Cha Cha Cha Caribbean Cafe. Pascal and Christine Chevillot's culinary pedigree is impeccable: Pascal's Uncle Charles owns New York's La Petite Ferme. So what have they done here? Created a chi-chi dive. Japanese gardens, gaudy colors, and a gaudier clientele have made this the island hot spot (the mouthwatering haute-Caribbean cuisine and reasonable prices don't hurt). Try the giant prawns in passion-fruit butter or grilled snapper with avocado, then wash it down with a "Grand Case Sunset." *Grand Case, tel. 590/87–53–63. MC, V. Moderate.*

St. Thomas/St. John

St. Thomas is the busiest cruise port of call in the world. As many as a dozen ships tie up in the two dock areas or just outside the harbor in a single day. Don't expect an exotic island experience: One of the three U.S. Virgin Islands (with St. Croix and St. John), St. Thomas is as American as any place on the mainland, complete with McDonald's franchises, HBO, and the U.S. dollar. The positive side of all this development is that there are more tours to choose from here than anywhere else in the Caribbean, and every year the excursions get better. Of course, shopping is the big draw in Charlotte Amalie, the main town, but experienced travelers remember the days of "real" bargains. Today, so many passengers fill the stores that it's a seller's market. One of St. Thomas's best tourist attractions is its neighboring island, St. John, with its beautiful national parks and empty beaches.

Passports and Visas U.S. and Canadian citizens need proof of citizenship; a passport is best. British citizens need a passport.

Telephones and Mail It's as easy to call home from St. Thomas as from any city in the United States. And public phones are all over the place, including right on the dock. Postal rates are the same as elsewhere in the States: 29¢ for a letter, 19¢ for a postcard.

Shore Excursions *Not all excursions are offered by all cruise lines. All times and prices are approximate.*

Adventure **Scuba Diving:** This excursion to one or two choice sites via boat or off a beach may be limited to certified divers or open to novices who have been taking lessons on the ship. *3 hrs. Cost: $38–$75.*

Helicopter Tour: An exciting aerial tour of St. Thomas and surrounding islands. *2 hrs. Cost: $50–$100.*

Boats and Beaches **Coki Beach Snorkeling:** A shallow reef just offshore next to Coral World, this busy locale has a large population of fish, coral, and snorkelers. Good for novices who want to learn snorkeling and see a variety of wildlife. *3 hrs. Cost: $21–$22.*

Kon Tiki Party Tour: This booze-cruise barge picks up passengers at the ship, with a steel band blazing lively calypso and the bar already open. Then it's off to Brewer's Bay for a beach party that includes limbo contests, dancing, and swimming. *3 hrs. Cost: $27.*

Sailing and Snorkeling Tour: A romantic sail, a snorkeling lesson, and an attractive snorkeling site make this an excellent excursion for experiencing the true beauty of the Virgin Islands. The boat may be a modern catamaran, a single-hull sailing yacht, or a sailing vessel done up to look like a pirate ship. *3¹/₂–4 hrs. Cost: $32–$40.*

Submarine Tour: A surface boat ferries you out to a submarine with large picture windows that dives to explore the underwater world, with good accompanying narrative. If your ship doesn't offer this tour, or if theirs is filled, you can book directly with **Atlantis Submarine** (Havensight Mall, tel. 809/776–5650). *2 hrs. Cost: $68 adults, $34 children under 13.*

Scenic **Island Tour & Coral World:** In addition to the island tour described above, you'll stop at Coral World, where an underwater observatory offers a fascinating view of native fish and coral. *3 hrs. Cost: $23–$28.*

St. John Island Tour: Either your ship tenders you in to St. John in the morning before docking at St. Thomas, or you take a bus from the St. Thomas docks to the St. John ferry. On St. John, an open-air safari bus winds through the national park to a beach for snorkeling, swimming, and sunbathing. (If you have the option, go to Honeymoon Bay instead of Trunk Bay.) All tours end with a ferry ride back to St. Thomas. *4–4 1/2 hrs. Cost: $22–$40.*

Getting Around The best place to dock is along Havensight, a shopping mall that has the same merchandise at similar prices as that sold in downtown Charlotte Amalie. Many passengers don't even bother going into town if their ship is at Havensight. A newer dock has been built at the old submarine base (about about a 10-minute taxi ride from town).

By Car Driving is on the left side of the road, though steering wheels are on the left side of the car. Car rentals are available from numerous agencies, including **ABC Rentals** (By Havensight Mall, tel. 809/776–1222), **Budget** (104 West St., tel. 809/776–7575), and **Hertz** (Near the Airport, tel. 809/774–1879). Rates for one day range from $55 to $70.

By Ferry You can get to St. John on your own via ferry from Charlotte Amalie. Get ferry schedules and information from the tourist information offices at Havensight or in Charlotte Amalie.

By Taxi Taxis meet every ship. They don't have meters, so check with the shore-excursion director for correct fares; establish the fare before getting in the cab. Most taxis are minivans, which take multiple fares and charge per person. Many of them will give you a guided tour of the island for far less than you'd pay for a ship-sponsored excursion.

Exploring St. *Numbers in the margin correspond to numbered points of in-*
Thomas *terest on the St. Thomas map.*

Charlotte Amalie **Charlotte Amalie** is a hilly, overdeveloped shopping town.
❶ There are plenty of interesting historical sights here, and much of the town is quite pretty. But the most scenic parts of the island will require a car or taxi. To tour downtown on foot, first
❷ take a taxi to **Frenchtown** (about a half-mile southwest of the town center). Here Frenchies—descendants of emigrants from St. Barts—sell fish from their boats. The island offshore is **Hassel Island,** now a Virgin Island national park in the process of building an infrastructure to accommodate visitors. Take a moment to walk west through some of Frenchtown's winding streets.

Cross Veterans Drive (also called Waterfront Highway) and walk east past the **Windward Passage Hotel** to Kronprindsen's Alley and turn left. At the top of the alleyway is the Roman Catholic **Cathedral of St. Peter and St. Paul,** consecrated in 1848. Head east on Main Street and take the second left onto Strand Gade. On the left is **Christ Church Methodist,** which dates back to 1700. Across the street are the open-air stalls of **Market Square,** a busy produce bazaar that was an infamous slave market two centuries ago. You're now at the west end of

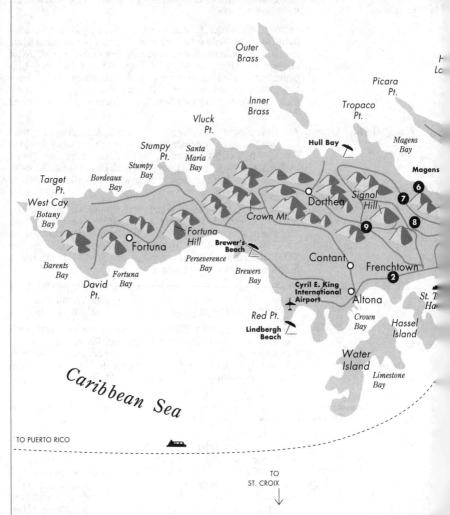

Charlotte Amalie, **1**
Coral World, **4**
Drake's Seat, **6**
Fairchild Park, **8**
Four Corners, **9**
Frenchtown, **2**
Mountain Top, **7**
Red Hook, **3**
Tillet's Gardens, **5**

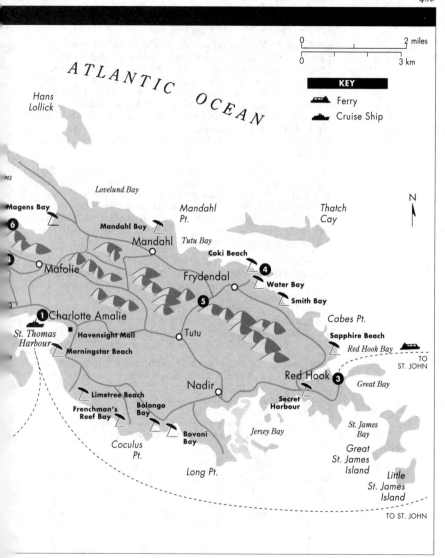

ATLANTIC OCEAN

Hans
Lollick

Lovelund Bay

Magens Bay

6

3

Mafolie

ns

*Mandahl
Pt.*

Mandahl Bay

Mandahl

Tutu Bay

Frydendal

Coki Beach

4

Water Bay

Smith Bay

*Thatch
Cay*

5

N

1 Charlotte Amalie

*St. Thomas
Harbour*

Havensight Mall

Morningstar Beach

Tutu

Cabes Pt.

Sapphire Beach

Red Hook Bay

TO
ST. JOHN

Red Hook **3**

Great Bay

Nadir

**Secret
Harbour**

Limetree Beach

**Frenchman's
Reef Bay**

**Bolongo
Bay**

**Bovoni
Bay**

Jersey Bay

*St. James
Bay*

*Great
St. James
Island*

*Little
St. James
Island*

*Coculus
Pt.*

Long Pt.

TO ST. JOHN

| 0 | | 2 miles |
| 0 | | 3 km |

KEY

Ferry

Cruise Ship

Charlotte Amalie's feverish duty-free shopping district, which stretches along and between **Main Street** and the waterfront.

Stroll east on Main Street among the shops until you reach the **Pissarro Building,** in the block between Store Tvaer Gade and Trompeter Gade. A plaque around the block, on Back Street, identifies the location as where the French Impressionist painter Camille Pissarro was born in 1830, upstairs from what is now the Tropicana Perfume Shop. Turn left on Raadet's Gade and go up the hill to Crystal Gade. Across the street to the left is the **St. Thomas Synagogue,** the second oldest in the Western Hemisphere; the sand on the floor commemorates the biblical Exodus.

Head west along Crystal Gade and wander up the steps on the right that lead to the old Greek Revival **Danish Consulate Building** (1830) and **Villa Santana** (1858). Return to Crystal Gade and walk east to the 1844 **Dutch Reformed Church,** which was founded in 1744, burned in 1804, and rebuilt to its present austere loveliness in 1844. From here Nye Gade leads to the **All Saints Anglican Church,** built in 1848.

Head back down the hill, and take the steps to Kongen's Gade and ahead to the beautiful Spanish-style **Hotel 1829,** whose restaurant (*see* Dining, *below*) is one of the best on St. Thomas. To the right is the base of the **99 Steps,** a staircase "street" built by the Danes in the 1700s. Go up the steps (there are more than 99) and continue to the right to **Blackbeard's Castle,** originally Ft. Skysborg and now a small hotel and restaurant (*see* Dining, *below*). The massive five-story watchtower was built in 1679.

With gravity now on your side, head back down the steps. To the left down Kongen's Gade is **Government House** (1867), the official residence of the governor of the U.S. Virgin Islands. Inside are murals and paintings by Pissarro. Continue down the steps in front of Government House to Norre Gade and turn right to reach the **Frederick Lutheran Church,** the second-oldest Lutheran church in the Western Hemisphere. Its walls date to 1793.

Walk down Tolbod Gade toward the water to **Emancipation Garden,** a park that honors the 1848 freeing of the slaves and features a smaller version of the Liberty Bell. As you stand in the park facing the water, you'll see a large red building to your left, close to the harbor; this is **Ft. Christian,** St. Thomas's oldest standing structure (1627–87) and a U.S. national landmark. The building was used at various times as a jail, governor's residence, town hall, courthouse, and church; its dungeons now house a museum featuring artifacts of Virgin Islands history. The clock tower was added in the 19th century. To your far right, on the waterfront, is a visitor information center and lounge, with rest rooms.

If you continue toward the water and cross Veterans Drive, you'll be at **Kings Wharf.** To the left is the lime-green **Legislature Building** (1874), the seat of the 15-member U.S.V.I. Senate since 1957.

The South Shore   Leaving Charlotte Amalie, head east along the waterfront on
and East End   Veterans Drive (Route 30), which becomes Route 32, called Red Hook Road as it passes **Benner Bay, East End Lagoon,** and
❸ **Compass Point.** Staying on Route 32 brings you into **Red Hook,** which has grown from a sleepy little town, connected to the rest

of the island only by dirt roads, into an increasingly self-sustaining village. There's luxury shopping at American Yacht Harbor, or you can stroll along the docks and visit with sailors and fishermen, stopping for a beer at Piccola Marina Cafe or Larry's Warehouse. Above Red Hook, the main road swings toward the north shore and becomes Route 38, or Smith Bay
❹ Road, taking you past Sapphire Beach and on to **Coral World,** with its three-level underwater observatory, the world's largest reef tank, and an aquarium with more than 20 TV-size tanks providing capsulized views of sea life. *Tel. 809/775–1555. Admission: $14 adults, $9 children. Open daily 9–6.*

❺ Farther west on Route 38 is **Tillett's Gardens** (*see* Shopping, *below*), where local artisans craft stained glass, pottery, and ceramics. Tillett's paintings and fabrics are also on display.

North Shore/ In the heights above Charlotte Amalie is **Drake's Seat,** the
Center Islands mountain lookout from which Sir Francis Drake was supposed
❻ to have kept watch over his fleet and looked for enemy ships of the Spanish fleet. Magens Bay and Mahogany Run are to the north, with the British Virgin Islands and Drake's Passage to the east. Off to the left, or west, are Fairchild Park, Mountain Top, Hull Bay, and smaller islands, such as the Inner and Outer Brass islands.

❼ West of Drake's Seat is **Mountain Top,** not only a tacky mecca for souvenir shopping, but also the where the banana daiquiri was supposedly invented. There's a restaurant here and, at 1,500 feet above sea level, some spectacular views. Below
❽ Mountain Top is **Fairchild Park,** a gift to the people of the U.S.V.I. from philanthropist Arthur Fairchild.

If you head west from Mountain Top on Crown Mountain Road
❾ (Rte. 33), you'll come to **Four Corners.** Take the extreme right turn and drive along the northwestern ridge of the mountain through **Estate Pearl, Sorgenfri,** and **Caret Bay.** There's not much here except peace and quiet, junglelike foliage, and breathtaking vistas.

Shopping There are well over 400 shops in Charlotte Amalie alone, and near the Havensight docks there are at least 50 more, clustered in converted warehouses. Even diehard shoppers won't want to cover all the boutiques, since a large percentage peddle the same T-shirts and togs. Many visitors devote their shopping time on St. Thomas to the stores that sell handicrafts and luxury items.

Although those famous "give-away" prices no longer abound, shoppers on St. Thomas can still save money. Today, a realistic appraisal puts prices on many items at about 20% off stateside prices. What's more, there is no sales tax in the U.S. Virgin Islands, and visitors can take advantage of the $1,200-per-person duty-free allowance and the additional 5% discount on the next $1,200 worth of goods. Remember to save receipts.

You won't need to spend a lot of time comparison shopping, since some luxury items—perfumes, cosmetics, liquor—are uniformly priced throughout the U.S. Virgin Islands. Prices on almost everything else, from leather goods to leisure wear, vary very little from shop to shop. The prices on jewelry do vary quite a bit, however, and it's here that you'll still run across some real "finds." Major credit cards are widely accepted.

Shopping Districts The major shopping area is Charlotte Amalie, in centuries-old buildings that once served as merchants' warehouses and that for the most part have been converted to retail establishments. Both sides of **Main Street** are lined with shops, as are the side streets and walkways between Main Street and the Waterfront. These narrow lanes and arcades have names like Drake's Passage, Royal Dane Mall, Palm Passage, Trompeter Gade, Hibiscus Alley, and Raadet's Gade. The **Bakery Square Shopping Mall** (one block north of Main St. off Nye Gade) has about 15 boutiques. The streets adjacent to Bakery Square, notably Back Street, Nye Gade, Garden Street, Kongen's Gade, and Norre Gade, are also very good areas for browsing. At **Havensight Mall,** near the deep-water port where many cruise ships dock, you'll find branches of downtown stores, as well as specialty shops and boutiques.

Charlotte Amalie Unless otherwise noted, the following stores have branches both downtown and in Havensight Mall and are easy to find. If you have any trouble, shopping maps are available at the tourist offices and often from your ship's shore-excursion desk. U.S. citizens can carry back a gallon or six "fifths" of liquor duty-free.

A.H. Riise Gift Shops: Waterford, Wedgwood, Royal Crown, Royal Doulton, jewelry, pearls, ceramics, perfumes, watches, art, books, historical prints; liquors, cordials, and wines, including rare vintage Cognacs, Armagnacs, ports, and Madeiras; tobacco and imported cigars; fruits in brandy; barware from England. **Al Cohen's Discount Liquor** (across from Havensight Mall only): discount liquors. **Amsterdam Sauer** (downtown only): one-of-a-kind fine jewelry. **Aperiton** (downtown only): Greek and Italian jewelry. **Blue Diamond** (downtown only): 14K and 18K jewelry crafted by European goldsmiths. **Boolchand's:** cameras, audio-video equipment.

The Caribbean Marketplace (Havensight Mall only): Caribbean handicrafts, including Caribelle batiks from St. Lucia; bikinis from the Cayman Islands; Sunny Caribee spices, soaps, teas, and coffees from Tortola. **The Cloth Horse** (downtown only): pottery from the Dominican Republic; wicker and rattan furniture and household goods from Hispaniola; pottery, rugs, and bedspreads from all over the world. **Cosmopolitan:** Gortex swimsuits; 300 different styles of bikinis, maillots, and "constructed" one-piece suits; men's Italian knit sport shirts; sea-island cotton shirts from London. **Dilly D'Alley** (downtown only): more than 20 lines of swimwear; comfortable, tie-dyed cotton wraparound dresses. **Down Island Traders** (downtown only): hand-painted calabash bowls; jams, jellies, spices, and herbs; herbal teas made of rum, passion fruit, and mango; high-mountain coffee from Jamaica; Caribbean handicrafts. **The English Shop:** china and crystal from Spode, Limoges, Royal Doulton, Royal Crafton, Royal Worcester, Villeroy & Boch.

The Gallery (downtown only): Haitian and local oil paintings, metal sculpture, wood carvings, painted screens and boxes, figures carved from stone, oversize papier-mâché figures. **G'Day** (downtown only): umbrellas, artwork, sportswear. **Gucci:** wallets, bags, briefcases, totes, shoes. **H. Stern:** gems and jewelry. **Ilias Lalaounis** (downtown only): 18K and 22K gold jewelery by the Greek designer. **Janine's Boutique:** women's and men's apparel and accessories from European designers and manufacturers, including Louis Feraud, Valentino, Christian Dior,

Pierre Cardin. **Java Wraps** (downtown only): Indonesian batik, swimwear, leisure wear, sarongs, ceremonial Javanese puppets. **The Leather Shop:** Fendi, Bottega Veneta, other fine leather goods. **Lion in the Sun** (downtown only): men's and women's designer fashions. **Little Switzerland:** Lalique, Bacarat, Waterford, Swarovski, Riedel, Orrefors, other crystal; Villeroy & Boch, Aynsley, Wedgwood, Royal Doulton, other china; Rolex watches. **Louis Vuitton** (downtown only): scarves, umbrellas, leather briefcases and steamer trunks, other fine goods. **Luisa:** leather shoes and bags from Italy.

Purse Strings (downtown only): leather handbags by Christian Dior, Carlo Fiori, Lesandro Saraso; straw and canvas Caribbean goods; eelskin and snakeskin bags and accessories. **Red Fort** (downtown only): antique boxes and textiles; lapis, turquoise, ruby, and emeralds in unusual gold or silver settings. **Royal Caribbean:** cameras, cassette players, audio-video equipment. **Sea Wench** (Havensight Mall only): swimwear, lingerie. **Shoe Tree** (downtown only): women's shoes by Bandolino, Pierre Cardin, Evan Picone, Liz Claiborne, others. **Travelers Haven** (Havensight Mall only): leather bags, backpacks, vests, money belts. **Tropicana Perfume Shoppes** (downtown only): fragrances for men and women. **Virgin Islands Pot Pourri Company** (downtown only): batik and tie-dyed works, other Virgin Islands fabric creations.

Tillett Gardens **Tillett Gardens and Craft Complex** (Estate Tutu, tel. 809/775–1405) is more than worth the cab fare to reach it. Jim Tillett's artwork is on display, and you can watch craftsmen and artisans produce watercolors, silk-screened fabrics, pottery, enamel work, candles, and other handicrafts.

St. John Opportunities for duty-free shopping are more limited and the prices a bit higher on St. John than on the other islands. One popular spot is **Wharfside Village,** an attractive, compact mall of some 30 shops overlooking Cruz Bay Harbor. **Mongoose Junction,** just north of Cruz Bay across from the Park Service Visitor Center, is one of the most pleasant places to shop in the Caribbean. Built from native stone, the graceful staircases and balconies wind among the shops, a number of which sell handicrafts designed and fashioned by resident artisans.

Sports Call **American Yacht Harbor** at Red Hook (tel. 809/775–6454)
Fishing if you're interested in some serious angling.

Golf Scenic **Mahogany Run** (tel. 809/775–5000), north of Charlotte Amalie, has a par-70 18-hole course and a view of the British Virgin Islands. Rates for 18 holes are $75, cart included.

Water Sports The **St. Thomas Diving Club** (tel. 809/776–2381), at Bolongo Bay, caters to scuba divers. **Underwater Safaris** (tel. 809/774–1350 or 809/774–4044) is at the Ramada Yacht Haven Motel and Marina, near Havensight. Other reliable scuba and snorkeling operators are **Joe Vogel Diving Co.** (tel. 809/775–7610) and **Aqua Action** (tel. 809/775–6285).

Beaches All beaches in the U.S. Virgin Islands are public, but occasion-
St. Thomas ally you'll need to stroll through a resort to obtain access. Government-run **Magens Bay** is lively and popular because of its spectacular loop of white beach, more than a half-mile long, and its calm waters. Food, changing facilities, and rest rooms are available. **Secret Harbour** is a pretty cove for superb snorkeling; go out to the left, near the rocks. **Morningstar Beach,**

close to Charlotte Amalie, has a mostly sandy sea bottom with some rocks; snorkeling is good here when the current doesn't affect visibility. **Sapphire Beach** has a fine view of St. John and other islands. Snorkeling is excellent at the reef to the east, near Pettyklip Point, and all kinds of water-sports gear can be rented. Be careful when you enter the water; there are many rocks and shells in the sand.

St. John **Trunk Bay** is the main beach on St. John, mostly because of its underwater snorkeling trail. However, experienced snorkelers may find it tame and picked over, with too little coral or fish. Lifeguards are on duty.

Dining *Some restaurants add a 10%–15% service charge to the bill.*

Hotel 1829. Candlelight flickers over old stone walls and across the pink table linens at this restaurant on the gallery of a lovely old hotel. The award-winning menu and wine list are extensive, from Caribbean rock lobster to rack of lamb; many items, including a warm spinach salad, are prepared tableside. The restaurant is justly famous for its dessert soufflés: chocolate, Grand Marnier, raspberry, coconut. *Government Hill, a few steps up from Main St., Charlotte Amalie, tel. 809/776–1829. Reservations required. AE, MC, V. No lunch. Expensive.*

Gladys' Cafe. Even if the food were less tasty and the prices higher, it would be worth visiting just to see Gladys smile. Antiguan by birth, she won a local following as a waitress at Palm Passage before opening her own restaurant for breakfast and lunch in a courtyard off Main Street in Charlotte Amalie. Try the Caribbean lobster roll, the barbecue ribs, Gladys' hot chicken salad, or one of the filling salad platters. *Tel. 809/774–6604. AE. Inexpensive.*

San Juan, Puerto Rico

Although Puerto Rico is part of the United States, no other city in the Caribbean is as steeped in Spanish tradition as San Juan. Old San Juan has restored 16th-century buildings, museums, art galleries, bookstores, 200-year-old houses with balustrade balconies overlooking narrow, cobblestoned streets—all within a seven-block neighborhood that's an easy, though hilly, stroll from the cruise-ship piers. In contrast, San Juan's sophisticated Condado and Isla Verde areas have glittering hotels, flashy Las Vegas–style shows, casinos, and discos.

Out in the countryside is the 28,000-acre El Yunque rain forest, with more than 240 species of trees growing at least 100 feet high. You can also visit dramatic mountain ranges, numerous trails, vast caves, coffee plantations, old sugar mills, and hundreds of beaches. No wonder San Juan is one of the busiest ports of call in the Caribbean. Like any other big city, San Juan has its share of crime, so guard your wallet or purse, and avoid walking in the area between Old San Juan and the Condado.

Passports and Visas U.S. citizens do not need passports. British citizens must have a passport and, in some cases, a visa—Brits should check to see if the ship they're on is part of the visa-waiver program. Canadians need proof of citizenship (preferably a passport).

Telephones and Mail Use the long-distance telephone-service office in the cruise-ship terminal at the recently built and extremely clean and attractive Pier. Postal rates are the same as in the United States.

Shore Excursions *Not all excursions are offered by all cruise lines. All times and prices are approximate.*

Beach Party Many ships arrange to drive their passengers to a beach (often Luquillo) where changing rooms and deck chairs (sometimes at an extra charge) are provided. The trip may include a buffet lunch and/or rum punch. *3–5 hrs. Cost: $15–$27.*

Scenic **Old and New San Juan City Tour:** Bus tour includes a visit to El Morro Fortress, a drive through town, and sightseeing in modern residential areas. *2–3 hrs. $14–$19.*

El Yunque Rain Forest: A 45-minute drive heads east through picturesque villages to the Caribbean National Forest, where you may walk along various trails, see waterfalls, and climb the observation tower. The trip may include a stop at Luquillo Beach. *4 hrs. Cost: $20.*

Sightseeing **Bacardi Rum Distillery:** After seeing how it is made, you can buy some Bacardi rum and/or visit the family museum. *2 hrs. Cost: $15.*

San Juan Nightlife Tour: Several major hotels (like the Condado Plaza) have very exciting revues, especially those that feature flamenco or Latin dancers. Includes a drink or two. *3 hrs. Cost: $26–$34.*

Getting Around Pier 1, the cruise-ship terminal farthest left if you are facing away from the water, is close to a tourist information booth and a long-distance telephone office.

By Bus The **Metropolitan Bus Authority** operates buses that thread through San Juan. The fare is 25¢, and the buses run in exclusive lanes, against traffic, on all major thoroughfares, stopping at yellow posts marked *Parada* or *Parada de Guaguas.* The main terminal is Intermodal Terminal, at Marina and Harding streets in Old San Juan.

By Car U.S. driver's licenses are valid in Puerto Rico. All major U.S. car-rental agencies are represented on the island. Contact **Avis** (tel. 809/721–4499 or 800/331–1212), **Budget** (tel. 809/791–3685 or 800/654–3131), **Hertz** (tel. 809/791–0840 or 800/527–0700), or **L & M Car Rental** (tel. 809/725–8416). Prices start at $30 a day (plus insurance), with unlimited mileage. If you plan to drive across the island, arm yourself with a good map and be aware that many roads up in the mountains are unmarked, and many service stations require cash. To keep you on your toes, speed limits are posted in miles, distances in kilometers, and gas prices are per liter.

By Taxi Taxis line up to meet ships. The docks are in Old San Juan; a 10- to 15-minute taxi ride to New San Juan costs $8–$10, and a five- minute ride to the Condado costs $3–$4. Metered cabs authorized by the Public Service Commission charge an initial $1 and 10¢ for each additional ¹⁄₁₀ mile. Waiting time is 10¢ for each 45 seconds. Demand that the meter be turned on, and pay only what is shown, plus a tip of 10%–15%.

By Trolley If your feet fail you in Old San Juan, climb aboard the free open-air trolleys that rumble through the narrow streets. They meet the ships, or you can board them anywhere along the route.

Exploring Old San Juan *Numbers in the margin correspond to numbered points of interest on the Old San Juan map.*

Casa de los Contrafuertes, **6**
City Hall, **5**
Cruise ship port, **1**
Dominican Convent, **9**
El Morro (Fuerte/San Felipe del Morro), **10**
La Fortaleza, **13**
La Intendencia, **4**
Pablo Casals Museum, **7**
Plaza de Armas, **3**
Plazuela de la Rogativa, **12**
San Cristóbal, **2**
San José Church, **8**
San Juan Cathedral, **11**

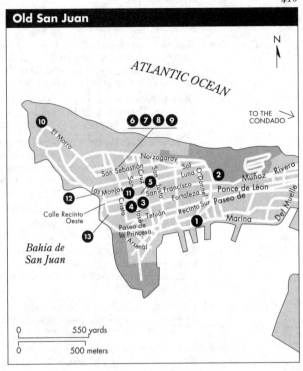

Old San Juan

Old San Juan, the original city founded in 1521, contains authentic and carefully preserved examples of 16th- and 17th-century Spanish colonial architecture. Graceful wrought-iron balconies decorated with lush green hanging plants extend over narrow cobblestoned streets. Seventeenth-century walls still partially enclose the old city. Designated a U.S. National Historic Zone in 1950, Old San Juan is packed with shops, open-air cafés, private homes, tree-shaded squares, monuments, plaques, pigeons, people, and traffic jams. It's faster to walk than to take a cab. Nightlife is quiet, if spooky during the low-season; you'll find more to do in New San Juan, especially the Condado area.

1 The **cruise-ship port** is within a couple of blocks of Old San Juan. Across from piers, local artisans display their wares at the **Plazoleta del Puerto.** From here, stroll along the **Paseo de la Princesa,** a tree-lined promenade beneath the city wall, featuring local crafts and refreshment kiosks.

2 Walk up the hill along Calle O'Donnell past the Tapia Theater and the bus terminal. A right onto Calle San Francisco leads to **San Cristóbal,** the 18th-century fortress that guarded the city from land attacks. Larger than El Morro (*see below*), San Cristóbal was known as the Gibraltar of the West Indies and offers spectacular views of both Old San Juan and the new city. *Tel. 809/729–6960. Admission free. Open daily 9:15–6.*

3 Return along Calle San Francisco; three to four blocks past **St. Francis Church** and the **Museum of the Puerto Rican Family/Museum of Colonial Architecture** is the **Plaza de Armas,** the original main square of Old San Juan. The plaza has a lovely fountain with statues representing the four seasons. West of

❹ the square stands **La Intendencia,** a handsome three-story neo-classical building that was home to the Spanish Treasury from 1851 to 1898. *Calle San José at Calle San Francisco. Admission free. Open weekdays 8–noon and 1–4:30.*

❺ On the north side of the plaza is **City Hall,** called the *alcaldía.* Built between 1604 and 1789, it was fashioned after Madrid's city hall, with arcades, towers, balconies, and a lovely inner courtyard. A tourist information center and an art gallery are on the first floor. *Tel. 809/724–7171, ext. 2391. Open weekdays 8–noon and 1–4.*

❻ Turn right onto Calle San José. Here, the **Casa de los Contrafuertes**—also known as the Buttress House because buttresses support the wall next to the plaza—is one of the oldest remaining private residences in Old San Juan. Inside is the Pharmacy Museum, a re-creation of an 18th-century apothecary shop. *101 Calle San Sebastián, Plaza de San José, tel. 809/724–5949. Admission free. Open Wed.–Sun. 9–4:30.*

❼ The **Pablo Casals Museum,** farther down the block, contains memorabilia of the famed Spanish cellist, who made his home in Puerto Rico for the last 20 years of his life. *101 Calle San Sebastián, Plaza de San José, tel. 809/723–9185. Admission free. Open Tues.–Sat. 9:30–5:30, Sun. 1–5.*

❽ In the center of Plaza San José is the **San José Church.** With its series of vaulted ceilings, it is a fine example of 16th-century Spanish Gothic architecture. *Calle San Sebastián, tel. 809/725–7501. Admission free. Open daily 8:30–4; Sun. mass at 12:15.*

❾ Next door is the **Dominican Convent.** Also built in the 16th century, the building now houses an ornate 18th-century altar, religious manuscripts, artifacts, and art. *98 Calle Norzagaray, tel. 809/724–0700. Admission free. Chapel museum open Wed.–Sun. 9–noon and 1–4:30.*

❿ Follow Calle Norzagaray to **El Morro** (Fuerte San Felipe del Morro), set on a rocky promontory on the northwestern tip of the old city. Rising 140 feet above the sea, the massive six-level Spanish fortress is a labyrinth of dungeons, ramps, turrets, and tunnels. Built to protect the port, El Morro has a commanding view of the harbor and Old San Juan. Its small museum traces the history of the fortress. *Tel. 809/729–6960. Admission free. Open daily 9:15–6:15.*

⓫ Leaving El Morro, head for **San Juan Cathedral** on Calle Cristo. This great Catholic shrine of Puerto Rico had humble beginnings in the early 1520s as a thatch-top wood structure that was destroyed by a hurricane. It was reconstructed in 1540, when the graceful circular staircase and vault ceilings were added, but most of the work on the church was done in the 19th century. The remains of Ponce de León are in a marble tomb near the transept. *153 Calle Cristo. Open daily 8:30–4.*

⓬ Go west alongside the Gran Hotel El Convento on Caleta de las Monjas toward the city wall to the **Plazuela de la Rogativa.** In the little plaza, statues of a bishop and three women commemorate a legend that the British, while laying siege to the city in 1797, mistook the flaming torches of a religious procession for Spanish reinforcements and beat a hasty retreat.

⑬ One block south on Calle Recinto Oeste is **La Fortaleza,** on a hill overlooking the harbor. The Western Hemisphere's oldest executive mansion in continuous use, La Fortaleza was built as a fortress. The original 16th-century structure has seen numerous changes, including the addition of marble and mahogany, medieval towers, and stained-glass galleries. Guided tours are conducted every hour on the hour in English, on the half-hour in Spanish. *Tel. 809/721–7000. Admission free. Open weekdays 9–4.*

New San Juan In Puerta de Tierra, a half-mile east of the pier, is Puerto Rico's white marble **Capitol,** dating from the 1920s. Another mile east, at the tip of Puerta de Tierra, tiny **Ft. San Jeronimo** perches over the Atlantic like an afterthought. Added to San Juan's fortifications in the late 18th century, the structure barely survived the British attack of 1797.

Santurce, the district between Miramar on the west and the Laguna San José on the east, is a busy mixture of shops, markets, and offices. The classically designed **Sacred Heart University** is home of the **Museum of Contemporary Puerto Rican Art** (tel. 809/268–0049).

San Juan Environs From San Juan, follow Route 2 west toward Bayamón and you'll spot the **Caparra Ruins,** where, in 1508, Ponce de León established the island's first settlement. The ruins are those of an ancient fort. Its small **Museum of the Conquest and Colonization of Puerto Rico** contains historic documents, exhibits, and excavated artifacts. *Km 6.6 on Rte. 2, tel. 809/781–4795. Admission free. Open weekdays 9–5, weekends 10–6.*

Continue on Route 2 to **Bayamón.** In the Central Park, across from the city hall, are some historic buildings and a 1934 sugarcane train that runs through the park. Along Route 5 from Bayamón to Catano, you'll see the **Barrilito Rum Plant.** On the grounds is a 200-year-old plantation home and a 150-year-old windmill, which is listed in the National Register of Historic Places.

The **Bacardi Rum Plant,** along the bay, conducts 45-minute tours of the bottling plant, museum, and distillery, which has the capacity to produce 100,000 gallons of rum a day. (Yes, you'll be offered a sample.) *Km 2.6 on Rte. 888, tel. 809/788–1500. Admission free. Tours Mon.–Sat. 9:30–3:30; closed Sun. and holidays.*

Shopping San Juan is not a free port, and you won't find bargains on electronics and perfumes. In fact, many Puerto Ricans go to Miami to do their shopping, and their savings usually pay for the trip. However, shopping for native crafts can be fun. Popular souvenirs and gifts include *santos* (small, hand-carved figures of saints or religious scenes), hand-rolled cigars, handmade lace, carnival masks, Puerto Rican rum, and informal men's shirts called *guayaberas.*

Old San Juan is filled with shops, especially on **Calles Cristo, La Fortaleza,** and **San Francisco.** You can get discounts on Hathaway shirts and clothing by Christian Dior and Ralph Lauren at **Hathaway Factory Outlet** (203 Calle Cristo, tel. 809/723–8946) and on raincoats at the **London Fog Factory Outlet** (156 Calle Cristo, tel. 809/722–4334). For one-of-a-kind local crafts, head for **Puerto Rican Arts & Crafts** (204 Calle La Fortaleza, Old San Juan, tel. 809/725–5596), **Plazoleta del Puerto**

(Calle Marina, Old San Juan, tel. 809/722–3053), **Don Roberto** (205 Calle Cristo, tel. 809/724–0194), and **M. Rivera** (107 Calle Cristo, Old San Juan, tel. 809/724–1004).

Sports There are two 18-hole courses shared by the **Hyatt Dorado**
Golf **Beach Hotel** and the **Hyatt Regency Cerromar Beach Hotel** (Dorado, tel. 809/796–1234). You'll find 18-hole courses at **Palmas del Mar Resort** (Humacao, tel. 809/852–6000), **Club Riomar** (Rio Grande, tel. 809/887–3964), and **Punta Borinquen** (Aquadilla, tel. 809/890–2987).

Hiking Dozens of trails lace **El Yunque.** Information is available at the Sierra Palm Visitor Center (Km 11.6, Rte. 191).

Water Sports Virtually all the resort hotels on San Juan's Condado and Isla Verde strips rent paddleboats, Sunfish, and Windsurfers.

Beaches By law, all of Puerto Rico's beaches are open to the public (except for the Caribe Hilton's artificial beach in San Juan). The government runs 13 public beaches (*balnearios*), which have lockers, showers, and picnic tables; some have playgrounds and overnight facilities. *Admission free; parking $1. Open Tues.–Sun. 8–5 in summer; 9–5 in winter.*

Isla Verde is a white sandy beach close to metropolitan San Juan. Backed by several resort hotels, the beach offers picnic tables and good snorkeling, with equipment rentals nearby.

Dining *A 10%–15% tip is expected in restaurants.*

La Chaumière. Reminiscent of a French inn, this intimate yet bright white restaurant serves a respected onion soup, oysters Rockefeller, rack of lamb, and veal Oscar, in addition to daily specials. *327 Calle Tetuán, tel. 809/722–3330. Reservations advised. AE, DC, MC. Closed Sun. Expensive.*
Amadeus. The atmosphere of this restaurant is gentrified Old San Juan, with an ever-changing menu of 20 appetizers, including *tostones* with sour cream and caviar, plantain mousse with shrimp, and arrowroot fritters with gauva sauce. Entrées on the nouvelle Caribbean menu range from grilled mahimahi with cilantro butter to creamy pasta dishes, and chicken and steak sandwiches. Most nights, you'll dine among locals. *106 Calle San Sebastián, tel. 809/722–8635. Reservations recommended. AE, MC, V. Closed Mon. Moderate.*

Nightlife Almost every ship stays in San Juan late or even overnight to give passengers an opportunity to enjoy the nightlife—the most sophisticated in the Caribbean.

Casinos By law, all casinos are in hotels. Alcoholic drinks are not permitted at the gaming tables, although free soft drinks, coffee, and sandwiches are available. The atmosphere is quite refined, and many patrons dress to the nines, but informal attire is usually fine. Casinos set their own hours, which change seasonally, but generally operate from noon to 4 AM. Casinos are located in the following hotels: **Condado Plaza Hotel, Caribe Hilton, Caribe-Inn, Clarion Hotel, Dutch Inn, El San Juan, Ramada,** and **Sands.**

Discos In Old San Juan young people flock to **Neon's** (203 Tanca St., tel. 809/725–7581) and to **Lazers** (251 Cruz St., tel. 809/721–4479). In Puerta de Tierra, Condado, and Isla Verde, the 30-something crowd heads for **Amadeus** (El San Juan Hotel, tel. 809/791–1000), **Juliana's** (Caribe Hilton Hotel, tel. 809/721–

0303), **Isadora's** (Condado Plaza Hotel, tel. 809/721–1000), and **Mykonos** (La Concha Hotel, tel. 809/721–6090).

Nightclubs The Sands Hotel's **Calypso Room** has a flamenco show nightly except Monday. El San Juan's **Tropicoro** presents international revues and occasionally top-name entertainers. The Condado Plaza Hotel has the **Copa Room,** and its **La Fiesta** sizzles with steamy Latin shows. Young professionals gather at **Peggy Sue** (tel. 809/722–4750), where the design is 1950s and the music mixes oldies and current dance hits.

The Hawaiian Islands

It's hard to believe such a gentle paradise sprang from such a violent beginning—mighty volcanic explosions. Over the centuries, crashing surf, strong sea winds, and powerful rivers carved and chiseled the great mountains and lush valleys that are Hawaii's pride.

Polynesian explorers stumbled upon these islands in the 4th century AD while navigating the South Pacific in their huge voyaging canoes. A succession of native rulers began in 1795 with King Kamehameha I and ended with the deposition of Queen Liliuokalani in 1893, when a provisional government was installed. In 1900 Hawaii was established as a U.S. territory, and in 1959 it became the 50th state. Today the islands retain a mystique that makes Hawaii America's most exotic state, with 132 islands and atolls stretching across 1,600 miles of ocean.

At one time many a ship brought travelers to the Hawaiian Islands, but when Pan Am's amphibious *Hawaii Clipper* touched down on Pearl Harbor's waters in 1936, it marked the beginning of the end of regular passenger-ship travel. Since then, visitors have been flown in, and only a few cruise ships now pass through the islands. For details, check with such cruise lines as Cunard, Holland America, and Royal Cruise Line (*see* Chapter 3).

Travelers can, however, experience the lure of Hawaii's waters by cruising among the Hawaiian Islands on American Hawaii Cruises' 800-passenger twin ships, the SS *Constitution* and the SS *Independence* (*see* Chapter 3). Both leave Honolulu on seven-day cruises that visit the Big Island, Maui, and Kauai; shorter three- and four-day cruises, which make fewer stops, are also available.

When to Go   Hawaii is always temperate, sunny, and a pleasure. Although rainfall is slightly greater from December through February the sun is rarely hidden behind the clouds for a solid 24-hour period. Summer is big with families, as are holidays. February and March are also busy cruising months.

Passport and Visas   Canadians need only prove their place of birth, with a passport, birth certificate, or similar document. Other foreign citizens require a passport and visa.

Shopping   Retail outlets abound in the Aloha State, from major tourist centers to small villages. Shopping malls are prevalent. One of the largest on Oahu is the **Ala Moana Center,** which is just west of Waikiki—home of the **Royal Hawaiian Shopping Center.** Outside Waikiki are **Ward Warehouse,** the **Kahala Mall,** and **Pearlridge Center.**

On the Neighbor Islands smaller strips of shops are the rule, but larger stores exist in Kauai's **Kukui Grove Center** in Lihue, Maui's **Kahului Shopping Center,** and the Big Island's **Prince Kuhio Plaza** in Hilo. Kauai is known for its mom-and-pop shops and family-run boutiques. Exclusive shops are abundant in the luxury hotels.

Distinctively Hawaiian gifts include Aloha shirts and muu-muus, rich roasted Kona coffee, Macadamia nuts, pineapples, and hand- carved wood. In general, major stores and shopping

The Hawaiian Islands

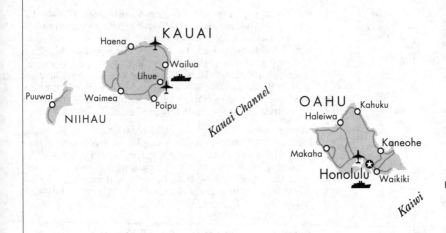

KAUAI

Haena

Wailua

Lihue

Puuwai

Waimea

Poipu

NIIHAU

Kauai Channel

OAHU

Kahuku

Haleiwa

Kaneohe

Makaha

Honolulu

Waikiki

Kaiwi

H

P A C I F I C   O C E A N

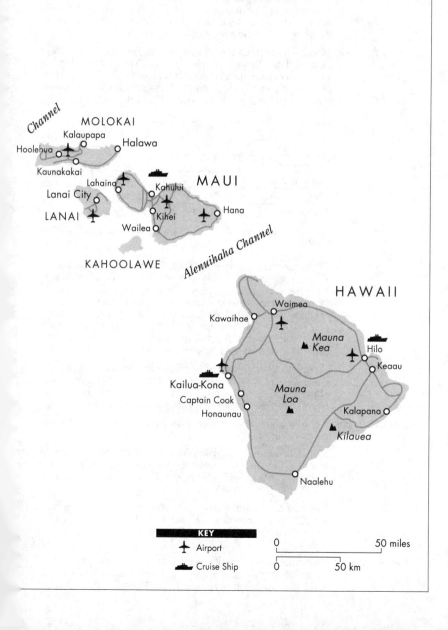

N

Channel
MOLOKAI
Kalaupapa
Hoolehua
Halawa
Kaunakakai
Lahaina
Kahului
MAUI
Lanai City
LANAI
Kihei
Hana
Wailea
KAHOOLAWE
Alenuihaha Channel

HAWAII
Waimea
Kawaihae
Mauna
Kea
Hilo
Keaau
Kailua-Kona
Captain Cook
Mauna
Loa
Honaunau
Kalapana
Kilauea
Naalehu

KEY
✈ Airport
🚢 Cruise Ship
0   50 miles
0   50 km

centers are open from 9 or 10 AM to 4:30 or 5 PM; some have
evening hours.

Dining   Hawaii's melting-pot population accounts for its great variety
of epicurean delights. You can dine on Japanese sashimi, Thai
curry, Hawaiian *laulau*, or Chinese roast duck and a mouth-
watering array of French, German, Korean, American, Mexican, Indian, Italian, and Greek dishes.

There are, of course, a few uniquely tropical tastes, especially
when it comes to fruit. Bananas, papayas, and pineapples grow
throughout the year, while the prized mangos, watermelons,
and litchis appear in summer. Seafood is equally exotic, with
such delicacies as *mahimahi* (dolphin fish), *opakapaka* (pink
snapper), *ulua* (crevelle), and *ahi* (yellowfin tuna).

Many tourists rate a trip to a luau among the highlights of their
stay. At these feasts, you're likely to find the traditional *kalua*
pig, often roasted underground in an *imu* (oven); *poi*, the star-
chy, bland paste made from the taro root; and *laulau*—fish,
meat, and other ingredients wrapped and steamed in ti leaves.

Category	Cost*
Very Expensive	over $60
Expensive	$40–$60
Moderate	$20–$40
Inexpensive	under $20

*per person, excluding drinks, service, and sales tax (4%)

Oahu

The person who dreamed up Oahu's nickname, "The Gathering
Place," was prophetic. Hawaii's most populated island boasts
an eclectic blend of people, places, customs, and cuisines. Its
geography ranges from peaks and plains to rain forests and
beaches. The sands of Waikiki brim with honeymooners, couples celebrating anniversaries, Marines on holiday, and every
other type of tourist imaginable. Beaches to the west and north
are surprisingly unspoiled and uncrowded.

Since cruises originate and terminate in Honolulu, you can visit
Oahu as part of your pre- or post-cruise vacation. American
Hawaii Cruises offers hotel packages and a variety of Oahu
shore excursions for those wishing to linger on Oahu.

Shore Excursions   *Not all excursions are offered on every cruise. All times and
prices are approximate.*

Pearl Harbor and Punchbowl Tour: A comprehensive excursion
includes the *Arizona* memorial and the National Memorial
Cemetery of the Pacific ("Punchbowl"), the most visited site in
the Pacific. *Cost: $25–$30.*

Polynesian Cultural Center: A trip to the 42-acre "living museum," which chronicles the folklore and history of Polynesia
in seven re-created South Pacific villages. *11 hrs. Daily except
Sun. Cost: $54 adults, $26.75 children.*

Getting Around   American Hawaii passengers with air supplements will be
picked up at the airport by shuttle. Ships leave from the upper
level of Aloha Tower in Honolulu. The **Hawaii Visitors Bureau**

(2270 Kalakaua Ave., 8th floor, Honolulu, tel. 808/923–1811) has information on the area.

For those arriving independently, taxis wait outside the airport exit; the fare to Waikiki is about $20. Or **Terminal Transportation** (tel. 808/836–0317) runs an airport shuttle to Waikiki. Municipal buses cost 60¢, but you are allowed only one bag, which must fit on your lap.

By Car Don't bother renting a car unless you're sightseeing outside Waikiki, in which case a number of highly competitive car-rental companies offer deals and discounts. When making hotel or plane reservations, ask if there's a car tie-in. At peak times—summer, Christmas vacation, and February—reservations are a must.

Avis (tel. 800/331–1212), **Hertz** (tel. 800/654–3131), and **Budget** (tel. 800/527–0700) are among the many national agencies available. For an inexpensive local budget renter, try **Tropical** (tel. 808/836–1041).

By Bus Fare anywhere on the island is 60¢, including one free transfer per fare; ask when boarding.

By Taxi Rates are $1.75 at the drop of the flag, plus 25¢ each additional ⅐ mile. The two biggest cab companies are **Charley's** (tel. 808/531–1333) and **SIDA of Hawaii, Inc.** (tel. 808/836–0011).

Beaches **Waikiki** is a 2½-mile chain of beaches extending from the Hilton Hawaiian Village to the base of Diamond Head. The sands are harder, coarser, and more crowded than some of the less-frequented beaches out of town, but food stands and equipment rentals are more accessible here. A protective reef keeps **Ala Moana Beach Park**'s waters calm. Other than Waikiki, this is the most popular beach in Honolulu. Amenities include playing fields, changing houses, indoor and outdoor showers, lifeguards, concession stands, and tennis courts.

Dining **Orchids.** You can't beat this eatery's seaside setting: Diamond Head looms in the distance, and fresh orchids are everywhere. The popovers are huge, the salads light and unusual. The Sunday brunch buffet is a big hit. *Halekulani Hotel, 2199 Kalia Rd., Waikiki, tel. 808/923–2311. AE, DC, MC, V. Expensive.*

Golden Dragon. Local Chinese consider this the best Chinese food in town. Set right by the water, it has stunning red-and-black decor. Best bets are stir-fried lobster with *haupia* (coconut) and Szechuan beef. *Hilton Hawaiian Village, 2005 Kalia Rd., Waikiki, tel. 808/949–4321. AE, DC, MC, V. Moderate.*

The Willows. Thatched dining pavilions set amid ponds filled with prized *koi* (carp) make The Willows a cherished landmark in Oahu. Sautéed opakapaka with spinach sauce is excellent, as are lamb medallions in brandy and honey. *901 Hausten St., Honolulu, tel. 808/946–4808. AE, DC, MC, V. Moderate.*

Kauai

Nicknamed "the Garden Isle," Kauai is Eden epitomized. In the mountains of Kokee, lush swamps ring with the songs of rare birds, while the heady aroma of ginger blossoms sweetens the cool rain forests of Haena. Time and nature have carved elegant spires along the remote northern shore, called the Pali Coast, while seven powerful rivers give life to the valleys where ancient Hawaiians once dwelled.

Shore Excursions *Not all excursions listed are offered on every cruise. All times and prices are approximate.*

Scenic **Helicopter Tour:** A bird's-eye view of Kauai. *50–60 mins. Thurs. and Fri. only. Cost: $129.*

Waimea Canyon and Olu Pua Gardens: Includes a visit to the majestic Waimea Canyon, known as the "Grand Canyon of the Pacific," followed by a stroll through the Ola Pua Botanical Gardens and Estate. *Half-day. Cost: $25 adults, $17.50 children.*

Getting Around Nawiliwili is Kauai's major port. A branch of the **Hawaii Visitors Bureau** (3016 Umi St., Lihue Plaza, Lihue, tel. 808/245–3971) is nearby in Lihue.

By Car It's easy to get around since one major road almost encircles the island. Daily rental-car rates average $25–$30. Try **Dollar** (tel. 800/367–7006) or **Westside U-Drive** (tel. 808/332–8644).

By Taxi A cab will take you islandwide, but you'll pay dearly, at $1.60 a mile. A trip from Lihue to Poipu costs $25 plus tip. Major companies are **Akiko's** (tel. 808/822–3613) and **Kauai Cab** (tel. 808/246–9544).

Beaches The Garden Isle is embraced by stretches of magnificent ivory sand, many with breathtaking mountains as a backdrop. Water is clean, clear, and inviting. Although some of the most scenic beaches are on the north shore, the surf there can be treacherous in winter. Beaches are free.

Brennecke's Beach, on the south shore near Poipu, is a bodysurfer's paradise. Showers, rest rooms, and lifeguards are on hand. **Kalapaki Beach,** fronting the Kauai Lagoons Resort in Nawiliwili, is a sheltered bay ideal for swimming. There are rest rooms and showers. **Lumahai Beach,** near Hanalei on the north coast, is one of the most scenic beaches. Its majestic cliffs, black lava rocks, and hala trees were the setting for the film *South Pacific.* There are no lifeguards, showers, or rest rooms, and swimming is not recommended.

Dining **Gaylord's.** A gracious 19th-century plantation is the charming setting in which to enjoy venison in blueberry-juniper sauce, or pan-blackened and highly spiced fresh salmon. The alfresco dining area opens to extensive gardens. *Kilohana Plantation, 3–2087 Kaumualii Hwy., 1 mi south of Lihue, tel. 808/245–9593. Reservations recommended. AE, D, DC, MC, V. Moderate.*

The Big Island of Hawaii

Nearly twice the size of the other Hawaiian Islands combined, the Big Island is also the most diverse. With 266 miles of coastline of black-lava, white-coral, and green-olivine beaches, and with cliffs of lava and emerald gorges slashing into jutting mountains, the Big Island is so large and so varied that ships stop at two ports, Hilo and Kona.

Shore Excursions *Not all excursions listed are offered on every cruise. All times and prices are approximate.*

Boat and Beach **Deep-Sea Fishing:** Fish the waters around Kona, renowned for their abundance of billfish. Blue marlin and yellowfin tuna are other prizes here. Bait, tackle, and ice are provided. *3 or 6 hrs. Cost: $95 half-day, $159 full day.*

Fairwind Snorkel Sail: Sail aboard a trimaran to Kealakekua Bay along the Kona Coast, then glide down a 16-foot water slide and begin exploring. Snorkeling equipment, instruction, and barbecue lunch are included; bring your own towel. A glass-bottom boat allows nonswimmers to join in the viewing. *4¹/₂ hrs. Cost: $54 adults, $30 children 5–12, $16 children 2–4.*

Scenic **Garden Delight/Lyman House Museum:** After visiting the Japanese Yedo Garden in Liliuokalani Park, you'll drive through Hilo to the historic Lyman Museum and Mission House. Stops are made at Rainbow Falls and the Nani Mau Gardens. *Half-day. Cost: $21 adults, $14.50 children.*

Volcano National Park/Macadamia Nut Farm: A bus takes you to Hawaii Volcanoes National Park, the Big Island's most popular attraction. A tour of the Macadamia Nut Factory and the Akatsuka Orchid Nursery follows. *Half-day. Cost: $21 adults, $14.50 children.*

Volcanoes by Helicopter: Hover over the still-active craters. If you're lucky, they'll be oozing lava. *50–60 mins. Cost: $145.*

Getting Around Ships dock at Hilo and at Kailua-Kona.

By Bus A locally sponsored **Hele-On Bus** operates Monday–Saturday between Hilo and Kailua-Kona ($6 one way).

By Car If you choose to tour the Big Island on your own, you'll need a car. **Avis** (tel. 800/327–9633), **Dollar** (tel. 800/800–4000), and **Harper's** (tel. 808/969–1478) are good choices.

By Taxi Several companies advertise guided tours by taxi, but it is an expensive way to travel: The trip around the island costs about $300. Meters start at $2, with $1.60 charge for each additional mile. In Hilo, call **Ace Taxi** (tel. 808/935–8303) or **Hilo Harry's** (tel. 808/935–7091). In Kona, try **Paradise Taxi** (tel. 808/329–1234) or **Marina Taxi** (tel. 808/329–2481).

Beaches Don't believe anyone who tells you the Big Island lacks beaches; it actually has 80 or more. Small but beautiful, swimmable white-sand beaches dot the Kohala coastline. The surf is rough in summer, and few public beaches have lifeguards. In Hawaii beaches change constantly; a new black-sand beach, **Kamoamoa,** was formed in 1989 by molten lava encountering cold ocean waters, then was closed in 1992 by lava flow from Kilauea, which has been erupting since 1983. Lava also covered the Harry K. Brown and Kaimu beaches in 1990.

Hapuna State Recreation Area, north of Kailua-Kona, is a half-mile crescent of glistening sand framed by rocky points. Children enjoy the shallow cove with tidal pools at the north end, and adventuresome swimmers jump from the sea cliffs to the south. State cabins and public facilities are available nearby, but no lifeguards are available in the winter when the waters are rough. **Kauanoa Beach** at Mauna Kea Beach Resort competes with neighboring Hapuna for the title of most beautiful island beach. The amenities are hotel-owned. **Punaluu Beach Park** is 27 miles from Volcanoes National Park on the south side of the island. Turtles swim in the bay and lay their eggs in the black sand. Fish ponds are just inland. There are rest rooms across the road.

Dining **The Garden at Mauna Kea Beach Hotel.** Table settings of Hawaiian koa and teak alongside French and Belgian crystal accent the beautiful Polynesian decor. Every item on the menu is grown or raised in Hawaii. Lamb chops smoked in coffee, breast of pheasant, and Pacific lobster and prawns with melon-and-ginger sabayon are among the imaginative offerings guaranteed to please. *1 Mauna Kea Dr., Kohala Coast, tel. 808/882-7222. AE, MC, V. Expensive.*

Harrington's. At this popular and reliable steak and seafood restaurant, two outstanding dishes are fresh ono or mahimahi *meunière*, served with brown butter, lemon, and parsley; and Slavic steak, thinly sliced and slathered with garlic butter. *135 Kalanianaole St., Hilo, tel. 808/961-4966. MC, V. Inexpensive-Moderate.*

Maui

Maui, say the locals, is *no ka oi*—the best, the most, the top of the heap. To those who know Maui well, there's good reason for superlatives. The second-largest island in the Hawaiian chain, the Valley Isle has made an international name for itself with its tropical allure, heady nightlife, and miles of perfect-tan beaches.

Shore Excursions *Not all excursions listed are offered on every cruise. All times and prices are approximate.*

Adventure **Bike Trip:** Whiz more than 38 miles downhill from the summit of Mt. Haleakala. Bikes, helmets, windbreakers, and gloves are supplied. Continental breakfast and lunch included. Bring eye protection. This trip can be dangerous; must be 16 or older. *7½ hrs. Cost: $93.*

Scenic **Haleakala Crater:** A motorcoach takes you through Maui's beautiful interior to the Haleakala crater at 10,000 feet, where you'll enjoy spectacular views. *Half-day. Cost: $21 adults, $14.50 children.*

Hana Drive: This drive along the rugged Hana Coast is beautiful but long and winding. Lunch in Hana is provided. *Full day. Cost: $75 adults, $52 children.*

Getting Around Ships dock at the industrial town of Kahului; a $15 shuttle takes you to the Kaanapali Beach Resort and the historic whaling town of Lahaina on Maui's west coast.

By Car Those wishing to venture outside Lahaina, which is small enough to explore on foot, should rent a car. Ships can arrange for car rentals. Try **Budget** (tel. 800/527-0707), **Dollar** (tel. 800/367-7006), or **National** (tel. 800/CAR-RENT).

By Taxi For short hops, this can be a convenient way to go, but you'll have to call ahead—even busy West Maui lacks curbside taxi service. Try **Alii Cab** (tel. 808/661-3688), **Kihei Taxi** (tel. 808/879-3000), or **West Maui Taxi** (tel. 808/667-2605).

Beaches Maui has more than 100 miles of coastline. Not all of this is beach, but striking white crescents do seem to be around every bend. **D.T. Fleming Beach,** just north of the Kapalua Resort, is better for sunbathing than for swimming because the current can be quite strong. There are rest rooms, picnic tables, and grills. **Makena** offers two fine swimming beaches, Big Beach and Little Beach. Nudists frequent Little Beach, though officially, nude sunbathing is illegal in Hawaii. **Kaihalulu Beach** is a gorgeous cove with good swimming and snorkeling on the Hana Coast. Though a bit hard to access, this red-sand beach is worth the hike. No facilities are available.

Dining **Mama's Fish House.** Looking for the best seafood on Maui? Head to this Old Hawaii restaurant a mile from Paia in a lovely oceanfront setting. Try the stuffed fish Lani, a fresh fillet baked with shrimp stuffing. *799 Kaiholo Pl., Paia, tel. 808/579–8488. AE, MC, V. Expensive.*

Avalon Restaurant and Bar. The decor at this most trendy spot is 1940s Hawaii. The "Pacific Rim" cuisine features dishes from Hawaii, California, Mexico, Indonesia, Thailand, Vietnam, and Japan. *Mariner's Alley, 844 Front St., Lahaina, tel. 808/667–5559. AE, D, DC, MC, V. Moderate.*

David Paul's Lahaina Grill. Cap off a day of sightseeing and shopping with dinner at this amiable grill. Chef David Paul revises the menu regularly, marrying imaginative sauces and side dishes to poultry, meat, and seafood. Vanilla-bean rice, for example, is an innovative complement for grilled opakapaka. *127 Lahainaluna Rd., Lahaina, tel. 808/667–5117. AE, DC, MC, V. Moderate.*

Mexican Riviera

Along the Mexican Riviera's 2,000-mile, sun-bleached coast, most travelers find a pleasing mixture of the exotic and the familiar. Among the McDonald's and Pizza Huts and the Fords and Chevys are adobe cantinas, washerwomen at the streams, breathtaking parasailing, and high-cliff divers. While Spanish and various Indian dialects predominate, most Mexicans involved in tourism speak some English. Although you can sample tacos, burritos, and other south-of-the-border fare, you may just as easily order a steak or lobster dinner.

The transformation of once sleepy fishing villages—most notably, Acapulco, Puerto Vallarta, and Mazatlán—into booming cities has been a direct response to the demands of a rapidly expanding tourist industry. And the growth has not been gentle. Although the area's recorded history stretches back more than 400 years, cruise passengers will find few significant landmarks or archaeological sites. Tour guides make up for this lack with their own wild embellishments of local events. If it's authentic history and genuine culture you want, go elsewhere. But for sun, sea, and sports, the colorful Mexican west coast is a fine choice. Indeed, Mexico's beaches compare favorably with the best in the world. Their talcum-powder sands are white, wide, and beckoning; the water is warm and clear. The most accessible beaches, unfortunately, are overrun by persistent vendors. Women shouldn't wear short shorts, bathing suits, or halter tops beyond bathing areas.

When to Go November through March is the Mexican Riviera's cruising season—most ships sail to Alaska for the summer. Still, it is possible to cruise here year-round, and prices are lowest from April through October. June has the best weather, though it is remarkably good almost all year, with daytime temperatures averaging from 82°F–90°F. During the June–October rainy season, very brief showers can be expected.

Currency In the 1980s, Mexico's inflation soared to more than 160% and the peso (P$) tumbled against the dollar. But since 1988, the government has worked to reduce inflation and slowly devalue the peso against the dollar. At press time, the rate was about P$3.20 to U.S. $1. (In January 1993, Mexico created the "new peso," knocking three zeros off the old unit.) U.S. dollars and credit cards are accepted at many restaurants and large shops. There is no advantage to paying in dollars, but there may be an advantage to paying in cash. To avoid having to change unused pesos back to dollars, change just enough to cover what you'll need for public transportation, refreshments, phones, and tips. Use up your Mexican coins; they can't be changed back to dollars.

Passports and Visas Although U.S. and Canadian citizens do not need a passport or visa to enter or leave Mexico, they must fill out a *tarjeta de tourista* (tourist card), issued by the cruise line, a Mexican embassy or consulate, or any airline flying to Mexico. This is free, but you must show proof of citizenship (passport or birth certificate) to have it validated. British travelers need a passport and a tourist card.

Telephones and Mail Phoning home from the Mexican Riviera can be frustrating because lines are few and the sound quality can be poor. Calling

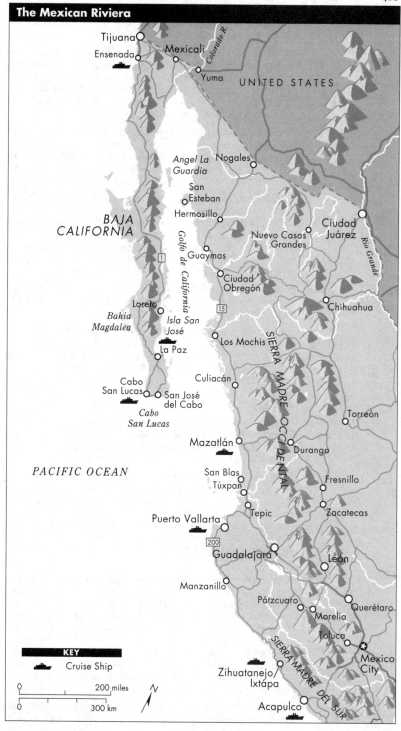

The Mexican Riviera

KEY
Cruise Ship

0 — 200 miles
0 — 300 km

from the ship can be much more expensive and every bit as frustrating. A sizable dose of patience and a sense of humor will keep you from getting ulcers.

Pay phones that connect to the United States are found on the dock in Mazatlán and Acapulco. Better than the phone booth is the phone building, *caseta de larga distancia*, where operator assistance is available, though English is seldom spoken. International calls can also be placed from major hotels and resorts; most add a 35% minimum service charge.

To call the United States from Mexico, dial 95, the area code, and the phone number, or dial 09 for an English-speaking international operator. Collect calls, which are not subject to hefty Mexican taxes, are less expensive than calling direct, but you must pay a service charge if the call is not accepted.

The Mexican postal system is notoriously slow and unreliable; *never* send packages, as they may simply vanish without a trace. There are numerous post offices (*oficinas de correos*) in the larger cities. Always use airmail for overseas correspondence; it will take anywhere from 10 days to two weeks or more. Rates are quite low: P\$2 for a letter (up to 20 grams) or postcard to the United States, and P\$2.50 to Europe.

Tipping Everyone wants a dollar; not everyone expects one. It's wise to carry some pesos for those times when a dollar tip is too much. Don't tip less than P\$2.

For taxi rides, tips are usually included in the negotiated rate. Good taxi tours, however, merit a small tip; about P\$5 for a three-hour tour is average. If you stop for a cold beer or a soda, you are expected to buy your driver a bottle. Bus-tour guides expect a tip of about \$1 per person per half-day tour. In restaurants a service charge of 15% is occasionally included; otherwise tip 10%–15%.

Shore Excursions Not surprisingly, some of the best excursions are those that take advantage of the area's wonderful beaches, where passengers indulge in parasailing, waterskiing, snorkeling, and windsurfing. Sunset sails and booze cruises are also popular.

Deep-sea fishing has long drawn sport-fishing fans hoping to land trophy-size marlin and sailfish, as well as tuna, wahoo, and bonito. Most ships sailing the Mexican Riviera offer half-day or full-day fishing at rates comparable to what it would cost to charter a boat on your own. Be careful about chartering your own boat: The locals' relaxed sense of time is not shared by cruise-ship captains, who will—and do—leave without late passengers.

And be wary of land tours. A substantial percentage of the bus tours range from mediocre to indifferent. Too often, guides speak poor English, the vehicles are in poor repair, and the tour itself is of limited interest. Typically, a bus tour of the *ciudad* (city) will drive past the *malecón* (sea wall), stop briefly at the central cathedral on the *zócalo* (main town square)—and then, bypassing the few historic sites or authentic native markets, pull up at various hotels and time-share properties, where passengers are subjected to a sales pitch. Finally, passengers will be taken for an extended stop at a shopping area or crafts shop.

Other bus tours rush passengers through a brewery or distillery, where you'll sample tequila or rum, and can buy bottles of the local brew. Or you'll be dragged to the ubiquitous folkloric show, usually at a resort hotel or in a shopping area. While a few superb folkloric shows exist, most dance companies seen on bus tours are either young amateurs or jaded semiprofessionals who merely go through the motions.

Taxis are a worthwhile alternative to the bus tour. They are numerous and relatively cheap, and every driver accepts dollars. Taxis are not metered, however, nor are there fixed rates to specific destinations. Don't get in until you've negotiated exact fare (including tip), and never pay the driver in advance. The cruise director usually knows the appropriate fare to various destinations, or how much it costs to hire a taxi by the hour. Not all taxi drivers are qualified to act as tour guides, however, and cabs almost never have air-conditioning.

Shopping It's possible to get great bargains and souvenirs, even in those ports where cruise ships call. Haggling is the rule of thumb in markets and with street vendors, but most boutiques have fixed prices. Start by offering no more than half the asking price, then raise your price very slowly but pay no more than 70%. For silver, first offer about one-quarter the asking price, and beware of disreputable shops that hawk *faux* silver—always check for the stamp ".925," which must by law appear on all sterling.

Most Mexican shops open at 9 or 10 AM, break between 2 and 4 for siesta, then reopen until 7 or 8 PM. Street vendors generally start packing up at 6 PM or when dusk falls, whichever comes first.

Dining Mexican restaurants run the gamut from humble, hole-in-the-wall shacks, street stands, and chairs and tables in the markets, to *taquerías* (taco stands), American-style fast-food joints, and acclaimed gourmet restaurants.

Ceviche—raw fish and shellfish (*mariscos*) marinated in lime juice and topped with cilantro, onion, and chili—is almost a national dish, though it originated in Acapulco. Shrimp, lobster, and oysters can be huge and succulent; the safest time to eat oysters is October–March. Avoid all foods sold by street vendors—especially meat and fruit—no matter how tempting. *Tacos al pastor*—thin pork slices grilled on a revolving spit and garnished with cilantro, onions, and chili—are delicious but dangerous for most non-Mexican stomachs. If you're not keen on spiciness, ask that your food be prepared *no muy picante.* Stick to bottled beverages, and ask for your drinks *sin hielo* (without ice).

Category	Cost*
Very Expensive	over $35
Expensive	$25–$35
Moderate	$15–$25
Inexpensive	under $15

per person, excluding drinks, service, and sales tax (15%)

Acapulco

As the ship enters the harbor, passengers look out on Acapulco's gently curving, high-rise-studded waterfront backed by a series of dramatic hills. Distant mountains are shrouded in haze. As the ship passes Roqueta Island, a pillar of rock jutting almost straight up in the air, you see hundreds of boats and a sprawling fort. The municipal pier, where cruise ships dock, is alive with food hawkers, souvenir vendors, taxi drivers, and small boys ready to dive for coins. Acapulco, the largest city on the Mexican Riviera, bustles with crowded markets, trendy discos, fashionable restaurants, and spectacular gardens and scenery.

Shore Excursions None of the guided tours in Acapulco can be recommended; it is preferable to decide in advance what to see, then hire a taxi for a personal tour (about $25 for 3 hours, plus a 10% tip). If you prefer, the following bus tour is available:

Acapulco City Tour: This overview wends through the commercial area, passes celebrity homes and the Las Brisas hotel, and stops at the Acapulco Princess Hotel. Included is a visit to see the cliff divers at La Quebrada and a shopping stop. *3¹/₂ hrs.*

Getting Around Acapulco sprawls for miles along the waterfront and far into the hills. However, most of the action occurs within a few hundred yards of Costera Miguel Alemán, the main boulevard that wraps around the harbor from Old Acapulco to Icacos Beach. The pier where cruise ships dock opens onto Costera Miguel Alemán; across the boulevard is the Fuerte de San Diego.

By Bus Public buses are cheap (about 20¢). The bus marked HORNOS follows the Costera from the pier to the Strip. New ACATUR-BUSES, with air-conditioning and reclining seats, make the trip from the Hyatt to Caleta and cost about 60¢.

By Carriage Buggy rides are available up and down the Strip on weekends. Bargain before you get in—fares are about $20 for a half- hour.

By Taxi Taxis are cheap and plentiful. Negotiate the fare; a ride to town shouldn't cost more than $5. Volkswagen Beetles are cheapest. Flagging a cab in the street costs less than at a hotel.

Exploring Acapulco *Numbers in the margin correspond to numbered points of interest on the Acapulco map.*

Though it is within walking distance of the docks, in Old Acapulco you'll find more Mexicans than tourists. Colors are earthier, odors more pungent, and air-conditioning almost non-
❶ ❷ existent. Close to the **municipal pier** is the **zócalo,** a pleasant plaza crisscrossed with shaded promenades and alive with shoe-shine stands, vendors, children, and old men ogling a new generation of lovers. Sunday means music in the grandstand. The church of **Nuestra Señora de la Soledad** is a modern oddity, with a stark white facade and blue and yellow spires.

❸ Opposite the pier and towering over it is **El Fuerte de San Diego,** built in the 18th century as protection from pirates. An earlier fort, finished in 1616, was destroyed by an earthquake. Today the fort's air-conditioned rooms offer archaeological, historical, and anthropological exhibits, covering early Mexican exploration and Spanish trade. *Admission: about $3.50. Open Tues.–Sun. 10:30–4:40.*

❹ Take a $3 taxi ride along the Strip to the **Continental Plaza**
❺ **Hotel** and stroll back along the harbor boulevard toward **Papagayo Park.** Most tourist interests are on or near this section
of Costera Miguel Alemán—shops, hotels, and restaurants.
Tackiness prevails, but there's no reason you can't enjoy it.

❻ A few blocks away is the **Mercado Municipal,** where locals buy
everything from fresh vegetables and candles to plastic buckets and love potions; much of the merchandise is trucked in from
Guadalajara and Mexico City. Try to go between 10 and 1. If
coming by taxi, ask to get out near the *flores* (flower stand)
closest to the souvenir-and-crafts section. From here, turn
right and head into the market.

❼ **La Quebrada,** where world-famous cliff divers perform daily, is
a 15–20 minute walk west, up a rather steep hill, so consider a
taxi (the fare is about $3). A $2 entrance fee gives you access
to a platform beside the **Plaza las Glorias El Mirador Hotel,** an
excellent vantage point, or you can see the cliffdiving show
while having drinks and dinner at the hotel's **La Perla** nightclub
(four shows nightly, 7:30–10:30 PM).

Shopping The best bargains are found in the public markets. In places
like **El Mercado de Artesanías** on the Strip, **Noa Noa** near the
docks, and any of the several open-air markets set up around
town, you can haggle for woven blankets, puppets, colorful
wood toys, leather, baskets, hammocks, and handmade wood
furniture.

The **Galeria Rudic,** across from the Continental Plaza, has
great prices on authentic Mexican fine art. For silver jewelry
and flatware, go to **Taxco El Viejo** (La Quebrada 830) or, for
better pieces, **Joya** in the Acapulco Plaza. Custom-made Mexican blouses and skirts are sold at **Samy's** (Calle Hidalgo 7). The
expensive and formal **Esteban's,** the most glamorous shop in
Acapulco, is on the Costera near the Club de Golf.

Sports Try the **Pesca Deportiva,** the dock across from the zócalo. Boats
Fishing accommodating four to eight people cost $150 to $500 a day, or
$40 a chair. Excursions leave about 7 AM and return at 2 PM.
Most fishing operations get a license for you; otherwise, go to
the **Secretaria de Pesca,** above the central post office at Costera
Miguel Alemán 215.

Golf Two great 18-hole golf courses are shared by the **Princess and
Pierre Marques hotels.** Greens fees are $84. At the public nine-
hole course on the Costera Miguel Alemán, next to the Centro
Internacional Acapulco, the fee is $30.

Water Waterskiing (about $20 per half-hour), Broncos (one-person
Sports motorboats; $30 per half-hour), and parasailing—an Acapulco
highlight ($15 for eight minutes; tel. 74/82–20–56)—can be ar-
ranged at the beach. Windsurfing is available on the beaches
of all the major hotels along the Costera.

Beaches Acapulco's beaches are legendary. Every water sport is available, but think twice about swimming: There is a dangerous
undertow at some beaches, and the water is polluted. Smack in
the middle of Acapulco Bay, **Playa Condesa** is a tourist-riddled
stretch of sand that's especially popular with singles. The
beachside restaurants are convenient. Between the Paraíso
Radisson and Las Hamacas hotels, **Playa Hornos** is crammed
with Mexican tourists who know a good thing: Graceful palms
shade the sand, and scads of casual eateries are within walking

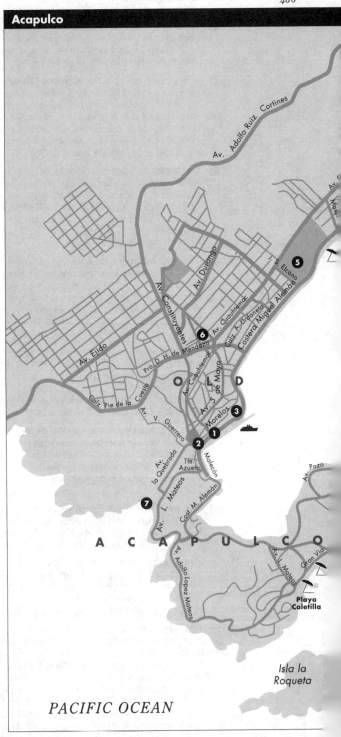

Acapulco

Continental Plaza
Hotel, **4**
El Fuerte de
San Diego, **3**
La Quebrada, **7**
Mercado Municipal, **6**
Municipal pier, **1**
Papagayo Park, **5**
Zócalo, **2**

PACIFIC OCEAN

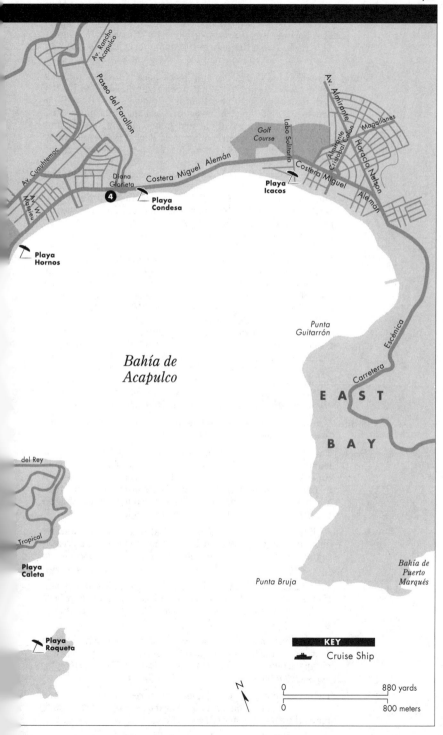

Av. Rancho Acapulco

Paseo del Farallon

Av. Cuauhtémoc

Av. W. Massieu

Diana Glorieta

4

Costera Miguel Alemán

Golf Course

Lobo Solitario

Av. Almirante

Almirante Cristóbal Colón

Horacio Nelson

Magallanes

Costera Miguel Alemán

Playa Icacos

Playa Condesa

Playa Hornos

Bahía de Acapulco

Punta Guitarrón

Carretera Escénica

E A S T

B A Y

del Rey

Tropical

Playa Caleta

Punta Bruja

Bahía de Puerto Marqués

Playa Roqueta

KEY

Cruise Ship

N

0   880 yards

0   800 meters

distance. Stretching from the naval base to El Presidente, **Playa Icacos** is less populated than other beaches on the Strip. The morning waves are especially calm. Mexicans frequently day-trip to **Playa Roqueta;** a 10-minute ferry ride to Roqueta Island and visit to the small zoo costs about $4 round-trip.

Dining **Blackbeard's.** The pirate-ship motif here translates to walls decked with fishing nets and wood figureheads, and booths with maps on the tables. Photos of movie stars, from Bing Crosby to Liz Taylor, who've eaten here hang in the much-used lounge. A luscious salad bar and jumbo shrimp, lobster, and steak portions keep 'em coming back. Part of the restaurant is a disco. *Costera Miguel Alemán, tel. 74/84–25–49. Reservations advised. AE, MC, V. Expensive.*

Beto's. By day you can eat and enjoy live music beachside; by night, this palapa-style restaurant is transformed into a dim and romantic dining area lighted by candles and paper lanterns. Whole red snapper, lobster, and ceviche are recommended. *Costera Miguel Alemán, tel. 74/84–04–73. Reservations not needed. AE, MC, V. Moderate.*

Carlos 'n Charlie's. This is *the* happening eatery in Acapulco; the line forms well before the doors open at 6:30 PM. An atmosphere of controlled craziness is cultivated through prankster waiters, a joky menu, and the eclectic decor. Ribs, stuffed shrimp, and oysters are among the best offerings. *Costera Miguel Alemán 999, tel. 74/84–12–85 or 74/84–00–39. No reservations. AE, DC, MC, V. No lunch. Moderate.*

Mimi's Chili Saloon. Posters of Marilyn Monroe and caged tropical birds make this place popular with all ages. Gorge on Tex-Mex, onion rings, and quality burgers, and wash it all down with peach and mango daiquiris. Expect to wait for a table at night, or you can order from Blackbeard's next door, operated by the same owner. *Costera Miguel Alemán, tel. 74/84–25–49. No reservations. AE, MC, V. Closed Mon. Moderate.*

Nightlife Cruise ships often dock in Acapulco late into the night or for two days to take advantage of the city's discos and nightclubs.

Discos The discos open late, around 10:30 PM, and diehards are still at it at sunrise. Most places have a cover charge of $10–$20. Sometimes you get a drink or two with that, perhaps even access to an open bar; sometimes you don't. Lines are common but usually move quickly. Since many discos are bunched together on the Strip, you can easily hop from one to another.

As if the spectacle of a crowded, pulsating dance floor weren't enough, a huge glass wall at **Extravaganzza** provides a breathtaking wraparound view of the harbor. *Carretera Escénica to Las Brisas, next to Los Rancheros restaurant, tel. 74/84–71–64.*

For stargazing, Hollywood-style, go to **Fantasy's;** it's expensive, exclusive, and one of the few places in Acapulco where you're supposed to dress to the nines. *On Scenic Hwy., next to Las Brisas, tel. 74/84–67–27.*

News is billed as a "disco and concert hall." It's enormous, with seating for 1,200 in booths and love seats. Theme parties and competitions are offered nightly. *Costera Miguel Alemán, across from the Hyatt Regency, tel. 74/84–59–02.*

Baby O, one of the best singles discos, resembles a cave in a tropical setting. A big 18-to-30 crowd of mostly tourists dominates the scene. *Costera Miguel Alemán 22, tel. 74/84–74–74.*

The decor of **Magic** is black, and the place has a fabulous after-midnight light show. As many as 500 vivacious nightcrawlers compete for the tables and chairs arranged on three levels overlooking the dance floor. *Across the Costera from Baby O, tel. 74/84–88–15.*

Entertainment One of Acapulco's best folkloric shows is performed nightly at 7:30 at the **Acapulco International Center**, also called the convention center. For $42 per person you receive a full-course dinner and a rousing show with dancers, singers, and a mariachi band.

Tourists love watching the cliff divers at **La Quebrada** plunge into floodlighted waters. Where better to watch than from a boat below, sipping champagne and listening to strumming guitars? Several companies sell sunset cruises that end up at La Quebrada; you can find out which boats are going, and at what price, by calling **Divers de Mexico** (tel. 74/82–13–98).

Cabo San Lucas

Cabo San Lucas sits at the southern tip of Baja California, where the Gulf of California and the Pacific Ocean meet. Here, the surf has shaped the dun-colored cliffs into bizarre jutting fingers and arches of rock. The desert ends in white-sand coves, with cacti standing at their entrances like sentries under the soaring palm trees. Big-game-fishing fans are lured from all over the world for marlin and sailfish. Although Cabo San Lucas and its neighboring town of San José del Cabo have little to offer in the way of sophistication, their isolation and beauty make them superb cruise destinations.

Shore Excursion *The following excursion may not be offered by all cruise lines. Time and price are approximate.*

Best of Cabo San Lucas: A glass-bottom boat cruise of Los Arcos sails past Lovers Beach and offers an overview of the area. *1–2 hrs. Cost: $7.*

Getting Around The shallow harbor makes it necessary for ships to anchor in the bay and tender passengers in. A flea market is on the wharf, and the tour boats to Los Arcos and Lovers Beach are to the left on the pier. Downtown is a few blocks away and small enough for you to get anywhere on foot. San José del Cabo is 23 miles away.

By Bus Public transportation is spotty at best. Minivans between Cabo San Lucas and San José del Cabo charge about $4 per person.

By Taxi Fares are standardized, but check before getting in. It should cost $2 from the pier to the entrance to Cabo San Lucas, $25 between the two towns.

Exploring Cabo *Numbers in the margin correspond to numbered points of in-*
San Lucas *terest on the Cabo San Lucas map.*

❶ The main downtown street of Cabo San Lucas, Avenida Lázaro Cárdenas, passes a small **zócalo.** Most shops, services, and restaurants are between the avenida and the waterfront, two blocks east. Downtown businesses have suffered a bit as a re-
❷ sult of the marina's new **Handicrafts Market.** From the marina
❸ you can see the spectacular natural rock arches called **Los Arcos,** but they are more impressive from the water.

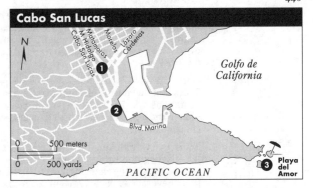

About 15 minutes from town is a dramatic desert, populated by wild horses and incredible cacti. A taxi out here costs $20 an hour, or you can take a five-hour bus tour for $32.

Shopping Along the waterfront and on its side streets, Cabo San Lucas is a shopper's mecca; the selection of handicrafts and sportswear is especially good. Sportswear shops—**Amarras, Ferrioni, Bye-Bye, Fila,** and **Benetton**—cluster at the **Plaza Cabo San Lucas,** on Avenida Madero near the waterfront, and at **Plaza Bonita,** at the Marina. **Temptations,** in the building also occupied by the Giggling Marlin restaurant, has some chic and original designs for women, including the Maria de Guadalajara line. On the waterfront is a **Tianguis,** a maze of thatched booths selling mediocre silver jewelry, mass-produced wood sculptures, T-shirts, and other souvenirs. **La Paloma** in town sells some better-quality souvenirs, and the boutiques in the **Mexican Village** at the Hacienda Hotel are popular with tourists. **El Dorado Gallery,** across from the marina, is a must. Its two rooms are filled with sculptures in ceramic, papier-mâché, brass, and copper; the creations of Mario Gonzalez; and contemporary Mexican paintings and handicrafts.

Sports The best fishing on the Baja is to be had here. You can charter
Fishing a 28-foot cruiser for about $280 a day from the Cabo San Lucas marina. Contact **Pesca Deportiva Solmar** (Hotel Solmar, tel. 684/3–0022).

Scuba Diving Los Arcos is the prime diving and snorkeling area, but several good rocky points are off the coast. Contact **Amigos del Mar** (near the sportfishing docks, tel. 684/3–0022), **Cabo Acuadeportes** (at the Cabo San Lucas, Hacienda, Plaza Las Glorias, and Pueblo Bonito hotels, tel. 684/3–0117), and **Cabo Divers** (Blvd. Marina and Av. Madero, tel. 684/3–0747).

Beaches **Playa del Amor** is in a very small cove at the end of the peninsula, with the Golfo de California on one side and the Pacific on the other. The beach and nearby arches are some of the most romantic spots along the Mexican Riviera. The surf on the Pacific side is too rough for swimming. A water taxi ferries passengers out to the cove for $16 round-trip.

The crowded 2-mile **Playa Medano,** just north of town, is the most popular stretch of beach for sunbathing and people-watching. **Playa Hacienda,** in the inner harbor by the Hacienda Hotel, has calm waters and good snorkeling around the rocky point. A water taxi from the marina to the hotel costs about $2.50 per person.

Dining   **El Galeón.** The choice seats at this posh eatery across from the marina are on terraces facing the water. The interior is an assemblage of heavy wood furniture. Seafood and traditional Italian fare are prepared expertly. Drop in for the piano music, which starts at 6:30 PM. *By the road to the Finesterra Hotel, tel. 684/3–0443. AE, MC, V. Very Expensive.*

The Giggling Marlin. Five large color TVs broadcast major sporting events and other U.S. programs at this bar-restaurant, raking in a huge crowd during the Super Bowl, World Series, and other important spectacles. Though the menu is extensive—burgers, sandwiches, tostadas, burritos, steaks—regulars advise sticking with tacos, appetizers, and drinks. *Av. Matamoros and Blvd. Marina, tel. 684/3–0606. MC, V. Expensive.*

Las Palmas. Playa Medano's most popular hangout is headquarters to beach-vollcyball competitors, dune-buggy enthusiasts, and beach bums of all types. The barbecued ribs are great; better is the quail, lobster, and steak combo, or the tequila-marinated abalone. *Tel. 684/3–0447. MC, V. Moderate.*

Mazatlán

Mazatlán (an Aztec word meaning "place of the deer") is the only major city on the Mexican Riviera that has a *raison d'être* other than welcoming droves of tourists. With 500,000 inhabitants, it's a thriving seaport, home to a large shrimp fleet and other commercial-fishing boats. Long before the first cruise ships called and the tourist hotels were built, Mazatlán was a year-round mecca for sportfishermen and hunters in search of sailfish and marlin, duck and quail. Hunting is on the wane now as time-share condos and high rises pop up, but Mazatlán still has the feel of a working fishing town rather than a tourist resort.

Shore Excursions   *Not all excursions listed are offered by all cruise lines. All times and prices are approximate.*

Mazatlán City Tour: A quick overview of the city includes a stop to watch cliff divers (who don't have quite the panache of those in Acapulco), followed by a stop at a shopping area, where a folkloric show is often staged. *3 hrs. Cost: $20.*

Isla de la Piedra Tour: Stone Island, opposite Olas Altas beach, has for now been spared a huge redevelopment plan, and one and all can still enjoy the island's 10 miles of palm-fringed beaches. The tour, by catamaran, usually includes food and drink. *6 hrs. Cost: $30.*

Sierra Madre Tour: Go inland, up into the mountains, to visit the ancient towns of Copala and Concordia, with their baroque houses, wonderfully unspoiled plazas, a deserted silver mine, and shopping stopovers. Lunch is served in a local cantina that frequently features amateur musicians. *4–5 hrs. Cost: $30.*

Getting Around   Mazatlán, on a peninsula, is flanked by the harbor on one side and the Pacific on the other. Unfortunately, its attractions are spread far and wide, and walking from one section of town to another can take hours. The zócalo, however, with the cathedral and the *mercado municipal* (flea market), is just a few blocks from the pier.

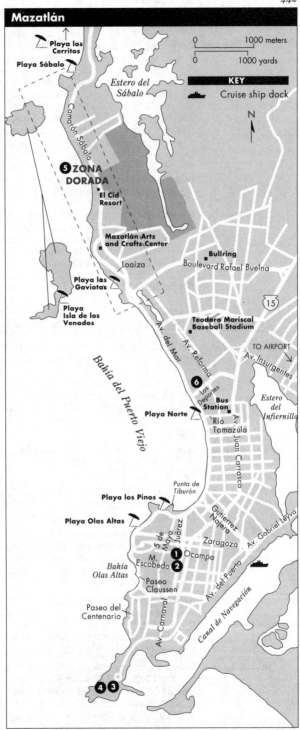

442

Mazatlán

Acuario Mazatlán, **6**
Cerro del Crestón, **3**
El Faro, **4**
Mazatlán Catedral, **1**
Zócalo (Plaza
Revolución), **2**
Zona Dorada, **5**

0   1000 meters
0   1000 yards

KEY
Cruise ship dock

N

Playa los
Cerritos

Playa Sábalo

*Estero del
Sábalo*

Camarón Sábalo

5 **ZONA
DORADA**

**El Cid
Resort**

**Mazatlán Arts
and Crafts Center**

Bullring
Boulevard Rafael Buelna

Loaiza

Playa las
Gaviotas

Playa
Isla de los
Venados

Bahía del Puerto Viejo

Av. del Mar

15

**Teodoro Mariscal
Baseball Stadium**

Av. Reforma

TO AIRPORT

Av. Insurgentes

6

Los
Deportes

**Bus
Station**

*Estero
del
Infiernilla*

Playa Norte

Río
Tamazula

Av. Juan Carrasco

Punta de
Tiburón

Playa los Pinos

Playa Olas Altas

5 de Mayo

Juárez

M.
Escobedo

Ocampo

1
2

Gutierrez
Nájera

Zaragoza

Av. Gabriel Leyva

*Bahía
Olas Altas*

Paseo
Claussen

Av. del Puerto

Paseo del
Centenario

Av. Carnaval

Canal de Navegación

4 **3**

By Bus Air-conditioned minibuses, marked SABALO-CENTRO, run along the coastal road up to the town plaza. The fare is about 50¢.

By Scooter *Pulmonías* (pneumonias), hybrids of a golf cart and a motorized rickshaw, will shuttle you around town. The fare starts at about $2 for three passengers. It's fun, but some people object to the traffic fumes.

By Taxi Taxis are cheap and readily available and will take you almost everywhere along the hotel strip for no more than $4. The Golden District, or Zona Dorado, with its shops, boutiques, and hotels, is about 15 miles from the pier; a taxi ride there costs about $5.

Exploring *Numbers in the margin correspond to numbered points of in-*
Mazatlán *terest on the Mazatlán map.*

Downtown is four blocks from the pier; its center is where Calle Juárez and Calle Cinco de Mayo intersect with Avenida del Mar. Here the streets are filled with buses and locals rushing to and from work and the market. Many travelers never see this part of Mazatlán, but it's worth a visit.

❶ Head for the blue and gold spires of the **Mazatlán Catedral,** at Calles Juárez and Ocampo. The cathedral, built in 1890 and made a basilica in 1935, has an ornate triple altar, with murals of angels overhead and many small altars along the sides. Dress appropriately (no shorts or tank tops) to enter. Steps away, at the Plazuela Machado, peek in at the newly restored **Angela Peralta Theater,** Mazatlán's former opera house.

❷ Across the street is the **zócalo, Plaza Revolución,** with a fascinating gazebo: It looks like a '50s diner inside the lower level, with a wrought-iron bandstand on top. The green and orange tile on the walls, the ancient jukebox, and the soda fountain serving shakes, burgers, and hot dogs couldn't make a more surprising sight. Facing the zócalo are the City Hall, banks, the post office, and a telegraph office.

❸ Continuing south to the end of the peninsula, you mount **Cerro**
❹ **del Crestón** (Summit Hill). At the top is **El Faro,** the second-tallest lighthouse in the world.

❺ If you take a taxi to the **Zona Dorada,** north of the center, stop
❻ by the **Acuario Mazatlán,** an aquarium with tanks of sharks, sea horses, eels, lobsters, and multicolor saltwater and freshwater fish. *Av. de los Deportes 111, tel. 69/81–7815. Admission: $2. Open daily 9–7, 9:30–6:30.*

Shopping Most tourists head for the **Mazatlán Arts and Crafts Center** in the Zona Dorada, then migrate to **Sea Shell City** next door. The quality and variety of Mazatlán's handicrafts are mediocre, and the prices high. But in town, at the **Plaza Nueva**—any cab driver knows where it is—you're likely to find worthwhile shopping. **La Carreta,** at the El Cid and Costa de Oro hotels, is probably the best handicrafts center in town. The enormous **Mercado Central,** between Calles Juárez and Serdan, sells produce, meat, fish, and handicrafts at the lowest prices in town. Outside, street-side stalls have the best crafts.

Sports Mazatlán has the largest charter fishing fleet in the region.
Fishing Contact **Bill Heimpel's Star Fleet** (tel. 69/82–2665), **De Oro** (tel. 69/82–3130), **El Dorado** (tel. 69/81–6204), **Estrella** (tel. 69/82–3878), or **Flota Faro** (tel. 69/81–2824).

Golf The spectacular Robert Trent Jones course at **El Cid** is reserved for resort guests and their guests.

Water Sports Rent Jet Skis, Hobie Cats, and Windsurfers from most hotels, and look for parasailing along the Zona Dorado. Mazatlán has no good diving spots.

Beaches **Playa los Cerritos,** the northernmost beach on the outskirts of town, runs from Camino Real Resort to Punta Cerritos, and is cleanest and least populated. It's too rough for swimming but great for surfing. The two most popular beaches are along the Zona Dorado—**Playa Sábalo** and **Playa las Gaviotas.** Here you'll find as many vendors selling blankets, pottery, lace tablecloths, and silver jewelry as you will sunbathers. Boats, Windsurfers, and parasailers line the shores. Boats make frequent departures from the Zona Dorado hotels for **Playa Isla de los Venados** on Deer Island. It's only a 10-minute ride, but the difference is striking: The beach is pretty, uncluttered, and clean, and you can hike around the southern point of the island to small, secluded coves covered with shells.

Dining **Sr. Peppers.** This is an elegant yet unpretentious place, with ceiling fans, lush foliage, candlelit tables, and choice steaks and lobsters cooked over a mesquite grill. You can bop around the dance floor to live music. *Av. Camarón Sábalo, across from the Camino Real Hotel, tel. 69/84–0120. AE, DC, MC, V. Expensive.*
El Marinero. At the region's best seafood house, try the generous seafood platter, grilled on a hibachi at your table and piled high with frogs' legs, turtle, shrimp, oysters covered with melted cheese, and fresh fish. Also good is the shrimp *machaca*, sautéed in olive oil with tomatoes, chives, and chilis. *Calle Cinco de Mayo 530, tel. 69/82–7682. AE, MC, V. Moderate.*
Señor Frog. Almost every gringo eventually ends up here. Bandidos waiters carry tequila bottles and shot glasses in their bandoliers, and patrons stand on tables to sign their names on the ceiling. Barbecued ribs and chicken, served with corn on the cob, and heaping portions of standard Mexican dishes are the specialties. The tortilla soup is excellent. *Av. del Mar, tel. 69/82–1925. DC, MC, V. Moderate.*

Puerto Vallarta

Puerto Vallarta was an unknown fishing village until John Huston filmed *Night of the Iguana* here in 1964 with Richard Burton, who brought along his girlfriend Liz Taylor. The torrid romance made international headlines and launched Puerto Vallarta as one of the most popular resorts on the Riviera.

The area between the airport and Old Town, including the new Marina Vallarta complex, is overdeveloped; luxury high-rise hotels block sea views and mar the landscape. Downtown and the area south of the Río Cuale, however, have avoided the raw boomtown look that afflicts so many Mexican towns. Here, efforts are made to retain the image of the charming fishing village that once was: You'll still find the traditional whitewashed houses with red-tile roofs and lush bougainvillea, cobblestone streets, and fleets of colorful fishing boats hauling in their afternoon catches.

Shore Excursions *Not all excursions listed are offered by all cruise lines. All times and prices are approximate.*

Banderas Bay Cruise: Sail along the coast to a beach for swimming and sunning. Drinks and snacks may be included. *3 hrs. Cost: $25.*

Vallarta Horseback Riding: Ride along the shore to a private beach club for a swim. *2¹/2 hrs.. Cost: $30.*

Puerto Vallarta City Tour: An overview of the city includes a visit to Gringo Gulch, where Taylor and Burton built a bridge over the street to join their houses; Mismaloya Beach, where *Night of the Iguana* was filmed; and a stop in the downtown shopping district. *3 hrs. Cost: $18.*

Getting Around The wharf is nearly 3 miles from downtown. Taking a bus tour or hiring a taxi is recommended if you want to see all of the large, sprawling town, but you can easily cover the downtown area on foot.

By Bus Buses are cheap and crisscross the city, but figuring out which goes where is too much effort for most passengers with only a few hours. A better bet is the Volkswagen *combis* or vans that whiz between town, the beaches, and the major hotels; prices average about $1.50.

By Car Rental cars and motorbikes are expensive, but they may be the only practical way to visit the beaches at Boca de Tomatlán if you can't catch a convenient van or taxi (*see* Beaches, *below*). Contact **Avis** (Carretera Aeropuerto Km 2.5, tel. 322/2–1412), **Budget** (Carretera Aeropuerto Km 5, tel. 322/2–2980), **Dollar** (Lucerna 105, tel. 322/4-0001), **Hertz** (Lucerna 109–A, tel. 322/2–0024), **National** (Carretera Aeropuerto Km 1.5, tel. 322/2–1107), and **Quick** (Carretera Aeropuerto Km 1.5, tel. 322/2–3505).

By Taxi Cabs are the best way into town. Union cabs found at the hotel and wharf are more expensive and not necessarily more reliable than the taxis you pick up on the street outside the fence. Negotiate your fare before getting in; it should be about $3.50 to the center of town. A tour should cost $20 per hour, and a good guide should be able to show you the town and the outskirts in a few hours.

Exploring Puerto *Numbers in the margin correspond to numbered points of in-*
Vallarta *terest on the Puerto Vallarta map.*

There are three major regions: the northern hotels and resorts, the downtown, and the Río Cuale and Playa de los Muertos. Exploring downtown is best done on foot. Along the
❶ *malecón,* or sea wall, is the bronze sea horse that has become the town's trademark. The street is peppered with touristy sing-along bars, open-air restaurants, and boutiques.

Walk a few hundred yards, keeping the sea on your right, and you will cross a bridge. Halfway across, descend a staircase to
❷ **Río Cuale Island,** where you'll find purveyors of paintings, folk art, stuffed iguanas, and other interesting handmade wares.
❸ The **Museo Arqueológico** displays pre-Columbian artifacts that are hardly worth seeing. More appealing are the restaurants on the island and the view of the sea. Return to the bridge and continue walking south to reach the beginning of the residential district, which has a warren of shops, small hotels, and cantinas where the locals go.

Head back over the bridge, past Río Cuale Island, to return to Old Town. The three streets that parallel the malecón are lined

446

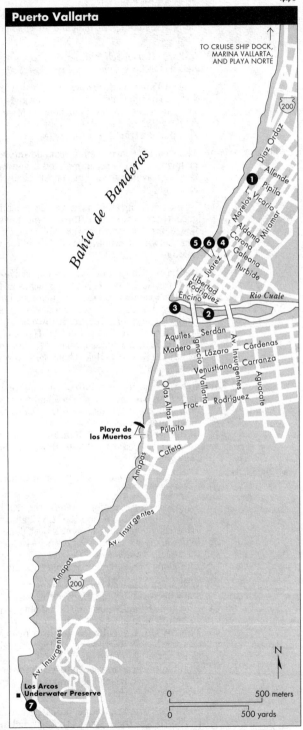

Puerto Vallarta

TO CRUISE SHIP DOCK,
MARINA VALLARTA,
AND PLAYA NORTE

Bahía de Banderas

Díaz Ordaz
Allende
Pipila
Morelos
Vicario
Miramar
Aldama
Corona
Galeana
Iturbide
Juárez
Libertad
Rodríguez
Encino
Río Cuale
Aquiles
Serdán
Madero
Ignacio Lázaro
Av. Insurgentes
Cárdenas
Venustiano
Vallarta
Carranza
Olas Altas
Frac. Rodríguez
Aguacate
Playa de
los Muertos
Púlpito
Cafeta
Amapas
Av. Insurgentes
Amapas
Av. Insurgentes
Los Arcos
Underwater Preserve
N
0   500 meters
0   500 yards

with shops, boutiques, and car-rental agencies. Several blocks

❹ beyond is **La Iglesia de Nuestra Señora de Guadalupe** (Our Lady of Guadalupe Cathedral), with the distinctive crown on its clock tower and an impressive interior. The steps are always crowded with vendors and women weaving colored shawls and

❺ bags. A cathedral dominates the **Plaza de Armas,** the zócalo.

❻ On the north side is **City Hall,** where a colorful mural painted by the town's most famous artist, Manuel Lepe, depicts Puerto Vallarta before the tourist boom.

❼ Hop in a cab to go the 8 miles to **Playa Mismaloya,** where *Night of the Iguana* was filmed. The drive south passes spectacular homes, some of the town's oldest and most refined resorts, and a slew of condo and time-share developments. Somewhat spoiled by the huge hotel complex La Jolla de Mismaloya, the pretty Mismaloya cove is backed by rugged, rocky hills and affords a good view of Los Arcos, a rock formation in the water. Motor launches leave from here for the more secluded beaches of Los Arcos, Las Animas, Quimixto, and Yelapa for about $3.50 an hour per person.

Shopping The downtown is filled with shops, boutiques, and stalls charging inflated prices. Better prices can be found in the **Mercado Municipal,** a large public market at Avenida Miramar and Libertad, in front of the inland bridge (the one farthest from the sea). Among stalls of fish, meat, chicken, fruit, and vegetables, you will find serapes, cotton dresses, silver jewelry, and leather goods. The late Manuel Lepe's primitive interpretations of Puerto Vallarta life are sold at several shops and galleries around town, including **Arte Antigua** (Hotel Pelícanos), **Arte Mágico Huichol** (Corona 164), **Galería Indígena** (Juárez 168), **Nevaj** (Morelos 223), **Querubines** (Juárez and Galeana), and **St. Valentin** (Morelos 574).

Sports Head over to the **Fishermen's Association** shack at the north
Fishing end of the malecón to find out about fishing trips. Large group boats cost about $60 per person; private charters start at $150 for up to six passengers.

Golf **Los Flamingos Country Club** (tel. 322/8–0280) has an 18-hole course; reservations should be made a day in advance and include transportation. **Club de Golf Marina** (tel. 322/1–0171) is also good course.

Water Sports Snorkeling and diving are best at **Los Arcos,** a natural underwater preserve on the way to Mismaloya.

Beaches **Playa Norte** stretches from the wharf to downtown and changes according to the character of the hotel it fronts. It's particularly pleasant by the Fiesta Americana and Krystal hotels. Within walking distance of town, **Playa de los Muertos** (Beach of the Dead) is said to have been the site of a battle between pirates and Indians. Budget travelers hang out here, along with myriad vendors selling kites, blankets, and jewelry. If you plan to go to one of the beautiful beaches south of the city, be prepared to pay about $10 each way for a taxi, $2 for a van, or P$1 for a city bus from town. However, be aware that return taxis are impossible to find.

Dining **El Dorado.** This is popular one with American expatriates. The eclectic menu includes spaghetti, burgers, and crepes, but stick with Dorado-style fish, broiled with a thick layer of melted cheese. *Amapas and Pulpito, tel. 322/2–1511. AE, DC, MC, V. Moderate.*

Andale. A Playa de los Muertos hangout and a popular spot for an afternoon beer with the locals, this restaurant serves good fettuccine with scallops, garlic bread, and an unusual chicken *Mestizo* with white wine, pineapple juice, and jalapeño peppers. *Paseo de Velasco 425, tel. 322/2–1054. AE, D, MC, V. Inexpensive.*

Ixtápa/Zihuatanejo

Few Mexican resorts can claim the graceful balance between old and new offered by the twin resort towns of Ixtápa ("ees-TAH-pah") and Zihuatanejo ("see-wha-tah-NAY-ho"). Until the early 1970s Zihuatanejo was just another sleepy fishing village and neighboring Ixtápa was a swampy coconut plantation. But with some of the most beautiful beaches anywhere, the area could not go undiscovered by tourism. Developers would like to turn Ixtápa into another Cancún, but growth has been pleasantly slow. Ixtápa today is an isolated oasis of about a dozen hotels, and Zihuatanejo a charming village of small hotels and restaurants less glitzy than Ixtápa's. Hoping to boost tourism, investors are spending $500 million on a marina tourist complex at the end of Ixtápa's hotel row. For now, at least, the area has something Cancún lacks: a quiet, easy pace and a way of life that more closely resembles that of a fishing village than a resort.

In this wild, rugged part of Mexico, Spanish colonization was never very successful. As a result, many natives speak one of five Indian dialects. But the people are friendly, and despite the language barrier, it's somehow easier to make yourself understood here (even if communication is in sign language) than in other Riviera ports.

Shore Excursions *Not all excursions are offered by all cruise lines. All times and prices are approximate.*

Beach Tour: Spend the day at Playa Las Gatas or Ixtápa Island, where vendors are more gracious, the beach is cleaner, and the water is more inviting than at the other ports. *3–5 hrs. Cost: $30.*

Ixtápa City Tour: A guided bus ride to Ixtápa to see the hotels and shopping district. A taxi ride is cheaper, and you'll see the same things. *3 hrs. Cost: $20.*

Getting Around Ships anchor in Zihuatanejo's harbor and tender passengers to the pier. The town covers about 2 square miles of cobblestone streets to the right of the dock, and the main shopping area is concentrated in a few blocks near the pier. If you're lost, just walk to the sea and turn right. Ixtápa is 10 minutes away via the main highway. At present, Ixtápa is only a narrow 3-mile-long strip of hotels, restaurants, and shopping centers.

By Bus Buses and minibuses run between the Ixtápa Hotel Zone and Zihuatanejo approximately every hour for about 15¢; they're often late. Stops are clearly marked.

By Taxi You can easily walk around Zihuatanejo or Ixtápa, but you must take a bus or taxi to get from one to the other. Fare between the two is about $4, and $3 to the popular beach at Playa la Ropa in Zihuatanejo. Getting anywhere within the Ixtápa Hotel Zone is about $2. You may also flag down a "collective" taxi, which will pick up as many people as it can fit, at about half the price of a private cab.

Exploring Zihuatanejo's charm lies in its narrow sun-baked streets, its
Ixtápa/Zihuatanejo little shops and boutiques. A small museum and a folk-art store are beside the cathedral.

Ixtápa is strictly a resort town, with hotels strung for miles along the beach. Aside from the main boulevard, there is little to explore. However, with seven malls clustered together, it's a shopping nirvana.

Shopping Budget an hour here. Unlike elsewhere on the Riviera, mer-
Zihuatanejo chants leave you alone and let you browse. Locally produced goods include wood carvings, ceramics, weavings, and leather goods. Indians display handicrafts in a **street market** on Juan Alvarez. **El Embarcadero,** on the waterfront, has a large selection of indigenous embroidered clothing made of hand-loomed cotton, wool rugs, and wall hangings. **Coco Cabaña,** the folk-art store on Vicente Guerrero, behind Coconuts restaurant, is fabulous. Artwork from the Yucatán, hand-embroidered clothing, and masks are sold at **Galería Maya,** at Hermenegildo Galeana 5.

Ixtápa In Ixtápa browse at the **La Puerta** shopping mall along the Hotel Zone. It has more mainstream boutiques than Zihuatanejo, with pricey merchandise by such designers as Ralph Lauren, Christian Dior, and Calvin Klein, as well as a number of shops selling handicrafts and casual clothing and beachwear by local designers. Five other malls are beside it—**Ixpamar, Los Patios, Plaza Bugambilias, Galerías Ixtápa,** and the bright, white **Los Fuentes. Luisa Conti,** at Los Patios, uses interesting combinations of materials for her unique line of costume jewelry. **Xochitl Bazar/Hyacinth,** at Plaza Bugambilias, has one-of-a-kind handmade dresses, jewelry, and an unusual selection of art and handicrafts.

Sports You can rent a boat at the **Municipal Beach**'s Zihuatanejo Pier
Fishing and at **Playa Quieta** in Ixtápa. Rates range from $80 to $250 per day.

Water Sports Waterskiing, windsurfing, snorkeling, diving, and sailing can be arranged at the Hotel Zone beaches in Ixtápa. Waterskiing costs about $25 a half-hour.

Beaches A few steps from downtown, **Municipal Beach** curves around
Zihuatanejo Zihuatanejo Bay. It's lined with restaurants and hotels.

Ixtápa **Playa Quieta** is one of the best beaches, famous for its clear waters and lush vegetation. It's a five-minute taxi ride from the Ixtápa Hotel Zone. **Ixtápa Island** requires a 15-minute boat ride from the Hotel Zone. This nature preserve delivers pleasant snorkeling, swimming, scuba diving, and several small restaurants. **Playa Las Cuatas,** a half-moon cove bordered by craggy rocks, offers waterskiing and other sports equipment. Snacks are available 11:30–4:30. **Playa Palmar** is a 2½-mile stretch of beach in the Hotel Zone.

Dining **Garrobus.** This delightful restaurant specializes in seafood and
Zihuatanejo Mexican cuisine. The house paella is tops—and too much for one person to eat. *Juan N. Alvarez 52, near the church, tel. 753/4–2977. MC, V. Moderate.*
Zi Wok. At this hilltop restaurant with a great panoramic view of the bay, stir-fried seafood with a Mexican accent is the fare.

A touch of chile peppers spices up the specialty of the house: fresh tuna with broccoli. *Carr. Escénica a Playa La Ropa, tel. 753/4–4510. MC, V. Moderate.*

La Bocana. This favorite with locals and visitors has been here for ages. Service is good, and so's the food. Musicians sometimes stroll through. *Juan Alvarez 13, tel. 753/4–3545. MC, V. Inexpensive.*

Puntarenas. Home-cooked, authentic Mexican food in a no-nonsense setting makes this a favorite with locals and visitors in the know. *Across the bridge at the end of Juan Alvarez, no phone. No credit cards. Closed Easter–mid-Dec.; no dinner. Inexpensive.*

Ixtápa **Las Esferas.** This is a complex of two restaurants and a bar in the Hotel Camino Real. **Portofino** specializes in Italian cuisine and is decorated with multicolor pastas and scenes of Italy. In **El Mexicano** you get Mexican food along with Mexican ambience—bright pink tablecloths, Puebla jugs, and a huge "tree of life." *Playa Vista Hermosa, tel. 753/3–2121, ext. 3444. AE, DC, MC, V. Expensive.*

Carlos 'n Charlie's. Hidden away at the end of the beach is an outpost of the famous Anderson's chain. Pork, seafood, and chicken are served in a Polynesian setting. *Next to Posada Real Hotel, tel. 753/3–0035. AE, DC, MC, V. Moderate.*

Da Baffone. Italian dishes are the specialties of this restaurant, one of three eateries in La Puerta mall. *Tel. 753/3–11–22. AE, MC, V. Moderate.*

Nueva Zelanda. At this fast-moving cafeteria with good food that you order by number, try the chicken enchiladas with green sauce, *sincronizadas* (flour tortillas filled with ham and cheese), and healthy fruit drinks. *Behind the bandstand at Plaza Bugambilias, no phone. No credit cards. Inexpensive.*

Panama Canal

Transit of the Panama Canal takes only one day. The rest of your cruise will be spent on islands in the Caribbean or at ports along the Mexican Riviera. Most Panama Canal cruises are one-way trips, lasting 10–14 days, between the Atlantic and Pacific oceans. Shorter loop cruises enter the canal from the Caribbean, sail around Gatun Lake for a few hours, and return to the Caribbean.

The Panama Canal is best described as a water bridge that "raises" ships up and over Central America, then down again, using a series of locks or water steps. Artificially created Gatun Lake, 85 feet above sea level, is the canal's highest point. The route is approximately 50 miles long, and the crossing takes eight to 10 hours. Ships pay an average of $30,000 in cash for each transit, which is less than half of what it would cost them to sail around Cape Horn, at the southern tip of South America.

Just before dawn, your ship will line up with dozens of other vessels to await its turn to enter the canal. Before it can proceed, two pilots and a narrator will come on board. The sight of a massive cruise ship being raised dozens of feet into the air by water is so fascinating that passengers will crowd all the forward decks at the first lock. If you can't see, go to the rear decks, where there is usually more room and the view is just as intriguing. Later in the day you won't find as many passengers in the front.

A running commentary is heard over the loudspeaker almost all day, imparting facts and figures as well as anecdotes about the history of the canal. The canal stands where it does today not because it's the best route but because the railroad was built there first, making access to the area relatively easy. The railway had followed an old Spanish mule trail that had been there for more than 300 years.

Frenchman Ferdinand de Lesseps, builder of the Suez Canal, was determined to construct a sea-level canal here, as he had done at Suez, instead of an easier lock canal. Disease, scandal, corruption, rain, mud, and jungle took their toll, including 16,000–20,000 lives, and the French company went bankrupt. (One worker during 1886–87 was an unknown French painter named Paul Gauguin.)

By 1900 it was apparent that only the United States had the resources to complete the huge project. After the Panamanian revolution, the United States was able to negotiate a favorable treaty with the Panamanians rather than trying to deal with Colombia, which held the isthmus at that time. The main obstacle to building the canal was disease, which was rampant in the Panamanian jungle. In 1904 Colonel William Gorgas undertook one of the great sanitation campaigns in history, clearing brush, draining swamps, eliminating areas where mosquitoes bred and swarmed. Within two years yellow fever had been wiped out and bubonic plague and malaria were on the decline.

The canal was completed in 1914, and, with constant dredging, it still functions smoothly. If you would like to learn more about its history, pick up a copy of David McCullough's *The Path Between the Seas.*

Panama Canal

KEY

Cruise Ship

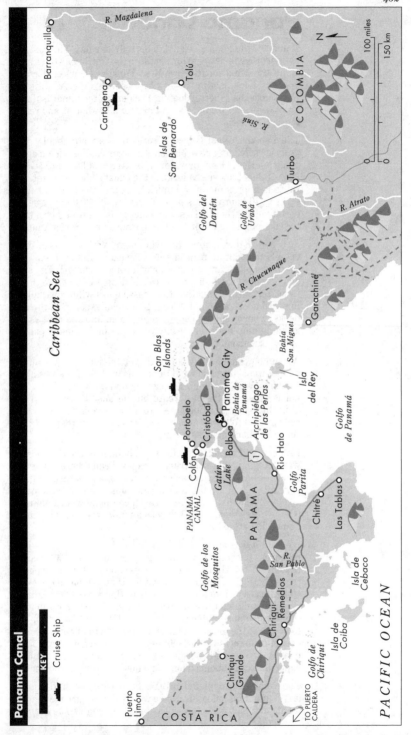

When to Go In spring and autumn a number of cruise ships use the Panama Canal to reposition between the Caribbean and Alaska, Mexico and Europe, Canada and the South Pacific. However, several ships offer regular transcanal and loop cruises throughout the winter season.

Currency Passengers won't need to change money to transit the canal, but some ships stop in the San Blas Islands, off Panama, and at Cartagena, Colombia. The balboa and the U.S. dollar are regular currency in Panama, and both have the same value. The monetary unit in Colombia is the peso. Currently, one U.S. $1 is worth about 580 pesos.

Passports and Visas No visas are necessary to transit the Panama Canal because passengers do not disembark. For ships that stop at the San Blas Islands, a valid passport is needed. U.S. and Canadian citizens don't need visas; they can travel with $3 tourist cards, but must carry proof of citizenship, such as a birth certificate or a passport. British citizens only need a passport. Canadian passengers visiting Cartagena, Colombia, require a valid passport and a visa or tourist card; U.S. and British citizens need only a passport.

San Blas Islands and Cartagena

The beautiful islands of the **San Blas** archipelago are home of the Cuna Indians, whose women are famous for hand-worked stitching. These women are a charming sight with their embroidered *molas,* strings of necklaces, gold jewelry in their noses, and arm and ankle bracelets. If you are wavering between two Panama Canal cruises, take the one that stops at San Blas.

Cartagena, Colombia, is one of the Western Hemisphere's most fascinating cities. With a population of 850,000, Cartagena deals largely in platinum and timber from the headwaters of the Atrato and San Juan rivers, coffee from the Sierra Nevada, and oil products piped from Barrancabermeja. Seventeenth-century walls divide Cartagena into the "old" and "new" city. In the old city, houses are in the Iberian style: thick walls, high ceilings, central patios, gardens, and balconies. The streets are narrow and crooked, designed for protection during assault. Filled with historical sites, forts, museums, and stores, it is a pleasant alternative to the typical Caribbean port.

Northeastern United States and Canada

The region between New York, Boston, Nova Scotia, and Québec is rapidly becoming one of the hottest cruise destinations. Less crowded and less expensive than Alaska, it offers beautiful scenery, historical sights, and wildlife (including whales). Prime attractions of a cruise in this area are tiny Maine fishing villages, the historic St. Lawrence Seaway, and hillsides ablaze with autumn colors.

When to Go Cruises in the area are available summer through early autumn. The best cruising time is autumn, when the leaves are turning color, or summer if you enjoy jazz and arts festivals. Some ships offer only a couple of cruises between their summer season in Europe and their Caribbean season, so the number of berths is limited. For that reason, no bargains are offered during any part of the season.

Boston

Boston is a popular terminus and port of call for cruises to the north. Over the past decade, however, it has become increasingly difficult to find the "real" Boston. What was once thought of as the most staid and settled of American cities now defies such easy stereotyping. The historic shrines along the Freedom Trail (which remains an excellent walking tour) are surrounded today by forests of skyscrapers that many critics say represent the "Manhattanization" of Boston. The old Italian North End is slowly "going condo." The Back Bay is now known more for its shopping and chic restaurants than for its quiet residential blocks with their superlative architecture. For many travelers it is this dynamism that has come to express the essence of Boston. Those who want something older may have to use their imaginations, but the traditional city remains for those who search.

For these traditionalists, then, a walk through Boston should start on **Beacon Hill,** taking in all the little side streets; then wind past **Government Center,** heading for the back corners of the North End, where landmarks like **Paul Revere's House** and the **Old North Church** reveal themselves at every turn. Continue through the downtown streets, through the Common and the Public Garden and along a Beacon Street that still belongs to the ghost of Oliver Wendell Holmes. As afternoon shadows lengthen, walk along the Charles River toward **Harvard Square,** as Archibald MacLeish did on the night he decided to become a poet rather than a lawyer. Cross the river into **Cambridge** and consider what possessed men to build a college in what in 1636 was the wilderness.

Newport

In contrast to Boston, the genteel community of Newport, Rhode Island, offers a very manageable day of exploring. Newport is best known for its high-society splendor: Million-dollar yachts can still be seen skimming across Narragansett Bay, with or without the America's Cup in sight. Along Bellevue Avenue and Ocean Drive you can see the **summer mansions**

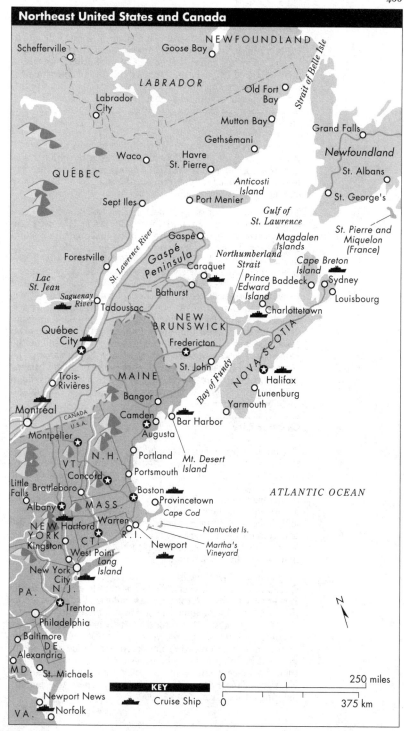

Northeast United States and Canada

NEWFOUNDLAND

Schefferville

Goose Bay

LABRADOR

Strait of Belle Isle

Labrador City

Old Fort Bay

Mutton Bay

Grand Falls

Gethsémani

Newfoundland

Waco

Havre St. Pierre

St. Albans

QUÉBEC

Anticosti Island

St. George's

Sept Iles

Port Menier

Gulf of St. Lawrence

St. Pierre and Miquelon (France)

Gaspé

Magdalen Islands

St. Lawrence River

Forestville

Gaspé Peninsula

Caraquet

Northumberland Strait

Cape Breton Island

Lac St. Jean

Bathurst

Prince Edward Island

Baddeck

Sydney

Saguenay River

Tadoussac

NEW BRUNSWICK

Charlottetown

Louisbourg

Québec City

Fredericton

St. John

NOVA SCOTIA

Trois-Rivières

MAINE

Bay of Fundy

Halifax

Montréal

Bangor

Lunenburg

CANADA
U.S.A.

Camden

Bar Harbor

Yarmouth

Montpelier

Augusta

Mt. Desert Island

VT.

N.H.

Portland

Concord

Portsmouth

ATLANTIC OCEAN

Little Falls

Brattleboro

Boston

Albany

MASS.

Provincetown

Cape Cod

NEW

Hartford

Warren

Nantucket Is.

YORK

Kingston

CT.

R.I.

Newport

Martha's Vineyard

West Point

Long Island

New York City

N.J.

PA.

Trenton

Philadelphia

Baltimore

DE.

Alexandria

M.D.

St. Michaels

KEY	
🚢	Cruise Ship

0 — 250 miles

0 — 375 km

Newport News

VA.

Norfolk

N

(several sumptuous ones open as museums) that accompany the yachts and society balls. Newport is famous also as a navy town, and a visit to the **Naval War College Museum** will help to explain Rhode Island's historic involvement with naval strategists and fighting ships. Newport's **Colonial waterfront** boasts more restored 18th-century homes than Williamsburg or Boston, first-rate restaurants, jazz and folk festivals, a lively nightlife, and special events throughout the year.

Halifax

Halifax, Nova Scotia, has one of the finest harbors in the world, with a history of shipping and understated hospitality that makes it a wonderful port of call. If you are on one of the very few cruises that actually start or stop here, a pre- or post-cruise stay is highly recommended.

The combination of old and new in Halifax is nowhere more apparent than in and around the area known as **Historic Properties,** on the waterfront. High-rise office and apartment buildings spear the skyline downtown, yet the low, 19th-century profile of Historic Properties is only a few steps away. In the 1800s, the area was the center of business for the young city. The stone **Privateer's Warehouse** housed the cargoes captured by Nova Scotia privateers until the captured ships and cargoes could be auctioned off by the Admiralty. The area's historic buildings now hold boutiques, restaurants, nightclubs, and souvenir shops. Between June and October, you can hear the town crier, take helicopter and stern-wheeler tours, and sail on the *Bluenose II.* Other sites worth visiting are the **Citadel** and the **Nova Scotia Museum** on Summer Street, the excellent **Marine Museum of the Atlantic** on Lower Water Street, **Ft. Needham** off Gottingen Street, and the many sidewalk cafés frequented by university students.

Québec City

The birthplace of French-colonial North America, Québec City is a jewel. Perched high on a cliff overlooking the St. Lawrence River, it is rich in charm and history. Extremely proud of their heritage, Québecois have preserved dozens of buildings (many dating back to the 17th century), battle sites, and monuments. The result is a charming blend of winding cobblestone streets and old houses reminiscent of Europe. In fact, Québec is so full of architectural treasures that in 1985 UNESCO declared it a World Heritage Treasure site, ranking it with Egypt's pyramids and India's Taj Mahal.

Ships dock below the cliffs, within walking distance of **Vieux Québec,** the old walled city. Walk the couple of blocks to the **Lower City** to browse through art galleries and superb boutiques. Then take the funicular, or elevator tram, into the upper city (for about CAN $1) to stand on the boardwalked **Dufferin Terrace,** with its panoramic view of the waterway below. To your right is the **Château Frontenac,** probably the most photographed building in Canada. Street musicians and jugglers turn the **Place d'Armes** into an open-air theater in summer. Nearby is **Trésor Street,** the artists' alley, where you can buy paintings priced from $5 to $5,000.

Montréal

In contrast to Québec, Montréal is a thoroughly modern city, though also with a French accent. Your ship will dock within a few blocks of the old part of town. A nearby pier has been transformed into a flea market worth a visit, but you'll need a taxi or the subway to explore much farther afield. Montréal is clean and organized, so most visitors feel safe and comfortable as they wander its many vibrant neighborhoods, or *quartiers*.

Downtown are the boutiques, department stores, and museums, such as the **Montreal Museum of Fine Arts,** on Sherbrooke. The gigantic **Place Montréal Trust** shopping complex has 120 trendy boutiques featuring Canadian and international designers and adventure-travel exotica. Buildings linked by the underground city include Place Ville-Marie, the Château Champlain and Queen Elizabeth hotels, Place de la Cathédrale, the Montreal Trust complex, Les Terrasses and the Montreal Eaton Centre, and Les Cour Mont-Royal. Close to the docks, the **Latin Quarter** has a Metro station at Berride Montigny on St-Denis. Lower St-Denis has a typical student-quarter atmosphere, with bookstores, art galleries, and bistros. In summer, musicians in town for the Jazz Festival gather for jam sessions. Off St-Denis, 19th-century homes on **St-Louis Square** surround a fountain and flower market. The square's west side leads to the **Prince Arthur pedestrian mall,** lined with restaurants (many of them inexpensive) and outdoor cafés. A healthy walk will lead you to **Place Jacques-Cartier** in Old Montreal, where you will see many historic sites.

Other Ports

Other possible ports or places of interest in this cruising region include the historic French fortress city of Louisbourg, Nova Scotia; the quaint but upscale island of Nantucket, Massachusetts; Maine fishing villages; the scenic St. Lawrence Seaway; and Campobello Island on the Bay of Fundy, site of President Franklin D. Roosevelt's summer home. More than any other major cruising area, the northeastern United States and Canada remain relatively unscathed, full of charm and history, and offer a fresh perspective on very beautiful lands.

South America

Several cruise lines now offer itineraries that wind through the Caribbean and then up the Amazon. Others sail down to Rio de Janeiro to coincide with Carnival; a few even head farther south, rounding the tip of the continent at Tierra del Fuego.

The Amazon region has figured so prominently in novels and films that most people arrive with several preconceived notions. Most often they expect an impenetrable jungle, herds of animals, flocks of swooping birds, and unfriendly Indians. In reality, ground cover is sparse, trees range from 50 to 150 feet in height, little animal life can be spotted, and the birds nest in the tops of the high trees. However, the natural romance of the Amazon River, the free-flowing water, and the hint of mystery remain.

Most of the Amazon basin has been explored and charted. The river itself is 3,900 miles long—the second-longest in the world—and has 17 tributaries, each over 1,000 miles long. About one-third of the world's oxygen is produced by the vegetation, and one-fifth of all the fresh water in the world is provided by the Amazon. Although more than 18,000 plant species thrive here, the extremely heavy rainfall leaches the soil of its nutrients and makes organized cultivation impractical. Poor in agricultural possibilities, the Amazon is rich in other products, including gold, diamonds, lumber, rubber, oil, and jute.

Listed below are brief overviews of South America's major cruise ports; your shore excursion director will have detailed information on getting around these ports, choosing excursions, and exchanging currency. For additional information on specific South American ports, contact the following consulates or tourist offices: The **Argentine Consulate General** (12 W. 56th St., New York, NY 10019, tel. 212/603–0400); **Argentine International Trade Market** (2 Canal St., Suite 915, New Orleans, LA 70130, tel 504/523–2823); the **Brazilian Consulate General,** (630 5th Ave., Suite 2720, New York, NY 10011, tel. 212/757–3080); the **Chilean Consulate General** (866 United Nations Plaza, Suite 302, New York, NY 10017, tel. 212/980–3366); **LAN-Chile** (630 5th Ave., Suite 809, New York, NY 10011, tel. 212/582–3254); the **Consulate General of Ecuador** (18 E. 41st St., 18th floor, New York, NY 10017, tel. 212/683–7555); the **Ecuador Tourism Office** (1390 Brickell Ave., Miami, FL 33131, tel. 305/577–0522 or 800/553–6673); the **Consulate General of Peru** (805 3rd Ave, 14th floor, New York, NY 10022, tel. 212/644–2850); the **Peruvian Tourism Promotion Board** (444 Brickell Ave., Suite M-126, Miami, FL 33131, tel. 305/375–0885); the **Uruguayan Consulate General** (747 3rd Ave., 37th floor, New York, NY 10017, tel. 212/753–8193).

When to Go South America's cruising season is short—from the end of December or early January to the end of February or early March. Therefore, the few ships going there tend to be booked quickly. Make your reservations early.

Health Travelers to the Amazon, and other South American rural areas and small cities are advised to get vaccinated against yellow fever and to take medication against malaria. There are no formal vaccination requirements for entry, but the **Centers for**

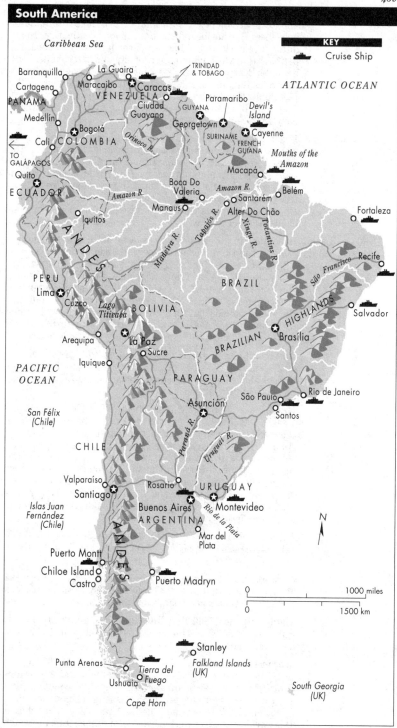

Disease Control (tel. 404/639–2572) in Atlanta, offers up-to-the-minute advice on health precautions. Call their **International Travellers Hotline** for information on your destination. In addition to malaria and yellow fever; you'll be warned about hepatitis A (for which immune serum globulin is recommended), hepatitis B, typhoid fever, and cholera. Contact your health department for immunization information. Local offices of the **U.S. Public Health Service** (a division of CDC) handle inquiries. There are branches in Chicago, Hawaii, Los Angeles, Miami, New York, San Francisco, and Seattle.

Passports and Visas Brazil requires valid passports and tourist visas of visitors whose countries demand visas of Brazilians. This includes the United States and Canada, but not the United Kingdom. A tourist visa, valid for 90 days, is free and easily obtainable from a Brazilian consulate if you apply in person and bring your passport, a 2"-by-3" passport photo, and a round-trip ticket. Check requirements with your cruise line if your itinerary includes other countries.

Local Cruise and Tour Operators In addition to the cruise lines reviewed in Chapter 3 that offer cruises in and around South America (*see* individual reviews of Clipper, Crystal, Cunard, Fantasy, Marquest, Princess, Regency, Royal, Royal Viking, Seabourn, Special Expeditions, and Sun Line), a number of U.S.-based tour operators match up prospective visitors with local cruise companies offering Galápagos Islands and Amazon River expeditions, with either fixed departure dates or "à la carte" tours with flexible itineraries. Listed below are some of the more reputable operators:

Abercrombie & Kent (1520 Kensington Rd., Oak Brook, IL 60521, tel. 708/954–2944 or 800/323–7308) offers a variety of cruises aboard an 18-passenger trimaran, the *Lammar Law*, and aboard two small cruise ships.

Brazil Nuts (1150 Post Rd., Fairfield, CT 06430, tel. 203/259–7900 or 800/553–9959) offers excursions on the Amazon River that vary greatly in accommodation. Seven-day cruises on the *Amazon Clipper*, a deluxe riverboat with eight air-conditioned cabins, each with private bath, start and end with a stay in the luxurious Tropical Hotel in Manaus. Or you can rough it a bit sailing aboard an expedition boat, sleeping on hammocks on the lower deck. And for the truly adventurous, there's a "cruise-it-yourself" option: Passengers paddle their own canoe and camp in the jungle.

F&H Brazil Travel Service (2441 Janin Way, Solvang, CA 93463, tel. 805/688–2441 or 800/544–5503) arranges Amazon River cruises.

First Mango Adventures (415 Herondo St., Box 151, Hermosa Beach, CA 90254, tel. 310/798–6468 or 800/397–3482) arranges trips to the Galápagos Islands and along the Amazon.

Galápagos Inc. (7800 Red Rd., Suite 112, South Miami, FL 33143, tel. 305/665–0841 or 800/327–9854) tours the Galápagos Islands by ship or yacht.

Ivaran Lines (111 Pavonia Ave., Jersey City, NJ 07310, tel. 201/798–5656 or 800/451–1639) operates a freighter-cum-cruise ship, the MV *Americana*. This high-tech container-vessel carries cargo and up to 88 passengers between Port Elizabeth, New Jersey, and Buenos Aires. Passengers aboard this working cargo vessel have the unique opportunity to watch cargo as its loaded and unloaded. Surprisingly, accommodations and public areas are comparable to most upscale ships: Staterooms are equipped with a private bath, a minibar, a VCR, and ample closet space. The 45-day round-trip voyages operate year-round, 16- and 28-day segments are available. Rates for the 45-day voyage begin at $7,875 for an Inside Single Cabin and $11,610 per person for the Owner's Suite.

Marco Polo Vacation (16776 Bernardo Center Dr., Suite 106A, San Diego, CA 92128, tel. 619/451–8406 or 800/421–5276) charters yachts and ships along the Amazon and in the Galápagos Islands.

Maupintour (1515 St. Andrews Dr., Box 807, Lawrence, KS 66407, tel. 913/843–1211 or 800/255–4266) offers Galápagos Islands cruises.

Metropolitan Touring (c/o Adventure Associates, Suite 110, 13150 Coit Rd., Dallas, TX 75240, tel. 214/907–0414 or 800/527–2500) sails around the Galápagos Islands and along the Amazon.

Mountain Travel–Sobek (The Adventure Company, 6420 Fairmount Ave., El Cerrito, CA 94530, tel. 510/527–8100 or 800/227–2384) arranges Amazon River rafting; Ecuador white-water rafting; Angel Falls (Venezuela) canoe trips; Galápagos sailboat or yacht cruises; and Bio-Bio (Chile) white-water rafting.

Overseas Adventure Travel (349 Broadway, Cambridge, MA 02139, tel. 617/876–0533 or 800/221–0814) offers Galápagos Island and Amazon River cruises.

Tara Tours (6595 N.W. 36th St., Miami Springs, FL 33166, tel. 305/871–1246 or 800/327–0080) runs six-day round-trip cruises aboard the MV *Rio Amazonas* between Iquitos (Peru) and Tabatinga (Brazil). The MV *Delfin* cruises remote rivers and lakes upriver from Iquitos. Several ships and yachts sail around the Galápagos Islands.

Travcoa (Box 2630, Newport Beach, CA 92658, tel. 714/476–2800, 800/992–2003, or 800/992–2004 in CA) has trips to the Galápagos Islands and along the Amazon River.

Alter do Chão/Santarém, Brazil

Cruise ships that call at Alter do Chão generally spend half the day here and half at nearby Santarém—they're both on the Amazon about halfway between Belém and Manaus. Shopping for such local handicrafts as masks, blowguns, earrings, necklaces, and straw baskets is a major pastime. You'll find the same wares sold by literally the same merchants in both towns.

There are no formal shore excursions in Alter do Chão, a small village on the Tapajós River with lush vegetation and fine river swimming. After tendering ashore, passengers can shop, visit the **Museum of Indigenous Art**, with exhibits and artifacts representing 58 Amazonian Indian tribes, or watch folk dances performed by local children. For a small fee ($2–$4), local fishermen will row you across the little harbor to a small but very clean beach.

Santarém, founded in 1661, is a city of 250,000 people. It's notable for its riches of timber, bauxite, and gold, and the colorful

waterfront makes for an engaging stroll. There are no formal excursions here, either. The ship runs shuttle buses to the **Mercado Modelo** (handicrafts market) for about $10 per person, but taxis are readily available and cheaper at $3–$5 per carload.

Belém, Brazil

The Brazilian city of Belém is the gateway to the Amazon, 90 miles from the open sea. It has ridden the ups and downs of Amazon booms and busts since 1616, alternately bursting with energy and money and slumping into relative obscurity. This is evident in the city's architecture: Ultramodern high rises mingle with older red-tile-roof buildings, Colonial structures survive alongside rubber-era mansions and ostentatious monuments.

In the "old city" you will find the **Our Lady of Nazare** church, with its ornate interior; the former **city palace;** and the **Bolonha Palace.** Walk to the **Praca da Republica,** facing the Municipal Theatre, to see the Victorian marble statues. Nearby is the **handicrafts center** run by the state tourism office; at this daily fair you will find wood, leather, and straw objects, plus handmade Indian goods and examples of the region's colorful and distinctive pottery, called *marajoara.* In addition to the **Goeldi Museum**'s extensive collection of Indian artifacts and excellent photographs, there is a **zoo** with many local animals in their natural surroundings. The **Ver-o-Peso** market is short on cleanliness but long on local color, with vendors offering medicinal herbs, regional fruits, miracle roots from the jungle, alligator teeth, river fish, and good-luck charms for body and soul.

Shore Excursions *Not all shore excursions are offered by all cruise lines.*

Belém City and the Goeldi Museum. Includes visits to the Ver-o-Peso market, the Goeldi Museum, the marble, turn-of-the-century Basilica of Our Lady of Nazareth, and a stop at the enormous, neoclassical Teatro de la Paz. *Half-day. Cost: $35.*

Brazilian Jungle River Cruise. Cruise in riverboats into creeks and channels of the Guama River. Stop at Santa Maria Island for a walk into the Amazon rain forest, which can be muddy and is always hot and humid. *Half-day. Cost: $50.*

Boca de Valeria, Brazil

Calling tiny, undeveloped Boca de Valeria a port is a bit generous. In fact, cruise ships set up inflatable docks for disembarkation at this village east of Manuas. There are only about 50 Indians in Boca de Valeria, so passengers can outnumber them by as many as ten to one. The big draw here is a chance to capture on film little boys holding their pet monkeys, sloths, and alligators and little girls selling beaded necklaces. If you're one of the first ashore you'll get a fascinating, though somewhat contrived, picture of an Amazon village.

Buenos Aires, Argentina

Buenos Aires has been called the most sophisticated city in South America. Most cruise lines recognize its late-night appeal by calling here overnight. Spending the evening in this city that never sleeps gives you the chance to see an Argentine folk dance or even venture out to a tango parlor on your own! Pre- or post-cruise packages in Buenos Aires or to nearby Iguazú Falls are extremely popular.

Shore Excursions *Not all shore excursions are offered by all cruise lines.*

Buenos Aires City Tour. The drive through Buenos Aires gives you a feel for this sprawling city, with its broad boulevards, narrow colonial streets, and famous landmarks, such as the Casa Rosada (the pink "White House"), the tomb of Evita Perón, the Obelisk, and the Teatro Colón. *Half-day. Cost: $25.*

Steak Dinner and Tango Show. Combines an Argentine steak dinner at one of the city's barbecue and *parilla* (grill) restaurants with a stage show of tango Argentino and gaucho (cowboy) folk dancing. *5 hrs. Cost: $70–$89.*

A Day in the Pampas. Drive out of the city into the nearby pampas to visit an *estancia* (ranch). Watch a performace of traditional gaucho guitar music and a show of horsemanship. A barbecue lunch is served. *7 hrs. Cost: $60–$80.*

Devil's Island, French Guiana

Many cruises that advertise a stop at Devil's Island may actually put ashore at another of French Guiana's three Iles du Salut, of which Devil's Island is one. All three were prisons, and today tourism is unwilling—and unable—to push back the rampant jungle. Typically, passengers tender ashore to Ile Royale to explore the remains of the penal colony and follow the footpath that encircles the island. The area is picturesque, lush, and haunting, so don't forget your camera.

Fortaleza, Brazil

Several hundred miles southeast of Belém, Fortaleza is Brazil's fifth largest city. A long drought devasted this agrarian region during the 1980s, and only in recent years has Fortaleza begun to recover. On the Atlantic, you'll find wonderful beaches and some of the best lobster in South America. Its famed lace industry is fast turning Fortaleza into one of the nation's top fashion centers. Within walking distance of the port you can stroll along the crowded beaches and watch vendors parade by, dangling live crabs from sticks.

Shore Excursions. *Not all shore excursions are offered by all cruise lines.*

City tour. Includes the gothic-style cathedral, the Monument to former president of Brazil Castello Branco, the Fortress, and a visit to an artisan's center—in the old city jail—to shop for such local handicrafts as lacework, leather, wooden figures, and sand paintings in bottles. *Half-day. Cost: $35.*

Galápagos Islands, Ecuador

Ecuador's "Enchanted Isles", the Galápagos archipelago includes 13 major islands and dozens of islets. Travel in expedition boats and *pangas* (rubber motor-rafts) to view remote bays and hidden coves and over land with local guides who describe the flora and fauna. This 3-million-year-old cluster of volcanic islands is home to giant tortoises (after which Galápagos Islands are named), marine iguanas, sea lions, and such rare birds as the blue-footed boobies, cormorants, and albatross. Travelers either reach the Galápagos by air from Quito or Guayaquil to pick up the local cruise or by ship from Esmeraldas, Ecuador.

Manaus, Brazil

A sprawling city of nearly 1.5 million people, Manaus is built in the densest part of the jungle some 1,000 miles up the Amazon. After years of dormancy, it has reestablished its role as the key city of the Amazon. A number of cruise lines use it as the embarkation or disembarkation port, making Manaus an ideal jumping off point for a pre- or post-cruise overnight jungle experience (*see* Local Cruise and Tour Operators, above). Vestiges of Manaus's opulent rubber-boom days remain, including the famous **Teatro Amazonas Opera House** where Jenny Lind once sang and the Ballets Russes once danced. Completed in 1910 and restored to its former splendor, the building is adorned with French ironwork and works of art and chinaware.

The **Custom House** and **Lighthouse** were imported piece by piece from England and reassembled alongside the floating dock, built to accommodate the annual 40-foot rise and fall of the river. Take a taxi to the suburbs to the **Salesian Mission Museum** to see a documentary on the now vanished "Floating City"; also visit the **Indian Museum** operated by the same religious order. For insight into the rubber-boom period, visit a **rubber plantation.** For shopping, try the **Credilar Teatro,** an imposing edifice of native redstone and glass.

Of excursions listed below, the two river tours are most worthwhile. Because it's possible to tour the Opera House by day, you may wish to skip the fabricated evening-perfomance. You can hire a taxi to show you the sights described in the city shore excursion. Some jewelry companies, such as **H. Stern** and **Amsterdam Sauer,** give free taxi tours (stopping only upon request) provided you agree to end with a showroom visit.

Shore excursions *Not all shore excursions are offered by all cruise lines.*

Cultural **Manaus City Tour.** Visit the art deco–style Municipal Market, housing meat, fruit, hats, and herb vendors; the turn-of-the-century Teatro Amazonas Opera House; the Indian Museum; and the Natural Science Museum, which showcases piranhas, electric eels, butterflies, beetles, and tarantulas. *3 hrs. Cost: $38.*

An Evening Perfomance at Teatro Amazonas (Manaus Opera House). Attend a 50-minute folklore performance, designed especially for cruise passengers, which provides a historic overview of Indian nations and Manaus's rubbery past and firm future. *1 1/2 hours. Cost: $45.*

Amazon River Tour. A local riverboat plies the the black-tinted Rio Negro, until it meets the caramel-color Solimoes River; they eventually blend to form the Amazon. At Lake January, motorized canoes whisk you via small *igarpés* (creeks) into the jungle. Water levels permitting, you'll walk over a wooden bridge to a point overlooking the Victoria Regia water lilies. *4 1/2–7 hrs. Cost: $48–$55 per person.*

Alligator Spotting. A nighttime version of the Amazon River tour, motorized canoes venture into alligator-infested creeks. Guides search for gators with a strong flashlight, picking up the creatures' gleaming red eyes. Hypnotized by the bright light, the alligator is lifted by the guide for photographs and then released unharmed. *3 hrs. Cost: $55.*

Montevideo, Uruguay

An increasing number of cruise ships has begun calling at this sprawling capital city of nearly 2 million. Although Montevideo has no medieval history or regal colonial past, it is a pleasant place to relax and a well-laid-out metropolis. The best way to see the sights is on a ship-arranged city tour:

From the harbor, a drive takes you by the downtown's art deco- and nouveau-style buildings, the **Prado district,** past **monuments,** and down the **Rambla** (the riverfront drive). You can combine the city tour with a visit to an *estancia* (ranch) for a traditional barbecue of beef, chicken, and sausages, then watch a *gaucho* (cowboy) show of folkloric music and horsemanship. Another popular option is spending the day at the South American resort Punta Del Este, on the Atlantic Ocean.

Port Stanley, Falkland Islands (United Kingdom)

Although there are no formal shore excursions, some cruise ships call here for a day. The islands (of which there are several hundred) are located 350 miles east of Cape Horn. The war in 1982 between Great Britain and Argentina put the Falkland Islands on the map.

Puerto Madryn/Ushuaia, Argentina

These two ports, several hundred miles apart, on Argentina's east coast are becoming increasingly popular with cruise ships.

A day in Puerto Madryn might be spent driving around **Peninsula Valdes** to observe the some 13,000 sea elephants reclining on the pebbled beaches. Another option is a drive to Punta Tombo through the Patagonian countryside to watch the thousands of migrating birds, including tuxedo-clad Magellan penguins, that gather here annually.

From Ushuaia, the southernmost town in the world (population 20,000), visit **Tierra del Fuego National Park,** take a catamaran ride to see the wildlife of the **Beagle Channel,** or spend a full day on **Fagnano Lake,** where you'll see beaver dams, peat bogs, and have lunch in a country inn.

Rio de Janeiro, Brazil

Rio is blessed with deep green, mountainous jungles; a profusion of birds, butterflies, and flowers; and long stretches of soft sandy beaches lined with tall palm trees. People have added to these natural blessings promenades in black-and-white mosaics, colonial buildings vying for space with dramatic skyscrapers, and music everywhere—from honking automobile horns to soft singing voices to the thump of recorded drums accompanying street dancers. Several ships offer cruises that coincide with Carnival (four days before Ash Wednesday) and reserve grandstand seats for their passengers; if you enjoy crowds and pageantry, nowhere is more exciting.

Anytime, the city offers many museums and historical sites, distinctive coffeehouses, and remarkable districts where shopping is good and affordable: You can buy a fine leather coat for less than a cloth one would cost back home. At the beaches you can watch barely clothed youths sunbathing and playing volleyball. Or head up to **Pão de Açúcar** (Sugar Loaf) for a rousing samba show. Be aware, however, that Rio is home to a great many poor settlers living in a country rife with economic problems. Watch your valuables, and don't walk down empty streets.

Shore Excursions *Not all shore excursions are offered by all cruise lines.*

Rio's Beaches and Sugar Loaf. Drive through the Reboucas Tunnel (the longest in Brazil) and along the famous beaches of Leblon, Ipanema, and Copacabana. Ride the cable car to the peak of Pão de Açúcar (Sugar Loaf). A stop is made for shopping. *Half-day. Cost: $35.*

Salvador, Brazil

With a rich colonial past evident in its churches, forts, and other historical buildings, Salvador is known to Brazilians as the most Brazilian of their cities. For this it draws not only upon its history (Salvador was the country's first capital), but also upon its colors, tastes, sounds, and aromas—a blend of African, Native Indian, and European cultures. Salvador moves to its own rhythm, slow and sensual, more at ease than Rio and blessed with miles of practically untouched beaches. Plunge into the **Upper City,** home to Brazil's best-preserved colonial architecture. Don't miss a folk show of Bahian dances and other folklore, and enjoy the special Bahian cuisine.

Shore Excursions *Not all shore excursions are offered by all cruise lines.*

City tour. Includes visits to the *Mercado Modelo* (public market), the Upper City and colonial section, the Church of São Francisco and Carmo church (Salvador has nearly 200 churches), and Largo do Pelourinho—a plaza of Latin America's finest colonial buildings. Shops near the Plaza sell Bahian costumes and jewelry. *Half-day. Cost: $35.*

Santos/São Paulo

Santos is São Paulo's port; they're about 40 miles apart. São Paulo, overflowing with more than 14 million residents, is one of the largest cities in the world. It's the richest area in South America, the fastest growing, and the pride of all Brazilians. Sprawling over 589 square miles, São Paulo is covered by a semipermanent blanket of smog. Skyscrapers dominate the horizon in jagged concrete clusters. Coffee plantations made São Paulo what it is today; now a variety of industries thrive.

Santos, which has the largest dock area in South America, is a lovely tropical retreat of sun-worshipping and swimming. Apart from the historic basilica of Santo Andre, the city offers little in the way of culture. Locally, there's shopping (for coffee and handicrafts) at the port area.

Shore Excursions *Not all shore excursions are offered by all cruise lines.*

São Paulo city tour. From Santos a two-hour bus ride passes banana plantations and oil refineries before glimpsing the skyscrapers of downtown São Paulo. A stop is made at Butanta Institute, where snakes are raised for anti-venin. Lunch is included. *6–7 hrs. Cost: $100.*

Santos Beach Party. A trip to the resort island of Ilha Porchat. Swimmers can choose from among two swimming pools or the beach. *Half-day. Cost: $45.*

Less Visited Ports

Brazil A few cruise ships call at Recife on the east coast of Brazil or, as part of an Amazon River itinerary, Macapá, Parintins, or the Anavilhanas archipelago.

Chile Ships visiting **Santiago,** the capital, call at **Valparaíso,** two to three hours away. Further south, from **Puerto Montt,** passengers can explore the lake country of southern Chile. Down around Chile's tip, **Punta Arenas** provides an opportunity for adventurous travelers to board a flightseeing plane to view the White Continent, **Antarctica,** to take a drive up to Observation Point for a panoramic view of the city of the **Strait of Magellan,** or to drive alongside Otway Bay to the **Penguin Caves.**

Peru Calls may include **Callao,** the port city of **Lima,** the capital, which is 30 minutes away. From Lima, passengers can visit **Machu Picchu,** the ancient fortress of the Incas, high in the Andes Mountains. Calls are contingent upon Peru's unstable political conditions. Check with your travel agent or cruise line.

Index

Announcing the only guide to explore a Disney World you've never seen before:

The one for grown-ups.

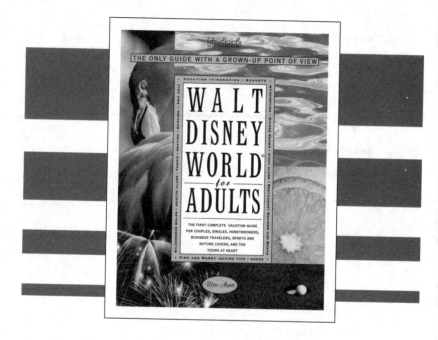

This terrific new guide is the only one written specifically for the millions of adults who visit Walt Disney World each year <u>without</u> kids. Upscale, sophisticated, packed full of facts and maps, *Walt Disney World for Adults* provides up-to-date information on hotels, restaurants, sports facilities, and health clubs, as well as unique itineraries for adults, including: a Sporting Life Vacation, Day-and-Night Romantic Fantasy, Singles Safari, and Gardens and Natural Wonders Tour. Get essential tips and everything you need to know about reservations, packages, annual events, banking service, rest stops, and much more. With *Walt Disney World for Adults* in hand, you'll get the most out of one of the world's most fascinating, most complex playgrounds.

At bookstores everywhere, or call 1-800-533-6478

Fodor's

Personal Itinerary

Departure *Date*

Time

Transportation

Arrival *Date*   *Time*

Departure *Date*   *Time*

Transportation

Accommodations

Arrival *Date*   *Time*

Departure *Date*   *Time*

Transportation

Accommodations

Arrival *Date*   *Time*

Departure *Date*   *Time*

Transportation

Accommodations

Personal Itinerary

Arrival *Date*   *Time*

Departure *Date*   *Time*

Transportation

Accommodations

Arrival *Date*   *Time*

Departure *Date*   *Time*

Transportation

Accommodations

Arrival *Date*   *Time*

Departure *Date*   *Time*

Transportation

Accommodations

Arrival *Date*   *Time*

Departure *Date*   *Time*

Transportation

Accommodations

Personal Itinerary

Arrival *Date*   *Time*

Departure *Date*   *Time*

Transportation

Accommodations

Arrival *Date*   *Time*

Departure *Date*   *Time*

Transportation

Accommodations

Arrival *Date*   *Time*

Departure *Date*   *Time*

Transportation

Accommodations

Arrival *Date*   *Time*

Departure *Date*   *Time*

Transportation

Accommodations

Personal Itinerary

Arrival *Date* *Time*

Departure *Date* *Time*

Transportation

Accommodations

Arrival *Date* *Time*

Departure *Date* *Time*

Transportation

Accommodations

Arrival *Date* *Time*

Departure *Date* *Time*

Transportation

Accommodations

Arrival *Date* *Time*

Departure *Date* *Time*

Transportation

Accommodations

Addresses

Name	*Name*
Address	*Address*
Telephone	*Telephone*
Name	*Name*
Address	*Address*
Telephone	*Telephone*
Name	*Name*
Address	*Address*
Telephone	*Telephone*
Name	*Name*
Address	*Address*
Telephone	*Telephone*
Name	*Name*
Address	*Address*
Telephone	*Telephone*
Name	*Name*
Address	*Address*
Telephone	*Telephone*
Name	*Name*
Address	*Address*
Telephone	*Telephone*
Name	*Name*
Address	*Address*
Telephone	*Telephone*

Addresses

Name	*Name*
Address	*Address*
Telephone	*Telephone*
Name	*Name*
Address	*Address*
Telephone	*Telephone*
Name	*Name*
Address	*Address*
Telephone	*Telephone*
Name	*Name*
Address	*Address*
Telephone	*Telephone*
Name	*Name*
Address	*Address*
Telephone	*Telephone*
Name	*Name*
Address	*Address*
Telephone	*Telephone*
Name	*Name*
Address	*Address*
Telephone	*Telephone*
Name	*Name*
Address	*Address*
Telephone	*Telephone*

Fodor's Travel Guides

Available at bookstores everywhere, or call 1–800–533–6478, 24 hours a day.

U.S. Guides

Alaska	Las Vegas, Reno, Tahoe	Philadelphia & the Pennsylvania Dutch Country	The Upper Great Lakes Region
Arizona	Los Angeles		USA
Boston	Maine, Vermont, New Hampshire	The Rockies	Vacations in New York State
California		San Diego	
Cape Cod, Martha's Vineyard, Nantucket	Maui	San Francisco	Vacations on the Jersey Shore
The Carolinas & the Georgia Coast	Miami & the Keys	Santa Fe, Taos, Albuquerque	Virginia & Maryland
	New England	Seattle & Vancouver	Waikiki
Chicago	New Orleans	The South	Walt Disney World and the Orlando Area
Colorado	New York City	The U.S. & British Virgin Islands	
Florida	Pacific North Coast		Washington, D.C.
Hawaii			

Foreign Guides

Acapulco, Ixtapa, Zihuatanejo	The Czech Republic & Slovakia	Japan	Provence & the Riviera
Australia & New Zealand	Eastern Europe	Kenya & Tanzania	Rome
Austria	Egypt	Korea	Russia & the Baltic Countries
The Bahamas	Euro Disney	London	Scandinavia
Baja & Mexico's Pacific Coast Resorts	Europe	Madrid & Barcelona	Scotland
Barbados	Europe's Great Cities	Mexico	Singapore
Berlin	Florence & Tuscany	Montreal & Quebec City	South America
Bermuda	France	Morocco	Southeast Asia
Brazil	Germany	Moscow & St. Petersburg	Spain
Brittany & Normandy	Great Britain	The Netherlands, Belgium & Luxembourg	Sweden
Budapest	Greece	New Zealand	Switzerland
Canada	The Himalayan Countries	Norway	Thailand
Cancun, Cozumel, Yucatan Peninsula	Hong Kong	Nova Scotia, Prince Edward Island & New Brunswick	Tokyo
Caribbean	India		Toronto
China	Ireland	Paris	Turkey
Costa Rica, Belize, Guatemala	Israel	Portugal	Vienna & the Danube Valley
	Italy		Yugoslavia

Special Series

Fodor's Affordables

Caribbean

Europe

Florida

France

Germany

Great Britain

London

Italy

Paris

Fodor's Bed & Breakfast and Country Inns Guides

Canada's Great Country Inns

California

Cottages, B&Bs and Country Inns of England and Wales

Mid-Atlantic Region

New England

The Pacific Northwest

The South

The Southwest

The Upper Great Lakes Region

The West Coast

The Berkeley Guides

California

Central America

Eastern Europe

France

Germany

Great Britain & Ireland

Mexico

Pacific Northwest & Alaska

San Francisco

Fodor's Exploring Guides

Australia

Britain

California

The Caribbean

Florida

France

Germany

Ireland

Italy

London

New York City

Paris

Rome

Singapore & Malaysia

Spain

Thailand

Fodor's Flashmaps

New York

Washington, D.C.

Fodor's Pocket Guides

Bahamas

Barbados

Jamaica

London

New York City

Paris

Puerto Rico

San Francisco

Washington, D.C.

Fodor's Sports

Cycling

Hiking

Running

Sailing

The Insider's Guide to the Best Canadian Skiing

Skiing in the USA & Canada

Fodor's Three-In-Ones (guidebook, language cassette, and phrase book)

France

Germany

Italy

Mexico

Spain

Fodor's Special-Interest Guides

Accessible USA

Cruises and Ports of Call

Euro Disney

Halliday's New England Food Explorer

Healthy Escapes

London Companion

Shadow Traffic's New York Shortcuts and Traffic Tips

Sunday in New York

Walt Disney World and the Orlando Area

Walt Disney World for Adults

Fodor's Touring Guides

Touring Europe

Touring USA: Eastern Edition

Fodor's Vacation Planners

Great American Vacations

National Parks of the East

National Parks of the West

The Wall Street Journal Guides to Business Travel

Europe

International Cities

Pacific Rim

USA & Canada

WHEREVER YOU TRAVEL, HELP IS NEVER FAR AWAY.

From planning your trip to

providing travel assistance along

the way, American Express®

Travel Service Offices* are

always there to help.

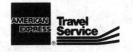

© 1992 American Express Travel Related Services Company, Inc.

* Comprises Travel Service locations of American Express Travel Related Services Company, Inc., its affiliates and Representatives worldwide.